Ebersole and Hess'
Gerontological Nursing &
Healthy Aging in Canada

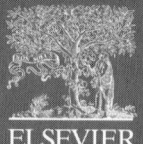

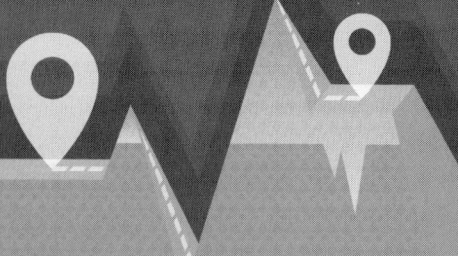

Ebersole and Hess'
Gerontological Nursing & Healthy Aging in Canada

▪ ▪

Third Edition

VERONIQUE BOSCART, RN, MScN, MEd, PhD

CIHR/Schlegel Industrial Research Chair for Colleges in Seniors Care
Executive Director, Canadian Institute for Seniors Care
Executive Dean, School of Health and Life Sciences
Conestoga College Institute of Technology and Advanced Learning
Kitchener, Ontario

LYNN McCLEARY, RN, PhD

Associate Professor
Department of Nursing
Brock University
St. Catharines, Ontario

LINDA SHEIBAN TAUCAR, RN, BSc, BScN, MSc

Schlegel Associate Research Chair, Canadian Institute for Seniors Care
Conestoga College Institute of Technology and Advanced Learning
Kitchener, Ontario

US 6th Edition Authors

THERIS A. TOUHY, DNP, CNS, DPNAP

Emeritus Professor
Christine E. Lynn College of Nursing
Florida Atlantic University
Boca Raton, Florida

KATHLEEN F. JETT, PhD, GNP-BC

Gerontological Nurse Practitioner, Board Certified
Memphis, Tennessee

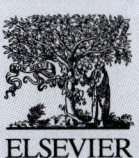

ELSEVIER

Managing Director, Global Content Partners: Kevonne Holloway
Senior Content Strategist (Acquisitions, Canada): Roberta A. Spinosa-Millman
Director, Content Development Manager: Laurie Gower
Content Development Specialists: Tammy Scherer, Courtney Thorne
Publishing Services Manager: Deepthi Unni
Project Manager: Thoufiq Mohammed
Design Direction: Margaret Reid
Cover art credits: Clouds Over the Escarpment, 1 through 4 are courtesy
of Lynn McCleary, RN, PhD

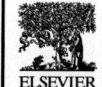

Working together
to grow libraries in
developing countries

www.elsevier.com • www.bookaid.org

Last digit is the print number: 9   8   7   6   5   4   3   2   1

To my exquisite grandmothers, for instilling a healthy respect for older adults and teaching me that a person's wisdom, interest, and enthusiasm can keep a passion alive. To Dr. Dorothy Pringle and Dr. Katherine McGilton, for their knowledge, guidance, and untold support in guiding me in my gerontological career. I share this accomplishment with them.

VERONIQUE BOSCART

To Elsa Marziali, Lynn McDonald, and Dot Pringle. Thank you for introducing and welcoming me to gerontological nursing and social work.

LYNN McCLEARY

To my Jiddos and Tetas, and my parents, thank you for your endless love and support. To my husband Christopher and children Chloé and Benedict, who continue to inspire me daily. Thank you, Dr. Paul Stolee, for introducing me to a career in gerontology. Thank you, Dr. Veronique Boscart, for your continued mentorship in gerontological nursing.

LINDA SHEIBAN TAUCAR

REVIEWERS

HEIDI MATARASSO BAKERMAN, RN, BA (COMMUNITY NURSING), MScN
Faculty Member, Nursing
Vanier College
Montréal, Quebec

DR. DEANNA BICKFORD, RN, PhD
Instructor
College of Nursing
University of Saskatchewan
Saskatoon, Saskatchewan

JAN CINNAMON, RN, BScN
Practical Nursing Instructor
Bow Valley College
Calgary, Alberta
Prairie College
Three Hills, Alberta

SARA CONNELLY, RN, MN, SANE-A
Professor
School of Health and Life Sciences
Conestoga College
Kitchener, Ontario

KATHLEEN M. DAVIDSON, RN, BScN, MN
Senior Instructor
Faculty of Nursing
University of Calgary
Calgary, Alberta

JOANNE GULLISON, RN, BScN
Coordinating Instructor
School of Health and Wellness
New Brunswick Community College
Fredericton, New Brunswick

NADINE RAE HENRIQUEZ, RN, BN, MN
Assistant Professor
Faculty of Health Studies
Brandon University
Brandon, Manitoba

KRISTA HEWITT, BN, RN
Practical Nursing Instructor
College of the North Atlantic
Stephenville, Newfoundland and Labrador

DAWN INMAN-FLYNN, RN, BScN, MN
Clinical Nursing Instructor
Faculty of Nursing
University of Prince Edward Island
Charlottetown, Prince Edward Island

IRENE KOREN, HBA, BScN, MSc
Assistant Professor
Faculty of Health, School of Nursing
Laurentian University
Sudbury, Ontario

CATHY MACDONALD, PhD
Associate Dean, Academic Affairs
Associate Professor
Rankin School of Nursing
St. Francis Xavier University
Antigonish, Nova Scotia

SUSAN MARTIN KALLER, RN, BScN, GDCT
Faculty of Nursing
Champlain College—Saint-Lambert
Saint-Lambert, Quebec

HOLLY MCSHANE, RN, BScN, MN
Professor of Nursing
Loyalist College
Belleville, Ontario

EVA PEISACHOVICH, RN, PhD
Director, Simulated Person Methodology Lab
Assistant Professor
School of Nursing
York University
Toronto, Ontario

JOCELYN REMPEL, RN, BN, MN, GNC(C)
Associate Professor
School of Nursing and Midwifery
Mount Royal University
Calgary, Alberta

PAMELA SCHEVECK, MEd, RN
Faculty, Practical Nursing Instructor
Health and Human Services
Assiniboine Community College
Winnipeg, Manitoba

DIANA SNELL, MN, RN
Senior Instructor
Faculty of Nursing
University of Calgary
Calgary, Alberta

DR. CATHERINE THIBEAULT, RN, PhD, CCNE
Associate Professor
Trent/Fleming School of Nursing
Trent University
Peterborough, Ontario

ELIZABETH UBALDI, RN, BA, MN, CCNE
Nursing Professor
Department of Health Sciences
Sault College of Applied Arts and Technology
Sault Ste. Marie, Ontario

PREFACE

Gerontological nurses have always led the way in promoting health and well-being and improving health care for older adults. Gerontological nursing continues to grow in influence and importance, with practice competencies recognized as essential educational requirements for all nurses. All nurses need to be knowledgeable about aging and health. The majority of our clients are older, regardless of where we work, be it in the community, in acute care hospitals, or in retirement or long-term care homes. This text provides the knowledge that nurses need to promote healthy aging and well-being and to meet the complex health care needs of a growing number of older Canadians.

We are delighted to bring you this Third Canadian Edition of *Ebersole and Hess' Gerontological Nursing & Healthy Aging in Canada*. This well-respected, established, and valued textbook has been thoroughly revised for Canadian students, nurses, and educators, providing the most current Canadian and international evidence for gerontological nursing practice. The content is consistent with the Canadian Gerontological Nursing Association's Standards of Practice.

ORGANIZATION

The organization of the Second Canadian Edition and the recently revised Sixth US Edition is retained in this Third Canadian Edition. The content is organized in four parts. In **Section I**, the foundations of healthy aging and the foundations of gerontological nursing are examined. Healthy aging, culture and aging, communication, and documentation in health and illness are described. Historical and current trends in gerontological nursing are explained. In **Section II**, changes associated with normal aging are presented, including the challenges older adults may experience as they adapt to these changes. The nurse's role in health promotion and implications for working in partnership with older adults to maintain or restore wellness are described. **Section III** focuses on common health problems experienced by older adults. Implications for practice are described, including how nurses can help older adults living with persistent health problems that are more common in older age. This section does not provide the in-depth coverage of health problems that one would find in a medical-surgical nursing textbook. The emphasis is on the unique experiences of older adults and the implications for nursing with older adults experiencing health problems. In **Section IV**, social, psychological, economic, and legal issues that affect healthy aging are presented. Health and social policies that affect how health care is delivered and the continuum of care are described. Challenges related to mental health and sexual well-being are examined. Transitions in relationships, roles, loss, grief, and death are discussed.

The text is organized for optimal student learning. Each chapter begins with the phenomenological consideration of the lived experience of the older adult. Key concepts, glossaries, learning activities, and discussion questions summarize the chapter and relate directly to the objectives of the chapter. Sources of additional information and reputable websites are provided at the end of each chapter.

NEW TO THIS EDITION

- New fully revised design makes it easier to locate pertinent pedagogical learning and teaching tools.
- Revised chapter structure provides clarity and greater solo emphasis on key topics:
  - Cognitive impairment (Chapter 21) and neurological disorders (Chapter 22) are addressed

in their own chapters to highlight the important differences between these chronic illnesses.

- Mental Health and Wellness in Later Life (Chapter 23) has been moved into Section III (Coping with Chronic Illness in Later Life) to better align this critical topic with other chapters in this section.
- A new chapter, Sexual Health and Well-being (Chapter 26), has been created to highlight this important aspect of healthy aging. Topics include biological changes that impact intimacy and sexuality in later life; impacts of aging on sexual health; how intimacy and sexuality are affected by cohort, culture, and environment (such as long-term care homes); and the unique needs of LGBTQ2 older adults.
- New Healthy Aging Care Plans in Chapters 8, 9, 11, 21, and 22 relate back to the "Lived Experience" feature at the start of these chapters. Based on real-life situations, these features engage the student by providing a glimpse into how learned concepts are applied.
- Scenarios and "Questions to Consider" appear at the beginning of each chapter, and responses to these questions conclude each chapter.
- New content related to the COVID-19 pandemic and the SARS-CoV-2 virus is incorporated throughout, focusing on its impacts on nurses and patients alike (including how policies affect care priorities, opportunities for optimization in long-term care homes, and the effects of social isolation on older adults).
- New and updated photos and illustrations throughout the textbook add interest and enhanced learning opportunities for visual learners.
- Up-to-date comprehensive inclusion of Canadian statistics, research, references and resources, clinical guidelines, assessment and screening tools, and more!
- Use of current and inclusive terminology regarding Indigenous Peoples and a commitment to eliminating gender bias and cis-normative language. Healthy Aging Care Plans include preferred pronouns and employ initials in place of full names.
- New enhanced coverage of cultural care, cultural assessment, and cultural safety to increase cultural competence and delivery of care when addressing the unique needs of the older adult.

- New in-depth discussion of the Truth and Reconciliation Commission's Calls to Action and the impact on nursing and health care delivery for Indigenous older adults.
- New expanded discussion of LGBTQ2 aging considerations throughout the text.

A WORD ON TERMINOLOGY

The authors and contributors of the text recognize and acknowledge the diverse histories of the First Peoples of the lands now referred to as Canada. It is recognized that individual communities identify themselves in various ways; within this text, the term *Indigenous* is used to refer to all First Nations, Inuit, and Métis people within Canada.

In the text, gender-neutral language is used to be respectful of and consistent with the values of equality recognized in the *Canadian Charter of Rights and Freedoms*. Using gender-neutral language is professionally responsible and mandated by the Canadian Federal Plan for Gender Equality. Knowledge and language concerning sex, gender, and identity are fluid and continually evolving. The language and terminology presented in this text endeavour to be inclusive of all peoples and reflect what is, to the best of our knowledge, current at the time of publication.

EVOLVE WEBSITE

Located at http://evolve.elsevier.com/Canada/Ebersole/gerontological/, the Evolve website for this textbook includes these materials for instructors and for students:

For Instructors

- **Next-Generation NCLEX™ (NGN)-Style Case Studies:** New to the third edition!
- **PN Case Studies for Clinical Judgement**
- **TEACH for Nurses:** TEACH for Nurses Lesson Plans that focus on the most important content from each chapter and provide innovative strategies for student engagement and learning. These new lesson plans include strategies for integrating nursing curriculum standards, concept-based learning examples, relevant student and instructor resources, and an original instructor-only case study in most chapters.

- **PowerPoint Presentations:** PowerPoint lecture slides consisting of 28 chapters of customizable text slides for instructors to use in lectures.
- **Test Bank:** ExamView® Test Bank, featuring examination-format test questions, with rationales and answers for all 28 chapters. The robust ExamView® testing application, provided at no cost to faculty, allows instructors to create new tests; edit, add, and delete test questions; sort questions by category, cognitive level, and nursing process step; and administer and grade tests online, with automated scoring and gradebook functionality.
- **Image Collection:** Illustrations and photos that can be used in a presentation or as visual aids.

For Students

- **Examination Review Questions:** Approximately 390 review questions for exam preparation, practice, and self-assessment, designed to reinforce content from each textbook chapter.
- **Next-Generation NCLEX™ (NGN)-Style Case Studies**
- **PN Case Studies for Clinical Judgement**
- **Glossary**

Next-Generation NCLEX™ (NGN)

The National Council for the State Boards of Nursing (NCSBN) is a not-for-profit organization whose members include nursing regulatory bodies. In empowering and supporting nursing regulators in their mandate to protect the public, the NCSBN is involved in the development of nursing licensure examinations, such as the NCLEX-RN®. In Canada, the NCLEX-RN® was introduced in 2015 and is, as of the writing of this text, the recognized licensure exam required for practising RNs in Canada.

As of 2023, the NCLEX-RN® will be changing in order to ensure that its item types adequately measure clinical judgement, critical thinking, and problem-solving skills on a consistent basis. The NCSBN will also be incorporating into the examination what they call the Clinical Judgement Measurement Model (CJMM), which is a framework the NCSBN has created to measure a novice nurse's ability to apply clinical judgement in practice.

These changes to the examination come as a result of findings indicating that novice nurses have a much higher than desirable error rate with patients (errors causing patient harm) and, upon NCSBN's investigation, discovering that the overwhelming majority of these errors were caused by failures of clinical judgement.

Clinical judgement has been a foundation underlying nursing education for decades, based on the work of a number of nursing theorists. The theory of clinical judgement that most closely aligns with what NCSBN is basing their CJMM on is the work of Christine A. Tanner.

The new version of the NCLEX-RN® is identified loosely as the "Next-Generation NCLEX," or "NGN," and will feature the following:

- Six key skills in the CJMM: recognizing cues, analyzing cues, prioritizing hypotheses, generating solutions, taking actions, and evaluating outcomes.
- Approved item types as of March 2021: multiple response, extended drag and drop, cloze (drop-down), enhanced hot-spot (highlighting), matrix/grid, bowtie, and trend. More question types may be added.
- All new item types are accompanied by mini-case studies with comprehensive patient information—some of it relevant to the question, and some of it not.
- Case information may present a single, unchanging moment in time (a "single episode" case study) or multiple moments in time as a patient's condition changes (an "unfolding" case study).
- Single-episode case studies may be accompanied by one to six questions; unfolding case studies are accompanied by six questions.

For more information and details regarding the NCLEX-RN® and changes coming to the exam, visit the NCSBN website: https://www.ncsbn.org/11447.htm and https://ncsbn.org/Building_a_Method_for_Writing_Clinical_Judgment_It.pdf.

For further NCLEX-RN® examination preparation resources, see *Elsevier's Canadian Comprehensive Review for the NCLEX-RN Examination*, Second Edition, ISBN 9780323709385.

Before preparing for any nursing licensure examination, please refer to your provincial or territorial nursing regulatory body to determine which licensure examination is required in order for you to practise in your chosen jurisdiction.

ACKNOWLEDGEMENTS

We would like to thank Priscilla Ebersole and Patricia Hess, the creators of the first edition of this book, for entrusting us to continue their legacies as we share their beautiful words and passion for gerontological nursing. We hope that our work honours them and the specialty we all love. It has been a real privilege for us to be a part of the work of two gerontological nurses from whom we have learned to care.

We would also like to thank the people at Elsevier who helped produce this book, including Sandy Clark, Billie Sharp, Laurel Shea, and Carol O'Connell.

THERIS A. TOUHY
KATHLEEN JETT

We are, likewise, honoured and privileged to have had the opportunity to author this Third Canadian Edition. We are grateful for the opportunity to contribute to the continued growth of gerontological nursing in Canada.

VERONIQUE BOSCART
LYNN MCCLEARY
LINDA SHEIBAN TAUCAR

CONTENTS

Ebersole and Hess' Gerontological Nursing & Healthy Aging in Canada

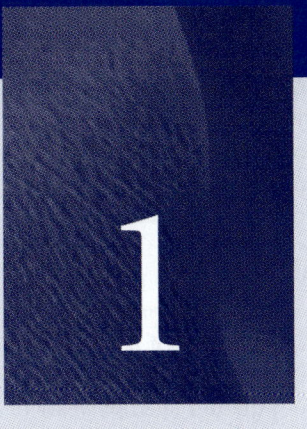

1 INTRODUCTION TO HEALTHY AGING

LEARNING OBJECTIVES

Upon completion of this chapter, the reader will be able to:

- Identify factors that influence the aging experience.
- Define *health* and *wellness* within the context of aging and chronic illness.
- Describe the trends seen in global aging today.
- Apply the principles of primary health care to gerontological nursing.

GLOSSARY

Centenarian   A person who is at least 100 years old.

Cohort   A group whose members share some common experience.

Determinants of health   Factors and conditions that influence the health status of individuals, communities, and populations.

Fertility rate   The average number of children born to a woman in her lifetime; reported for countries and global regions.

Holistic health care   Care in which the whole person is considered, as well as the interaction with and between the various components of a person's life.

Interprofessional collaboration   Collaboration among individuals in different professions, including health professions and other professions.

Life expectancy   The average number of years a person is expected to live. Life expectancy is based on mortality rates and can be calculated for newborns (life expectancy at birth) or for people who have survived to a particular age (e.g., life expectancy at age 65).

Old Age Security pension   A Canadian federal government pension provided to persons who are aged 65 years and older and have lived in Canada for at least 10 years.

Sector   A part of the economy (for example, the health care sector, the education sector, and the social services sector).

Social determinants of health   Specific groups of social and economic factors, such as income, education, and employment, that lie within broader determinants of health and can reflect an individual's status within society.

Wellness   A state of health (including physical, psychological, spiritual, and economic well-being) that is optimal for an individual at any point in time.

THE LIVED EXPERIENCE

"20 or 30 years ago, I might have listed some of the usual terms associated with the expression 'good quality of life': good health, an adequate income, a reliable social network, good friends, and an enjoyable and encouraging job. Today, at the age of 86, my definition is different. With a growing absence of those pleasures, I now see a good 'quality of life' as the ability to adapt to an increasingly difficult situation without letting problems interfere with gratitude and joyfulness; to experience fine literature and music, and as far as one can manage, to be useful and encouraging towards other people. In other words, a good 'quality of life' is the ability to endure no matter what."

From van Leeuwen, K. M., van Loon, M. S., van Nes, F. A., et al. (2019). What does quality of life mean to older adults? A thematic synthesis. *PLOS One*, *14*(3), e0213263. doi:10.1371/journal.pone.0213263.

Providing nursing care to older adults is a rewarding, life-affirming vocation. Through this textbook, we hope to provide students with the basics of starting a career as a gerontological nurse. Most nurses care for older adults. This chapter presents an overview of aging, the health care needs of older adults, and the vital and exciting role of the nurse in facilitating healthy aging.

AGING IN CANADA

Although all of us begin aging at birth, both the meaning of aging and those who are identified as older adults are determined by society and culture and are influenced by history and gender. For example, in ancient times, Eastern cultures influenced by Confucianism and Taoism revered older people, but in ancient Western civilizations this was not the case. Older people were sometimes valued for their wisdom, but the physical decline of old age was viewed as a disease (Oxman, 2018). Achenbaum notes that while people as young as 40 years may have been viewed as "old" in some ancient societies, "old age" was typically perceived to start much later. Since 1700 in Europe and North America, "old age" has started "at around 65, give or take 15 years either way" (Achenbaum, 2005, p. 24).

The terms *senior* and *elderly* refer to older people. In this book, the preferred term is *older adult*. As discussed in Chapters 6 and 7, there is no absolute threshold age at which a person becomes "old." In Canada, one standard for the designation of *old* is the age of eligibility for the **Old Age Security pension**—eligibility began at 70 years when Old Age Security was established in 1952, and was reduced to 65 years in the 1960s. Currently, people as young as 60 years of age can apply for Old Age Security. Retirement age, another marker of "old age," varies considerably; some people are able to retire in their fifties, while others continue to work into their eighties. Most Canadian statistical summaries define *older people* as those aged 65 years and older.

Psychologists and researchers have divided the "old" into three groups: the "young-old," roughly 65 to 74 years old; the "middle-old," 75 to 84 years old; and the "old-old," over 85 years old. A fourth group, persons aged 100 years and older (**centenarians),** is growing rapidly. Currently, about 1.5% of the Canadian population is at least 100 years old. The total number is expected to increase from 8,230 persons in 2016 to 40,000 persons in 2051. The majority of centenarians will continue to be women (Statistics Canada, 2017).

The proportion of the population aged 65 years or older has been steadily increasing since the early 1970s. In 1966, older adults accounted for 7.7% of the population; in 2015, 16.1% of the population was aged 65 years and older. This increase is due to a relatively low **fertility rate** of about 1.6 children per woman and an increased **life expectancy** in the 1900s (Statistics Canada, 2016a). Female Canadians born today have a life expectancy of 83.9 years, and males have a life expectancy of 79.8 years (Statistics Canada, 2018).

Life expectancy varies across the country. Life expectancy in the territories and in Newfoundland and Labrador is lower than that in other regions of Canada, and the highest life expectancy is in British Columbia (Statistics Canada, 2020a). Lower life expectancy among Inuit and First Nations people accounts for at least some of these geographic differences (Statistics Canada, 2020b). The proportion of older adults in the Canadian population is expected to increase dramatically over the coming years as "baby boomers" born between 1946 and the early 1960s retire (Statistics Canada, 2020c). Fig. 1.1 shows the projected increase in the population aged 65 years and older by region in Canada.

Those born within the same decade and country may share a common historical context and are usually referred to as a **cohort.** For example, men born between 1920 and 1930 were very likely to have been active participants in World War II or the Korean War. In comparison, men born between 1940 and 1950 are not likely to have been in the military. That these two groups of men have different perspectives and different health problems is not surprising. Likewise, privileged women born between 1920 and 1930 were raised with what are known as traditional values and roles; they may never have worked outside the home, or they were limited to what was considered "women's

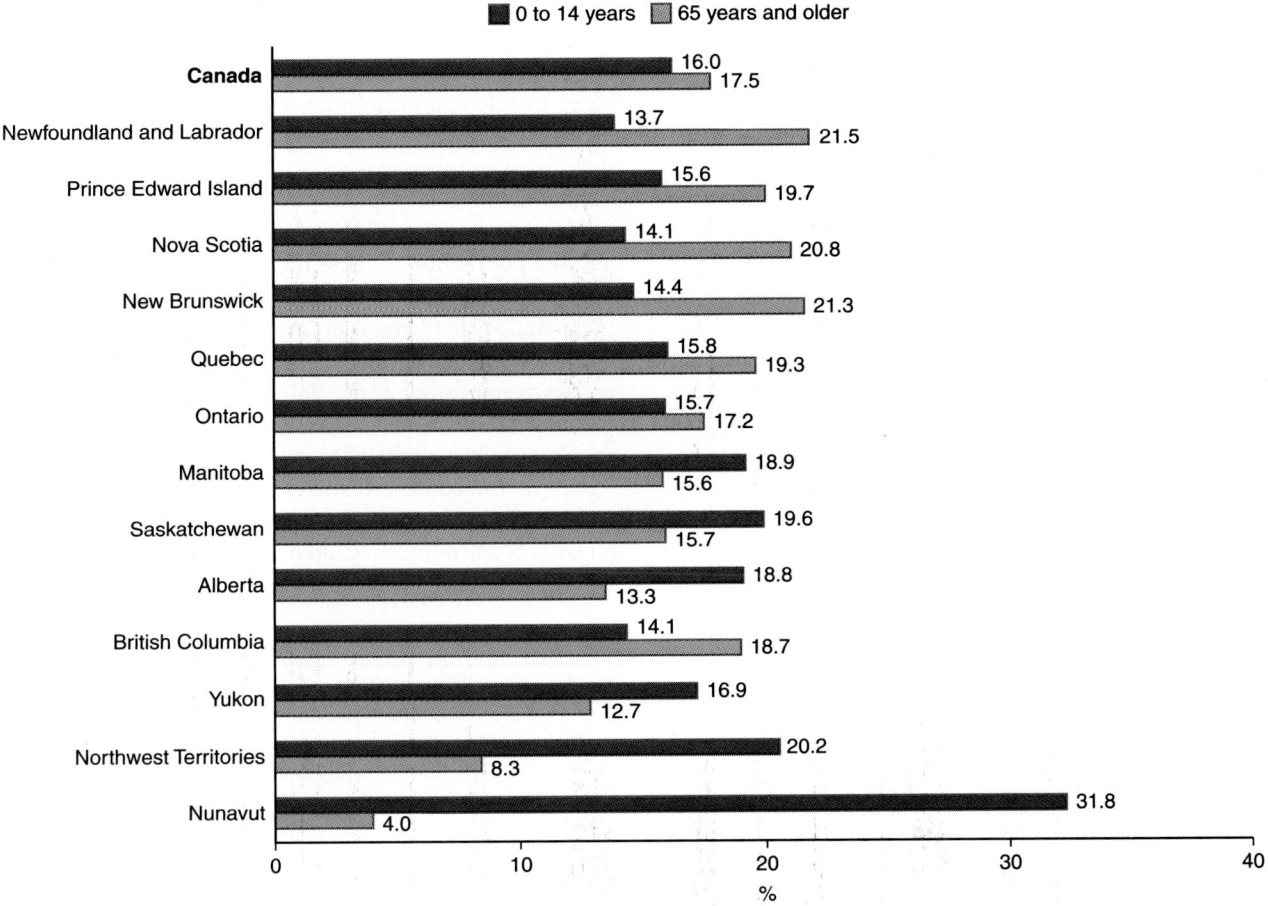

Fig. 1.1 ■ Percentage of population aged 0 to 14 and 65 years and older, July 1, 2019, Canada, provinces and territories. (***Source:*** Statistics Canada. (2019). *Proportion of the population aged 0 to 14 and 65 and older, July 1, 2019, Canada, provinces and territories (Chart 4).* https://www150.statcan.gc.ca/n1/daily-quotidien/190930/cg-a004-eng.htm.)

work," such as housekeeping, teaching, and nursing. In contrast, similar women born between 1940 and 1950 experienced social pressure to work outside of the home and had considerably more career opportunities as adults, partially as a result of the feminist revolution of the 1960s and 1970s.

Gender can have a significant effect on various aspects of aging. Women usually live longer than men, and they live alone in widowhood. Men who survive their wives often remarry. Women's social networks outside the work environment are usually larger than those of men, which can potentially reduce women's social isolation after the death of a spouse

or partner. The social construct of gender is discussed in Chapter 26.

Finally, Canada is home to a large cohort of ethnically diverse older adults. By 2031, at least 1 in 4 Canadians will be an immigrant, and about 1 in 3 will belong to a visible minority (Statistics Canada, 2015). Only a relatively small proportion (8%) of Indigenous peoples are seniors (Statistics Canada, 2016b). However, Indigenous seniors have a high prevalence of chronic health conditions and poor access to services (Fruch et al., 2016). Increasing the number of health care providers from different cultures, as well as ensuring the cultural competence of all health care providers, is essential to meeting the needs of a rapidly growing and ethnoculturally diverse aging population (see Chapter 4).

GLOBAL AGING

Historically, as little as 2% of the world's population were older adults (Achenbaum, 2005). Life expectancy increased dramatically in the 1900s. At the same time, the global fertility rate decreased substantially (Fig. 1.2) and is projected to continue to decrease, from 2.5 children per woman in 2010–2015 to 2.2 children per woman in 2050 (United Nations, 2020). As a result of these two trends, the ratio of older adults to younger people is increasing. Western countries have the highest percentage of the population over 60 years of age; more than 25% of people in Germany, Italy, and Japan are over age 60 (United Nations, 2017).

Worldwide, the number of older adults is expected to double by 2050, reaching about 2.1 billion of those aged 60 years or older (United Nations, 2017). By 2030, older people will outnumber children under 10 years of age worldwide (United Nations, 2017). Although developed countries have a higher proportion of older adults within their populations, the majority (67%) of older adults in the world live in less-developed regions, and the population in these regions is aging at a much faster rate (United Nations, 2017). These changes pose major challenges in meeting the needs of a globally aging community.

Africa stands out as the only major region in which the population is still relatively young and where the number of older adults, although increasing, will remain relatively low compared with the number of younger persons. By 2050, 9% of the population in Africa will be 60 years of age or older (United Nations, 2017).

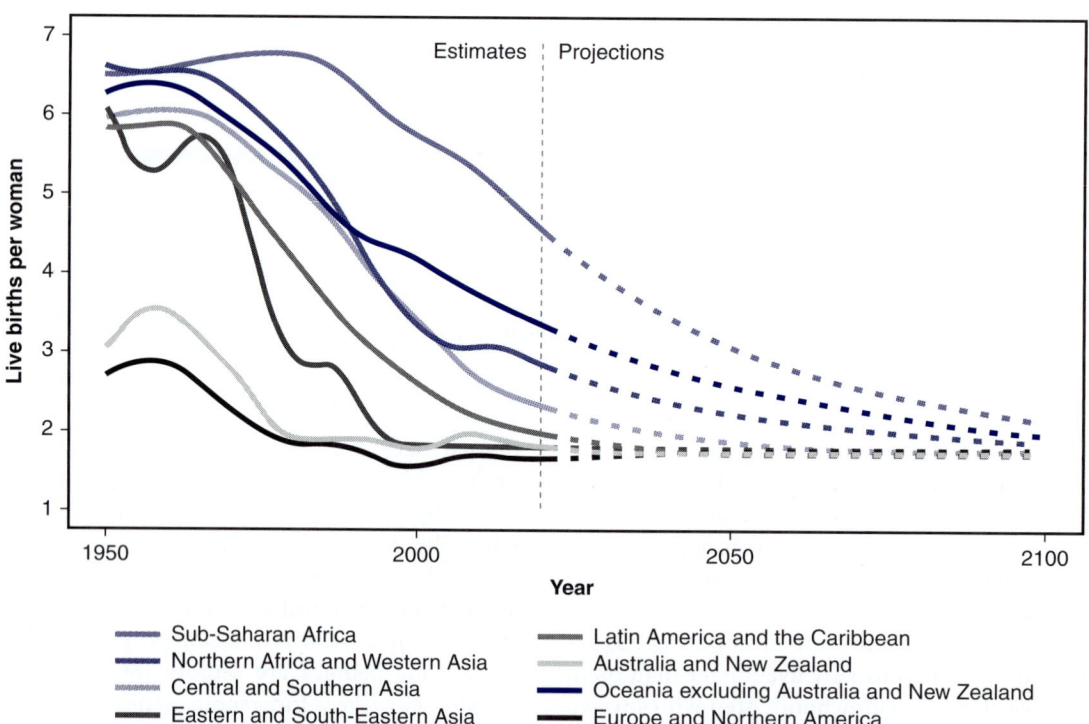

Fig. 1.2 ■ Total fertility rate by region, estimates and projections, 1950–2100. (*Source*: United Nations Department of Economic and Social Affairs. (2020). *World fertility and family planning 2020, highlights* (p. 9). Author. https://www.un.org/development/desa/pd/sites/www.un.org.development.desa.pd/files/files/documents/2020/Aug/un_2020_worldfertility familyplanning_highlights.pdf.)

HEALTH, WELLNESS, AND AGING

The definitions of *health* vary greatly and are influenced by culture. The strong emergence of the **holistic health care** movement has resulted in even broader definitions of health and **wellness.** Wellness involves one's whole being—its physical, emotional, mental, and spiritual components, all of which are vital (Fig. 1.3). In his classic work, Dunn defined the holistic approach to health as "an integrated method of functioning which is oriented toward maximizing the potential of which the individual is capable within the environment where he is functioning" (Dunn, 1961, p. 4). A holistic view of health incorporates the components shown in Fig. 1.3. Wellness involves achieving a balance between one's internal and external environments and one's emotional, spiritual, social, cultural, and physical processes.

Wellness is a state of being and feeling that one strives to achieve through effective health practices. It involves the realization of the individual's full potential physically, psychologically, spiritually, and economically and is "the fulfillment of one's role expectations in the family, community, place of worship, workplace and other settings" (Smith et al., 2006). In working toward wellness, an individual may reach plateaus in their ascension to higher-level wellness. The person may also regress because of an illness,

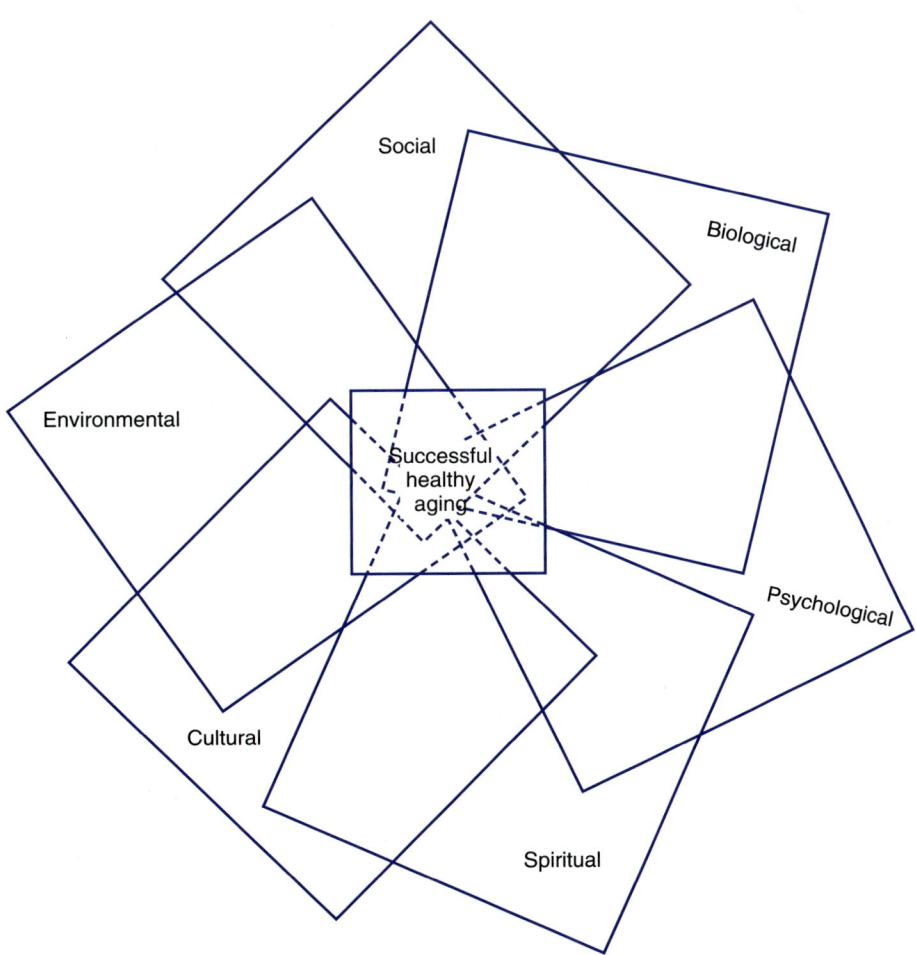

Fig. 1.3 ▪ Healthy aging. Developed by Patricia Hess.

acute event, or crisis, but these events can be a potential stimulus for growth and a return to moving along the wellness continuum (Fig. 1.4).

According to Dunn, health in later life is often thought of in terms of functional ability rather than the absence of disease—that is, the ability to do what is important to a given person (Dunn, 1961). In approaching aging from a viewpoint of health, a person's strengths, resilience, resources, and capabilities are emphasized rather than the person's existing pathological conditions. A wellness perspective is based on the belief that every person has an optimal level of health independent of their situation or functional ability. Even in the presence of persistent illness, potentially disabling conditions, or impending death, it is possible to move toward higher wellness. This can be attained as long as the emphasis of care is placed on the promotion of well-being in the least restrictive environment, with support and encouragement for the person to find meaning in the situation.

PROMOTING HEALTHY AGING

Well-being for those older than 60 years is related to functional status but is also affected by **determinants of health**—the underlying causes of illness or wellness. Determinants of health have long been recognized as important in Canada. In 1974, the Minister of Health, Marc Lalonde, argued that socioeconomic, environmental, and biological factors are equally or more important than health care in their influence on the health of the Canadian population. The Government of Canada (2020) has identified 12 determinants of health, describing the range of personal, economic, and environmental factors that influence individual and population health: (1) income and social status; (2) employment and working conditions; (3) education and literacy; (4) childhood experiences; (5) physical environments; (6) social supports and coping skills; (7) healthy behaviours; (8) access to health services; (9) biology and genetic endowment; (10) gender; (11) culture; and (12) race/racism.

Social determinants of health refer to specific groups of factors, both social and economic, that lie within the broader determinants of health outlined in the previous paragraph. Social determinants of health can reflect a person's place in society (such as income, education or employment). Experiences of racism, discrimination, and historical trauma can affect social determinants of health for populations such as LGBTQ2, Indigenous peoples, and visible minorities (Government of Canada, 2020). All of these determinants of health have an effect on older adults and are discussed in more detail throughout this book. To promote healthy aging and individualize nursing care for older adults, gerontological nurses must assess and address the impact of determinants of health.

Primary Health Care Principles

A primary health care approach is a way to build health and attend to determinants of health. This approach was adopted by the World Health Organization in 1978 (World Health Organization & United Nations Children's Fund, 1978). The principles of primary health care are accessibility, public participation, health promotion, appropriate technology, and intersectoral collaboration. Box 1.1 provides questions related to each principle. Nurses can use these questions to strengthen their practice in any setting where they work with older adults and their families.

Accessibility refers to the availability of health services to all Canadians regardless of their age or geographic location (Canadian Nurses Association [CNA], 2005). Accessibility to services for older adults is limited in rural and remote regions. There is a need to improve accessibility for older ethnocultural minorities and for those who do not speak English or French.

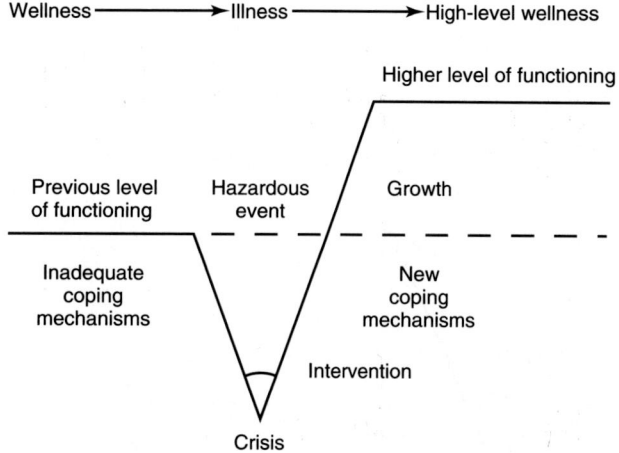

Fig. 1.4 ▪ Growth potential: Crisis as a challenge.

BOX 1.1
QUESTIONS TO CONSIDER FOR PRINCIPLES OF PRIMARY HEALTH CARE

Accessibility: What issues (e.g., hours, transportation, disability, cultural, economic factors) affect the ability of older adults to access your services? How can your services be made more accessible?

Health promotion: What are the effects of social, economic, and environmental factors on the health of older adults? Do you take these factors into account when you develop your interventions?

Interprofessional, interdisciplinary, and intersectoral collaboration: Do you work as a team with other health care providers or professionals from nonhealth disciplines? Could services or support from outside the health

sector make a difference for older adults? Do you work as a team with people who work outside the health sector? What could be done to make these relationships more effective?

Use of appropriate skills and technology: Are the skills of different health care and social service providers used in the most effective way to support older adults? Are models of service provision based on the best evidence?

Public participation: Does the community you work with have input into the kinds of programs you offer or the way in which these programs are delivered? Do older adults and their families have a say in how services are organized and delivered in their community?

Source: Adapted from Canadian Nurses Association. (2005). *Primary health care: A summary of the issues* (p. 4). Author. https://www.cna-aiic.ca/~/media/cna/page-content/pdf-en/bg7_primary_health_care_e.pdf?la=en.

Health promotion is "the process of enabling people to increase control over and to improve their health" (CNA, 2005, p. 1). Health promotion addresses the determinants of health; it includes health education, public education, nutrition, sanitation, and the prevention and control of diseases. Most chapters in this book include examples of strategies to promote the health of older adults.

In gerontological nursing practice, *public participation* refers to individual older adults and their communities being "active partners in making decisions about their health care and the health of their communities" (CNA, 2005, p. 1). Partnership with individuals is important in all nursing care. Public participation goes beyond nurse–community partnership. It means that citizens are involved in the identification of the health needs of the community.

Appropriate technology "includes methods of care, service delivery, procedures and equipment that are socially acceptable and affordable" (CNA, 2005, p. 1). An example of an innovative model of care for older adults, based on research evidence, is the Hospital Elder Life Program described in Chapter 21 (Hospital Elder Life Program, 2016).

Intersectoral collaboration "recognizes that health and well-being are linked to both economic and social policy. Intersectoral collaboration means experts in the health **sector** working with experts in other sectors such as education, housing, employment, immigration, etc. It also means that health care professionals

from various disciplines collaborate and function interdependently to meet the needs of Canadians" (CNA, 2002, p. 3). Gerontological nurses work in collaboration with health care providers from many disciplines. The Age-Friendly Communities initiative described in Chapter 28 is an example of a model that depends on collaboration across multiple sectors and incorporates all principles of primary health care.

IMPLICATIONS FOR GERONTOLOGICAL NURSING AND HEALTHY AGING

Nurses are responsible for assisting older adults with achieving the highest level of wellness possible in a given situation. Through knowledge and affirmation, the nurse can empower, enhance, and support the older adult's movement toward the highest level of wellness possible. The nurse assesses and explores the underlying situations that may be interfering with the achievement of wellness and works with the person and significant others to develop appropriate plans of care. The nurse and the older adult collaborate on interventions to achieve individual goals and evaluate effectiveness. Gerontological nurses often work with other health care providers to support the health of older adults. **Interprofessional collaboration,** interdisciplinary collaboration, and intersectoral collaboration are important parts of gerontological nursing. By incorporating the principles of primary health care into their practice, nurses can improve older adults' access to health promotion and health care services.

KEY CONCEPTS

- Gerontological nursing is an opportunity to make a significant difference in the lives of older adults.
- The meaning of aging is influenced by many factors.
- Nurses have a responsibility to contribute to accessible health care and the reduction of health disparities.
- Health, history, and gender are among the major factors influencing the aging experience.
- Each age cohort is distinctly different from others.
- Individual persons become more unique the longer they live. Nurses must be cautious in attributing any specific characteristics of older adults to "old age."
- All persons, regardless of age, illness, or life situation, can be supported to achieve a higher level of wellness that is uniquely and personally defined.
- Primary health care principles can be used as an organizing framework for health promotion, regardless of a person's age or situation.
- Gerontological nurses have key roles in providing the highest quality of care to older adults in a wide range of settings and situations.

ACTIVITIES AND DISCUSSION QUESTIONS

1. Discuss the ways in which older adults contribute to society today.

2. Interview an older person and ask them how they have changed since they were 25 years old.

3. Discuss health and wellness with your peers. Develop a definition of aging.

4. Discuss the dimensions of wellness and which ones you think may be most important.

5. Explain wellness in the context of chronic illness.

6. Discuss how you seek wellness in your own life.

7. Discuss what you can do to enhance the quality of life for the older adults to whom you provide care.

8. Discuss how older adults are portrayed in popular TV shows, commercials, and movies.

RESOURCES

Age pyramid of the population of Canada, 1956–2006
*http://www12.statcan.gc.ca/census-recensement/2011/dp-pd/
pyramid-pyramide/his/index-eng.cfm*
Canadian Association of Retired Persons (CARP)
http://www.carp.ca
Health Canada. Healthy living: Seniors.
*https://www.canada.ca/en/health-canada/services/healthy-living/
seniors.html*
Registered Nurses' Association of Ontario: Best Practice Guidelines.
https://rnao.ca/bpg

**For additional resources, please visit *https://evolve.elsevier.com/
Canada/Ebersole/gerontological/***

REFERENCES

Achenbaum, W. A. (2005). Ageing and changing: International perspective on ageing. In M. L. Johnson, V. L. Bengtson, P. G. Coleman, & T. B. L. Kirkwood (Eds.), *The Cambridge handbook of age and ageing* (pp. 21–29). Cambridge University Press.

Canadian Nurses Association (CNA). (2002). *Primary health care: A new approach to health care reform.* Author. https://www.cna-aiic.ca/~/media/cna/page-content/pdf-fr/phc_presentation_kirby_6602_e.pdf?la=en.

Canadian Nurses Association (CNA). (2005). *Primary health care: A summary of the issues.* Author. https://www.cna-aiic.ca/~/media/cna/page-content/pdf-en/bg7_primary_health_care_e.pdf?la=en.

Dunn, H. L. (1961). *High-level wellness.* Beatty.

Fruch, V., Monture, L., Prince, H., & Kelley, M. L. (2016). Home to die: Six Nations of the Grand River Territory develops community-based palliative care. *International Journal of Indigenous Health, 11*(1), 50–74. doi:10.18357/ijih111201615303.

Government of Canada. (2020). *Social determinants of health and health inequalities.* https://www.canada.ca/en/public-health/services/health-promotion/population-health/what-determines-health.html.

Hospital Elder Life Program. (2016). *Hospital Elder Life Program.* http://www.hospitalelderlifeprogram.org/.

Lalonde, M. (1974). *A new perspective on the health of Canadians: A working document.* Ministry of Supply and Services Canada. https://www.phac-aspc.gc.ca/ph-sp/pdf/perspect-eng.pdf.

Oxman, T. E. (2018). Reflections on aging and wisdom. *American Journal of Geriatric Psychiatry, 26*(11), 1108–1118. doi:10.1016/j.jagp.2018.07.009.

Smith, B. J., Tang, K. C., & Nutbeam, D. (2006). WHO health promotion glossary: New terms. *Health Promotion International, 21*(4). doi:10.1093/heapro/dal003.

Statistics Canada. (2015). *Analysis of results.* https://www150.statcan.gc.ca/n1/pub/91-551-x/2010001/ana-eng.htm.

Statistics Canada. (2016a). *Fertility: Fewer children, older moms.* http://www.statcan.gc.ca/pub/11-630-x/11-630-x2014002-eng.htm.

Statistics Canada. (2016b). *Aboriginal peoples in Canada: First Nations People, Métis and Inuit.* https://www12.statcan.gc.ca/nhs-enm/2011/as-sa/99-011-x/99-011-x2011001-eng.cfm.

Statistics Canada. (2017). *A portrait of the population aged 85 and older in 2016 in Canada.* https://www12.statcan.gc.ca/census-recensement/2016/as-sa/98-200-x/2016004/98-200-x2016004-eng.cfm.

Statistics Canada. (2018). *Health-adjusted life expectancy in Canada.* https://www150.statcan.gc.ca/n1/pub/82-003-x/2018004/article/54950-eng.htm.

Statistics Canada. (2020a). Life expectancy, at birth and at age 65, by sex, three-year average, Canada, provinces, territories, health regions and peer groups. https://www150.statcan.gc.ca/t1/tbl1/en/tv.action?pid=1310038901.

Statistics Canada. (2020b). *Projections of the Aboriginal Populations, Canada, provinces and territories – ARCHIVED.* https://www150.statcan.gc.ca/n1/en/catalogue/91-547-X.

Statistics Canada. (2020c). *Distributions of household economic accounts for income, consumption, saving and wealth of Canadian households, 2019.* https://www150.statcan.gc.ca/n1/daily-quotidien/200626/dq200626a-eng.htm.

United Nations. (2017). *World population ageing.* https://www.un.org/en/development/desa/population/publications/pdf/ageing/WPA2017_Highlights.pdf.

United Nations. (2020). *World fertility and family planning 2020.* https://www.un.org/en/development/desa/population/publications/pdf/family/World_Fertility_and_Family_Planning_2020_Highlights.pdf.

World Health Organization & United Nations Children's Fund. (1978). *Report of the International Conference on Primary Health Care.* Author. http://whqlibdoc.who.int/publications/9241800011.pdf.

2

GERONTOLOGICAL NURSING HISTORY, EDUCATION, AND ROLES

■ ■

LEARNING OBJECTIVES

Upon completion of this chapter, the reader will be able to:

- Discuss the history of gerontological nursing and the factors influencing the development of this practice.
- Identify elements of the Canadian Gerontological Nursing Association Nursing Competencies and Standards of Practice.
- Examine the recommended competencies for gerontological nursing practice.
- Recognize and discuss the importance of certification.
- Discuss the professional nursing leadership role in the care of older adults across the continuum of care settings.
- Describe several gerontological nursing roles and the educational preparation for practising them.
- Discuss formal gerontological organizations and their significance to the gerontological nurse.

GLOSSARY

Almshouse   A historic charitable home providing accommodation for frail older adults. Also known as a poorhouse.

Alternate level of care (ALC)   Care for patients in hospital who no longer require acute care services but who remain in hospital awaiting a suitable discharge destination, such as a long-term care home or a home in the community with home care services.

Knowledge translation   The process of moving knowledge from research to practice, which includes synthesizing, disseminating, exchanging, and providing an ethically sound application of knowledge (Canadian Institutes of Health Research [CIHR], 2020). Examples include the creation and dissemination of research syntheses and practice guidelines.

Unregulated care provider (UCP)   A member of the health care team who is not part of a regulatory body. The term is used in this book to refer to nursing assistants, personal support workers, health care assistants, and continuing care assistants.

THE LIVED EXPERIENCE

"The person I [cared for], she lived her life and it didn't matter what happened; she looked forward, she didn't dwell on what was happening to her . . . her outlook was amazing and you learn a lot from them I think."

Undergraduate nursing student. From Moquin, H., Seneviratne, C., & Venturato, L. (2018). From apprehension to advocacy: A qualitative study of undergraduate nursing student experience in clinical placement in residential aged care. *BMC Nursing, 17,* 8. doi:10.1186/s12912-018-0277-z.

"To know that I have made them feel they are human, that they're loved . . . that someone still cares about them. I believe that lots of times they feel ignored and as if they have no value. It's very important to me that older people feel valued and they know that they still contribute, not only to society but to the personal growth of everyone that comes into contact with them."

Gerontological nurse working in a long-term care home.

CARE OF OLDER ADULTS: A NURSING IMPERATIVE

Older adults make up a significant and growing proportion of the population worldwide. Older adults today are healthier, better educated, and expect a much higher quality and greater quantity of life as they age than did the previous generation of older adults. Healthy aging is an achievable goal for many, and it is essential that nurses have the knowledge and skills to help people of all ages, races, orientations, and cultures achieve this goal.

Most nurses will care for older adults during the course of their careers. In addition, the public looks to nurses to be professional care providers with the knowledge and skills to help people age well. Every older adult should be able to receive care provided by nurses who have competence in gerontological nursing. Gerontological nursing is not only for a specialty group of nurses. Knowledge of aging and gerontological nursing is core knowledge for the entire profession of nursing (Garbrah et al., 2017).

Care of older adults is the fastest-growing employment segment in the health care sector and industry. Older adults are the core consumers of health care, having higher rates of outpatient visits, hospitalizations, as well as home, retirement and long-term care (LTC) service use than any other age group. Despite this high demand, the number of health care workers who are interested in and prepared to care for older adults remains low. Less than 1% of registered nurses (RNs) are certified in gerontology (Chai et al., 2019).

It is essential to enhance the interest and increase the recruitment of students and practising nurses to care for older adults across the continuum of health care settings. Factors that motivate nurses to specialize in gerontological nursing often include positive interactions with older adults over the course of a nurse's life, faculty and strong practice role models, a deep commitment to caring, and an appreciation of how a nursing model of care contributes to the well-being of older adults. Nurses also realize the importance of understanding each individual's needs and preferences, and how nursing practice can be tailored to support older adults' unique circumstances and opportunities. Box 2.1 presents the views of some gerontological nursing pioneers, as well as of current leaders, on the practice of gerontological nursing and what drew them to the care of older adults.

History of Gerontological Nursing

Historically, nurses have always been on the front lines of caring for older adults. They have provided individuals and communities with compassionate and competent care, leadership, administration, advocacy, program development, education, support, and research, and are to a great extent responsible for the rapid advance of gerontology and gerontological nursing. Nurses have been and continue to be the mainstay of care of older adults, and most nurses will work with older adults at some point in their careers.

Gerontological nurses have made substantial contributions to the body of knowledge guiding evidence-informed practices in the care of older adults. In examining the history of gerontological nursing, one must marvel at the advocacy and perseverance of nurses who have remained deeply committed to the care of older adults despite struggling against insurmountable odds over the years. Box 2.2 presents a timeline of significant accomplishments in the history of gerontological nursing and gerontology in Canada.

The history and development of gerontological nursing in Canada is tied to the history and development of the field of gerontology in Canada, as well as to the development of gerontological nursing and gerontology in the United States and internationally. Canadian nurses have benefited from leadership in gerontological nursing in the United States and from collaboration between American and Canadian nursing scholars and nursing bodies. For example, gerontological nursing textbooks, journals, and graduate education programs were available in the United States long before they were available in Canada. Since 1996, the John A. Hartford Foundation has substantially funded gerontological nursing research, **knowledge translation,** and educational initiatives, resulting in significant development in the field of gerontological nursing.

Gerontological nursing originated when Florence Nightingale, the founder of modern nursing, accepted a position as superintendent in an institution similar to what we would think of as an early version of an LTC home, the Institution for the Care of Sick Gentlewomen in Distressed Circumstances (Wykle & McDonald, 1997).

BOX 2.1

REFLECTIONS ON GERONTOLOGICAL NURSING FROM GERONTOLOGICAL NURSING PIONEERS AND CURRENT LEADERS IN THE FIELD

VERA MCIVER, CANADIAN GERONTOLOGICAL NURSING PIONEER

"A transformation took place in my psyche as I began working at the St. Mary's Priory. I saw needless degradation and knew changes had to be made to enrich the lives of these unfortunate patients. I kept striving for excellence, not only in efficiency and economy but also in improvements to the patient's environment and daily living experience. This feeling was so profound I simply had to express it . . . Latent forces and talents must have come to the fore as my consciousness expanded and I came alive with this new endeavour . . . I was single-minded. I was consumed by a passion to bring humanity to all those who became my responsibility." (Mantle & Funke-Furber, 2003, pp. xi–xii)

ELAINE GALLAGHER, CANADIAN GERONTOLOGICAL NURSING PIONEER

"I chose to go to Duke University in 1975 because of a woman named Stone, Virginia Stone, and she was going around the world and was quite influential in Canada in terms of talking about personalizing care; giving people autonomy; treating them like people, like human beings as opposed to cases or patients or whatever. And was really optimistic about the fact that, you know, if you developed a really individualized care plan for someone, and encouraged them to get active and to get involved that you could actually reverse some of what people thought were some of the negative changes of aging." (Roberts, 2008, p. 27)

TERRY FULMER, DEAN OF THE COLLEGE OF NURSING AND CO-DIRECTOR OF THE JOHN A. HARTFORD FOUNDATION INSTITUTE FOR GERIATRIC NURSING, NEW YORK UNIVERSITY

"I soon realized that in the arena of caring for the aged, I could have an autonomous nursing practice that would make a real difference in medical outcomes. I could practice the full scope of nursing. It gave me a sense of freedom and accomplishment. With older patients, the most important component of care, by far, is nursing care. It's very motivating." (Ebersole & Touhy, 2006, p. 129)

MATHY MEZEY, INDEPENDENCE FOUNDATION PROFESSOR OF NURSING EDUCATION, DIVISION OF NURSING, STEINHARDT SCHOOL OF EDUCATION, AND DIRECTOR OF THE JOHN A. HARTFORD FOUNDATION INSTITUTE FOR GERIATRIC NURSING, NEW YORK UNIVERSITY

"Because geriatric nursing especially offers nurses the unique opportunity to dramatically impact people's lives for the better and for the worst, it demands the best that you have to offer. I am very optimistic about the future of geriatric nursing. Increasing numbers of older adults are interested in marching into old age as healthy and involved.

Geriatric nursing offers a unique opportunity to help older adults meet these aspirations while at the same time maintaining a commitment to the oldest and frailest in our society." (Ebersole & Touhy, 2006, p. 142)

DOROTHY PRINGLE, RN, PHD, PROFESSOR AND DEAN EMERITUS, FACULTY OF NURSING, UNIVERSITY OF TORONTO

"When I started out in gerontological nursing, it was in its early days. We all came to it from other specialties. I was the mental health nursing coordinator in an acute care teaching hospital and essentially none of the professions was interested in older people. When we had an older person with dementia or psychotic depression, none of the psychiatrists or the social workers was very interested so it was left to the nurses and, frankly, we didn't know what to do. I thought, 'I need to go back to school. Somebody has to know how to work with these people.' I learned gerontology in my PhD education, where I worked with good practitioners and researchers who were an inspiration in terms of what was possible. Now gerontological nursing has matured enormously into a very clearly defined area of expertise, with nurses who take pride in what they are doing, and a community of interprofessional practitioners working together. Demographics dictate that all graduating nurses need to know about aging and age-related changes. They need to know what the research says and what best practices are, and be able to adapt that knowledge to the unique context of each older person. All nurses take into account the uniqueness of the people they work with, but with older people there's so much more life history influencing their values, their goals, and the kind of care they want. That's the special contribution of gerontology, and gerontological nurses bring that orientation to all the care they provide." (Dorothy Pringle, personal communication, December 2010)

SANDRA HIRST, RN, PHD, DIRECTOR OF THE BRENDA STRAFFORD CENTRE FOR EXCELLENCE IN GERONTOLOGICAL NURSING AND ASSOCIATE PROFESSOR AT THE FACULTY OF NURSING, UNIVERSITY OF CALGARY

"I started working in gerontological nursing by chance. I was inspired by the stories I heard from my older patients. The people I cared for had serious health challenges and a sense of humour that inspired me. It also gave me opportunities to reflect upon my own attitudes and behaviours towards older adults. I gained tremendous respect and value for seniors. Being a gerontological nurse has given me wonderful opportunities to grow—in community practice, educating students, creating programs, working with older adults to prevent falls, leadership initiatives, and so many other ways. The range of possibilities for making a real difference

---

BOX 2.1
REFLECTIONS ON GERONTOLOGICAL NURSING FROM GERONTOLOGICAL NURSING PIONEERS AND CURRENT LEADERS IN THE FIELD—cont'd

is huge. To me, gerontological nursing is what nursing is really about; taking knowledge to the bedside, drawing on everything you've learned, connecting with people in a real way, caring, and commitment. It's like a puzzle. The sense of satisfaction you get from completing a puzzle is the same as when you work with older adults. That frustration you have when there is a missing puzzle piece is solved with nursing knowledge. Gerontological nursing knowledge is unique and special and makes it possible to feel like you're not just

doing a good job; you're influencing quality of life. One of the important changes I've seen recently is that we're beginning to overcome ageism in nursing and nursing education. We're the largest specialty group within CNA [Canadian Nurses Association]. Individual faculty members are taking initiative to improve curriculum. Students are interested in gerontological nursing. We still have a way to go, but it's a big improvement." (Sandra Hirst, personal communication, January 2011)

Sources: Ebersole, P., & Touhy, T. (2006). *Geriatric nursing: Growth of a specialty.* Springer; Mantle, J. H., & Funke-Furber, J. (2003). *The forgotten revolution: The priory method.* Trafford Publishing; Roberts, E. (2008). *Developing gerontological nursing in British Columbia: An oral history study* [Unpublished master's thesis.] The University of British Columbia. https://open.library.ubc.ca/soa/cIRcle/collections/ubctheses/24/items/1.0066969.

BOX 2.2
GERONTOLOGICAL NURSING IN CANADA: A TIMELINE

1950	International Association of Gerontological Societies (currently International Association on Gerontology and Geriatrics [IAGG]) founded
1950s	Home care programs established by the Victorian Order of Nurses (VON)
1967–1968	The Priory Method Restorative Care Model created by Vera McIver
1971	Canadian Association on Gerontology (CAG) founded
1974	Gerontological Nursing Association Ontario, the first provincial gerontological nursing association, founded
1976	*Perspectives* (formerly *The Journal of the Gerontological Nursing Association Ontario*) established
1983	First Canadian gerontological nursing conference held in Victoria, British Columbia
1985	Canadian Gerontological Nursing Association (CGNA) founded
1987	Standards of Gerontological Nursing established by GNAO and subsequently adopted by CGNA
1993	*Promoting Healthy Aging: A Nursing and Community Perspective* published
1995	Standards of Practice for gerontological nursing established by CGNA
1999	Canadian Nurses Association adds Gerontological Nursing Specialty Certification
2004	Sandra Hirst the first nurse elected president of CAG
2008	Brenda Strafford Centre for Excellence in Gerontological Nursing established at the University of Calgary
2010	Nursing Competencies and Standards of Practice for gerontological nursing established by CGNA

Historically in Canada, the care of older adults and the care of the ill were provided by female family members at home. In the early years of the transition to hospital treatment for illness, inhumane hospital conditions could be avoided by the wealthy, who hired nurses to care for older adults at home.

Awareness of the need for education in gerontological nursing, as well as the need for improvement in the care of older adults in **almshouses,** first appeared in the American nursing literature in the early 1900s. In a 1903 article published in the *American Journal of Nursing,* Bassell wrote about the care of older adults in Labrador

(Hirst et al., 1996). An *American Journal of Nursing* editorial in 1908 focused on the need for better training in the care of older adults (Dock, 1908). The first book on gerontological nursing was written by Newton and Anderson in 1950 in the United States (Newton & Anderson, 1950). In the 1950s, several articles about the need to improve the nursing care of older adults appeared in the *Canadian Nurse*, and another two appeared in the *Alberta Association of Registered Nurses* newsletter, contributing to the emergence of gerontological nursing in Canada (Hirst et al., 1996; Dahlke, 2011).

In 1967, Vera McIver, who was to emerge as a leader in innovative gerontological nursing care and is discussed in Box 2.3, took a position at St. Mary's Priory Hospital in Victoria, British Columbia. In Canada, the first provincial gerontological nursing association was formed in Ontario in 1974, followed by the establishment of the Canadian Gerontological Nursing Association (CGNA) in 1985. A few years later, in 1987, gerontological nursing standards were established by the CGNA. In 1993, the first Canadian gerontological nursing textbook was published (Beckingham & DuGas, 1993). Whereas most specialties in nursing practice developed from those identified in medicine, this was not the case with gerontological nursing, since the health care of older adults was traditionally considered to fall within the domain of nursing (Davis, 1984).

Gerontological nurse educators, scholars, and clinicians continue their commitment to and advocacy for older adults. As will be seen throughout this book, gerontological nursing research provides a strong evidence base for practice across care settings. Gerontological nursing research has gained wide acceptance in the scientific community and has made significant contributions to improved care, as well to policy decisions that influence care and service outcomes.

Research has shown that better care for older adults is possible and should be expected. The task ahead of us is to communicate this knowledge to all nurses, leaders, decision makers, and policymakers who care for older adults and to create environments that support nurses' ability to use that knowledge in their practice and work settings (McCleary et al., 2017).

Standards of Gerontological Nursing Practice

In order to provide appropriate and informed nursing care, gerontological nursing organizations have

---

BOX 2.3
VERA MCIVER AND THE PRIORY MODEL

St. Mary's Priory Hospital in Victoria, British Columbia, was an LTC facility providing 24-hour nursing care to women. It followed a custodial care model typical of LTC facilities at that time. The model was based on acute care models in which "the care of the physical body received preference over the care of the person" (Mantle & Funke-Furber, 2003, p. 7). Patients were expected to be dependent; medications and restraints were used if patients were too active. In 1967, Vera McIver was appointed Director of Nursing. She came to this position from acute care and, like most nurses of the time, had no extra educational preparation for caring for older adults. She quickly came to believe that "the end result of custodial care [was] a cascade of effects set in motion," and that immobility and lack of attention to social, emotional, and spiritual needs caused further physical deterioration along with "mental deterioration and death of the human spirit" (Mantle & Funke-Furber, 2003, p. 8). McIver transformed care and management approaches at the Priory, creating a restorative care model that became known as the Priory Method. This approach was far ahead of its time and influenced care models in North America and farther afield (Roberts, 2008). As described by Mantle and Funke-Furber (2003), the five overall strategies of the Priory Method restorative care model are as follows:

- Attention to the whole person, not just the disability
- Environment and staff behaviours designed to "convey positive expectations of wellness and the maximum use of remaining abilities" (Mantle and Funke-Furber, 2003, p. 23)
- Humanized, deinstitutionalized environment
- Normalization of activities of daily living through environmental changes and physical strengthening, and
- Strengthening of residents' egos, owing to staff support of residents carrying out their own activities of daily living.

Sources: Mantle, J. H., & Funke-Furber, J. (2003). *The forgotten revolution: The priory method.* Trafford Publishing; Roberts, E. (2008). *Developing gerontological nursing in British Columbia: An oral history study* [Unpublished master's thesis.] The University of British Columbia. https://open.library.ubc.ca/soa/cIRcle/collections/ubctheses/24/items/1.0066969.

---

established standards of practice, thus upgrading the gerontological knowledge base, enhancing the image of gerontological nursing, and identifying the opportunities of caring for older adults. In Canada, nursing practice competencies and standards are regulated by provincial and territorial organizations. In 2006, provincial and territorial regulatory bodies collaboratively developed a national set of entry-to-practice competencies that are updated on a regular basis (Black et al., 2008). However, the regulatory bodies do not set out specific competencies for gerontological nursing. In 1989, the CGNA adopted the Standards of Gerontological Nursing developed by the Gerontological Nursing Association Ontario (GNAO). The GNAO then embarked on a consultative process to develop national standards for gerontological nursing and published these in 1996. In 2010, the *Gerontological Nursing Competencies and Standards of Practice* were published (Canadian Gerontological Nursing Association [CGNA], 2010). These were updated in 2020 (CGNA, 2020). There are six broad standards, each supported by a set of competencies. The standards are outlined in Box 2.4.

Certification

Certification is a means of assuring the public that an individual has pursued some specialized study in a given area, has successfully demonstrated the requisite knowledge and competencies, and has been awarded recognition of this achievement. Canadian Nurses Association certification in gerontological nursing for RNs, nurse practitioners (NPs), and registered practical nurses (RPNs) verifies professional competency and assures nursing colleagues, the public, and employers that the nurse possesses specialized knowledge that meets predetermined standards. In 2020, more than 2000 RNs, NPs, and RPNs were certified as gerontological

---

BOX 2.4
CANADIAN GERONTOLOGICAL NURSING ASSOCIATION STANDARDS OF PRACTICE AND COMPETENCIES

STANDARD I: RELATIONAL CARE

Gerontological nurses address: 1. Relationships of older persons and their care partners to optimize health and well-being, 2. Preferences of older persons and their care partners to reflect unique experiences, cultural contexts, and social determinants of health, and 3. All aspects of care as part of an inter-professional collaborative team.

STANDARD II: ETHICAL CARE

Gerontological nurses address: 1. Older persons and care partners as their advocates, 2. Human rights for autonomy, diversity, inclusion, 3. Self-determination and freedom of expression, 4. Ethical, moral and legal contexts of nursing practice, 5. Collaborative decision-making, 6. Access to and provision of care reflecting the person's preferences and cultural requirements, and 7. Promotion and support of autonomy and independence.

STANDARD III: EVIDENCE-INFORMED CARE

Gerontological nurses address: 1. All aspects of health and well-being, 2. Information and educational needs, 3. Assessment of health, functional and cognitive capacities, 4. Geriatric syndromes, 5. Pain and symptom management, 6. Acute illness and chronic health conditions management, 7. Medication management, 8. Behaviour and cognitive therapy, 9. Adaptive communication needs, 10. Advance care planning, 11. Coping and grieving, and 12. End-of-life care and Medical Assistance in Dying.

STANDARD IV: AESTHETIC/ARTFUL CARE

Gerontological nurses address: 1. Needs of older persons to share experiences and meanings, 2. Aesthetics of living/caring spaces, 3. Environmental design, 4. Need for music, warmth, comfort, food, artistic elements, presence of familiar people or objects, 5. Access to activities that address the need for cultural, creative and spiritual expressions through social/health resources, and 6. Appropriate skill mix, shared decision-making, shared power, effective staff relationships and supportive organizational systems.

STANDARD V: SAFE CARE

Gerontological nurses address: 1. Health literacy, 2. Culturally competent, safe and sensitive care, 3. Equipment requirements for maintaining safety, 4. Risk reduction and monitoring of risk over time, 5. Assessment, prevention and mitigation of all forms of abuse, 6. Safe interpersonal relationships, including relationships of intimacy, 7. Assessment of risk; reduction, mitigation, and monitoring of risk over time, 8. Food safety and security, and 9. Access to safe and affordable housing.

STANDARD VI: SOCIO-POLITICALLY ENGAGED CARE

Gerontological nurses address: 1. Ageism that limits health care delivery and stigmatizes older persons within society, 2. Care inequities across all sectors of health care delivery, 3. Health policy at the local, provincial and national levels, and 4. Advocacy needs of older persons within the healthcare system.

Source: Canadian Gerontological Nursing Association. (2020). *Gerontological nursing standards of practice and competencies* (4th ed.). Author.

nurses (Canadian Nurses Association [CNA], 2020). (For additional information on certification, see http://www.cna-aiic.ca).

GERONTOLOGICAL NURSING EDUCATION

Ensuring that all students graduating from a nursing program have competency in gerontological nursing is imperative for the improvement of health care for older adults. Adequate preparation of students and the need for improved gerontological nursing education in Canada have been discussed in the gerontological nursing literature for many years (Burns et al., 1986; Boscart et al., 2016; Hsu et al., 2019). The necessity of stand-alone courses, as provided for specialty practice areas such as maternal–child or mental health nursing, is under debate. Some educators advocate for standalone courses or the integration of gerontological content in other courses (McCleary et al., 2017). There is evidence that gerontological content in nursing education is insufficient (Boscart et al., 2016; McCleary et al., 2017; Hsu et al., 2019). The reasons for this deficiency may include unsupportive faculty; insufficient gerontological nursing expertise among faculty; gerontological content being regarded as an extra requirement that overloads the already extensive requirements for accreditation of nursing education programs; assumptions that such content is integrated throughout the program; and a lack of interest from students and faculty. Deficient gerontological content and coursework in the education of health care providers can be viewed as a form of ageism (see Chapter 3) and discrimination.

Some colleges and universities have incorporated dynamic courses in aging into their curricula (Boscart et al., 2016), and several resources to improve curricula and teaching are available. The John A. Hartford Foundation in the United States has been responsible for some of the most significant advances in gerontological nursing, education, and research. The foundation's nursing initiatives include the Institute for Geriatric Nursing at New York University and the Centers for Geriatric Nursing Excellence at nine universities in the United States. The clinical nursing website of the Hartford Institute for Geriatric Nursing (https://hign.org/consultgeri-resources/elearning) contains abundant evidence-informed resources for gerontological nurses

and nurse educators. The Canadian Institutes for Health Research (CIHR) has funded knowledge-exchange institutes for Canadian nursing faculty members (McCleary et al., 2009; McCleary, 2010). CIHR has provided faculty with Canadian and US evidence-informed resources to improve gerontological nursing education. A publicly accessible wiki has also been created to share resources (http://kumu.brocku.ca/geriatricnursingeducation/Main_Page). With such resources now available, nursing educators must seriously consider specific minimum requirements for the care of older adults to fulfill the responsibility of nurses to the public and the profession.

Beyond course curriculum development, a large amount of research and practice innovation is available to gerontological nurses. Considering the rate of expansion of this domain of knowledge and the fact that many nurses do not have sufficient knowledge about caring for older adults with complex needs, taking advantage of available continuing education resources is important. The resources listed on the previously cited wiki can be used for continuing education in health care facilities. Many colleges also offer continuing education courses and postgraduate certificates in gerontological nursing.

ROLES IN GERONTOLOGICAL NURSING

Gerontological nursing roles encompass many different venues and circumstances. The opportunities are limitless. The impact of gerontological nursing on the health and well-being of older adults and their families can be seen across various practice settings, in communities, in people's homes, and in care environments. Gerontological nurses work directly with older adults and their families, linking them to needed services. Through leadership and research, gerontological nurses influence improvements in services, care practices, and policies.

A gerontological nurse may be a generalist or a specialist. The generalist functions in a variety of settings (primary care, acute care, home care, rehabilitation and LTC homes, as well as in the community), providing nursing care and services to individuals and their families. The gerontological nursing specialist is an advanced practice nurse (APN) with education at the master's level.

Specialist Roles

APNs, sometimes referred to as clinical nurse specialists, perform all the functions of generalists but possess advanced clinical expertise, integrate health and social policy, and are proficient in planning, implementing, and evaluating health programs. NPs function in an extended nursing role. The NP scope of practice varies among provinces and territories in Canada. For example, in Ontario, upon graduating, NPs can work in four areas: primary health care, adult care, pediatric care, and anesthesia (Nurse Practitioner Association of Ontario [NPAO], 2020). In nine provinces and territories (Alberta, British Columbia, Manitoba, Newfoundland and Labrador, New Brunswick, Northwest Territories, Nova Scotia, Nunavut, Ontario, Prince Edward Island, and Saskatchewan), NPs can conduct advanced health assessments and diagnoses (Canadian Institute for Health Information [CIHI], 2020a). NPs can also prescribe pharmacotherapy in nearly all provinces and territories (except British Columbia) (CIHI, 2020a).

APNs and NPs have demonstrated their skills in improving health outcomes and cost effectiveness in primary, acute, and continuing care settings; community settings; retirement homes; hospices; LTC homes; and care settings that provide specialized care for older adults.

Research has demonstrated the positive outcomes associated with APNs and NPs, including increased satisfaction among patients, clients, and residents and their families and care partners, decreased costs, fewer hospitalizations and emergency room visits, and improved quality of care (Chavez et al., 2018). NPs in LTC homes provide primary care and advanced nursing care, resulting in improved quality of care (Chavez et al., 2018). Some Canadian universities offer graduate courses in gerontological nursing but none have specialty programs. Mezey and Fulmer have suggested that all graduate nursing programs be "gerontologized" so that all APNs and NP graduates would have gerontological nursing competencies to meet the health care needs of an aging population (Chavez et al., 2018).

Generalist Roles
Hospital-Based Care

Even though most nurses work in acute care with older adults and their families, many have not had specialized gerontological nursing in their nursing education programs. Between 2017 and 2018, older adults accounted for 51% of all injury-related hospitalizations in Canada (CIHI, 2019). In addition, older adults who experience episodic or acute illnesses often have multiple chronic conditions and comorbidities and therefore present with complex care needs.

Exacerbations of persistent, chronic illnesses and injuries are often the cause of hospitalization for older adults. The most common reasons for the admission of older adults to Canadian hospitals are chronic obstructive pulmonary disease, heart failure, knee and hip replacements, pneumonia, and myocardial infarction (CIHI, 2020b). Often, older adults experience iatrogenic complications while being hospitalized, including functional decline, new-onset incontinence, malnutrition, pressure ulcers, medication interactions and adverse effects, delirium, and falls. Many of these conditions are directly related to and influenced by nursing care, reinforcing the need for nurses to be competent in the care of older adults.

Because of problems accessing home care, rehabilitation, or LTC after hospitalization, some older adults are ready to be discharged but are unable to leave the hospital. This group of older adults are classified as needing an **alternate level of care (ALC).** In recent years, several acute care hospital beds have been designated as ALC beds (Health Quality Ontario, 2017). The vast majority of ALC patients are older adults, and a significant proportion of them live with dementia.

Nurses caring for older adults in hospitals may function as direct care providers, care coordinators, educators, and discharge planners. They may also work in leadership, research, quality improvement, and management positions. The complex needs of older adults who require hospital-based care means that, in order to provide competent care, all nurses in hospital settings need to have a depth of knowledge about the various conditions associated with aging, the ability to distinguish normal aging from pathology, and well-developed critical thinking, care planning, intervention, and evaluation skills.

Some health care organizations have made organization-wide commitments to excellent care for older adults. The Nurses Improving Care for Health System Elders (NICHE) program was developed by the Hartford Institute for Geriatric Nursing in 1992. It emphasizes institutional commitment, collaboration, and nursing leadership to achieve improved safety and outcomes for hospitalized older adults

(Fulmer & Mezey, 2019). More than 500 hospitals in the United States and 13 in Canada are involved in NICHE programs (http://www.nicheprogram.org).

A key component of the NICHE program is the geriatric resource nurse model, whereby nurses are trained by advanced practice gerontological nurses and then function as clinical resource experts on geriatric issues for other nurses. This is an innovative role for a hospital nurse interested in the care of older adults. The NICHE Acute Care of the Elderly Medical-Surgical Unit is based on patient- and family-centred approaches. The physical environment is adapted to meet the needs of older adults and to enhance functional independence. Staffing consists of an interprofessional team with expert knowledge in the care of older adults. Older adults are discharged to the least restrictive environment. Outcomes in hospitals using NICHE models include enhanced nursing knowledge and skills related to the management of common geriatric syndromes, improved patient satisfaction, decreased length of stay, reductions in admission rates, and reductions in hospital costs (Fulmer & Mezey, 2019).

Community- and Home-Based Care

The majority of older adults live in the community. Community-based care settings include home care, independent older-adult housing, retirement communities, adult day health programs, primary care clinics, and public health departments. The growth in home- and community-based health care is expected to continue, since older adults prefer to age in place, a perspective that is increasingly recognized in policy and planning. Several provinces have developed strategies to support aging in place (e.g., Manitoba Health [http://www.gov.mb.ca/health/aginginplace/] and the Ontario Ministry of Health and Long-Term Care [https://www.ontario.ca/page/aging-confidence-ontario-action-plan-seniors]), measures that are discussed in Chapters 26 and 28. However, access to publicly funded home care varies from province to province, and for some older adults, the cost of purchasing needed home care services further limits their accessibility (Davies et al., 2017).

Nurses in the home setting provide comprehensive assessments; may provide and supervise care for older adults who have a variety of care needs, including dementia care; and provide specific treatments such as wound care, catheter care, intravenous therapy, and tube feedings. Older adults requiring care at home include people living with unstable medical conditions, people with complex medication or care regimens, and those receiving rehabilitation, supportive, or palliative care services. Advances in technology for remote monitoring of health status and safety show promise in improving outcomes for older adults who want to age in place. These technologies present exciting opportunities for nurses in the management and evaluation of care (see Chapter 15). Gerontological nurses have opportunities to create practices in community-based settings with a focus not only on caring for those who are ill but also on promoting health and addressing determinants of health.

Long-Term Care

Formal settings for LTC include chronic-care hospitals, complex continuing care facilities, inpatient rehabilitation settings, and LTC homes (also referred to as nursing homes). About 7% of older Canadians live in LTC homes where most of the residents are older adults (Statistics Canada, 2018). As the health care system has evolved to support aging at home, the complexity and acuity of residents in LTC settings has increased considerably (Ontario Long Term Care Association, 2019). In addition, stringent regulations governing care practices, the interprofessional and cross-functional team models, the expanded use of nurses and **unregulated care providers (UCPs;** i.e., personal support workers), the innovative use of APNs and NPs, and the limited presence of physicians on site influence the role of professional nursing in these settings. Thus, it is essential that gerontological nurses in LTC homes possess excellent assessment skills; the ability to work in partnership with other team members and families; skills in acute, rehabilitative, and palliative care; and leadership, advocacy, management, collaboration, and delegation skills.

Professional nurses in LTC homes must be highly skilled in order to practise independently and collaboratively. This setting provides significant opportunities for independent decision making, nursing leadership, optimized integrated team models of care, and evaluation of resident and family outcomes, including well-being. Nursing roles may include those of administrator, manager, supervisor, coordinator, educator, case manager, quality improvement coordinator, and clinical nurse.

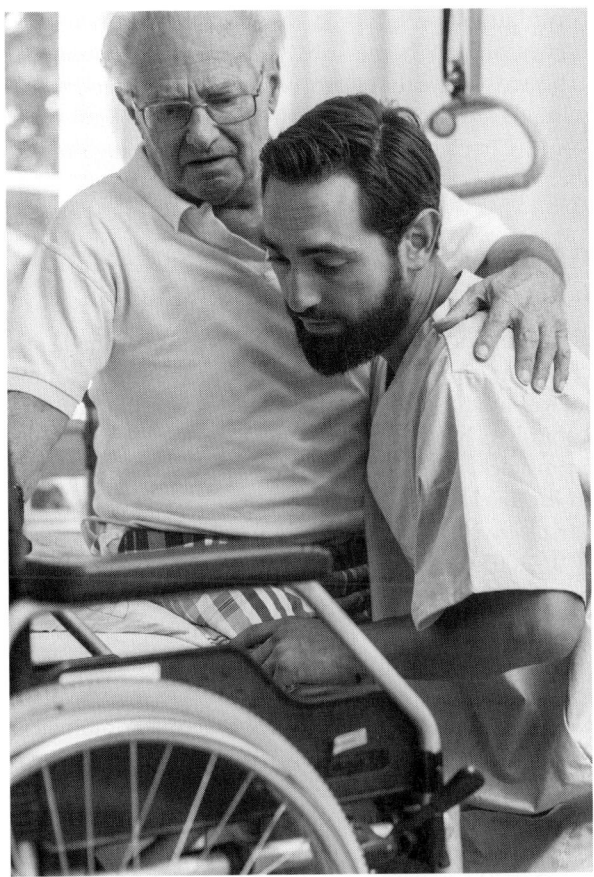

Nurses working in long-term care settings use both independent and interprofessional skill sets to address the complex and varied needs of residents. Copyright CanStock Photo Inc. / Kzenon.

LTC homes care for people who need skilled comprehensive nursing care but who may not need the intense care that is provided in complex continuing care hospitals. Such people include those who have had a severe stroke, those living with Alzheimer's disease and related dementias, those who have Parkinson's disease, and those who are in need of comfort and end-of-life care. About 30% of LTC home residents are aged 85 years or older (Statistics Canada, 2018). Residents of LTC homes represent the frailest of the older adult population; their need for 24-hour care cannot be met in the home or may have exceeded their families' abilities to provide care. A survey of Ontario LTC homes found that about two-thirds of residents have a diagnosis of dementia, and 61% of residents take 10 or more prescription medications (Ontario Long Term Care Association, 2019). Payment for LTC homes is subsidized by provincial governments. Residents pay for basic accommodations and for medications that are not covered by provincial drug plans.

In 2020, there were 2,039 LTC homes in Canada (CIHI, 2020c). As the population in Canada continues to age, the number of LTC homes is predicted to significantly increase. The hiring of an adequate number of competent staff continues to be of critical importance in these settings, especially in view of the acuity and complex needs of the residents. Provincial standards set staffing requirements by numbers of hours of care per resident, not by staff-to-resident ratios. Staffing levels have often been criticized as inadequate (Harrington et al., 2020), and many LTC homes do not consistently meet staffing requirements (Harrington et al., 2020). More time spent by RNs providing direct care to each resident in LTC is associated with better resident outcomes with respect to fall prevention, urinary tract infection, and hospitalization (Harrington et al., 2020). Despite increases in the acuity level of LTC home residents' conditions and the positive relationship between nurse staffing and quality of care, relatively few RNs work in LTC homes.

In 2020, the World Health Organization declared a global pandemic of severe acute respiratory syndrome coronavirus 2 (SARS-CoV-2, or COVID-19), which affected millions of people. Unfortunately, LTC homes were most affected in Canada, accounting for more than 80% of all COVID-19 deaths (CIHI, 2020d). This sparked an urgent need to reform the LTC system, including by addressing the need for a workforce mix in Canadian LTC homes (Estabrooks et al., 2020).

There are several new initiatives in LTC that nurses can be involved with to improve professional nursing practice and resident quality outcomes, including the Registered Nurses' Association of Ontario Spotlight Organization program for LTC homes and Sigma Theta Tau's Center for Nursing Excellence in Long-Term Care. The culture change movement, discussed in Chapter 28, provides many exciting opportunities for nurses to lead the change from an institution-centred culture to a person-centred culture in LTC homes.

Unregulated Care Providers (Personal Support Workers)

Although it is important to promote professional nursing care for older adults, UCPs, also known as personal support workers, provide the majority of care and services in LTC homes and home care settings (Zysberg et al., 2019), contributing significantly to quality of life for older adults and their care partners. The results of several studies confirm the deep commitment and passion that UCPs bring to their jobs and to the older adults whom they care for (Zysberg et al., 2019). The significance and importance of close personal relationships between UCPs and older adults (often described as "like family") form a central dimension of quality of care and positive outcomes (Thompson & McClement, 2019).

However, recruiting and retaining UCPs has been difficult to achieve in LTC homes as well as in home care (Boscart et al., 2019). In a Canadian study, UCPs in LTC homes reported being rushed in their care and not having sufficient time to complete needed tasks (Boscart et al., 2018). Several recent studies have investigated the relationship between factors such as turnover, work satisfaction, staffing, and power relations to the quality of care and positive outcomes in LTC homes. The results support the importance of developing a culture of respect in which the work of UCPs is understood and valued at all levels of the organization (Boscart et al., 2018). It is difficult to recruit and retain UCPs in LTC homes. Lack of fulltime work, pay, and benefits coupled with poor working conditions contribute to this difficulty (Estabrooks et al., 2020).

One of the most important components of the culture change movement in LTC homes is the creation of team models of care that value and honour the important work of UCPs, who are undervalued by society and the health care system (Hewko et al., 2015). Such models are consistent with the Priory Method pioneered by Vera McIver (see Box 2.3). Culture change is equally concerned about the needs of residents and the well-being of staff. According to Thomas and Johansson, "An organization that learns to give love, respect, dignity, tenderness, and tolerance to all members of the staff will soon find these same virtues being practiced by the staff" (Thomas & Johansson, 2003, p. 3). Until health care providers and society make a real commitment to providing adequate wages, providing individual supports (e.g., benefits, education, career ladders), and appreciating the significant

contribution by UCPs to the quality of care in LTC homes and in home care, these workers cannot be expected to have the energy or incentive to extend themselves fully to their work with older adults (Kash et al., 2007). Chapter 28 discusses the culture change movement in greater depth.

GERONTOLOGICAL NURSING AND GERONTOLOGY ORGANIZATIONS

Gerontological nursing organizations in Canada include the nationwide CGNA and provincial gerontological nursing associations in Newfoundland and Labrador, Nova Scotia, Prince Edward Island, New Brunswick, Ontario, Manitoba, Alberta, and British Columbia. The CGNA publishes a refereed journal, *Perspectives*, and holds a national biennial conference.

In 2003, the CGNA and the National Gerontological Nursing Association (NGNA) in the United States formed an alliance to exchange information and share mutual goals and opportunities for the advancement of both groups. Gerontological nursing associations in the United States include the NGNA, the Gerontological Advanced Practice Nurses Association, and the National Association of Directors of Nursing Administration in Long-Term Care. The NGNA publishes the journal *Geriatric Nursing*. The US Coalition of Geriatric Nursing Organizations represents more than 28,700 gerontological nurses from 8 organizations.

The Canadian Association on Gerontology (CAG) supports interdisciplinary and interprofessional collaboration in research and practice. The divisions of Health and Biological Sciences, Social Policy and Practice, Educational Gerontology, Psychology, and Social Sciences include members from myriad backgrounds and many disciplines who affiliate with CAG on the basis of their particular role and function rather than just their educational or professional credentials. The Association publishes the *Canadian Journal on Aging*. The CAG Student Connection is a national network for students interested in aging issues (http://cagacg.ca/student-connection/). Some provinces have provincial gerontology associations.

The Canadian Geriatrics Society (CGS) is devoted to promoting excellence in the medical care of older Canadians. Membership is open to all physicians with an interest in geriatrics. Nurses and other health care providers can join the CGS as associate members. The Canadian Academy of Geriatric Psychiatry is an association of physicians who have completed training in geriatric psychiatry or are in training. It provides leadership in the field of geriatric psychiatry and promotes the mental health of older adults. British Columbia and Ontario also have geriatric mental health associations.

International gerontology associations such as the Gerontological Society of America, the International Federation on Ageing, and the International Association of Gerontology and Geriatrics have interprofessional and interdisciplinary membership and offer the opportunity to study aging internationally.

IMPLICATIONS FOR GERONTOLOGICAL NURSING AND HEALTHY AGING

Nursing is a vital aspect of health care for older adults, and the practice of gerontological nursing provides a unique vantage point from which to make an impact. Nurses attracted to this field recognize that expertise in caring for older adults can make a significant difference in the quality of life of the older adult. Because of the complex needs of older adults with health problems, gerontological nursing is intellectually challenging. In times of illness, rehabilitation, and end-of-life care, outcomes for the older adult more often than not depend on the nursing care received. Through research, gerontological nurses have made substantial contributions to the body of knowledge of best practices in the care of older adults, and they are recognized as leaders in aging care.

Gerontological nurses have opportunities to provide care across the continuum of aging services, caring for everyone from the most ill and frail to those who are active and independent. As Mezey and Fulmer have pointed out, the commitment of gerontological nurses is to "tackle difficult but exceptionally meaningful issues that impact profoundly on the health and quality of life for older adults" (Mezey & Fulmer, 2002, p. 440). Gerontological nursing may be the most needed specialty in nursing, both now and in the future (Touhy et al., 2018).

KEY CONCEPTS

- Certification assures the public of nurses' commitment to specialized education and qualification for the care of older adults.
- All students graduating from nursing programs and all practising nurses caring for older adults should have competence in gerontological nursing.
- Major changes in health care delivery and the increasing number of older adults have resulted in numerous revised, refined, and emergent roles for nurses in the field of gerontological nursing. There is a critical shortage of competent and compassionate gerontological nurses.
- Advanced practice nurses and nurse practitioners have additional qualifications.
- Advanced practice opportunities for nurses offer more independence, are cost effective, and facilitate comprehensive care and improved outcomes for older adults.
- Nursing and interprofessional gerontological organizations support scholarship, the advancement and dissemination of new knowledge and best practices, and networking (including student member networking).

ACTIVITIES AND DISCUSSION QUESTIONS

1. Identify factors that have influenced the progress of gerontological nursing as a specialty practice.

2. Consider and discuss the various gerontological nursing roles that you find most interesting and stimulating.

3. Discuss what you consider the most important elements of the 2020 Canadian Gerontological Nurses Association Nursing Competencies and Standards of Practice.

4. Discuss the gerontological organizations of today and their significance to the practising nurse.

5. Discuss what you think are the most important issues in gerontological nursing education.

RESOURCES

Canadian Association on Gerontology (CAG)
http://www.cagacg.ca
Canadian Gerontological Nursing Association (CGNA)
http://www.cgna.net
Canadian Nurses Association (CNA) certification program
https://cna-aiic.ca/en/certification
Hartford Institute for Geriatric Nursing
https://hign.org/
National Gerontological Nursing Association (NGNA)
http://www.ngna.org

For additional resources, please visit *http://evolve.elsevier.com/ Canada/Ebersole/gerontological/*

REFERENCES

Beckingham, A. C., & DuGas, B. W. (1993). Promoting healthy aging: A nursing and community perspective. Mosby.

Black, J., Allen, D., Redfern, L., et al. (2008). Competencies in the context of entry-level registered nurse practice: A collaborative project in Canada. *International Nursing Review, 55*, 171–178. doi:10.1111/j.1466-7657.2007.00626.x.

Boscart, V., McCleary, L., Huson, K., et al. (2016). Integrating gerontological competencies in Canadian health and social service education: An overview of trends, enablers, and challenges. *Gerontology & Geriatrics Education, 38*(1), 17–46. doi:10.1080/02701960.2016.1230738.

Boscart, V., Sidani, S., Poss, J., et al. (2018). The associations between staffing hours and quality of care indicators in long-term care. *BMC Health Services Research, 18*(1), 750.

Boscart, V., d'Avernas, J., van der Horst, M., et al. (2019). Shared learning environments for unregulated care provider education in long-term care: Innovative approaches and key considerations. *Gerontology and Geriatrics Education, 18*, 1–9. doi:10.1080/02701960.2019/1645015.

Burns, L., MacLeod, F., MacTavish, M., et al. (1986). Career selection: Planting the seed for gerontological nursing. *Perspectives, 10*(8), 8–10.

Canadian Gerontological Nursing Association. (2010). *Gerontological nursing competencies and standards of practice.* Author.

Canadian Gerontological Nursing Association. (2020). *Gerontological nursing standards of practice and competencies* (4th ed.). Author.

Canadian Institute for Health Information (CIHI). (2019). *Injuries among seniors.* https://www.cihi.ca/en/injuries-among-seniors.

Canadian Institute for Health Information (CIHI). (2020a). *Nurse practitioner scopes of practice vary across Canada's provinces and territories.* https://www.cihi.ca/en/nurse-practitioner-scopes-of-practice-vary-across-canadas-provinces-and-territories.

Canadian Institute for Health Information (CIHI). (2020b). *Inpatient hospitalization, surgery and newborn statistics, 2018–2019.* Author.

Canadian Institute for Health Information (CIHI). (2020c). *Long-term care homes in Canada: How many and who owns them?* https://www.cihi.ca/en/long-term-care-homes-in-canada-how-many-and-who-owns-them.

Canadian Institute for Health Information (CIHI). (2020d). *Pandemic experience in the long-term care sector: How does Canada compare with other countries?* Author.

Canadian Institutes of Health Research (CIHR). (2020). *Knowledge translation.* https://cihr-irsc.gc.ca/e/29529.html.

Canadian Nurses Association (CNA). (2020). *Number of valid CNA certifications by specialty/area of nursing practice and province and/or territory.* https://www.cfmhn.ca/wp-content/uploads/2021/03/certification-statistics-2020-by-specialty-area-and-province_territory-en.pdf.

Chai, X., Cheng, C., Mei, J., et al. (2019). Student nurses' career motivation toward gerontological nursing: A longitudinal study. *Nurse Education Today, 76*, 165–171.

Chavez, K. S., Dwyer, A. A., & Ramelet, A. S. (2018). International practice settings, interventions and outcomes of nurse practitioners in geriatric care: A scoping review. *International Journal of Nursing Studies, 78*, 61–75.

Dahlke, S. (2011). Examining nursing practice with older adults through a historical lens. *Journal of Gerontological Nursing, 37*(5), 41–48. doi:10.3928/00989134-20110106-06.

Davies, L. A., Hirdes, J. P., & Mannell, R. (2017). When healthcare is delivered in your home, will you need to make economic trade-offs? In G. Joseph (Ed.), *Diverse perspectives on aging in a changing world* (pp. 145–166). Routledge.

Davis, B. (1984). Nursing care of the aged: Historical evolution. In S. Fondmiller (Ed.), *Conference proceedings: Historical basis of clinical nursing practice in the United States.* Chicago, IL: American Association for the History of Nursing. New Orleans, LA, June 26, 1984.

Dock, L. (1908). The crusade for almshouse nursing. *American Journal of Nursing, 8*(7), 520. doi:10.1097/00000446-190804000-00003.

Estabrooks, C. A., Straus, S., Flood, C. M., et al. (2020). *Restoring trust: COVID-19 and the future of long-term care.* Royal Society of Canada.

Fulmer, T., & Mezey, M. (2019). The compelling context for NICHE. In T. Fulmer, K. Glassman, S. Greenberg, P. Rosenfeld, M. Gilmartin, & M. Mezey (Eds). *NICHE: Nurses improving care for healthsystem elders* (pp. 3–10). New York: Springer. doi: 10.1891/9780826170828.0001.

Garbrah, W., Välimäki, T., Palovaara, M., et al. (2017). Nursing curriculums may hinder a career in gerontological nursing: An integrative review. *International Journal of Older People Nursing, 12*(3), e12152.

Harrington, C., Dellefield, M. E., Halifax, E., et al. (2020). Appropriate nurse staffing levels for US nursing homes. *Health Services Insights, 13.* doi:10.1177/1178632920934785.

Health Quality Ontario. (2017). *Measuring up 2017: A yearly report on how Ontario's health system is performing.* Queen's Printer for Ontario.

Hirst, S., King, T., & Church, J. (1996). The emergence of gerontological nursing education in Canada. *Geriatric Nursing, 17*(3), 120–122. doi:10.1016/S0197-4572(96)80093-0.

Hewko, S. J., Cooper, S. L., Huynh, H., et al. (2015). Invisible no more: A scoping review of the health care aide workforce literature. *BMC Nursing, 14*, 38. doi:10.1186/s12912-015-0090-x.

Hsu, M. H. K., Ling, M. H., & Lui, T. L. (2019). Relationship between gerontological nursing education and attitude toward older people. *Nurse Education Today, 74,* 85–90. doi:10.1016/j.nedt.2018.12.007.

Kash, B., Castle, N., & Phillips, C. (2007). Nursing home spending, staffing and turnover. *Health Care Management Review, 32*(3), 253–262. doi:10.1016/j.gerinurse.2008.01.005.

McCleary, L. (2010). Wiki supports excellence in gerontological nursing education. *Perspectives, 34*(1), 14–16.

McCleary, L., Boscart, V., Donahue, P., et al. (2017). Educator readiness to improve gerontological curricula in health and social service education. *Canadian Journal on Aging, 36*(4), 501–513.

McCleary, L., McGilton, K., Boscart, V., et al. (2009). Improving gerontology content in baccalaureate nursing education through knowledge transfer to nurse educators. *Nursing Leadership, 22*(3), 33–46. doi:10.12927/cjnl.2009.21153.

Mezey, M. D., & Fulmer, T. T. (2002). The future history of gerontological nursing. *Journal of Gerontology, 57A*(7), M438–M441. doi:10.1093/gerona/57.7.M438.

Newton, K., & Anderson, H. (1950). *Geriatric nursing.* Mosby.

Ontario Long Term Care Association. (2019). *This is long-term care 2019.* Author. https://www.oltca.com/OLTCA/Documents/Reports/TILTC2019web.pdf.

Nurse Practitioner Association of Ontario (NPAO). (2020). *What is a nurse practitioner?* https://npao.org/about-npao/what-is-a-np/.

Statistics Canada. (2018). *Transitions to long-term and residential care among older Canadians.* https://www150.statcan.gc.ca/n1/pub/82-003-x/2018005/article/54966-eng.htm.

Thomas, W., & Johansson, C. (2003). Elderhood in Eden. *Topics in Geriatric Rehabilitation, 19*(4), 282–289. doi:10.1097/00013614-200310000-00009.

Thompson, G. N., & McClement, S. E. (2019). Critical nursing and health care aide behaviors in care of the nursing home resident dying with dementia. *BMC Nursing, 18*(59). doi:10.1186/s12912-019-0384-5.

Touhy, T., Jett, K., Boscart, V., et al. (2018). *Ebersole and Hess' Gerontological nursing and healthy aging in Canada* (2nd ed.). Mosby Elsevier.

Wykle, M., & McDonald, P. (1997). The past, present, and future of gerontological nursing. In S. Klein (Ed.), *A national agenda for geriatric education.* Springer.

Zysberg, L., Band-Winterstein, T., Doron, I., et al. (2019). The health care aide position in nursing homes: A comparative survey of nurses' and aides' perceptions. *International Journal of Nursing Studies, 94,* 98–106.

3 COMMUNICATING WITH OLDER ADULTS

LEARNING OBJECTIVES

Upon completion of this chapter, the reader will be able to:

- Describe the importance of communication to the lives of older adults.
- Discuss how ageist attitudes affect communication with older adults.
- Describe interventions that facilitate communication individually and in groups.
- Understand the significance of the life story of an older adult.
- Discuss the modalities of reminiscence and life review.
- Identify effective communication strategies for older adults with speech, language, hearing, vision, and cognitive impairments.

GLOSSARY

Ageism   Ageism incorporates two concepts: "way[s] of thinking about older persons based on negative attitudes and stereotypes about aging; and a tendency to structure society based on an assumption that everyone is young, thereby failing to respond appropriately to the real needs of older persons" (Ontario Human Rights Commission, 2020, p. 1).

Aphasia   Loss of the ability to express and understand spoken and written language.

Apraxia   An impairment in the ability to manipulate objects or perform purposeful acts, including the ability to speak.

Communication   The exchange of information between individuals through a system of signs, symbols, speech, and behaviour.

Dysarthria   A speech disorder caused by weakness or incoordination of the muscles used for speech.

Elderspeak   A common speech style used when talking to older adults that presupposes their dependence, incompetence, and control by the speaker. Elderspeak includes baby talk, using terms like "honey" and "dear," and speaking louder and more slowly.

Life review   A critical analysis of a person's past life, with the goal of facilitating integrity.

THE LIVED EXPERIENCE

Listen to the aged for they will tell you about living and dying.

Listen to the aged for they will enlighten you about problem-solving, sexuality, grief, sensory deprivation, and survival.

Listen to the aged for they will teach you how to be courageous, loving, and generous.

They are a distinguished faculty without formal classrooms, tenure, sabbaticals. They teach not from books but from long experience in living.

From Burnside, I. M. (1975). Listen to the aged. *American Journal of Nursing, 75*(10), 1801. doi:10.2307/3423569.

Communication is the most important ability of human beings. Communication allows us to express our thoughts, feelings, likes, and dislikes through verbal and nonverbal means. Communicating allows us to exchange information through a system of signs, symbols, speech, or behaviour. Maslow's hierarchy of needs places the human need for affiliation second only to the need for safety and survival (Maslow, 1943). The need to communicate, to be listened to, and to be heard does not change with age or impairment. Meaningful communication and active involvement in society both contribute to healthy aging and could improve older adults' chances of living longer, responding better to health care interventions, and maintaining optimal function (Gasiorek et al., 2019).

Older adults may have fewer opportunities for social interaction owing to loss of family and friends; illnesses; and hearing, vision, and cognitive impairments. The ageist attitudes of the public, as well as those of health care providers, also present barriers to communicating effectively with older adults. Good verbal and nonverbal communication skills are the basis for accurate assessment, care planning, and the development of therapeutic relationships between the nurse and the older adult.

This chapter discusses the effect of health care providers' attitudes toward aging on their communication with older adults; verbal and nonverbal communication skills essential to interactions with older adults; and adapting communication for older adults with vision and hearing impairments, speech and language disorders, and cognitive impairment. The significance of life story, reminiscence, life review, and communication with groups of older adults is also discussed in this chapter. A discussion of age-related changes in hearing and vision is presented in Chapter 6; assessment of hearing, vision, and cognition in Chapter 13; diseases of the eye and ear in Chapter 19; and care of older adults with cognitive impairment in Chapter 21.

AGEISM AND COMMUNICATION

Ageist attitudes, myths, and stereotypical ideas about older adults can interfere with the nurse's ability to communicate with them effectively. For example, if the nurse believes that all older adults have memory problems or are unable to learn and process information, then the nurse will be less likely to engage in conversation, provide appropriate health information, or treat the person with respect and dignity. **Ageism** is a term used to express prejudice toward older adults through attitudes and behaviour (Ontario Human Rights Commission, 2020). Similar to other prejudices (e.g., racism, anti-Semitism, and sexism), ageism affects us all. Although ageism is cross-cultural, it is especially prevalent in the Western world, where aging is viewed with depression, fear, and anxiety (Rittenour & Cohen, 2016). Ageism leads to negative physical and mental health affects among older adults such as cardiovascular stress and lowered levels of self-efficacy (World Health Organization [WHO], 2020). Ageism toward older adults has also resulted in negatives attitudes about working in areas such as long-term care (LTC) homes, making it challenging to recruit and retain health care providers in this growing field (WHO, 2020). It is important for gerontological nurses to be aware of their own attitudes toward aging and to recognize how their beliefs may influence their verbal and nonverbal communication. The evaluation and enhancement of interpersonal communication skills form the foundation for therapeutic interactions with older adults.

Elderspeak, often referred to as "baby talk" directed toward older adults, is a form of ageism in which younger people alter their speech on the assumption that all older adults have difficulty comprehending what is said to them (Corwin, 2018). Although someone using elderspeak may intend to offer a supportive, warm, and friendly environment, this use of language may induce negative feelings of self-worth in the older adult (Zhang et al., 2020; Box 3.1).

Nurses may not be aware that they are using elderspeak. It is nonetheless important to note such speech style, as research has shown that this form of speech is offensive and patronizing and conveys the belief that older adults are dependent, incompetent, and controlled (Corwin, 2018). There is also evidence that elderspeak

---

BOX 3.1
CHARACTERISTICS OF ELDERSPEAK

- Speaking slowly or loudly or both
- Using a singsong voice
- Using the pronouns "we," "us," and "our" in place of "you"
- Using pet names such as "honey," "dearie," or "sweetheart"
- Answering questions for the older adult (e.g., "You would like your dinner now, wouldn't you?")

Source: Adapted from *Elderspeak: Babytalk directed at older adults.* http://changingaging.org/elderhood/elderspeak-babytalk-directed-at-older-adults/.

has a negative effect on the care of patients with dementia (Williams et al., 2017). Other examples of communication that convey ageist attitudes are ignoring the older adult, talking to family and friends as if the older adult were not present, and limiting interaction to task-focused communication only (Williams et al., 2017).

Therapeutic verbal and nonverbal communication strategies that apply to all situations in nursing—listening attentively, having an authentic presence and a nonjudgemental attitude, being culturally competent, clarifying, giving information, seeking validation of understanding, keeping focus, and using open-ended questions—are all applicable to communicating with older adults. It is important to respect older adults: address them by their surname and professional titles unless invited to address them in another manner. Older adults may need more time for giving information or answering questions simply because they have a larger life experience from which to draw. Sorting through thoughts requires intervals of silence; therefore, listening to older adults carefully and without rushing is very important. Retrieving words, particularly nouns and names, may be a slower process for them.

Open-ended questions are useful but difficult for some older adults. Those who wish to please, especially when feeling vulnerable or somewhat dependent, may wonder what it is you want to hear and may tell you what they think you want to hear rather than what they would like to say. The most productive communication will initially focus on the issue of major concern to the older adult, regardless of the priority of the nursing assessment. When using closed questioning to obtain specific information, the nurse should be aware that the older adult may feel pressured; thus, the appropriate information may not be immediately forthcoming. This is especially true when the nurse is asking questions to determine mental status. The older adult may develop a mental block because of anxiety or feel threatened if questions are asked in a quiz-like or demeaning manner. Furthermore, older adults may be reluctant to disclose information for fear of the consequences. For example, if older adults are having problems remembering things or are experiencing frequent falls, they may assume that sharing that information will result in their having to leave their home and move to a more protective place.

A substantial portion of our communication is nonverbal. Older adults respond to nurses' behaviours and nonverbal cues, including through posture, facial expression, eye gaze, gesture, and tone of voice. Nonverbal details can reveal feelings and attitudes and affect relationships with other persons. Therefore, nurses should be aware of their own nonverbal communication with older adults, as nurses' feelings and attitudes affect relationships with other persons (Wanko Keutchafo et al., 2020).

When communicating with older adults who are in a bed or wheelchair, it is important to position oneself at their level rather than talking over a side rail or standing above them. Nurses should pay attention to older adults' gazes, gestures, and body language, as well as to the pitch, volume, and tone of their voices to understand what they are trying to communicate. Thoughts left unstated are often as important as those that are verbalized. A nurse may ask, "What are you thinking about right now?" Clarification is essential to ensure that the older adult and the nurse have the same framework of understanding. Many generational, cultural, and regional differences in speech patterns and idioms exist. Thus, frequently seeking validation of what the nurse thinks they have heard is important.

IMPLICATIONS FOR GERONTOLOGICAL NURSING AND HEALTHY AGING

Every time a nurse communicates with someone, their words and actions affect the relationship in positive or negative ways, depending on the nurse's attitudes and skills (Wanko Keutchafo et al., 2020). Enhancing verbal and nonverbal communication with older adults is an important skill in gerontological nursing and is rewarding for both the nurse and the older adult. Communication with older adults provides the nurse with the opportunity to share in their wisdom and gain insight on life.

COMMUNICATION WITH OLDER ADULTS WHO HAVE SENSORY IMPAIRMENTS

Sensory impairments, such as hearing or vision deficits, place older adults at risk for communication difficulties. People rely on their senses to perceive the environment and to enjoy the pleasures of life. Sensory impairments, along with altered environmental stimuli, can contribute to delirium by causing sensory deprivation (see Chapter 21). Gerontological nurses need special knowledge and skills to promote effective communication with older adults who have these deficits. This section describes adaptations that enhance verbal and nonverbal communication with older adults who have hearing and vision impairments.

Hearing Impairment

While both vision and hearing impairments significantly affect all aspects of life, Oliver Sacks, in his book *Seeing Voices: A Journey Into the World of the Deaf*, presents the view that blindness may in fact be less serious than the loss of hearing (Sacks, 1989). Hearing loss interferes with communication with others. In addition, hearing loss limits a person's opportunity to be part of an interaction, and this can lead to a sense of not being engaged or involved in conversations. Hearing loss is a prevalent, persistent condition in older Canadians and is the most common sensory impairment in Canadians over 60 years of age. Hearing loss rises after the age of 40, with about 65% of adults aged 70 to 79 experiencing hearing loss (Canadian Hard of Hearing Association [CHHA], 2020).

Hearing loss diminishes quality of life and is associated with numerous negative outcomes, including decreased function, miscommunication, social isolation, depression, safety risks, and reduced income and employment opportunities (Nordvik et al., 2018). Also, a hearing impairment may cause older adults to become suspicious or distrustful or to display paranoid thoughts. Because older adults with hearing loss may not understand or respond appropriately to conversation, they may be inappropriately diagnosed with cognitive impairment. Older adults may be initially unaware of hearing loss because of the gradual manner in which it develops (Box 3.2). The *Try This* series from the Hartford Institute for Geriatric Nursing provides guidelines for screening hearing ability (https://hign.org/consultgeri-resources/try-this-series). The Better Hearing Institute provides an online hearing test for older adults who want to check their hearing (https://betterhearing.org/check-your-hearing/online-hearing-checks/). Additional information about hearing assessment can be found in Chapter 13.

Hearing impairment is underdiagnosed and undertreated in older adults. Although screening for hearing

---

BOX 3.2
DO I HAVE A HEARING PROBLEM?

- Do I sometimes feel embarrassed when I meet new people because I struggle to hear?
- Do I feel frustrated when talking to members of my family because I have difficulty hearing them?
- Do I have difficulty hearing or understanding co-workers, clients, or customers?
- Do I feel restricted or limited by a hearing problem?
- Do I have difficulty hearing when visiting friends, relatives, or neighbours?
- Do I have difficulty hearing in the movies or in the theatre?
- Does a hearing problem cause me to argue with family members?
- Do I have trouble hearing the television or radio at levels that are loud enough for others?
- Do I feel that any difficulty with my hearing limits my personal life or social life?
- Do I have trouble hearing family or friends when we are together in a restaurant?

Source: National Institute on Deafness and Other Communication Disorders. (2016). *Do you need a hearing test?* https://www.nidcd.nih.gov/health/do-you-need-hearing-test.

---

impairment and its appropriate treatment is considered an essential part of primary care for older adults, it is rarely done. Regular screening leads to earlier detection and intervention, which may increase one's quality of life (Statistics Canada, 2019). About 17% of persons with hearing impairments use a hearing aid (WHO, 2020). Research has shown that 90% of those who have hearing loss can improve their communication with hearing aids that are fitted properly (Canadian Hearing Society, 2017). Financial aid for older adults purchasing hearing aids in Canada varies among provinces and territories. The Canadian Hard of Hearing Association provides information about coverage at https://www.chha.ca/hearing-education/hearing-assistive-technology/.

The findings of a recent study (Box 3.3) indicate that hearing loss is an overlooked geriatric syndrome, and those with hearing loss tend to have a higher quality of life when using hearing aids (Hyams et al., 2018). Within LTC homes, lack of assessment and treatment of hearing loss is even more of a concern because the majority of residents have a hearing impairment.

The two major forms of hearing loss are conductive hearing loss and sensorineural hearing loss. Conductive

BOX 3.3
RESEARCH FOR EVIDENCE-INFORMED PRACTICE: HEARING AND QUALITY OF LIFE IN OLDER ADULTS

Problem: Researchers looked at quality of life (QoL) in older adults with and without hearing loss. They also looked to see whether hearing aids were associated with QoL.

Method: The study involved 100 participants aged 60 years or older (30 with normal hearing, 33 without hearing aids, and 37 with hearing aids). Hearing loss was measured in both ears by an audiologist. Those who had hearing loss were tested with hearing aids on and without hearing aids. Sociodemographic information (including sex, age, and hearing aid use) was measured. Three components of QoL were measured: general health, mental health, and physical functioning.

Findings: Hearing aids were associated with better QoL than having hearing loss and not using hearing aids. Those with hearing loss and who used hearing aids had equivalent QoL measures to those with normal hearing.

Implications for Nursing Practice: Hearing loss is an overlooked geriatric syndrome; a gap in assessment can have significant negative consequences. Nurses should be aware of the impact hearing aids may have on older adults who are experiencing hearing loss. Hearing aids may increase quality of life.

Source: Hyams, A.V., Hay-McCutcheon, M., & Scogin, F. (2018). Hearing and quality of life in older adults. *Journal of Clinical Psychology, 74,* 1874–1883. doi:10.1002/jclp.22648

hearing loss usually involves external and middle-ear abnormalities that reduce the transmission of sound to the middle ear. Otosclerosis, infection, perforated eardrum, fluid in the middle ear, or cerumen accumulation can all cause conductive hearing loss. Sensorineural hearing loss results from damage to any part of the inner ear or the neural pathways to the brain. *Presbycusis* is a form of sensorineural hearing loss that is related to aging. It is the most common form of hearing loss in Canada (Canadian Academy of Audiology, 2020) (see Chapter 13). Sensorineural hearing loss is treated with hearing aids and, in some cases, cochlear implants. Cerumen impaction, hearing aids, cochlear implants, and assistive listening and adaptive devices are discussed further in the following sections.

Cerumen Impaction

Cerumen impaction is the most common and easily corrected of all interferences in the hearing of older adults. Cerumen interferes with the conduction of sound through air in the eardrum. The reduction in the number and activity of cerumen-producing glands results in a tendency toward cerumen impaction. Longstanding impactions become hard, dry, and dark brown. At particular risk of impaction are people who wear hearing aids and older men with large amounts of ear canal tragi (hairs in the ear) that tend to become entangled with the cerumen. When hearing loss is suspected or a person with existing hearing loss experiences increasing difficulty, it is important to first check for cerumen impaction as a possible cause (Michaudet & Malaty, 2018).

Hearing Aids

A hearing aid is a personal amplifying system that includes a microphone, an amplifier, and a loudspeaker. The appearance and effectiveness of hearing aids have greatly improved in recent years, and many can be programmed to meet specific needs. Most people can obtain some hearing enhancement with a hearing aid. While hearing aids generally improve hearing by about 50%, they do not correct hearing deficits. It is important that hearing-impaired persons understand that the goal of hearing aid use is to improve communication, not to restore normal hearing.

Hearing aids contribute to higher quality of life for those who experience hearing loss (Hyams et al., 2018). Gallagher and Woodside (2018) completed a study looking at affective hearing aid adoption and use and asked participants about their experience adopting a hearing aid. In their study, one participant described how it will take time to adjust to his new hearing aids:

> *"The day that I got mine and I got into my car to go home I felt like driving my car to the nearest repair centre because I could hear the steering pump coming in I could hear all the bits and pieces from the engine that I didn't know was there. It takes a little while to adjust to it."* (M, 77, hearing aid user) (Gallagher & Woodside, 2018, p. 306)

Hearing aids necessitate a period of adjustment and training in their correct use. Most provinces and territories provide some financial assistance for purchasing a hearing aid. The financial investment in a good hearing aid is considerable, and a good fit is critical. A person must be assessed by an audiologist or a physician before being fitted for a hearing aid (CHHA, 2019). Prices of hearing aids are regulated by the Canadian government, and costs depend on an individual's degree of hearing loss as well as the brand and model prescribed. Batteries are changed every 1 to 2 weeks, adding to overall costs. It is important for nurses in hospitals, in LTC home settings, and in the community to be knowledgeable about the care and maintenance of hearing aids. In provinces and territories where financial assistance is available, assistance with replacement costs is limited. Many older adults experience unnecessary communication problems because their hearing aids are not inserted and working properly or are lost.

Cochlear Implants

Cochlear implants are increasingly being used for older adults who are profoundly deaf as a result of sensorineural hearing loss. Unlike a hearing aid, which magnifies sounds, a cochlear implant converts sound waves into electrical impulses and transmits them to the inner ear. A cochlear implant is surgically implanted in the mastoid bone behind the ear and electrically stimulates the cochlea, setting the cilia in motion and transmitting impulses along the auditory nerve to the brain's hearing centre. For persons whose hearing loss is so severe that amplification is of little or no benefit, the use of a cochlear implant is a safe and effective method of auditory rehabilitation.

Financial coverage of the cochlear implant procedure varies among provinces and territories. The transplant procedure carries some risk because the surgery destroys any residual hearing that remains. Therefore, cochlear implant users can never revert to using a hearing aid.

Assistive Listening and Adaptive Devices

Assistive listening devices (also called personal listening systems) are considered adjuncts to hearing aids or are used in place of hearing aids for people with hearing impairment. These devices are available commercially and can be used to enhance face-to-face communication, to understand speech better in large rooms such as theatres, to use the telephone, and to listen to the television.

Examples of assistive listening and adaptive devices are text messaging devices for telephones and closed-caption television (now required on all televisions with screens that measure 33 cm [13 inches] or more). Also available are alerting devices, such as vibrating alarm clocks (which shake the bed or activate a flashing light) and sound lamps that respond with lights to sounds such as those of doorbells and telephones. Assistive devices—such as pocket talkers, which amplify sound and send it to the user's ears through earphones, clips, or headphones—are helpful in health care situations in which privacy and accurate communication are essential. Nurses should be able to obtain appropriate devices to improve communication with hearing-impaired persons. (See the Resources section for additional information.)

A program called Hearing Dogs of Canada, run by the Lions Foundation of Canada, provides hearing dog guides throughout Canada (https://www.dogguides.com/hearing.html). A hearing dog guide serves to warn the hearing-impaired person of impending danger and to alert the person to audible signals, ringing telephones, fire and smoke alarms, emergencies, and intruders. Although other electronic means are available for dealing with these concerns, persons who have hearing dogs consistently comment on the alleviation of the sense of isolation that often accompanies hearing impairment. With a hearing dog companion, older adults may experience renewed courage, confidence, and freedom, as well as reduced tension, anxiety, and depression (Hall et al., 2017).

IMPLICATIONS FOR GERONTOLOGICAL NURSING AND HEALTHY AGING

Hearing impairment is extremely common among older adults and significantly affects communication, function, safety, and quality of life. Inadequate communication with an older adult who has a hearing impairment can also lead to misdiagnosis and affect the person's compliance with their medical regimen. Gerontological nurses must be able to assess hearing ability and use appropriate verbal and nonverbal communication skills and devices to help older adults minimize or even avoid problems. Box 3.4 presents communication strategies for older adults who have impaired hearing.

BOX 3.4

STRATEGIES FOR COMMUNICATING WITH OLDER ADULTS WHO HAVE HEARING IMPAIRMENTS

- Do not shout when speaking to an older adult, as shouting increases pitch and makes it more difficult for the person to hear.
- Never assume hearing loss is due to age until other causes (infection, cerumen buildup, etc.) are ruled out.
- Inappropriate responses, inattentiveness, and apathy may be symptoms of hearing loss.
- Face the person, stand or sit at the same level, and do not turn away to face a computer screen when using verbal and nonverbal approaches.
- Gain the person's attention before beginning to speak.
- Determine whether the person's hearing is better in one ear than in the other, and position yourself appropriately.
- If a hearing aid is used, make sure it is in place and that the batteries are functioning.
- Ask the person or a family member what helps the person to hear best.
- Keep your hands away from your mouth, and project your voice through controlled diaphragmatic breathing.

- Avoid conversations in which the speaker's face is in glare or darkness; orient the light source so that the light is on the speaker's face.
- Careful articulation and a moderate speed of speech are helpful.
- Lower your tone of voice and articulate clearly.
- Label the person's chart, and inform all caregivers that the person has a hearing impairment.
- Use nonverbal approaches: gestures, demonstrations, visual aids, and written materials.
- Pause between sentences or phrases to confirm the person's understanding of the communication.
- Restate with different words when you are not understood.
- When changing topics, preface the change by stating the topic.
- Reduce background noise (e.g., turn off the television, close the door).
- Use assistive listening devices, such as a pocket talker.
- Share resources with the hearing-impaired person, and refer to them as appropriate.

Vision Impairment

While vision decline occurs normally with age (see Chapter 6), the major causes of visual impairment and blindness among older adults are cataracts, macular degeneration, glaucoma, and diabetic retinopathy (see Chapter 19). About 1.5 million Canadians identify as having vision loss (Canadian National Institute for the Blind [CNIB], 2020a).

Visual impairment (low vision) is generally defined as a Snellen reading worse than 20/40 but better than 20/200. The definition of legal blindness can vary between countries. In Canada, legal blindness is defined as a Snellen reading equal to or worse than 20/200 with the best correction in the better eye or a visual extent of less than 20° in diameter (CNIB, 2020b). A reading of 20/50 may keep a person from obtaining a provincial or territorial driver's license or may restrict their driving to the daytime (Government of British Columbia, 2021). Vision loss is becoming a major public health issue and is projected to increase substantially as the population ages.

Vision can have a major effect on one's livelihood, contributing to limitations in the activities of daily living (Zult et al., 2020) (Box 3.5). A Canadian study by Aljied and colleagues (2018) found that visual impairment prevalence increases with age, from 2.7% in those aged 45 to 54 years old to 15.6% in those aged 75 to 84 years old. The researchers also found that women, those with less education, and those with lower income had higher rates of visual impairment. Those with health issues such as hypertension, diabetes (type 1 or 2), and memory problems were also more likely to experience visual impairment (Aljied et al., 2018). The WHO (2017) found that even with available cost-effective treatments, only 10% to 37% of older adults reported having an eye exam within the past year.

The prevalence of visual impairment among residents of LTC homes is estimated to be 3 to 15 times higher than that among adults of the same age who live in the community (Hawranik et al., 2016). The lack of routine eye care in LTC home settings may result in functional decline, decreased quality of life, and depression (Holloway et al., 2018).

Low-Vision Assistive Devices

Technological advances in the past decade have produced some low-vision devices that may be used successfully in the care of the visually impaired older adult. Persons with severe visual impairment may qualify for disability and

---

BOX 3.5

RESEARCH FOR EVIDENCE-INFORMED PRACTICE: LEVELS OF SELF-REPORTED AND OBJECTIVE PHYSICAL ACTIVITY IN INDIVIDUALS WHO HAVE AGE-RELATED MACULAR DEGENERATION

Problem: The prevalence of visual impairment, such as age-related macular degeneration, increases with age. It is known to be associated with decreased quality of life, as those with visual impairments live a less active lifestyle. This study compared older adults' self-reported physical activity levels with objective findings.

Methods: The study involved 23 individuals with age-related macular degeneration and 13 older adults with normal or corrected-to-normal vision. All participants completed a visual examination and responded to questions on the Global Physical Activity Questionnaire during a face-to-face interview. Objective findings were collected by asking the participant to wear an Actigraph accelerometer for 7 days on their hip. Researchers also looked at sedentary behaviour, light physical activity, moderate to vigorous physical activity, and step count.

Findings: Objective findings showed that those with age-related macular degeneration spent 33% to 34% less time completing moderate to physical activity compared to those with normal vision. Subjective findings indicated that both groups perceived themselves to be mostly engaged in walking and gardening. Those with normal vision engaged more often in other activities such as cycling. There were significant associations found between the amount of vision loss and objective measurement of physical activity.

Implications for Nursing Practice: Visual impairment contributes to less moderate to vigorous physical activity. It is important for the nurse to be aware of how vision changes may affect older adults and support a plan to help them maintain physical activity to ensure a high quality of life.

Source: Zult, T., Smith, L., Stringer, C., et al. (2020). Levels of self-reported and objective activity in individuals with age-related macular degeneration. *BMC Public Health, 20,* 1144. doi:10.1186/s12889-020-09255-7.

---

financial and social services assistance through government and private programs, including vision rehabilitation programs. An array of low-vision assistive devices are now available, including insulin delivery systems, talking clocks and watches, large-print books, audiobooks, podcasts, magnifiers, telescopes (handheld or mounted on eyeglasses), electronic magnification through closed-circuit television or computer software, and software that converts text into artificial voice output. The website of the Canadian National Institute for the Blind (http://www.cnib.ca) lists several resources that are specifically for older adults. Because each person's needs are unique, it is recommended that before investing in vision aids, the person should consult a low-vision centre or a low-vision specialist. (See the Resources section for additional information.)

IMPLICATIONS FOR GERONTOLOGICAL NURSING AND HEALTHY AGING

Vision impairment is common among older adults, occurring in connection with eye diseases and with changes resulting from aging. It can significantly affect communication, functional ability, safety, and quality of life. To promote healthy aging and quality of life,

nurses who care for older adults in all settings can improve outcomes for visually impaired older adults by assessing for vision changes and providing appropriate health teaching and referrals for the prevention and treatment of visual impairment. Suggestions for improving communication with and care for visually impaired older adults are presented in Box 3.6.

COMMUNICATION WITH OLDER ADULTS WHO HAVE NEUROLOGICAL DISORDERS

Three major categories of impaired verbal communication arise from neurological disturbances: (1) reception, (2) perception, and (3) articulation. Reception is impaired by anxiety or is related to a specific disorder, hearing deficits, or altered levels of consciousness. Perception is distorted by stroke, dementia, and delirium. Articulation is hampered by mechanical difficulties such as dysarthria, respiratory disease, destruction of the larynx, or cerebral infarction with neuromuscular effects. Specific difficulties can include the following:

- *Anomia:* Difficulty in retrieving words during spontaneous speech and naming tasks.

BOX 3.6

STRATEGIES FOR COMMUNICATING WITH OLDER ADULTS WHO HAVE VISUAL IMPAIRMENT

- Make sure you have the person's attention before you start talking.
- Always speak promptly, and clearly identify yourself and others with you. State when you are leaving, and make sure the person is aware of your departure.
- Get down to the person's level and face them when speaking.
- Speak normally but not from a distance. Do not raise or lower your voice, and continue to use gestures if doing so is natural to your communication.
- When others are present, address the visually impaired person by prefacing remarks with their name or a light touch on the arm.
- Use the analogy of a clock face to help locate objects (e.g., describe positions of food on a plate in relation to clock positions, such as meat at 3 o'clock, dessert at 6 o'clock).
- Ensure adequate lighting on your face and eliminate glare.
- Select rich, intense colours (e.g., red, orange) for paint, furniture, and pictures.

- Use large, dark, evenly spaced printing.
- Use contrast in printed material (e.g., black marker on white paper).
- Do not change the room arrangement or the arrangement of personal items without explanation.
- Use some means to identify persons who are visually impaired and include visual impairment in the plan of care.
- Screen for vision loss and recommend annual eye examinations for older adults.
- If a person is in an LTC home or a communal home, label their eyeglasses and have a spare pair, if possible.
- Be aware of low-vision assistive devices such as talking watches and books, and facilitate access to these resources.
- If the person is blind, offer your arm while walking. Pause before stairs or curbs and alert the person. When seating the person, place their hand on the back of the chair. Always let the person know their position in relation to objects. Never play with or distract a guide dog.

- *Aphasia*: A communication disorder that can affect a person's ability to use and understand spoken or written words. It results from damage to the side of the brain dominant for language; for most people, this is the left side. Aphasia usually occurs suddenly and often results from a stroke or head injury, but it can also develop slowly from a brain tumour, an infection, or dementia.
- *Dysarthria:* Impairment in the ability to articulate words as the result of damage to the speech mechanism controlled by either the central or peripheral nervous system.

Aphasia

The most common language disorder that occurs following a cerebral vascular accident, or stroke, is **aphasia.** Aphasia, in varying degrees, affects a person's ability to communicate in one or more ways, including speaking, understanding, reading, writing, and gesturing. Depending on the type and severity of aphasia, there may be little or no speech, speech that is fragmented or broken, or speech that is fluent but empty in content. When a stroke damages the dominant half of the brain, some

disruption will occur in the "word factory." Broca's and Wernicke's areas in the cerebral cortex are integral to the expression and understanding of language. The Heart and Stroke Foundation's (2018) *Canadian Stroke Best Practices* categorize two broad types of aphasia: expressive and receptive. Within these types, there are many subtypes of aphasia that nurses may encounter when caring for older adults:

- *Wernicke's aphasia* is the result of a lesion in the superior temporal gyrus, an area adjacent to the primary auditory cortex (Wernicke's area). Persons with Wernicke's aphasia speak easily and with many long runs of words, but the content does not make sense. There are word-finding problems and errors of word and sound substitution. Unrelated words may be strung together or syllables repeated. People with this type of aphasia also have difficulty understanding spoken language and may be unaware of their speech difficulties.
- *Broca's aphasia* typically involves damage to the posteroinferior portions of the dominant frontal

lobe (Broca's area). This type of aphasia is also called motor or anterior aphasia. Persons with Broca's aphasia usually understand others but speak very slowly and use a minimal number of words. They often struggle to articulate a word and seem to have lost the ability to voluntarily control the movements of speech. They experience difficulties in communicating orally and in writing.

- *Verbal apraxia* or *apraxia of speech* is a motor speech disorder that affects the ability to plan and sequence voluntary muscle movements. The muscles of speech are not paralyzed; instead, there is a disruption in the brain's transmission of signals to the muscles. When the person is thinking about what to say, they may struggle to say words or be unable to speak at all. In contrast, when not thinking about what to say, the person may be able to say many words or sentences correctly. **Apraxia** frequently occurs with aphasia.
- *Anomic* or *nominal aphasia* is associated with lesions of the dominant temporoparietal regions of the brain, although no single locus has been identified. Persons with anomic aphasia understand and speak readily but may have severe difficulty finding the words. They may be unable to remember crucial content words. This frequent form of aphasia is characterized by the inability to name objects. The individual struggles to come forth with the correct noun and often becomes frustrated at their inability to do so.
- *Global aphasia* is the result of large left-hemisphere lesions and affects most of the language areas of the brain. Persons with global aphasia cannot understand words or speak intelligibly. They may use meaningless syllables repetitively.

A speech-language pathologist (SLP) should be consulted for each type of aphasia to develop appropriate rehabilitation plans as soon as the affected person is physiologically stabilized. SLPs bring expertise in all types of communication disorders and are an essential part of the interprofessional team. The SLP can identify the areas of language that remain relatively unimpaired and can capitalize on the remaining strengths. Much can be done in aggressive speech-retraining programs to regain intelligible conversational ability. For those who do not regain meaningful speech, assistive and augmentative communication devices can be helpful. Hall and Gilliland (2019) have noted the importance of consulting with the SLP to create an appropriate care plan and have described the significance of well-equipped nursing staff caring for patients who are experiencing communication difficulties.

Alternative and Augmentative Speech Aids

Alternative or augmentative speech aid systems are frequently used, and communication tools exist for every imaginable type of language disability. These can be low-tech or high-tech systems. An example of a low-tech system is an alphabet or picture board that the individual uses to point to letters that spell out messages or to point to pictures of common objects and situations. High-tech systems include electronic boards and computers. Studies have shown that computer-assisted therapy can help people with aphasia improve speech. An example is speech-therapy software that displays a word or picture, speaks the word (using prerecorded human speech), records the user speaking it, and plays back the user's speech. Those with aphasia and their caregivers understand the benefits of text-to-speech technology (Hux et al., 2021).

For individuals with hemiplegic conditions, electronic devices and computers can be voice activated or have specially designed switches that can be activated by one finger or by slight contact with the ear, nose, or chin. Some experimental studies indicate that medications, in addition to speech therapy, may help manage aphasia in the acute phase of stroke and be of help following the acute situation and in persistent aphasia.

Dysarthria

Dysarthria is a speech disorder caused by poor coordination or weakness of the speech muscles. It occurs as a result of central or peripheral neuromuscular disorders that interfere with pronunciation and the clarity of speech. Dysarthria is second only to aphasia in incidence as a communication disorder in older adults and may be the result of stroke, head injury, Parkinson's disease, multiple sclerosis, or other neurological conditions. Dysarthria is characterized by weakness, slow movement, and a lack of coordination of the muscles associated with speech. Speech may be slow, jerky, slurred, quiet, lacking in expression, and difficult to understand. The disorder may involve several mechanisms of speech, such as respiration, phonation, resonance, articulation, and prosody (the metre or rhythm of speech). Weakness or a lack of coordination in any one of the speech-related systems can result in dysarthria. If the respiratory system is weak, then speech may be too quiet and produced one word at a time. If the laryngeal system is weak, speech may be breathy, quiet, and slow. If the articulatory system is affected, speech may sound slurred and be slow and laboured.

Treatment of dysarthria depends on the cause, type, and severity of the symptoms. An SLP works with the individual to improve communication abilities. Therapy for dysarthria focuses on maximizing the function of all systems. In cases of progressive neurological disease, it is important to begin treatment early and continue it throughout the course of the disease, with the goal being to maintain speech for as long as possible.

IMPLICATIONS FOR GERONTOLOGICAL NURSING AND HEALTHY AGING

Nurses are responsible for accurately observing and recording the speech and word recognition patterns of persons affected by aphasia or dysarthria and for consistently implementing the recommendations of the SLP. Communication with the older adult experiencing aphasia or dysarthria can be frustrating for both the affected person and the nurse as they struggle to understand each other. It is important to remember that in most cases of aphasia and dysarthria, the affected person retains normal intellectual ability. Therefore, verbal and nonverbal communication must always occur at an adult level but with special modifications. Furthermore, nurses need to be aware of their body language and other nonverbal behaviours when communicating with older adults. Hearing and vision losses can further contribute to communication difficulties for older adults with aphasia or dysarthria. Sensitivity and patience are essential to effective communication. It is helpful if staff members caring for the person remain consistent, so that they can come to know and understand the needs of the person and communicate these needs to others. It is exhausting for older adults to have to continually try to communicate their needs and desires to any number of staff members. Plans of care

should include specific helpful verbal and nonverbal communication strategies so that all staff members and patients' families and significant others know the most effective way to enhance communication. Suggestions for communicating with persons who have aphasia are presented in Box 3.7.

The gerontological nurse needs to be familiar with techniques that facilitate communication with the person who has aphasia or dysarthria, as well as with strategies that can be taught to the person to improve communication. Boxes 3.8 and 3.9 present suggestions for improving communication between the person who has dysarthria and the listener.

The nurse may encounter older adults who are in the acute or long-term phase of an illness that affects communication. Although early intensive rehabilitation efforts are most effective, all older adults with communication deficits should have access to state-of-the-art techniques and devices that enhance communication, a basic human need. In addition to being knowledgeable about appropriate communication techniques, nurses must be aware of equipment and resources that are available to the person with aphasia or dysarthria so that hope can be offered. Teaching families and significant others effective communication strategies is also an important nursing task. (See the Resources section at the end of the chapter.)

COMMUNICATION WITH OLDER ADULTS WHO HAVE COGNITIVE IMPAIRMENT

The experience of losing cognitive and expressive abilities is both frightening and frustrating. One type of cognitive impairment that affects memory, speech, and communication is dementia (see Chapter 21). Older adults who are experiencing dementia have difficulty expressing their personhood in ways that are easily understood by others. However, the need to communicate and the need to be treated as a person remain despite memory and communication impairments. No group of people is more in need of supportive relationships with skilled, caring health care providers. People with cognitive and communication impairments depend on emotional support from the relationships in their lives to aid in problem solving and coordinating complex activities (Young et al., 2017).

BOX 3.7
COMMUNICATING WITH INDIVIDUALS EXPERIENCING APHASIA

- Explain situations, treatments, and anything else that is pertinent to the person. Treat the person as an adult, and avoid patronizing and childish phrases. Talk to the person as though they understand what you are saying.
- Be patient and allow plenty of time to communicate in a quiet environment.
- Speak naturally. Speak slowly, ask one question at a time, and wait for a response. Do not shout. Repeat and rephrase as needed.
- Include the person in social gatherings and conversations. If needed, ensure that hearing aids are in place and that eyeglasses are being worn. Create an environment in which the person is encouraged to make decisions, offer comments, and communicate thoughts and desires.
- Ask questions that can be answered with a nod or the blink of an eye; if the person cannot respond verbally, instruct them in nonverbal responses. Use closed-ended questions so they can be answered with a "yes" or "no" response. Responses written on paper can be used so that the person can point to the correct response.
- Be honest. Let the person know if you cannot quite understand what they are telling you but that you will keep trying.
- When you have not understood what the person has said, it helps to repeat the part that you did understand as a question so that the person only has to

repeat the part that you did not understand. For example, you hear, "I would like an XX." Rather than saying "Pardon?" and getting the person to repeat what was said (which may sound the same to you and thus unclear), try asking, "You would like a . . . ?"
- Speak of things that are familiar and of interest to the person.
- Use visual cues, objects, pictures, gestures, and touch, as well as words. Have paper and pencil available so you can write down key words or even sketch a picture.
- If the person has Wernicke's aphasia, listen to and watch for the bits of information that emerge from the person's words, facial expressions, and gestures. Ignore the nonwords.
- Encourage all speech. Allow the person to try to complete their thoughts and to struggle with words. Avoid being too quick to guess what the person is trying to express.
- Use augmentative communication devices such as picture boards. These are useful to fill in answers to requests such as "I need" or "I want"; the person merely points to the appropriate picture.
- Try to keep staff who are caring for the person who has aphasia consistent, and make the care plan specific to the most helpful communication techniques.
- Turn off the television or radio when speaking with the person.

Communicating with older adults who are experiencing cognitive impairment requires special skills and patience. Dementia affects both receptive and expressive communication components and alters the way in which people speak. Early in the disease, finding words is difficult (a condition termed *anomia*), and remembering the exact facts of a conversation is challenging. The following reflection from a man with dementia illustrates this challenge:

> "I grasp for words. It is very common with people with dementia . . . I become descriptive. For example, "glass of water." I say, "it's something that you drink from" . . . If you think of it as a problem, it becomes an obstacle. But if you just laugh and say, "I'll remember it later. No big deal!" then, it is not a problem." (Angelo; Seetharaman & Chaudhury, 2020, p. 5).

As the disease progresses, the person has difficulty expressing thoughts and emotions and understanding verbal messages. In later stages, verbalization may be limited. Hughes and colleagues (2020) remind us that even in the later stages of dementia, the person may understand more than health care providers realize, and they still need opportunities for interaction and caring communication, both verbal and nonverbal. Often, health care providers do not communicate with older adults who have cognitive impairment or they communicate only task-focused information. To effectively communicate with a person experiencing cognitive impairment, one must believe that the person is trying to communicate something and that what the person is trying to communicate is important enough to make the effort to understand. As nurses, the best thing we can do is to treat everything the person says or tries to communicate in a nonverbal manner as important and as an

BOX 3.8
TIPS FOR THE PERSON WHO HAS DYSARTHRIA

- Explain to people that you have difficulty with your speech.
- Try to limit conversations when you feel tired.
- Speak slowly and loudly and in a quiet place.
- Pace out one word at a time while speaking.
- Take a deep breath before speaking so that there is enough breath for speech.
- Speak out as soon as you breathe out, to make full use of the breaths.
- Open the mouth more when speaking. Exaggerate tongue movements.
- Make sure you are sitting or standing in an upright posture; this will improve your breathing and speech.
- If you become frustrated, try to use other methods (such as pointing, gesturing, or writing), or take a rest and try again later.
- Practise facial exercises (blowing kisses, frowning, smiling) and massage your facial muscles.

Source: Adapted from American Speech-Language-Hearing Association. (n.d.). *Dysarthria.* http://www.asha.org/public/speech/disorders/dysarthria/.

BOX 3.9
TIPS FOR COMMUNICATING WITH INDIVIDUALS EXPERIENCING DYSARTHRIA

- Pay attention to the speaker; watch the speaker as they talk.
- Allow more time for conversation and conduct conversations in a quiet place.
- Be honest and let the speaker know when you have difficulty understanding.
- If the person's speech is very difficult to understand, repeat back what the person has said to make sure you understand.
- Remember that dysarthria does not affect a person's intelligence.
- Check with the person for ways in which you can help, such as guessing, finishing sentences, or writing.

Source: Adapted from *Dysarthria and coping with dysarthria.* Royal College of Speech and Language Therapists (http://www.rcslt.org) and the American Speech-Language-Hearing Association (http://www.asha.org).

attempt to tell us something. It is our responsibility to know how to understand and respond verbally or nonverbally. The person with cognitive impairment cannot change their communication; we must change ours.

Lanzi and colleagues (2017) have provided insight into communication strategies that are helpful in creating and maintaining a therapeutic relationship with people who are in the moderate to later stages of dementia. Their research has challenged some of the commonly held beliefs about communication with persons who have cognitive impairment. For example, one of those beliefs is that one should use closed-ended questions. Lanzi and colleagues (2017) offer suggestions for specific verbal and nonverbal communication strategies that are effective in various nursing situations, as well as hope for nurses trying to establish meaningful relationships that nurture the personhood of people who have cognitive impairments. Approaches to communication need to be adapted to suit the person's ability to understand and the purpose of the interaction (Hughes et al., 2020). To this end, the Hartford Institute for Geriatric Nursing's *Try This: Series* (https://hign.org/consultgeri-resources/try-this-series) has made available an evidence-informed practice guide for assessing communication abilities and for matching communication strategies to the communication abilities and challenges of older adults with dementia. Box 3.10 presents suggestions for communicating with persons experiencing cognitive impairment.

IMPLICATIONS FOR GERONTOLOGICAL NURSING AND HEALTHY AGING

Care and communication that value and show respect for the dignity and worth of all cared-for persons, including those with cognitive impairment, and the use of research-based communication techniques will enhance communication and affirm the patient's personhood. Buckwalter et al. (1995, p. 15) underscored this message as follows:

Gerontological nurses who are sensitive to communication and interaction patterns can assist both formal and informal caregivers in using more personal verbal and nonverbal communication strategies which are humanizing and show respect for the person. Similarly, they can monitor and

---

BOX 3.10
USEFUL STRATEGIES FOR COMMUNICATING WITH INDIVIDUALS EXPERIENCING COGNITIVE IMPAIRMENT

SIMPLIFICATION STRATEGIES—USEFUL WITH ACTIVITIES OF DAILY LIVING

- Give one-step directions.
- Speak slowly.
- Allow time for a response.
- Reduce distractions.
- Interact with one person at a time.
- Be aware of your nonverbal communication.
- Give clues and cues and use gestures or pantomime to demonstrate what you want the person to do—for example, if you want the person to sit, put the chair in front of the person, point to it, pat the seat, and say, "Sit here."

FACILITATION STRATEGIES—USEFUL IN ENCOURAGING EXPRESSION OF THOUGHTS AND FEELINGS

- Establish commonalities.
- Share self.
- Allow the person to choose subjects to discuss.
- Speak as if to an equal.
- Use broad openings, such as "How are you today?"
- Employ an appropriate use of humour.
- Follow the person's lead.

COMPREHENSION STRATEGIES—USEFUL IN ASSISTING WITH UNDERSTANDING OF COMMUNICATION

- Identify time confusion. (In what time frame is the person operating at the moment?)
- Find the theme. (What connection is there between apparently disparate topics?) Recognize an important theme such as fear, loss, or happiness.

- Recognize hidden meanings. (What did the person mean to say?)

SUPPORTIVE STRATEGIES—USEFUL IN ENCOURAGING CONTINUED COMMUNICATION AND SUPPORTING PERSONHOOD

- Introduce yourself and explain why you are there. Reach out to shake hands, and note the response to touch.
- If the person does not want to talk, go away and return later. Do not push or force.
- Sit closely and face the person at eye level.
- Limit corrections.
- Use multiple ways of communicating (nonverbal communication, gestures, touch).
- Search for meaning.
- Know the person's past life history as well as daily life experiences and events.
- Recognize and respond to feelings.
- Treat the person with respect and dignity.
- Show interest through body posture, facial expression, nodding, and eye contact. Assume a pleasant, relaxed attitude.
- Attend to vision and hearing losses.
- Do not try to bring the person to the present or use reality orientation. Go to where the person is and enjoy the conversation.
- When leaving, thank the person for their time and attention as well as for information.
- Remember that the quality of the interaction, rather than its content or quantity, is basic to therapeutic communication.

---

try to change object-oriented communication approaches, which are not only insensitive and dehumanizing, but also often lead to diminished self-image and angry, agitated responses on the part of the patient with cognitive impairment.

THE LIFE STORY

Older adults bring us complex stories derived from long years of living. In caring for older adults, listening to life stories is an important component of communication. The *life story* can tell us a great deal about the person and is an important part of the assessment process. Stories are "critical sources of information about etiology, diagnosis, treatment, and prognosis from the patient's point of

view" (Sandelowski, 1994, p. 25). Listening to memories and life stories requires time and patience and a belief that the story and the person are valuable and meaningful. A memory is an incredible gift given to the nurse, a sharing of a part of the patient when they may have little else to give. Personal memories are saved for persons who will patiently wait for their unveiling and who will treasure them. Stories are important. As Robert Coles (1989, p. 7) has stated, "The people who come to see us bring us their stories. They hope they tell them well enough so that we understand the truth of their lives. They hope we know how to interpret their stories correctly."

The life story—as constructed through reminiscence, journaling, life review, or guided autobiography—has held great fascination for gerontologists in the last quarter century. The universal appeal of the life story as a vehicle of culture, a demonstration of caring and generational continuity, and an easily stimulated activity has held allure for many care providers. The most exciting aspect of working with older adults is being a part of the emergence of the life story, the shifting and blending patterns. When one is young, looking forward and planning for the future are important for emotional health and growth. As one ages, it becomes more important to look back, talk over experiences, review and make sense of it all, and feel satisfied with one's life. This very important work, which Erik Erikson called ego integrity versus self-despair, is the major developmental task of older adulthood. Ego integrity is achieved when the person has accepted both the triumphs and disappointments of life and is at peace and satisfied with the life lived (Erikson, 1963).

Reminiscing

Reminiscing is an umbrella term that includes any recalling of the past. Reminiscing occurs from childhood onward, particularly at life's junctures and transitions. Reminiscing cultivates (1) a sense of security through the recounting of comforting memories, (2) a sense of belonging through sharing, and (3) self-esteem through the confirmation of uniqueness. Robert Butler (2002) pointed out that 50 years ago, reminiscing was thought to be a sign of senility or what we now call Alzheimer's disease. Older adults who talked about the past and told the same stories again and again were said to be boring and living in the past. Butler's seminal research showed that reminiscence is the most important psychological task of older adults (Butler, 1963). For the nurse, having the patient reminisce is a therapeutic intervention that is important for assessment and understanding.

Reminiscence can have many goals. It not only provides a pleasurable experience that improves quality of life but also increases socialization and connectedness with others, provides cognitive stimulation, improves communication, and can be an effective therapy for depressive symptoms (Woods et al., 2018). The therapeutic implications of reminiscence are discussed in Box 3.11.

The process of reminiscence can occur in individual conversations with older adults; can be structured, as in a nursing history; or can occur in a group in which each person shares their memories and listens to others sharing theirs, as discussed later in this chapter. The nurse

BOX 3.11
USES OF REMINISCENCE AS A DEVELOPMENTAL AND THERAPEUTIC STRATEGY

- Maintain continuity.
- Extract meaning.
- Define and develop personal philosophy.
- Identify cycles and themes.
- Recapitulate learning and growth.
- Enhance self-worth and feeling of accomplishment.
- Evolve identity.
- Provide insight and growth.
- Integrate and accept regrets and disappointments.
- Perceive universality.

can learn much about a person's history, communication style, relationships, coping mechanisms, strengths, fears, affect, and adaptive capacity by listening thoughtfully as the life story is constructed. Box 3.12 provides some suggestions for encouraging reminiscence.

Life Review

Robert Butler (1963) first noted and brought to public attention the review process that normally occurs in the older adult, as the realization of their approaching death creates a resurgence of unresolved conflicts. Butler called this process **life review.** Life review occurs quite naturally for many persons during periods of crisis and transition. Life review occurs most frequently as an internal review of memories, an intensely private and soul-searching activity.

Life review is considered more of a formal therapy technique than is reminiscence and takes a person through their life in a structured and chronological order. Life-review therapy (Rubin et al., 2018) and structured life review (Jeffers et al., 2020) are psychotherapeutic techniques based on the concept of life review. Gerontological nurses participate with older adults in both reminiscence and life review, and it is important to acquire the skills needed to be effective in achieving the purposes of both. Life review may be especially important for older adults facing death. Life review should occur not only when one is old or facing death but also frequently throughout one's life. This process can help one to examine where one is in life and to change course or set new goals. Life reviews

BOX 3.12
SUGGESTIONS FOR ENCOURAGING REMINISCENCE

- Listen without correction or criticism.
- Encourage older adults to reminisce about various ages and stages. Ask questions such as "What was it like growing up on that farm?," "What did teenagers do for fun when you were young?," and "What was school like for you?"
- Be patient with repetition. Sometimes people need to tell the same story often in order to come to terms with the experience, especially if it was very meaningful to them. If they have memory loss, it may be the only story they can remember, and it is important for them to be a member of the group and to contribute to it.
- Be attuned to signs of depression in conversation (e.g., dwelling on sad topics) or changes in physical status or behaviour, and provide appropriate assessment and intervention.
- If a topic arises that the person does not want to discuss, change to another topic.
- If people are reluctant to share because they do not feel their life has been interesting, reassure them that everyone's life is valuable and interesting, and tell them how important their memories are to you and others.
- Keep in mind that reminiscing is not an orderly process; one memory triggers another in a way that may not seem related. It is not important to keep things in order or verify accuracy.
- Keep the conversation focused on the person who is reminiscing, but do not hesitate to share some of your own memories that relate to the situation being discussed.
- Listen actively, maintain eye contact, and do not interrupt.
- Respond positively and give feedback by making caring and appropriate comments that encourage the person to continue.
- Use props and triggers, such as photographs, memorabilia (e.g., a childhood toy or antique), short stories or poems about the past, and favourite foods.
- Use open-ended questions to encourage reminiscing. You can prepare questions ahead of time, or you can ask the person to pick a topic that interests them. One question or topic may be enough for an entire session. Consider asking questions such as the following:

  How did your parents meet?
  What do you remember most about your mother? Father? Grandmother? Grandfather?
  What are some of your favourite memories from childhood?
  What was the first house you remember?
  What were your favourite foods as a child?
  Did you have a pet as a child?
  What do you remember about your first job?
  How did you celebrate birthdays or other holidays?
  What do you remember about your wedding day?
  What is your greatest accomplishment or joy in your life?
  What advice did your parents give you? What advice did you give your children? What advice would you give to young people today?

can contribute to a reduction in symptoms of depression and feelings of despair (Keisari & Palgi, 2017).

IMPLICATIONS FOR GERONTOLOGICAL NURSING AND HEALTHY AGING

One of the greatest privileges of nursing older adults is to accompany them in the final journey of life. As each person confronts mortality, there is a need for that person to integrate events and then transcend the self. Human experience, one's contributions, and the poignant anecdotes within the life story bind generations together, validate the uniqueness of each brief journey in this level of awareness, and provide the assurance that one will not be forgotten. The nurse who takes the time to listen to an older adult share memories and life stories communicates respect for the person and an appreciation of that person as an individual. What more can one ask for at the end of life than to know who one is and to know that what one has accomplished holds personal meaning as well as meaning for others? This is the essence of life's final tasks—achieving ego integrity and self-actualization.

Communication and Technology

Advances in technology have allowed for enhanced patient care and greater accessibility. For instance, technology now allows video conferencing between a patient and their health care provider or team, the retrieval of test results through online portals, and the use of other modes of conducting e-consults. According to a Canadian study by Jaana and Paré (2020), 70% of participants aged 65 years or older reported using on a daily basis an electronic device such as a smartphone or tablet that had access to the internet.

While uptake of technology is increasing among the older population, communication preferences still differ among age groups, with other factors also influencing preference. Younger adults tend to welcome new technology more often than older adults (Knowles & Hanson, 2018). Some older adults may not see technology as valuable and will prefer to engage with others face to face (Knowles & Hanson, 2018). It is important for health care providers to communicate all options for accessing health information and to respect the older adult's preferences. For example, if an older adult prefers not to access test results online, it is important to make note of that and to ensure that a follow-up phone call or appointment is made.

Group Structure and Special Considerations for Groups of Older Adults

Implementing a group intervention follows a thorough assessment of the environment, needs, and potential of various group strategies. Major decisions regarding goals will influence the strategy selected; for instance, several older adults with diabetes in an acute care setting may need health care teaching on diabetes.

The nurse sees the major goal of group work as education and the restoring of order (or control) in each person's lifestyle. The strategy best suited for that would be motivational or educational. People experiencing early-stage Alzheimer's disease may benefit from a support group in which to express feelings or a group that teaches memory-enhancing strategies. Successful group work depends on organization; attention to detail; agency support; assessment and consideration of the older adult's needs and status; and caring, sensitive, and skillful leadership. Group work with older adults is different from that with younger people; it requires special skills and training and extraordinary commitment on the part of the leader. However, these unique aspects may not apply to all types of older adult groups.

Reminiscing and Storytelling With Individuals Experiencing Cognitive Impairment

Cognitive impairment does not necessarily preclude older adults from participating in reminiscence or storytelling groups. Opportunities for telling their life stories, enjoying memories, and achieving ego integrity and self-actualization should not be denied to people on the basis of their cognitive status. Some modifications might be needed so that those with mild to moderate memory impairment can enjoy and benefit from group work focused on reminiscence and storytelling.

When the nurse is working with a group of cognitively impaired older adults in reminiscence groups, the emphasis is on sharing memories, however they may be expressed. There should be no pressure to answer questions such as "Where were you born?" or "What was your first job?" Rather, discussions may centre on places where people have lived. Additional props, such as music, pictures, and familiar objects (e.g., a Canadian flag or an old coffee grinder), can prompt many recollections and sharing. Many resources are available to guide these groups, including books such as *I Remember When* (Thorsheim & Roberts, 2000), which offer numerous ways to adapt the reminiscing process for those with cognitive impairment. (Other helpful resources are listed at the end of this chapter.)

Sullivan and colleagues (2018) have described a storytelling modality called TimeSlips, which is designed for people with cognitive impairment (http://www.timeslips.org). Group members, looking at a picture, are encouraged to use their imagination to create a story about the picture. The pictures can be fantastical and funny (like greeting cards) or more nostalgic (like Norman Rockwell paintings). All contributions are encouraged and welcomed—there are no right or wrong answers—and everything that the individuals say is included in the story and written down by the scribe. The stories that emerge are full of creativity and often include discussions about memories and reminiscing. John Killick (1999, p. 49), a writer-in-residence at an LTC home in Scotland, stated the following:

> *Having their words written down is empowering for people with dementia. It affirms their dignity and gives an assurance that their words still have value . . . One woman said, "Anything you can tell people about how things are for me is important. It's a rum do, this growing ancient . . . The brilliance of my brain has slipped away when I wasn't looking."*

SUMMARY

This chapter aimed to show the potential for respectful communication regardless of the impairment the older adult may be experiencing. Communicating with older adults calls for special skills, patience, and respect. As nurses, we must break through the barriers and continue to reach toward the humanity of these persons in the belief that communication is the most vital service we offer. This is the heart of nursing.

KEY CONCEPTS

- Communication is a basic need regardless of age, communication ability, or cognitive impairment. Respect for the person and a knowledge of therapeutic communication techniques are essential for gerontological nurses.
- Nurses need to develop and demonstrate effective communication strategies for older adults who have speech, language, hearing, vision, or cognitive impairment.
- Group work can meet many needs and can be valuable and rewarding for older adults.
- In a rapidly changing society, the shared life histories of older adults provide a sense of continuity among generations.
- The life history of a person is a story to be developed and treasured. This is particularly important toward the end of life.
- Gerontological nursing communication is mainly focused on using interpersonal communication techniques, providing necessary information, encouraging individuals to express personal interests and preferences, and, when function is impeded, ensuring that all needs are recognized, discussed, and met to the greatest extent possible.

ACTIVITIES AND DISCUSSION QUESTIONS

1. Using ear plugs or eyeglasses with the lenses covered in Vaseline, try performing some of your daily activities or engaging in conversation with your peers.

2. Discuss how you might provide medication instructions to a person who has hearing or vision loss.

3. Discuss adaptations to communication for individuals who have aphasia or dysarthria.

4. Discuss the ways in which you might respond to a person who has cognitive impairment and difficulty expressing their thoughts and feelings.

5. Role play in a simulated interaction with an older adult who is experiencing communication or cognitive impairments such as aphasia, dysarthria, or memory loss.

6. With a partner, plan and discuss an activity that would be appropriate for an individual who has cognitive impairment.

7. Watch the movie *Iris*, *The Notebook*, *Alice*, or *Away From Her*, and discuss the effective and ineffective communication strategies that nurses used to interact with persons who are experiencing cognitive impairment.

8. With your peers, form a small group and share memories about an event you have all experienced in your lives (e.g., first date, first day of school).

9. Interview an older adult and ask to hear their life story.

RESOURCES

Alzheimer Society of Canada. Daily Living: Communication.
https://alzheimer.ca/sites/default/files/files/national/brochures-day-to-day/day_to_day_communications_e.pdf
Canadian Association of the Deaf
http://www.cad.ca
Canadian Hearing Society
http://www.chs.ca
Canadian National Institute for the Blind (CNIB)
http://www.cnib.ca

Public Health Agency of Canada. Age-friendly communication: Facts, tips, and ideas.
https://www.canada.ca/en/public-health/services/health-promotion/aging-seniors/publications/publications-general-public/friendly-communication-facts-tips-ideas/introduction.html
Speech-Language and Audiology Canada
http://www.sac-oac.ca/
The Hartford Institute for Geriatric Nursing Try This: Series: Evidence-informed practice guide for assessing communication abilities and matching communication strategies.
https://hign.org/consultgeri-resources/try-this-series

The Heart and Stroke Foundation: Information on communication changes that can occur after a stroke.
https://www.heartandstroke.ca/
Vision Simulator: To experience visual impairment
http://www.visionsimulations.com/

For additional resources, please visit *http://evolve.elsevier.com/ Canada/Ebersole/gerontological/*

REFERENCES

Aljied, R., Aubin, M. J., Buhrmann, R., et al. (2018). Prevalence and determinants of visual impairment in Canada: Cross-sectional data from the Canadian longitudinal study on aging. *Canadian Journal of Ophthalmology, 53*(3), 291–297. doi:10.1016/j.jcjo.2018.01.027.

Buckwalter, K. C., Gerdner, L. A., Hall, G. R., et al. (1995). Shining through: The humor and individuality of persons with Alzheimer's disease. *Journal of Gerontological Nursing, 21*(3), 11–16. doi:10.3928/0098-9134-19950301-04.

Burnside, I. M. (1975). Listen to the aged. *American Journal of Nursing, 75*(10), 1800–1803. doi:10.2307/3423569.

Butler, R. (1963). The life review: An interpretation of reminiscence in the aged. *Psychiatry, 26*, 65–76. doi:10.1080/00332747.1963.11023339.

Butler, R. (2002). *Age, death and life review.* http://www.hospice-foundation.org.

Canadian Academy of Audiology. (2020). *Causes of hearing loss: Age-related hearing loss (presbycusis).* https://canadianaudiology.ca/for-the-public/causes-of-hearing-loss/.

Canadian Hard of Hearing Association (CHHA). (2019). *Types, cause & treatment.* https://www.chha.ca/hearing-education/types-cause-treatment/#suspect.

Canadian Hard of Hearing Association (CHHA). (2020). *Hearing loss in Canada.* https://www.chha.ca/about-us/advocacy/.

Canadian Hearing Society. (2017). *Facts and figures.* https://www.chs.ca/facts-and-figures.

Government of British Columbia. (2021). 22–Vision impairments–CCMTA Medical Standards. Retrieved from https://www2.gov.bc.ca/gov/content/transportation/driving-and-cycling/roadsafetybc/medical-fitness/medical-prof/med-standards/22-vision.

Canadian National Institute for the Blind (CNIB). (2020a). *Blindness in Canada.* https://cnib.ca/en/sight-loss-info/blindness/blindness-canada?region=on.

Canadian National Institute for the Blind (CNIB). (2020b). *What is blindness?* http://www.cnib.ca/en/sight-loss-info/blindness/what-blindness?region=on.

Coles, R. (1989). *The call of stories.* Houghton Mifflin.

Corwin, A. I. (2018). Overcoming elderspeak: A qualitative study of three alternatives. *The Gerontologist, 58*(4), 724–729. doi:10.1093/geront/gnx009.

Erikson, E. H. (1963). *Childhood and society* (2nd ed.). W.W. Norton.

Gallagher, N. E., & Woodside, J. V. (2018). Factors affecting hearing aid adoption and use: A qualitative study. *Journal of the American Academy of Audiology, 29*(4), 300–312. doi:10.3766/jaaa.16148.

Gasiorek, J., Fowler, C., & Giles, H. (2019). Communication and successful aging: Testing alternative conceptualizations of uncertainty. *Communication Monographs, 86*(2), 229–250. doi:10.1080/036377 51.2018.1538561.

Hall, K., & Gilliland, H. (2019). Changing the long-term care culture through interprofessional practice: A speech-language pathologist-led initiative. *Perspectives of the ASHA Special Interest Groups, 4*(2), 313–321. doi:10.1044/2019_PERS-SIG2-2018-0005.

Hall, S. S., MacMichael, J., Turner, A., et al. (2017). A survey of the impact of owning a service dog on quality of life for individuals with physical and hearing disability: A pilot study. *Health and Quality of Life Outcomes, 15*(59), 1–9. doi:10.1186/s12955-017-0640-x.

Hawranik, P., Bell, S., & McIntosh, D. (2016). Vision care services in long-term care facilities: Why are they overlooked? In G. Joseph (Ed.), *Diverse perspectives on aging in a changing world* (1st ed., pp. 130–142). Routledge.

Heart and Stroke Foundation. (2018). Canadian stroke best practices: Canadian stroke best practice recommendations: Acute stroke management: Prehospital, emergency department, and acute inpatient stroke care. https://www.heartandstroke.ca/-/media/1-stroke-best-practices/acute-stroke-management/csbpr2018-acute-stroke-module-final-17jul2018-en.ashx?rev=f57ce754098 04a98a1fdd7523c73bbd7.

Holloway, E. E., Constantinou, M., Xie, J., et al. (2018). Improving eye care in residential aged care facilities using the Residential Ocular Care (ROC) model: Study protocol for a multicentered, prospective, customized, and cluster randomized controlled trial in Australia. *Trials, 19*(1), 650. doi:10.1186/s13063-018-3025-5.

Hughes, S., Woods, B., Algar-Skaife, K., et al. (2020). Understanding quality of life and well-being for people living with advanced dementia. *Nursing Older People, 32*(1), 1–7. doi:10.7748/nop.2019.e1129.

Hux, K., Wallace, S. E., Brown, J. A., et al. (2021). Perceptions of people with aphasia about supporting reading with text-to-speech technology: A convergent mixed methods study. *Journal of Communication, 91*, 106098. doi:10.1016/j.jcomdis.2021.106098.

Hyams, A. V., Hay-McCutcheon, M., & Scogin, F. (2018). Hearing and quality of life in older adults. *Journal of Clinical Psychology, 74*(10), 1874–1883. doi:10.1002/jclp.22648.

Jaana, M., & Paré, G. (2020). Use of mobile health technologies for self-tracking purposes among seniors: A comparison to the general adult population in Canada. In *Proceedings of the 53rd Hawaii International Conference on System Sciences.* doi:10.24251/HICSS.2020.460.

Jeffers, S. L., Hill, R., Krumholz, M. F., et al. (2020). Themes of gerotranscendence in narrative identity within structured life review. *GeroPsych, 33*(2), 77–84. doi:10.1024/1662-9647/a000235.

Keisari, S., & Palgi, Y. (2017). Life-crossroads on stage: Integrating life review and drama therapy for older adults. *Aging & Mental Health, 21*(10), 1079–1089. doi:10.1080/13607863.2016.1199012.

Killick, J. (1999). "What are we like here?" Eliciting experiences of people with dementia. *Generations, 13*(3), 46–49.

Knowles, B., & Hanson, V. L. (2018). The wisdom of older technology (non) users. *Communications of the ACM, 61*(3), 72–77. doi:10.1145/3179995.

Lanzi, A., Burshnic, V., & Bourgeois, M. S. (2017). Person-centered memory and communication strategies for adults with dementia. *Topics in Language Disorders, 37*(4), 361–374. doi:10.1097/TLD.0000000000000136.

Maslow, A. (1943). A theory of human motivation. *Psychological Review, 50*, 370–396. doi:10.1037/h0054346.

Michaudet, C., & Malaty, J. (2018). Cerumen impaction: Diagnosis and management. *American Family Physician, 98*(8), 525–529.

Nordvik, Ø., Heggdal, P. O. L., Brännström, J., et al. (2018). Generic quality of life in persons with hearing loss: A systematic literature review. *BMC Ear, Nose and Throat Disorders, 18*(1), 1. doi:10.1186/s12901-018-0051-6.

Ontario Human Rights Commission. (2020). *Ageism and age discrimination (fact sheet).* http://www.ohrc.on.ca/en/ageism-and-age-discrimination-fact-sheet.

Rittenour, C. E., & Cohen, E. L. (2016). Age progression simulations increase young adults' aging anxiety and negative stereotypes of older adults. *International Journal of Aging and Human Development, 82*(4), 271–289. doi:10.1177/0091415016641690.

Rubin, A., Parrish, D. E., & Miyawaki, C. E. (2018). Benchmarks for evaluating life review and reminiscence therapy in alleviating depression among older adults. *Social Work, 64*(1), 61–72. doi:10.1093/sw/swy054.

Sacks, O. (1989). *Seeing voices: A journey into the world of the deaf.* University of California Press.

Sandelowski, M. (1994). We are the stories we tell. *Journal of Holistic Nursing, 12*(1), 23–33. doi:10.1177/089801019401200105.

Seetharaman, K., & Chaudhury, H. (2020). 'I am making a difference': Understanding advocacy as a citizenship practice among persons living with dementia. *Journal of Aging Studies, 52*, 100831. doi:10.1016/j.jaging.2020.100831.

Statistics Canada. (2019). *Unperceived hearing loss among Canadians aged 40 to 79.* https://www150.statcan.gc.ca/n1/pub/82-003-x/2019008/article/00002-eng.htm.

Sullivan, E., Sillup, G., & Klimberg, R. (2018). Reduction of agitation and anxiety observed in a case study of people with dementia using TimeSlips™ creative expression program. *International Journal of Behavioural and Healthcare Research, 6*(2). doi:10.1504/IJBHR.2018.091260.

Thorsheim, H., & Roberts, B. (2000). I remember when: Activity ideas to help people reminisce. Elder Books.

Wanko Keutchafo, E. L., Kerr, J., & Jarvis, M. A. (2020). Evidence of nonverbal communication between nurses and older adults: A scoping review. *BMC Nursing, 19*, 53. doi:10.1186/s12912-020-00443-9.

Williams, K. N., Perhounkova, Y., Herman, R., et al. (2017). A communication intervention to reduce resistiveness in dementia care: A cluster randomized controlled trial. *Gerontology, 57*(4), 707–718. doi:10.1093/geront/gnw047.

Woods, B., O'Philbin, L., Farrell, E. M., et al. (2018). *Reminiscence therapy for dementia. Cochrane Database of Systematic Reviews, 3*(3), CD001120. doi:10.1002/14651858.CD001120.pub3.

World Health Organization (WHO). (2017). *Evidence profile: Visual impairment.* https://www.who.int/ageing/health-systems/icope/evidence-centre/ICOPE-evidence-profile-visual.pdf?ua=1.

World Health Organization (WHO). (2020). *Ageing: Ageism.* https://www.who.int/ageing/features/faq-ageism/en/.

Young, K., Ng, P., Kwok, T., et al. (2017). The effects of holistic health group interventions on improving the cognitive ability of persons with mild cognitive impairment: A randomized controlled trial. *Clinical Interventions in Aging, 12*, 1543–1552. doi:10.214/CIA.S142109.

Zhang, M., Zhao, H., & Meng, F. P. (2020). Elderspeak to resident dementia patients increases resistiveness to care in health care profession. *INQUIRY: The Journal of Health Care Organization, Provision and Financing, 57*. doi:10.1177/0046958020948668.

Zult, T., Smith, L., Stringer, C., et al. (2020). Levels of self-reported and objective physical activity in individuals with age-related macular degeneration. *BMC Public Health, 20*, 1144. doi:10.1186/s12889-020-09255-7.

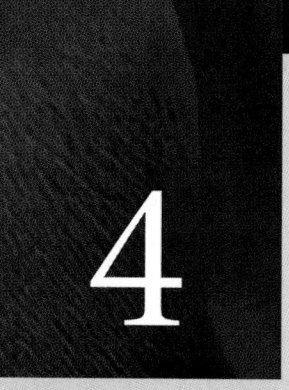

CULTURE, ETHNICITY, DIVERSITY, AND AGING

LEARNING OBJECTIVES

Upon completion of this chapter, the reader will be able to:

- Identify factors contributing to the nurse's cultural sensitivity and cultural competence.
- Identify factors contributing to older adults' cultural safety.
- Discuss approaches that facilitate an appreciation of diversity among older adults.
- Explain the prominent health belief systems.
- Identify nursing care interventions appropriate for ethnoculturally diverse older adults.
- Formulate a plan of care incorporating ethnoculturally sensitive interventions.

GLOSSARY

Culture Learned and transmitted knowledge, beliefs, values, and guidelines about living within a social group.

Determinants of health Factors and conditions that influence the health status of individuals, communities, and populations.

Ethnicity The cultural, racial, religious, or linguistic traditions of a people or country.

Ethnocentrism The belief in the inherent superiority of one's ethnic group, accompanied by the devaluation of other groups.

Family Class immigrant A Canadian Citizenship and Immigration term referring to immigrants who are eligible for sponsorship by a family member. Canadian citizens and permanent residents can sponsor a spouse, a common-law partner, a conjugal partner, dependent children, parents, grandparents, and certain other eligible relatives. The sponsor must promise to provide financial support to the immigrating relative for between 3 and 10 years.

Folk medicine Healing methods originating among the people of a given culture and primarily transmitted from person to person.

Health disparities Inequalities and differences in health status across population groups defined by characteristics such as socioeconomic status, geographic location (e.g., urban/rural, high-income/low-income neighbourhoods), ethnicity, gender, and other determinants of health.

Health literacy The degree to which individuals have the ability to obtain, process, and understand the basic information and services they need to make appropriate health decisions.

Interpreter A person who transmits the meaning of what is spoken in one language in another language.

Intersectionality "An understanding of human beings as shaped by the interaction of different social locations (e.g., 'race'/ethnicity, Indigeneity, gender, class, sexuality, geography, age, disability/ability, migration status, religion). These interactions occur within a context of connected systems and structures of power (e.g., laws, policies, state governments and other political and economic unions, religious institutions, media). Through such processes, interdependent forms of privilege and oppression shaped by colonialism, imperialism, racism, homophobia, ableism and patriarchy are created." (Hankivsky, 2014, p. 2)

Stereotype A belief applied to a group of persons on the basis of actual or assumed knowledge about an individual member of the group.

Translator A person who converts written materials from one language to another.

Visible minority A term referring to "persons of colour." As defined in Canadian federal data collection and official statistics, it refers to Chinese, South Asian, Black, Filipino, Latin American, Southeast Asian, Arab, West Asian, Korean, and Japanese people.

THE LIVED EXPERIENCE

"The beauty of working in the community is that you are in their setting. I can walk into someone's house and see important scripture, you know, a frame that's written on the wall or I can see a crucifix or I can see a Buddha. There are so many visual things in someone's home of what's important for them, where in the hospital you don't always see that."

From Reimer-Kirkham, S., Sharma, S., Grypma, S., et al. (2019). 'The elephant on the table': Religious and ethnic diversity in home health services. *Journal of Religion and Health, 58,* 908–925. doi:10.1007/210943-017-0489-7.

Attention to **culture** and health care is increasing. In the field of gerontology in Canada, interest in culture is stimulated to a great extent by three major issues: (1) the realization of a "gerontological explosion," (2) the impact of Canadian policies of multiculturalism that were established in 1971, and (3) the recognition of **health disparities** for members of minorities. *Gerontological explosion* refers both to the rapid increases in the total number of older adults, especially those over the age of 85 years, and to the relatively high proportion of older adults in most countries across the globe (see Chapter 1). *Health disparities* refers to the differences in disease burden between groups of people.

Nurses are expected to provide competent care to persons whose life experiences, cultural perspectives, values, languages, and styles of communication are different from their own. To competently assess and intervene, nurses must first develop cultural sensitivity through an awareness of their own **ethnocentrism.** Effective nurses develop cultural competence through knowing about **ethnicity,** culture, language, and health

belief systems and by acquiring the skills needed to optimize intercultural communication.

Culturally competent and culturally safe health care and health care systems are especially important in gerontological nursing, because many older adults are immigrants to Canada. Some have had limited opportunities to develop English or French language skills, increasing the risk for limited **health literacy** (see Chapter 7). Many other older adults, such as Indigenous persons, LGBTQ2+, and those who are part of an ethnic or racial minority, have experienced racism, discrimination, and exclusion in many areas of their lives, including health care. This chapter provides an overview of culture, diversity, and aging, as well as strategies that gerontological nurses can use to best respond to the changing face of aging and thus help to reduce health disparities.

THE GERONTOLOGICAL EXPLOSION

Multiculturalism is part of the Canadian identity and is valued by most Canadians (Thurairajah, 2017). Canada is officially a multicultural society, as multicultural policies were implemented by the federal government in 1971; the 1982 Canadian Charter of Rights and Freedoms states that the Charter "shall be interpreted in a manner consistent with the preservation and enhancement of the multicultural heritage of Canadians" (*Constitution Act, 1982,* s. 27). The population of Canada is rapidly becoming more diverse. It is projected that by 2036, between 25% and 30% of the Canadian population will be immigrants, between 35% and 40% of the population will be members of a **visible minority,** and the proportion of Canadians who identify as Christian will decline from about 67% (in 2011) to about 52% (Morency et al., 2017).

Currently, 13.6% of Canadians most often speak a language other than French or English, and 23% report a mother tongue other than English or French (Statistics Canada, 2019a, 2020). The proportion is higher for older Canadians. More than 7.6 million Canadians (22.3% of the population) are members of a visible minority, and an additional 1.6 million identify as Indigenous (First Nations, Inuit, or Métis) (Statistics Canada, 2019b).

Thirty percent of Canadians aged 65 years and older are immigrants (Statistics Canada, 2018). Most older immigrants live in Ontario, where 44% are immigrants, or in British Columbia, where 40% are immigrants. In the Atlantic provinces, Saskatchewan, and Nunavut, less than 10% of older adults are immigrants. Most older immigrants came to Canada before 2000 as young adults. Immigrants and refugees who arrived in Canada in the last 5 years are referred to as new immigrants. Just 3.3% of new immigrants are aged 65 or older (Employment and Social Development Canada, 2018). Among Canadians older than 65 years of age, the numbers of people who belong to ethnocultural minorities are not as dramatic, but growing numbers are being seen in all aspects of gerontological nursing. For example, 12.6% of Canadians over the age of 65 years are

members of visible minorities, but the number is increasing; among Canadians who are now between the ages of 45 and 64 years, 18.3% are members of a visible minority (Statistics Canada, 2019c). Table 4.1 shows the distribution of ethnic origins in the Canadian population and in subgroups of older or middle-aged Canadians.

HEALTH DISPARITIES

Significant health disparities exist in Canada and have been a concern in Canadian health policy for over 45 years. The most important factors associated with health disparities in Canada are Indigenous identity, low socioeconomic status, sexual and gender minority

TABLE 4.1
Population of Canada by Ethnic Origin and Age

Ethnic Origin*	Total Population	Population Aged 65 Years and Older
	N = 34,460,065 (% of Total)[†]	N = 5,479,910 (% of Age Group)[†]
Indigenous (First Nations, Inuit, and Métis)[‡]	2,130,520 (6.2%)	149,230 (2.7%)
Canadian	11,135,965 (32.3%)	1,589,010 (29.0%)
British Isles	11,211,850 (32.5%)	1,960,395 (35.8%)
European (excluding French)	12,472,490 (36.2%)	1,733,600 (31.6%)
French	4,680,815 (13.6%)	735,170 (13.4%)
East Asian, Southeast Asian	3,163,360 (9.2%)	321,400 (5.9%)
South Asian	1,963,330 (5.7%)	192,700 (3.5%)
West Central Asian, Middle Eastern	1,011,150 (2.9%)	76,015 (1.4%)
Caribbean	749,155 (2.2%)	72,700 (1.3%)
American	377,405 (1.1%)	56,970 (1.0%)
African	1,067,925 (3.1%)	49,790 (0.9%)
Latin, Central, and South American	674,640 (2.0%)	37,415 (0.7%)
Australian, New Zealander, Pacific Islander	85,465 (0.2%)	6,085 (0.1%)

*The census question was, "What were the ethnic or cultural origins of this person's ancestors?"
[†]Percentages add to more than 100% because people could specify as many origins as applicable.
[‡]Figures for Indigenous peoples are underestimates because they do not include data from one or more incompletely enumerated Indigenous reserves or settlements.
Source: Adapted from Statistics Canada. (2016). *Ethnic origin (264), single and multiple ethnic origin responses (3), generation status (4), age groups (10) and sex (3) for the population in private households of Canada, provinces, territories, Census Metropolitan Areas and Census Agglomerations, 2011 National Household Survey.* http://www12.statcan.gc.ca/nhs-enm/2011/dp-pd/dt-td/Rp-eng.cfm?LANG=E&APATH=3&DETAIL=0&DIM=0&FL=A&FREE=0&GC=0&GID=0&GK=0&GRP=0&PID=105396&PRID=0&PTYPE=105277&S=0&SHOWALL=0&SUB=0&Temporal=2013&THEME=95&VID=0&VNAMEE=&VNAMEF.

identity, racism, immigrant status, and living with a functional limitation. Other vulnerable populations include those with less than high school education, living in areas of high social and material deprivation, or living in rural or remote areas (Public Health Agency of Canada, 2018; Stinchcombe et al., 2018).

Indigenous peoples in Canada include First Nations, Inuit, and Métis. Addressing the health disparities experienced by Indigenous peoples in Canada requires an understanding of the differences and variability of disparities and inequities among and between First Nations, Inuit, and Métis peoples. Compared to non-Indigenous people in Canada, Indigenous peoples experience more chronic health conditions, disability, and death from injury, as well as lower life expectancy (Public Health Agency of Canada, 2018). Indigenous peoples are more likely to experience disadvantages related to other key **determinants of health** (see Chapter 1), including housing quality, access to safe drinking water, educational attainment, employment, income, and access to health services. Underlying health disparities for Indigenous peoples are rooted in colonialism, policies of assimilation, racism, and health systems and planning that do not incorporate Indigenous worldviews (Public Health Agency of Canada, 2018; Brooks-Cleator et al., 2019). Access to health services continues to be experienced as problematic, difficult, and limited for Indigenous people (Nguyen et al., 2020).

Health disparities persist for older Indigenous peoples. Many older Indigenous peoples in Canada attended residential schools (Box 4.1) and are still experiencing lasting health effects, including chronic health conditions, mental health issues, and poor self-rated health (Wilk et al., 2017). There are approximately 80,000 residential school survivors in Canada (Government of Ontario, 2021). Still more experienced a child welfare system that disrupted families, with lasting intergenerational traumatic impacts (Varley, 2017).

BOX 4.1
RESIDENTIAL SCHOOLS AND OLDER INDIGENOUS PERSONS IN CANADA

The residential school system in Canada existed from 1800 to 1997 (CBC News, 2021). The system peaked in 1930, when there were 80 schools. The schools were funded by the federal government and were operated mainly by churches. Residential schools were more common in the Prairies, British Columbia, and northern Canada, but they existed in all provinces except Newfoundland, Prince Edward Island, and New Brunswick. Indigenous children were often removed from their communities and separated from their families for 10 months of the year. The system was founded on the assumption that assimilation into mainstream culture would facilitate adaptation to a modernizing society. Students were not allowed to speak their first language or practise their traditions. The conditions in the schools and the skills taught there were substandard. Many students experienced malnutrition, emotional or physical abuse, and sexual abuse. Many students were ill-prepared for life in urban settings or in their home communities. Long-term negative effects include "lateral violence (when an oppressed group turns on itself and begins to violate each other), suicide, depression, poverty, alcoholism, lack of parenting skills, lack of capacity to build and sustain healthy families and communities" (Aboriginal Healing Foundation, 2010, p. 2). As with other forms of trauma, the traumatic effects of the residential school system pass between generations, affecting children, grandchildren, and future generations. "Furthermore, this trauma is consistently being reproduced and expressed in our current day and age: from homelessness, to violence, suicide and the pervasive use of alcohol and drugs" (Braganza et al., 2018, p. 3). The Prime Minister of Canada apologized in Parliament to Indigenous peoples on June 11, 2008. The Indian Residential Schools Settlement Agreement is a settlement package negotiated between the federal government, churches, the Assembly of First Nations, and lawyers representing former students (CBC News, 2021). It includes payments to former students and funding for healing funds, a truth and reconciliation commission, and commemoration. The Truth and Reconciliation Commission of Canada (2015) received statements from more than 6,750 people, including former students, families, and others. The Survivors Speak is a compilation of stories of residential school survivors, published as part of the Truth and Reconciliation Commission's report.

Sources: Aboriginal Healing Foundation. (2010). *FAQs*. http://www.ahf.ca/faqs; Braganza, B., McKinley, G. P., & Sibbald, S. L. (2018). The construction of "trauma" in Canadian residential school survivors and impacts on healing interventions and reconciliation initiatives. *The Canadian Journal of Native Studies*. 38(1), 1–18; CBC News. (2021, June 4). *Your questions answered about Canada's residential school system*. https://www.cbc.ca/news/canada/canada-residential-schools-kamloops-faq-1.6051632; Truth and Reconciliation Commission of Canada. (2015). *The survivors speak*. https://nctr.ca/records/reports/.

People who are members of a visible minority or who are immigrants tend to have worse health than the rest of the population (Public Health Agency of Canada, 2018). There is significant evidence for health disparities associated with ethnicity and race, particularly in the United States. However, health disparities among visible minorities have not been well researched in Canada, especially in older adults (Khan et al., 2017). People who are members of a visible minority tend to experience more poverty; visible minorities and Indigenous peoples fare the worst. There is considerable variety among visible minority and ethnocultural groups with respect to economic security and health status.

Most older immigrants have lived in Canada for decades and are less likely than younger and more recent immigrants to be members of visible minorities (Statistics Canada, 2019d). The ethnocultural composition of the older immigrant population reflects historical immigration policies. Thus, most older immigrants were born in Europe, and a significant minority were born in Asian countries. Older immigrants are more likely than nonimmigrants to live in urban areas. This is especially true for more recent immigrants and members of visible minorities, who are most likely to live in Toronto or Vancouver (Statistics Canada, 2019d).

Older adults who are immigrants to Canada may experience worse health than their Canadian-born counterparts. In a phenomenon known as the "healthy migrant effect," recent immigrants tend to have better health than long-term immigrants or nonimmigrants because of Canadian immigration policies. Over time, the health status of immigrants becomes more like that of their Canadian-born counterparts. There is evidence that the health of long-term immigrants is worse than that of their Canadian-born counterparts with respect to health conditions such as diabetes (Doyle et al., 2018) and mental illness (Davison et al., 2019, 2020). Although recent immigrants tend to have better health, age plays a role. Older recent immigrants, especially those who are refugees or who enter as **Family Class immigrants** sponsored by children or grandchildren, tend to have poorer health (Kwak, 2018). Most recent immigrants are not eligible for social security benefits such as Old Age Security until they have lived in Canada for at least 10 years. After 10 years of residence, immigrants who are aged 65 years or older are entitled to partial social security benefits (Government of Canada, 2020a) (see Chapter 24).

Barriers to accessing health care that may be experienced by older adults who are members of ethnic minorities include language barriers, cultural values and beliefs that can influence the seeking of health care, the lack of interpretation services, the absence of culturally specific programs, and the lack of health care providers who understand the culture (Wang et al., 2019; Koehn, 2020). Not only does racism create health inequities, but racism in the health care system is an important barrier to receiving adequate health care (Monchalin et al., 2020; Nwoke, 2020).

Reducing Health Disparities

Policies and practices that improve access to health care are important. However, reducing health disparities requires action and attention to the underlying causes of health disparities and determinants of health. This means considering not only single determinants of health but also **intersectionality**—the intersection of sources of inequity and older adults' multiple identities, such as age, race, ethnicity, Indigeneity, gender identity, sexual orientation, religion, language, disability, and religion and the power imbalances that perpetuate these inequities (Brotman et al., 2020).

For example, policies and practices related to socioeconomic status and poverty can have significant impacts on health. Canadian income protection and pension policies have resulted in poverty among older Canadians dropping from 29% in 1980 to 5.6% in 2018 (Government of Canada, 2020b). However, these policies have not had an equal effect for all older Canadians. Among older adults, the poverty rate is higher among those who identify as a visible minority (20%) and those who live alone (13%) (Statistics Canada, 2019e; Government of Canada, 2020b). Living alone is also a marker for other identities that are determinants of health for older adults, including being female, having lower education, and belonging to a sexual and gender minority (Srugo et al., 2020; Standing Committee on Health, 2019). Throughout the lifespan, LGBTQ2+ persons are also more likely to live in poverty and more likely to live alone (Standing Committee on Health, 2019). Thus, poverty among older adults is affected by experiences of inequity throughout the lifespan. As the example of poverty shows, effectively addressing health disparities and inequities for older adults requires political will and an intersectional approach.

INCREASING CULTURAL COMPETENCE AND CULTURAL SAFETY

Cultural competence means having the skills to put cultural knowledge to use in assessment, communication, negotiation, and intervention. As nurses move toward cultural competence, they increase their cultural awareness, knowledge, and skills. Nurses can become aware of their own personal biases, prejudices, attitudes, and behaviours toward persons who are different from themselves in race, ethnicity, age, sex, gender, sexual orientation, social class, economic situation, and many other factors. Through increased knowledge, nurses can better assess the strengths and needs of older adults within the context of their culture and know when and how to effectively intervene to support rather than hinder cultural patterns that enhance wellness and coping.

Responsibility for cultural competence rests mainly with individuals. However, health care organizations can support cultural competence through policies. Cultural competence is not enough to prevent unequal care and inequities experienced by older adults. Achieving equity requires cultural safety, where nurses and health care systems acknowledge the power differentials within organizations and in the relationships between nurses and patients that perpetuate inequities. Cultural safety means working to decrease bias, redress power imbalances, and achieve equity (Brooks-Cleator et al., 2019; Curtis et al., 2019) (Box 4.2).

Cultural Awareness

Increased awareness calls for openness and self-reflection. A White nurse needs to realize that their whiteness means having special privileges and freedoms in a predominantly White society. Older adults who are members of an ethnocultural or visible minority group may not have had the same advantages or experiences as the nurse. For example, many older Indigenous peoples in Canada experienced the residential school system (see Box 4.1), and many older Canadians who are members of a visible minority group have experienced racism and discrimination. Racism itself is an important determinant of health. Immigrants and members of visible minority groups continue to experience racism in the Canadian health care system (Boyer, 2017; Kitching et al., 2020). Many

---

BOX 4.2
RESEARCH FOR EVIDENCE-INFORMED PRACTICE: ELEMENTS OF CULTURALLY SAFE HEALTH INITIATIVES FOR INDIGENOUS PEOPLES IN CANADA

Problem: The impacts of colonization continue to impact the health of Indigenous peoples in Canada. Cultural safety can reduce health disparities, but there is limited information about its practical application.

Methods: The researchers conducted a scoping review of literature on using cultural safety in health care in Canada. The review followed established procedures.

Findings: Thirty publications were included. The following six key elements of a culturally safe health initiative were identified: (1) *Collaboration and partnerships* with members of Indigenous communities. Taking the time to establish trust and respect and embracing Indigenous knowledge were important. (2) *Power sharing* includes transferring power to patients, viewing patient strengths as a resource, and understanding that patients are the ones who define whether they experience cultural safety. (3) *Addressing the broader context of the patient's life* means understanding the endurance of colonialism and its traumatic effects, recognizing diversity among Indigenous groups, and respecting cultural values and community and family support. (4) *Safe environment* refers to emotionally and physically safe environments. This includes acceptance and welcoming attitudes of health care providers and space for Indigenous cultural practices. (5) *Organizational and individual level self-reflection* on and challenging of power dynamics, personal biases, and biases inherent in policies, practices, and standards is essential. (6) *Training for health care providers* is frequently part of cultural safety health initiatives.

Implications for Nursing Practice: Incorporating these six elements in cultural safety initiatives could improve cultural competence and cultural safety in health care. Accountability for working toward cultural safety rests with institutions. People experiencing health care are the only ones who can judge whether they experience cultural safety.

Source: Brooks-Cleator, L., Phillips, B., & Giles, A. (2018). Culturally safe health initiatives for Indigenous peoples in Canada—A scoping review. *Canadian Journal of Nursing Research, 50*(4), 202–213. doi:10.1177/0844562118770334.

older LGBTQ2+ persons have also experienced lifelong stigmatization and discrimination, both of which they have experienced within the health care system (Boulé et al., 2020). Transgender persons experience profound discrimination in the health care system (Kcomt, 2019). Being culturally aware means recognizing the presence of "isms," such as racism. It is imperative to understand how these "isms" affect not only the pursuing and receiving of health care but also the quality of life for older adults. Moreover, older adults may have to face ageism in addition to racism, sexism, classism, and other forms of discrimination.

The term *ageism* refers to discrimination and negative **stereotypes** that are based solely on age. Ageism may be at least partially determined by culture. For instance, in cultures where older adults are traditionally treated with special respect and honour, such as in Asian or Indigenous cultures, ageism may be less prevalent. However, there is great variability in ageist attitudes and behaviours within cultures, and personal values often differ from cultural norms (Vauclair et al., 2017). Indeed, at a societal level, ageism is more common when there are scarce resources and a high proportion of the population is older (Marques et al., 2020).

Some health care providers demonstrate ageism, undoubtedly in part because these providers tend to see many frail older adults and fewer older adults who are healthy and active. Ageism affects the quality of health care and limits access to health services for older adults (Wyman et al., 2018). The COVID-19 pandemic shone a light on structural ageism. For example, insufficient funding of long-term care homes has put older adults at greater risk for exposure to the virus; COVID-19 has been portrayed as an ageist problem of older adults, and ageist pandemic policies have disproportionally affected older adults (Ehni & Wahl, 2020; Rahman & Jahan, 2020). The experience of ageism is associated with psychological distress, which is amplified for older adults who have higher levels of concern about COVID-19 (Bergman et al., 2020).

Before the gerontological nurse provides quality care to older adults from ethnic or cultural backgrounds that are different from their own, it is essential that the nurse self-reflect by considering whether they hold any personal beliefs about such persons, how these beliefs affect the delivery of care, and whether these beliefs are based on facts rather than anecdotes.

Cultural Knowledge

Cultural knowledge is both what the nurse brings to a caring situation and what the nurse learns about older adults, their families, their communities, their behaviours, and their expectations. Essential knowledge includes knowledge of the person's way of life (i.e., ways of thinking, believing, and acting). This knowledge is obtained formally and informally through professional experience.

Some nurses prefer what can be called an "encyclopedic" approach to the details of a particular culture or ethnic group, such as proper name usage, touch, greeting, eye contact, gender roles, foods, and beliefs about relevant topics (e.g., health-promoting practices, expression of pain, end-of-life rituals, and caregiving). This information is available in many compendiums of cross-cultural information (see the Resources section at the end of this chapter). It is especially important for the nurse to know about the older adult's culturally based attitudes toward caregiving, decision making, and end-of-life rituals.

Although cultural knowledge is helpful and essential, it is just one component of cultural competence. Nurses should be cautious about potential stereotyping. In *stereotyping*, limited knowledge about one person with specific characteristics is applied to other persons with the same characteristics; negative characteristics are especially prone to this treatment. Stereotyping limits recognition of the heterogeneity of the group. Relying on a positive stereotype can be useful as a starting point in understanding, but it can also be used to limit understanding of the individual's uniqueness and impose unrealistic expectations. For example, a common way to stereotype older members of ethnic minority groups is to assume that religious organizations are a source of support to them or that adult children will be responsible for providing care at home. The nurse's assumption can easily lead to a negative outcome, such as fewer referrals for other forms of support (e.g., home-delivered meals, home care services, or respite care) or inadequate discharge planning.

Persons from a specific ethnocultural group may share a common geographical origin, migratory status, race, language or dialect, or religion. Traditions, symbols, literature, folklore, food preferences, and dress are expressions of ethnicity that are often adopted. This may be particularly true for older adults who have had no need to leave their culture-specific neighbour-hoods. Persons who identify with the same ethnic group may or may not be of the same race. For example, persons who consider themselves Latin Americans are members of a diverse ethnic group and may be of any race and from one of several countries. However, those who consider themselves Latin Americans often have in common the Catholic religion and the Spanish language.

Health beliefs and practices are usually a mixed expression of life experience and cultural knowledge. In most cultures, older adults are likely to treat themselves for familiar or chronic conditions in ways they have found to be successful in the past, practices that are referred to as domestic medicine, **folk medicine,** or folk healing. Much folk medicine is based on making the most of whatever is available.

The culture of nursing and health care in Canada advocates what is called the "Western" or "biomedical" system, which has its own set of beliefs about the cause of illness, the choice of treatments, and so on. In most settings, this belief system is considered superior to all others, an ethnocentric viewpoint. However, many of the world's peoples have different beliefs, such as belief in a personalistic (magico-religious) system or a naturalistic (holistic) system. Each system is complete, with beliefs about disease causation and recommendations for prevention and treatment. Nurses who are familiar with the range of health beliefs and realize the importance of those beliefs to followers will be able to provide more sensitive and appropriate care. In the absence of such understanding lies great potential for conflict.

Western or Biomedical System

In the Western or biomedical belief system, disease is thought to be the result of abnormalities in the structure and function of body organs and systems, often caused by an invasion of germs. The terms *disease* and *illness* are subjective; they are used by health care providers and are not always understood by others. In the biomedical system, assessment and diagnosis are directed at identifying the pathogen or the processes causing the abnormality using laboratory and other investigative procedures. Treatment consists of removing or destroying the invading organism or repairing, modifying, or removing the affected body part. In this belief system, prevention involves the avoidance of pathogens, chemicals, activities, and dietary agents known to cause abnormalities. Health has conventionally been considered the absence of disease, but Western conceptions of health are now more holistic (see Chapter 1).

Personalistic or Magico-Religious System

Those who follow the tenets of a personalistic or magico-religious system believe that illness is caused by the actions of supernatural entities such as gods or deities or by nonhuman beings such as ghosts, ancestors, or spirits. Health is viewed as a blessing or reward from these entities, and illness is seen as a punishment for breaching rules, breaking a taboo, or displeasing or failing to please the source of power. These beliefs may be more prevalent in the explaining of altered mental states, such as psychosis and dementia, and may influence the seeking of care for older adults with dementia. Personalistic or magico-religious systems are more common in certain cultures (for example, those of rural India) (Joshi & Vashist, 2018) and in remote, isolated communities (Fallon, 2017). Belief that illness and disease are caused by the wrath of God is prevalent among members of the Fundamentalist Baptist, Holiness, and Pentecostal churches. Examples of magical causes to which illness can be attributed are voodoo, hexing, and the "evil eye." Treatments may include religious practices such as praying, meditating, fasting, wearing amulets, burning candles, and establishing family altars.

Making sure that social networks of fellow humans are in good working order is viewed as the essence of prevention. It is therefore important to avoid angering a person's family, friends, neighbours, ancestors, and gods. This belief system can be traced back thousands of years to the ancient Egyptians and persists in its entirety or in part in many groups. Current practices include rituals such as prayer circles and the "laying on of hands." In this context, it is not uncommon to hear an older adult pray for a cure or ask, "What did I do to cause this?"

Naturalistic or Holistic Health System

The naturalistic or holistic health belief system is based on the concept of balance and stems from the ancient civilizations of China, India, and Greece (Fallon, 2017). Many people throughout the world view health as a sign of balance—the right amount of exercise, food, sleep, evacuation, interpersonal relationships, or the balance of the geophysical and metaphysical forces in the universe (e.g., chi). Disturbances in this balance results in disharmony and subsequent illness. Diagnosis calls for the determination of the type and extent of imbalance. The appropriate interventions, therefore, are methods of restoring balance and harmony.

Traditional Chinese medicine is based on the belief in the balance between yin and yang, darkness and light, and hot and cold. Older adults who were raised in one of the Pacific Rim countries (especially in Asia and the Pacific islands) or in a traditional Indigenous community frequently rely on these beliefs. The naturalistic system practised in India and some of its neighbouring countries is known as Ayurveda. Another such system is practised by those who follow hot–cold beliefs apart from traditional Chinese medicine; illness is believed to be the result of excess heat or cold that has entered the body and caused an imbalance. Hot and cold are generally metaphorical, although actual temperature is sometimes an aspect. Various foods, medicines, environmental conditions, emotions, and body conditions such as menopause may possess the characteristics of either hot or cold (Spector, 2017).

Selecting an appropriate treatment requires the identification of disease type—either hot or cold. Treatments are likewise divided, focused on using the opposite element; disease resulting from excess heat is treated with something that has cold properties, and vice versa. The treatments may take the form of teas, herbs, food, dietary restrictions, or medications (such as antibiotics) and therapies from Western medicine that have hot and cold properties, such as massage, poultices, cupping, or other treatments.

Naturalistic healers can be physicians, advanced practice nurses, or herbalists who specialize in symptomatic treatment and know which medicines will restore the body's equilibrium. Provincial nursing regulatory bodies offer guidance to nurses on providing complementary therapies (College and Association of Registered Nurses of Alberta, 2018). In Indigenous cultures, the healer is referred to as a medicine man or woman who combines naturalistic and magico-religious systems. Prevention is directed at protecting oneself from imbalance.

Cultural Skills

Skillful cross-cultural nursing entails mutual respect between the nurse and the older adult; it means working *with* the patient rather than *on* the patient. Providing the highest quality of care for ethnically diverse older adults and enhancing healthy aging calls for a refined set of knowledge and skills, including being able to listen carefully to the person (especially for their perception of the situation) and attending not just to the words but also to nonverbal communication and the meanings behind the stories. As well, the nurse needs to be able to hear the older adult's desired goals and ideas for treatment. Cultural skills required in gerontological nursing include the nurse's ability to explain their perceptions clearly and without judgement, acknowledging that there are both similarities and differences between the nurse's perceptions and goals and those of the older adult. Finally, cross-cultural skills include the ability to develop a plan of action that takes both perspectives into account and negotiates an outcome that is mutually acceptable (Almutairi et al., 2017).

Working With Interpreters

Working with persons in a cross-cultural nursing situation often includes working with an **interpreter**. *Interpretation* is the process of rendering oral expressions made in one language system into another in a manner that preserves the meaning and tone of the original without adding or deleting anything. The job of the interpreter is to work with two different linguistic codes in a way that will produce equivalent messages. The interpreter tells the older adult what the nurse has said and the nurse what the older adult has said, without adding any extra meaning or opinion, such that communication is as accurate as possible. This is often confused with *translation* (when interpreters are called **translators**), which instead deals with the written word.

Although it is always necessary, respectful communication is essential when the nurse works with people who have limited or no English proficiency and with older adults from cultures in which respectful communication is the norm. Respectful communication includes addressing the person in the appropriate manner (by their surname unless otherwise instructed by the person) and using acceptable body language. For example, people from most cultures other than those of northern Europe (including European Americans) consider direct eye contact to be disrespectful. To press for eye contact with an older adult may be particularly rude.

An interpreter is needed when the nurse and the older adult speak different languages, when the person has limited English proficiency, or when cultural tradition prevents the person from speaking directly to the nurse (for example, as a result of the nurse's being a specific gender). The more complex the decision to be made (such as when determining the person's wishes regarding life-prolonging measures or the family's plan for caregiving), the more important the skills of the interpreter are. Whenever possible, it is ideal to engage persons who are trained in medical interpretation and who are of the same age, gender, and social status as the older adult. Unfortunately, it is usually necessary to call on younger interpreters; the effectiveness of the exchange may be hampered by intergenerational boundaries. Children and grandchildren are often called on to act as interpreters. In this situation, the nurse may realize that the child or the older adult is "editing" comments because of cultural restrictions about the sharing of certain information (i.e., what is or is not considered appropriate to speak of to an older adult or to a child). For information on working with an interpreter, see Box 4.3.

IMPLICATIONS FOR GERONTOLOGICAL NURSING AND HEALTHY AGING

The contact between older adults and gerontological nurses often begins with a story and an assessment. During this process, the nurse and older adult have an opportunity to get to know each other. Listening is key to the assessment; the nurse needs to try to understand the meaning of the situation and the person's perception of it. A thorough assessment includes a cultural assessment. A comprehensive assessment takes time. Not all situations allow for this, but even if the assessment is done bit by bit over time, it will give the nurse a better understanding of how to work with and within the person's culture.

Several tools or instruments can assist the nurse in eliciting health care beliefs and help the nurse identify their own perceptions of alternative beliefs. Although Leininger's Sunrise Model (Giger & Haddad, 2021) is often recommended, alternative models may be more useful in today's fast-paced health care situations. The explanatory model developed by Kleinman et al. (1978) has become a classic and has helped nurses and other health care providers obtain the basic information needed in a culturally sensitive manner. Box 4.4 presents

> **BOX 4.3**
> ## WORKING WITH INTERPRETERS
>
> - Meet with the interpreter before an interview or session with an older adult to explain the purpose of the session.
> - Encourage the interpreter to meet with the older adult before the session in order to determine the person's educational level and attitudes toward health and health care and to determine the depth and type of information and explanation needed.
> - Look at and speak directly to the older adult, not the interpreter.
> - Be patient. Interpreted interviews take more time because long, explanatory phrases are often needed.
> - Use short units of speech. Long, involved sentences or complex discussions create confusion.
> - Use simple language. Avoid technical terms, professional jargon, slang, abbreviations, abstractions, metaphors, and idiomatic expressions.
> - Encourage interpretation of the person's own words rather than paraphrased professional jargon to get a better sense of the patient's ideas and emotional state.
> - Request that the interpreter avoid inserting their own ideas and avoid omitting information.
> - Listen to the older adult and be aware of nonverbal communications (facial expression, voice intonation, body movement) to learn about their emotions regarding a specific topic.
> - Clarify the older adult's understanding and the accuracy of the interpretation by asking the person to tell you what they understand, facilitated by the interpreter.
>
> *Source:* Adapted from Enslein, J., Tripp-Reimer, T., Kelley, L. S., et al. (2002). Evidence-based protocol: Interpreter facilitation for individuals with limited English proficiency. *Journal of Gerontological Nursing, 28*(7), 5–13. doi:10.3928/0098-9134-20020701-04.

an adaptation of this model that is used to obtain a meaningful cultural health assessment. Use of the LEARN model (Berlin & Fowkes, 1983) can increase the effectiveness of nursing interventions and is a helpful guide for nurses in the clinical setting. Through its use, the nurse can increase their cultural sensitivity and provide more culturally competent care, thus helping to reduce health disparities (Box 4.5).

With an understanding of basic cross-cultural communication and assessment, the nurse can reach a clear understanding of problems and solutions with the older adult or the older adult's identified support figure. The

BOX 4.4
EXPLANATORY MODEL FOR CULTURALLY SENSITIVE ASSESSMENT

1. How would you describe the problem that has brought you here? (*What do you call your problem? Does it have a name?*)
   a. Who is involved in your decision making about health concerns?
2. How long have you had this problem?
   a. When do you think it started?
   b. What do you think started it?
   c. Do you know anyone else with it?
   d. Tell me what happened to that person when dealing with this problem.
3. What do you think is wrong with you?
   a. How severe is it?
   b. How long do you think it will last?
4. Why do you think this happened to you?
   a. Why has it happened to the involved part?
   b. What do you fear most about your sickness?
5. What are the chief problems your sickness has caused you?
6. What do you think will help clear up this problem? (*What treatment should you receive? What are the most important results you hope to receive?*) (If specific tests or medications are listed, ask what they are and what they do.)
7. Apart from me, who else do you think can make you feel better?
   a. Are there therapies (*maybe in another discipline*) I do not know about that make you feel better?

Sources: Adapted from Kleinman, A. (1980). *Patient and healers in the context of culture: An exploration of the borderland between anthropology, medicine, and psychiatry.* University of California Press; Pfeifferling, J. H. (1981). A cultural prescription for mediocentrism. In L. Eisenberg & A. Kleinman (Eds.), *The relevance of social science for medicine* (pp. 197–222). D. Reidel.

BOX 4.5
THE LEARN MODEL

Listen carefully to what the older adult is saying. Attend not just to the words but also to the nonverbal communication and to the meaning of the stories. Listen to the person's perception of the situation, desired goals, and ideas for treatment.

Explain your perception of the situation and problems.

Acknowledge and discuss both the similarities and the differences between your perceptions and goals and those of the older adult.

Recommend a plan of action that takes both perspectives into account.

Negotiate a plan that is mutually acceptable.

Source: Adapted from Berlin, E. A., & Fowkes, W. C. (1983). A teaching framework for cross-cultural health care: Application in family practice. *Western Journal of Medicine, 139*(6), 934–938.

---

than one belief system, combining Western biomedical approaches with those that may be considered more culturally traditional. People choose among the health belief systems or include aspects of several of them to make sense of health, illness, and treatment. To optimize the healthy aging of the person who depends on the nurse for care, the nurse must be sensitive to the possibility that the person may hold one or more of these beliefs. When a patient refuses biomedical treatment because the health problem is viewed as destiny or as God's will, it is often particularly difficult for the nurse and other health care providers. Finding out more about the person's beliefs about the cause of disease and the type of treatments they believe are appropriate will allow the nurse to navigate the culture of the health care establishment and that of the patient in order to promote better health.

Nurses should not attempt to change the person's beliefs. This is difficult, if not impossible, and usually counterproductive, particularly when working with older adults who carry a lifetime of beliefs and illness experience. However, negotiating health, treatment, or prevention options can be helpful. The nurse can attempt to preserve helpful beliefs and practices, accommodate beliefs that are neither helpful nor harmful, or help patients give up beliefs or practices that have been shown to be harmful. The nurse who has little or no knowledge of the specific belief or practice will need to

nurse may then need to include consultation or collaboration with traditional or alternative healers if the older adult believes this is important. Religious leaders or Indigenous healers may provide essential consultation, support, and interventions of their own. Supporting cultural beliefs and practices conveys a sense of caring, and unbiased caring can surmount cultural differences.

Also critical to the cultural assessment is determining the person's health beliefs, as discussed earlier. Most people (nurses and patients alike) subscribe to more

learn about and evaluate the belief or practice to determine its helpfulness or potential harm. In this way, beliefs and practices can be preserved whenever possible. The nurse's respectfully explaining concern about potentially harmful practices, along with offering possible alternatives, may show the person that the nurse is considering the person's preferences. When care is provided in the home, nurses must adapt home care strategies to the beliefs and culture of the patient and family if they hope to promote healthy aging and wellness. Special attention should be given to caregivers who are conflicted about their acculturated beliefs with respect to long-term care homes, work–caregiver demands, and expectations of the role of the adult child. Nurses need to work with the person's family in attempting to find a solution to cross-cultural and intergenerational conflicts in caregiving and health care settings. The nurse must also focus on the older adult's overall health and help the person and family gain access to needed services. To do this, the nurse needs to ascertain the following: (1) affordability, efficacy, accessibility, and availability of services; (2) satisfaction with services; (3) availability of information; (4) perspective on illness; and (5) informal support systems. Respect for the person's health beliefs is paramount.

KEY CONCEPTS

- Population diversity will continue to increase rapidly for many years. Thus, nurses will be caring for a greater number of ethnoculturally diverse older adults than in the past.
- Recent research has revealed significant and persistent disparities in the outcomes of health for persons from minority groups, and members of these groups will bear the burden of morbidity and mortality in most areas.
- Nurses can contribute to the reduction of health disparities through increasing their own cultural awareness, knowledge, and skills.
- Negative stereotyping is never appropriate.
- Cultural awareness, knowledge, and skills are necessary to increase cultural competence.
- Nurses caring for ethnoculturally diverse older adults must be aware of and let go of their own ethnocentrism before they can give effective care.
- Ethnoculturally diverse older adults may hold health beliefs that are different from those of the biomedical or Western medical system used by most health care providers in Canada.
- Lack of awareness of the older adult's health beliefs can produce conflict in the nursing situation.
- The more complex the communication or decision-making needs in a given situation, the greater the need for skilled interpreter services for persons with limited English proficiency.
- Programs staffed by persons who reflect the ethnocultural background of the participants and speak their language may be preferred by older adults.
- The explanatory model and the LEARN model provide a useful framework for working with older adults from any ethnocultural background.

ACTIVITIES AND DISCUSSION QUESTIONS

1. Discuss your personal beliefs regarding health and illness and how they fit into the three major classifications of health systems. How can this knowledge affect culturally competent care for ethnoculturally diverse older adults?

2. Explain the types of questions that would be helpful in assessing an older person's health problems or challenges in a way that is respectful of the person and their cultural background and ethnic identity.

3. Propose strategies that would be helpful in planning care for older adults from different ethnocultural backgrounds.

4. Identify sensitive areas in which discussion is frequently needed with older adults and suggest how these areas would be affected by differences in the cultural backgrounds of the patient and the nurse.

5. After speaking with some of your own older family members, discuss your familial and culturally determined views of aging.

RESOURCES

Aboriginal Healing Foundation
http://www.ahf.ca/about-us
Canadian Nurses Association. *Position statement: Promoting cultural competence in nursing.*
https://www.cna-aiic.ca/-/media/cna/page-content/pdf-en/position_statement_promoting_cultural_competence_in_nursing.pdf?la5e n&hash54B394DAE5C2138E7F6134D59E505DCB059754BA9
Legacy of Hope Foundation. *Where are the children: Healing the legacy of residential schools* **(multimedia resource).**
http://www.wherearethechildren.ca/en/
Truth and Reconciliation Commission of Canada. *The survivors speak* **(report).**
https://nctr.ca/records/reports/

For additional resources, please visit *http://evolve.elsevier.com/ Canada/Ebersole/gerontological/*

REFERENCES

Almutairi, A. F., Adlan, A. A., & Nasim, M. (2017). Perceptions of the critical cultural competence of registered nurses in Canada. *BMC Nursing, 16*(1), 1–9. doi:10.1186/s12912-017-0242-2.

Bergman, Y. S., Cohen-Fridel, S., Shrira, A., et al. (2020). COVID-19 health worries and anxiety symptoms among older adults: The moderating role of ageism. *International Psychogeriatrics, 32*(11), 1371–1375. doi:10.1017/S1041610220001258.

Berlin, E. A., & Fowkes, W. C. (1983). A teaching framework for cross-cultural health care: Application in family practice. *Western Journal of Medicine, 139*(6), 934–938.

Boulé, J., Wilson, K., Kortes-Miller, K., et al. (2020). "We live in a wonderful country, Canada, but . . .": Perspectives from older LGBTQ Ontarians on visibility, connection, and power in care and community. *International Journal of Aging and Human Development, 91*(3), 235–252. doi:10.1177/0091415019857060.

Boyer, Y. (2017). Healing racism in Canadian health care. *CMAJ, 189*(46), E1408–E1409. doi:10.1503/cmaj.171234.

Brooks-Cleator, L. A., Giles, A. R., & Flaherty, M. (2019). Community-level factors that contribute to First Nations and Inuit older adults feeling supported to age well in a Canadian city. *Journal of Aging Studies, 48*, 50–59. doi:10.1016/j.jaging.2019.01.001.

Brotman, S., Ferrer, I., & Koehn, S. (2020). Situating the life story narratives of aging immigrants within a structural context: The intersectional life course perspective as research praxis. *Qualitative Research, 20*(4), 465–484. doi:10.1177/1468794119880746.

College and Association of Registered Nurses of Alberta. (2018). *Complementary and alternative health care and natural health products standards.* https://nurses.ab.ca/docs/default-source/document-library/standards/complementary-and-alternative-health-care-and-natural-health-products.pdf?sfvrsn=2480176b_36.

Constitution Act, 1982. s. 27. https://laws-lois.justice.gc.ca/eng/const/page-12.html#h-39.

Curtis, E., Jones, R., Tipene-Leach, D., et al. (2019). Why cultural safety rather than cultural competency is required to achieve health equity: A literature review and recommended definition. *International Journal for Equity in Health, 18*(1), 1–17. doi:10.1186/s12939-019-1082-3.

Davison, K. M., Lin, S., Tong, H., et al. (2020). Nutritional factors, physical health and immigrant status are associated with anxiety disorders among middle-aged and older adults: Findings from baseline data of the canadian longitudinal study on aging (CLSA). *International Journal of Environmental Research and Public Health, 17*(5), 1–19. doi:10.3390/ijerph17051493.

Davison, K. M., Lung, Y., Lin, S., et al. (2019). Depression in middle and older adulthood: The role of immigration, nutrition, and other determinants of health in the Canadian longitudinal study on aging. *BMC Psychiatry, 19*(1), 1–21. doi:10.1186/s12888-019-2309-y.

Doyle, M. A., Dutton, H., Brown, W., et al. (2018). Prevalence of diabetes among Canadian immigrants. *Canadian Journal of Diabetes, 42*(5), S41. doi:10.1016/j.jcjd.2018.08.124.

Ehni, H. J., & Wahl, H. W. (2020). Six propositions against ageism in the COVID-19 pandemic. *Journal of Aging & Social Policy, 32*(4–5), 515–525. doi:10.1080/08959420.2020.1770032.

Employment and Social Development Canada. (2018). *Social isolation of seniors.* https://open.alberta.ca/dataset/7fd7a9cd-0af5-4c6a-b4c1-a288b0ed108a/resource/6b60b4da-f20c-4b56-b6a4-dc5cfee453e6/download/social-isolation-new-immigrant-and-refugee-seniors.pdf.

Fallon, D. (2017). Understanding the theory of health and illness beliefs. In K. Holland (Ed.), *Cultural awareness in nursing and health care* (pp. 63–80). Routlege.

Giger, J. N., & Haddad, L. (2021). *Transcultural nursing: Assessment and intervention.* Elsevier.

Government of Canada. (2020a). *Old age security: Do you qualify.* https://www.canada.ca/en/services/benefits/publicpensions/cpp/old-age-security/eligibility.html.

Government of Canada. (2020b). *Persons in low income by age, sex and economic family type.* https://open.canada.ca/data/en/dataset/f80e7069-6974-4d93-a45f-f1d731ffa2eb.

Government of Ontario. (2021). *Ontario supporting the identification and commemoration of Indian residential school burial sites.* Queen's Printer for Ontario. https://news.ontario.ca/en/release/1000343/ontario-supporting-the-identification-and-commemoration-of-indian-residential-school-burial-sites.

Hankivsky, O. (2014). *Intersectionality 101.* The Institute for Intersectionality Research & Policy, Simon Fraser University.

Hendricks, J. (2012). Considering life course concepts. *Journals of Gerontology: Series B, 67B*(2), 226–231. doi:10.1093/geronb/gbr147.

Joshi, P. C., & Vashist, N. (2018). Illness, health and culture: Anthropological perspectives on ethno-medicine in India. In G. Misra (Ed.), *Psychosocial interventions for health and well-being* (pp. 227–240). Springer.

Kcomt, L. (2019). Profound health-care discrimination experienced by transgender people: Rapid systematic review. *Social Work in Health Care, 58*(2), 201–219. doi:10.1080/00981389.2018.1532941.

Khan, M. M., Kobayashi, K., Vang, Z. M., et al. (2017). Are visible minorities "invisible" in Canadian health data and research? A scoping review. *International Journal of Migration, Health, and Social Care, 13*(1), 126–143. doi:10.1108/IJMHSC-10-2015-0036.

Kitching, G. T., Firestone, M., Schei, B., et al. (2020). Unmet health needs and discrimination by healthcare providers among an Indigenous population in Toronto, Canada. *Canadian Journal of Public Health*, *111*(1), 40–49. doi:10.17269/s41997-019-00242-z.

Kleinman, A., Eisenberg, L., & Good, B. (1978). Culture, illness, and care: Clinical lessons from anthropologic and cross-cultural research. *Annals of Internal Medicine*, *88*(2), 251–258. doi:10.7326/0003-4819-88-2-251.

Koehn, S. (2020). "It is not a disease, only memory loss": Exploring the complexity of access to a diagnosis of dementia in a cross-cultural sample. In L. Garcia, L. McCleary, & N. Drummond (Eds.), *Evidence-informed approaches for managing dementia transitions* (pp. 29–52). Academic Press.

Kwak, K. (2018). Age and gender variations in healthy immigrant effect: A population study of immigrant well-being in Canada. *Journal of International Migration and Integration*, *19*(2), 413–437. doi:10.1007/s12134-018-0546-4.

Marques, S., Mariano, J., Mendonça, J., et al. (2020). Determinants of ageism against older adults: A systematic review. *International Journal of Environmental Research and Public Health*, *17*(7), 2560. doi:10.3390/ijerph17072560.

Monchalin, R., Smylie, J., & Nowgesic, E. (2020). "I guess I shouldn't come back here": Racism and discrimination as a barrier to accessing health and social services for urban Métis women in Toronto, Canada. *Journal of Racial and Ethnic Health Disparities*, *7*(2), 251–261. doi:10.1007/s40615-019-00653-1.

Morency, J. D., Malenfant, É. C., & MacIsaac, S. (2017). *Immigration and diversity: Population projections for Canada and its regions, 2011 to 2036*. https://www150.statcan.gc.ca/n1/pub/91-551-x/91-551-x2017001-eng.htm.

Nguyen, N. H., Subhan, F. B., Williams, K., et al. (2020). Barriers and mitigating strategies to healthcare access in Indigenous communities of Canada: A narrative review. *Healthcare*, *8*(2), 112. doi:10.3390/healthcare8020112.

Nwoke, C. N., & Leung, B. M. Y. (2020). Historical antecedents and challenges of racialized immigrant women in access to healthcare services in Canada: An exploratory review of the literature. *Journal of Racial and Ethnic Health Disparities*. doi:10.1007/s40615-020-00907-3.

Public Health Agency of Canada. (2018). *Key health inequalities in Canada: A national portrait—Executive summary*. https://www.canada.ca/en/public-health/services/publications/science-research-data/key-health-inequalities-canada-national-portrait-executive-summary.html.

Rahman, A., & Jahan, Y. (2020). Defining a "risk group" and ageism in the era of COVID-19. *Journal of Loss & Trauma*, *25*(8), 631–634. doi:10.1080/15325024.2020.1757993.

Spector, R. E. (2017). *Cultural diversity in health and illness* (9th ed.). Pearson.

Srugo, S. A., Jiang, Y., & de Groh, M. (2020). Living arrangements and health status of seniors in the 2018 Canadian Community Health Survey. *Health Promotion and Chronic Disease Prevention in Canada*, *40*(1), 18–22. doi:10.24095/hpcdp.40.1.03.

Standing Committee on Health. (2019). *The health of LGBTQIA2 communities in Canada: Report of the Standing Committee on Health*. House of Commons of Canada. https://www.ourcommons.ca/Content/Committee/421/HESA/Reports/RP10574595/hesarp28/hesarp28-e.pdf.

Statistics Canada. (2018). *Immigrant status and period of immigration by age and sex. Data table 98-402-X2016007-T1*. https://www12.statcan.gc.ca/census-recensement/2016/dp-pd/hlt-fst/imm/index-eng.cfm.

Statistics Canada. (2019a). *Language highlight tables, 2016 Census*. https://www12.statcan.gc.ca/census-recensement/2016/dp-pd/hlt-fst/lang/Table.cfm?Lang=E&T=11&Geo=00&SP=1&view=1&age=11.

Statistics Canada. (2019b). *Census profile, 2016 Census*. https://www12.statcan.gc.ca/census-recensement/2016/dp-pd/prof/details/page.cfm?Lang=E&Geo1=PR&Code1=01&Geo2=PR&Code2=01&SearchText=Canada&SearchType=Begins&SearchPR=01&B1=Visible minority&TABID=1&type=1.

Statistics Canada. (2019c). *Visible minority (15), generation status (4), age (12) and sex (3) for the population in private households of Canada, provinces and territories, census metropolitan areas and census agglomerations, 2016 Census—25% sample data*. https://www12.statcan.gc.ca/census-recensement/2016/dp-pd/dt-td/Rp-eng.cfm?TABID=2&Lang=E&APATH=3&DETAIL=0&DIM=0&FL=A&FREE=0&GC=0&GID=1341679&GK=0&GRP=1&PID=110531&PRID=10&PTYPE=109445&S=0&SHOWALL=0&SUB=0&Temporal=2017&THEME=120&VID=0&VNAMEE=&VNAMEF=&D1=0&D2=0&D3=0&D4=0&D5=0&D6=0.

Statistics Canada. (2019d). *Visible minority (15), immigrant status and period of immigration (11), age (12) and sex (3) for the population in private households of Canada, provinces and territories, census metropolitan areas and census agglomerations, 2016 census—25% sample data*. https://www12.statcan.gc.ca/census-recensement/2016/dp-pd/dt-td/Rp-eng.cfm?TABID=2&Lang=E&APATH=3&DETAIL=0&DIM=0&FL=A&FREE=0&GC=0&GID=1341679&GK=0&GRP=1&PID=110532&PRID=10&PTYPE=109445&S=0&SHOWALL=0&SUB=0&Temporal=2017&THEME=120&VID=0&VNAMEE=&VNAMEF=&D1=0.

Statistics Canada. (2019e). *Visible minority (15), individual low-income status (6), low-income indicators (4), generation status (4), age (6) and sex (3) for the population in private households of Canada, provinces and territories, census metropolitan areas and census agglomeration, 2016 census—25% sample data*. https://www12.statcan.gc.ca/census-recensement/2016/dp-pd/dt-td/Rp-eng.cfm?TABID=2&Lang=E&APATH=3&DETAIL=0&DIM=0&FL=A&FREE=0&GC=0&GID=1341790&GK=0&GRP=1&PID=110563&PRID=10&PTYPE=109445&S=0&SHOWALL=0&SUB=0&Temporal=2017&THEME=120&VID=0&VNAMEE=&VNAMEF=&D1=0&D2=0&D3=0&D4=0&D5=0&D6=0.

Statistics Canada. (2020). *Population by language spoken most often at home and geography, 1971 to 2016*. https://www150.statcan.gc.ca/t1/tbl1/en/tv.action?pid=1510000801.

Stinchcombe, A., Wilson, K., Kortes-Miller, K., et al. (2018). Physical and mental health inequalities among aging lesbian, gay, and bisexual Canadians: Cross-sectional results from the Canadian Longitudinal Study on Aging (CLSA). *Canadian Journal of Public Health*, *109*(5–6), 833–844. doi:10.17269/s41997-018-0100-3.

Thurairajah, K. (2017). The jagged edges of multiculturalism in Canada and the suspect Canadian. *Journal of Multicultural Discourses*, *12*(2), 134–148. doi:10.1080/17447143.2017.1319377.

Varley, A. (2017). "You don't just get over what has happened to you": Story sharing, reconciliation, and grandma's journey in the child welfare system. *First Peoples Child & Family Review*, *11*(2), 69–75.

Vauclair, C. M., Hanke, K., Huang, L. L., et al. (2017). Are Asian cultures really less ageist than Western ones? It depends on the questions asked. *International Journal of Psychology, 52*(2), 136–144. doi:10.1002/ijop.12292.

Wang, L., Guruge, S., & Montana, G. (2019). Older immigrants' access to primary health care in Canada: A scoping review. *Canadian Journal on Aging, 38*(2), 193–209. doi:10.1017/S0714980818000648.

Wilk, P., Maltby, A., & Cooke, M. (2017). Residential schools and the effects on Indigenous health and well-being in Canada—A scoping review. *Public Health Reviews, 38*, 8. doi:10.1186/s40985-017-0055-6.

Wyman, M. F., Shiovitz-Ezra, S., & Bengel, J. (2018). Ageism in the health care system: Providers, patients, and systems. In L. Ayalon & C. Tesch-Römer (Eds.), *Contemporary perspectives on ageism* (pp. 193–212). Springer.

5

NURSING DOCUMENTATION

LEARNING OBJECTIVES

Upon completion of this chapter, the reader will be able to:

- Describe the reasons for accurate and thorough documentation in gerontological nursing.
- Compare the major documentation methods used in acute care, residential and long-term care, and home care.
- Identify potential problems in documentation.
- Describe the responsibilities of the nurse in protecting the privacy of older adults.
- Identify the ways in which errors in documentation and communication are dangerous when older adults are being cared for.
- Identify ways to reduce the possibility of errors by making appropriate use of documentation when caring for older adults.

GLOSSARY

Activities of daily living (ADLs)   Routine activities that people tend to do every day without needing assistance. There are six basic ADLs: eating, bathing, dressing, toileting, transferring (walking), and continence.

Minimum data set (MDS)   The smallest number of a standardized data set that can be collected to identify essential, common, and core data elements of patients receiving nursing care.

***Personal Health Information Protection Act* (PHIPA)**   The *Personal Health Information Protection Act, 2004* (revised in 2016) legislates the handling of confidential patient information.

Resident Assessment Instrument (RAI)   A standardized approach to examining quality of care and improving regulation.

Resident assessment protocol (RAP)   A reference to documents that form part of the Resident Assessment Instrument. The resident assessment protocol provides a statement about the health problem; on the basis of that information, the minimum data set then triggers care planning.

THE LIVED EXPERIENCE

"I was so happy to be able to make a big difference in Mrs. Jones's life. She was 97 and had grown slowly confused over the years. She was also profoundly hard of hearing. She spent the majority of time calling for "Mary," her deceased sister. We really could not communicate effectively with her; we could only show her that we cared and kept her safe. Eventually she became acutely ill, and a decision had to be made about CPR [cardiopulmonary resuscitation]. When we tried to find out what her wishes were, we could not immediately find any record of them, and she had no living relatives or friends, just an attorney. I searched and searched and finally found documentation about her wishes. We were able to provide her the comfort she wanted because of a nurse's careful documentation years before."

Kathleen, a gerontological nurse

DOCUMENTATION

Nursing documentation is the mandatory practice of making a permanent record of nursing actions, the patient's conditions, and the patient's responses to nursing actions or the actions of others (College of Nurses of Ontario [CNO], 2020). All nurse-regulating bodies in Canada consider nursing documentation to be a mandatory practice. If nurses perform a specific nursing act but fail to document the action, it will appear as though the act was not performed.

Clinical documentation chronicles, supports, and communicates the condition of the person receiving care at all times. Appropriate and correct documentation helps the nurse to identify, implement, monitor, and evaluate treatments or interventions. The recorded assessment provides the information needed for the careful development of individualized care plans and the tracking and evaluation of outcomes. Documentation also ensures that the patient continues to be safe and receives the care needed regardless of shifts, health care providers, and care settings. At the same time, documentation is the major means by which nurses demonstrate the quality of care they provide (Larsson et al., 2019).

Detailed and accurate documentation is especially important in gerontological nursing. In the acute care setting, an older adult is often seriously ill and at higher risk for accidents, iatrogenic problems, and adverse reactions to interventions and treatments because the normal changes of aging are superimposed on acute and complex health problems. Furthermore, most older adults will require care across care settings at some point. Continuity of care within care facilities and from one setting to another (e.g., hospital to home) is especially important and is possible only with careful documentation. In long-term care (LTC) homes, residential facilities, and home care, health care aides or unregulated workers supervised by registered nurses and by registered or licensed practical nurses provide most of the care. In these settings, documentation often serves as a basis for calculating the overall quality of care and for justifying funding for care resources.

In Canada, advance directives—collectively known as advanced care planning—fall under provincial and territorial jurisdictions (Heckman et al., 2021) and are documented in the health record (see Chapter 27). They are put in place for the benefit of a substitute decision maker from whom nurses must receive consent if an older adult cannot give their own consent. On June 17, 2016, the federal government passed Bill C-14, which outlines the requirements that all patients must meet to be eligible to receive medical assistance in dying. Bill C-14 also "establishes safeguards that a doctor

or nurse practitioner must follow to legally provide medical assistance in dying" (Ministry of Health and Long-Term Care, 2017). Nursing records supplement this documentation with more details about patients' wishes, including who they want involved in their care and who they want to have access to their records, as well as the use of cardiopulmonary resuscitation (CPR) and the handling of their bodies after death. Older adults often discuss these wishes with nurses during conversations while receiving care. By recording these conversations in the nursing records, nurses are making sure that this important information can be shared with other members of the care team and that the older adult's wishes are respected.

DOCUMENTATION ACROSS CARE SETTINGS

Documentation begins as soon as a person enters the health care system. Ongoing documentation provides not only the basis for care and the evaluation of any interventions and treatments but also the basis for providing care continuity when a person moves from one care setting to another (including the home). The use of electronic health records allows for real-time record keeping of patient information to support comprehensive, timely access to the person's history, care plan, and treatment while ensuring confidentiality and privacy (Niazkhani et al., 2020). In LTC homes and other settings, platforms such as PointClickCare provide cloud-based electronic health record software that tracks resident progress and improves care planning (PointClickCare, 2020).

This chapter provides an overview of how nursing documentation is used to optimize the care of vulnerable older adults in a variety of care settings. A description of standardized assessment tools can be found in Chapter 13.

Acute Care Setting

Documentation in the acute care setting has undergone significant change in recent years. Computers and tablets can be found at the bedside, in nurses' pockets, and at strategic locations on the unit. Individual patient and nurse bar codes are scanned both for access to records and for the administration of treatments and medications. The use of electronic checklists, flow sheets, and standardized tools has become the norm (see Chapter 13). In some settings, "lower-tech" approaches may still be used, and some documentation is manually completed in the form of notes in the clinical record.

Mandatory nursing documentation includes findings from the patient's assessment (usually with a checklist), identified nursing diagnoses, and care plans. When the nurse needs to document a particular event in the course of a patient's stay, a SOAP (Subjective, Objective, Assessment, Plan) note may be used. The subjective section of the note represents the patient's perspective on how they are feeling. The objective section includes data on what the nurse can measure, observe, see, feel, touch, or smell. The assessment is the result of the nurse's analysis, considering both subjective and objective data. The care plan then includes nursing interventions to address the chief complaint. The education section includes the patient and family teaching needed (Box 5.1). The SOAP approach is useful for the succinct communication of information related to a specific problem. However, if the person has multiple problems, as do many older adults, this form can be complicated and lengthy.

Other approaches to nursing documentation include the DARE (document Data, Action, Response, and Evaluation) approach; FOCUS charting (which integrates narrative notes with the care plan and records relevant patient information in a systematic, accessible fashion) (British Columbia College of Nurses and Midwives, 2021); the SBAR (Situation, Background, Assessment, and Recommendation) approach; the IDRAW (Identify patient, Diagnosis, Recent changes, Anticipated changes, and What to watch for) approach; and narrative charting (nursing interventions and the impact of these interventions on patient outcomes, recorded in chronological order and covering a specific time frame) (British Columbia College of Nurses and Midwives, 2021).

Residential Care Settings

In LTC homes, assisted living facilities, and retirement homes, documentation is generally done only if a care provider or nurse has been providing care to the older adult. In retirement homes, nursing services are optional and are usually limited to the administration of medications and treatments or to assistance with **activities of daily living (ADLs)** by health care aides. Some health care aides are not allowed to document their care in the nursing record, as this is beyond their scope of practice; however, the level and type of documentation required varies by setting and by province or territory. If nurses chart on the health care aides' behalf, it is important that they follow their provincial professional regulatory organization's documentation guidelines for secondhand charting.

When older adults move to LTC homes, they often face challenges that are functional, cognitive, or both, and they may experience the onset or exacerbation of an acute or chronic problem. They are dependent on assistance for their ADLs (see Chapter 13).

Documentation in LTC homes encompasses the recording of day-to-day ADL care as well as vital signs, periodic assessment, medication and treatment administration, assessment of any unusual event or change in condition, and quarterly mandated comprehensive assessments. Documentation includes narrative progress notes, flow sheets, checklists, and mandated standardized and comprehensive instruments. Timely and correct documentation is a requirement for all registered and health care aides providing care. The nurse is ultimately responsible for the quality of care provided and for the completeness and accuracy of the documentation.

Resident Assessment Instrument

The **Resident Assessment Instrument (RAI)** is a standardized approach used to gather comprehensive assessment information on a person's functioning. The RAI

BOX 5.1

EXAMPLE OF A SUBJECTIVE, OBJECTIVE, ASSESSMENT, AND PLAN (SOAP) NOTE

S "I have to go to the toilet a lot, and when I urinate, it burns . . . It started last week and is getting worse."

O 72-year-old, Indian woman. Temp 99, pulse 94, blood pressure 140/86, respirations 18. Urine is dark yellow with strong foul odour, skin slightly damp, face flushed, abdomen tender.

A Altered elimination, elevated temperature, mild distress, possible infection.

P Call nurse practitioner with report. Provide treatment as prescribed. Ask patient to increase fluid intake, hourly. Check vital signs every 4 hours until resolved.

consists of different **minimum data sets (MDSs)**, each of which is specific to a care setting (e.g., LTC, home care, mental health). As of 2018–2019, 7 provinces and territories are using the RAI-MDS version 2.0 or the LTCF in all LTC homes (New Brunswick, Newfoundland and Labrador, Ontario, Saskatchewan, Alberta, British Columbia, and Yukon). Manitoba has a partial commitment, and participation is voluntary in Nova Scotia (Canadian Institute for Health Information [CIHI], 2020). The core component of the RAI-MDS 2.0 and the LTCF enables the care team to assess multiple key domains such as function, health, social support, and service use. **Resident assessment protocols (RAPs)** are additional assessments that are completed depending on the information gleaned from the initial assessment. RAPs are structured, problem-oriented frameworks for the organization and direction of care. The RAP provides a statement about the health problem; on the basis of that information, the MDS then triggers care planning.

In most provinces and territories, nurses are responsible for the coordination of the RAI-MDS 2.0 or LTCF within 14 days of a resident's admission, at quarterly intervals, and any time there is a significant change in the resident's status. The reassessments allow the care team to document and track the progress toward the resolution of identified problems and to make changes to the care plan as necessary. This type and level of documentation facilitates reliable and measurable communication and, when used properly, improves outcomes for residents (Dash et al., 2018). The resulting picture of the resident is as clear as possible. For persons who will benefit from active rehabilitation, the outcomes include discharge to a lower level of care. For persons whose condition is one of progressive decline, the RAI can lead to increased comfort and appropriate care. Although the MDS is completed in collaboration with all members of the care team, the nurse is responsible for verifying its accuracy and completion.

In Canada, data from the RAI-MDS 2.0 and LTCF are subsequently submitted to the Continuing Care Reporting System database for ease of analysis and communication of resident profiles. This information is then shared with the Canadian Institute for Health Information and becomes part of an aggregate national database that allows researchers to better respond to the needs of residents in Canadian LTC homes. This thorough assessment and documentation requirement

in LTC is an attempt to improve and standardize the quality of care provided and to help LTC residents achieve the highest level of functioning and the highest quality of life possible.

Home Care

Personal care at home is often provided informally by family and friends (see Chapters 23 and 26); yet the requisite professional care is provided through home visits from nurses, health care aides, occupational therapists, physiotherapists, or others. These services are delivered by provincial and territorial governments and, in some instances, by municipal governments (Government of Canada, 2019). For example, Ontario's Local Health Integration Networks (LHINs) (currently being transitioned to Ontario Health Teams) coordinate these services through Ontario's Ministry of Health and Long-Term Care. Alberta health care is organized through Alberta Health Services.

Home care services use the RAI system to collect an MDS for home care clients and determine the care required. Clinical Assessment Protocols (CAPs), used for documenting assessments, inform and guide comprehensive care and service planning in the home care setting. These CAPs are intended as a companion resource for RAI-Home Care (van Solm et al., 2017). Family and other care partners often develop documentation systems of their own to track appointments, medication administration, and instruction from health care providers. This system increases the continuity of care. Nurses may need to assist the family in developing and using effective systems.

As with all other documentation systems, home care documentation is used to improve both quality of care and the communications about the older adult. In addition, the RAI system serves as a guide for quality care, resource allocation, and reimbursement. The documentation is completed in the person's home, recorded directly on portable or handheld computers, and later transferred to a central database.

IMPLICATIONS FOR GERONTOLOGICAL NURSING AND HEALTHY AGING

Health care documentation, whether written or electronic, contains highly personal and private information about patients or residents. For many years, the confidentiality of health and medical information was protected through professional codes of ethics (Canadian Nurses Association, 2017). The expectation has always been that nurses and other health care providers would be able to access only information that relates to a specific person in their care. Nursing students are taught to avoid talking about their patients or residents in any public space or with persons outside their clinical groups, such as friends and family members. The nurse who notes that a friend or neighbour has been admitted to a care setting cannot review that person's health and medical information unless the nurse is assigned to provide care or services to that person.

However, not all health care providers are as respectful of people's privacy as they should be. The use of social media, coupled with the electronic exchange of personal health information, has significantly increased the risk for breaches of confidentiality. While the influence of social media on professional practice varies depending on the user and the context of their practice, the central concern for all nurses is patient confidentiality and privacy (Yousuf et al., 2017).

The *Personal Health Information Protection Act, 2004* **(PHIPA),** which was significantly amended in 2020, outlines the rules for the collection, use, and disclosure of personal health information. PHIPA also requires that all personal health information be kept confidential and secure. The Office of the Privacy Commissioner of Canada has the responsibility for enforcing privacy legislation. Patients and residents may request that all reasonable steps be taken to ensure that their verbal communications are confidential and that they have complete control as to who has access to their information. In the case of guardianship or in the case of a person who is not capable of making health care decisions, information can be shared with the guardian or with whoever has power of attorney, respecting the PHIPA rules. It is expected that nursing actions to protect privacy include closing the patient's or resident's door before having health-related conversations and not discussing a patient's or resident's needs or condition in a location where the discussion could be overheard, such as hallways or some nurses' stations.

Communication through documentation has become critical to ensuring patients' rights and adequate care and to providing data for policy and funding decisions. It is the responsibility of the nurse to make sure that communication and documentation are of the highest quality so as to provide error-free and appropriate care and continuity and to maximize both patient and resident outcomes and accurate reimbursement.

KEY CONCEPTS

- Excellence in documentation sets the stage for excellence in care.
- Standardized instruments for care outcomes and evaluation are integral to the consistent determination of the needs and the health and wellness status of older adults, as well as appropriate funding.
- Documenting the patient's status and needs is a key responsibility of the nurse.
- Nurses have a responsibility to protect patient confidentiality at all times, both in spoken communication and in the clinical record.

ACTIVITIES AND DISCUSSION QUESTIONS

1. Discuss the origins and purpose of the development of standardized documentation systems.

2. Discuss incomplete data or poor documentation practices you have experienced in a health care setting.

3. Discuss the potential uses of the RAI-MDS 2.0.

4. Discuss the ways in which patient confidentiality is breached and what the nurse can do to prevent such breaches.

5. Explain why documentation is critical to care.

RESOURCES

Canadian Nurses Association. Code of Ethics, 2017.
https://www.cna-aiic.ca/html/en/Code-of-Ethics-2017-Edition/files/assets/basic-html/page-4.html

Canadian Patient Safety Institute: Enabling patient safety.
https://www.patientsafetyinstitute.ca/en/toolsresources/patient-safety-culture-bundle/pages/enabling.aspx

Personal Health Information Protection Act, 2004 (PHIPA) and the Office of the Privacy Commissioner of Canada
https://www.ontario.ca/laws/statute/04p03
http://www.priv.gc.ca/

RAI-MDS 2.0 User's Manual, Canadian version, February 2012
https://secure.cihi.ca/estore/productSeries.htm?pc=PCC127&_ga=2.152358202.288636455.1586974399-1416417948.1586974399

Documentation Standards by Province and Territory

Alberta:
https://nurses.ab.ca/docs/default-source/document-library/standards/documentation-standards-for-regulated-members.pdf?sfvrsn=ec1cd2ea_12

British Columbia:
https://www.bccnm.ca/NP/PracticeStandards/Pages/documentation.aspx

Manitoba:
https://www.crnm.mb.ca/support/quality-practice-consultation/documentation

New Brunswick:
http://www.nanb.nb.ca/practice/standards

Newfoundland and Labrador:
https://crnnl.ca/site/uploads/2021/09/documentation-principles.pdf

Northwest Territories and Nunavut:
https://rnantnu.ca/professional-practice/documentation-guidelines/

Nova Scotia:
https://www.nscn.ca/professional-practice/practice-support/practice-support-tools/documentation/documentation-guidelines-nurses

Ontario:
https://www.cno.org/en/learn-about-standards-guidelines/educational-tools/learning-modules/documentation-2010/

Prince Edward Island:
https://crnpei.ca/wp-content/uploads/2020/12/Practice-Directive-Documentation-Standards-2020-12-10-CRNPEI-Edition.pdf

Quebec:
https://www.oiiq.org

Saskatchewan:
https://www.srna.org/wp-content/uploads/2021/02/Documentation-Guideline.pdf

Yukon:
https://www.yrna.ca/standards

For additional resources, please visit *http://evolve.elsevier.com/Canada/Ebersole/gerontological/*

REFERENCES

British Columbia College of Nurses & Midwives. (2021). Documentation. Retrieved from https://www.bccnm.ca/RN/PracticeStandards/Pages/documentation.aspx.

Canadian Institute for Health Information (CIHI). (2020). *Continuing care reporting system data users guide, 2018–2019.* Author.

Canadian Nurses Association. (2017). *Code of ethics for registered nurses.* https://www.cna-aiic.ca/html/en/Code-of-Ethics-2017-Edition/files/assets/basic-html/page-4.html.

College of Nurses of Ontario (CNO). (2020). *Documentation.* https://www.cno.org/en/learn-about-standards-guidelines/educational-tools/learning-modules/documentation-2010/.

Dash, D., Heckman, G. A., Boscart, V. M., et al. (2018). Using powerful data from the interRAI MDS to support care and a learning health system: A case study from long-term care. *Healthcare Management Forum, 31*(4), 153–159. doi:10.1177/0840470417743989.

Government of Canada. (2019). *Core community supports to age in community.* https://www.canada.ca/en/employment-social-development/corporate/seniors/forum/core-community-supports.html.

Heckman, G.A., Boscart, V., Quail, P., et al. (2021). Applying the knowledge-to-action framework to engage stakeholders and solve shared challenges with person-centred advance care planning in long-term care homes. *Canadian Journal on Aging,* 1–11. doi:10.1017.S0714980820000410.

Larsson, H., Handanovic, D., & Rosengren, K. (2019). Simplifying the care plan documentation procedure – An interview study with nurses at a medical ward at a university hospital in Sweden. *Journal of Hospital Administration, 8*(4), 54–64. doi:10.5430/jha.v8n4p54.

Ministry of Health and Long-Term Care. (2017). *Medical assistance in dying.* http://health.gov.on.ca/en/pro/programs/maid/.

Niazkhani, Z., Esmaeel, T., Cheshmekaboodi, M., Georgiou, A., & Pirejad, H. (2020). Barriers to patient, provider, and caregiver adoption and use of electronic personal health records in chronic care: A systematic review. *BMC Medical Informatics and Decision Making, 20* (153).

PointClickCare. (2020). *Why choose PointClickCare.* https://pointclickcare.com/why-pointclickcare/.

van Solm, A., Hirdes, J., Eckel, L., et al. (2017). Using standard clinical assessments for home care to identify vulnerable populations before, during, and after disasters. *Journal of Emergency Management, 15*(6), 355–366. doi:10.5055/jem.2017.0344.

Yousuf, R., Bakar, S., Haque, M., et al. (2017). Medical professional and usage of social media. *Bangladesh Journal of Medical Science, 16*(4), 606–609. doi:10.3329/bjms.v16i4.33622.

6

BIOLOGICAL THEORIES AND PHYSICAL CHANGES OF AGING

LEARNING OBJECTIVES

Upon completion of this chapter, the reader will be able to:

- Identify the normal physical changes associated with aging.
- Begin to differentiate normal age-related changes from those that are potentially pathological.
- Incorporate prevention and health promotion in a plan of care for an older adult.

GLOSSARY

Glomerular filtration rate   The rate at which the kidneys filter blood.

Hypercapnia   High levels of carbon dioxide in the blood.

Hypoxia   Low levels of oxygen supply to body tissues.

Kyphosis   C-shaped curvature of the cervical vertebrae.

Presbycusis   Progressive, bilateral, and symmetrical age-related hearing loss.

Presbyopia   Reduced near vision that normally occurs with age, usually resulting in improved distance vision.

Proprioception   The body's sense of movement and position in space, independent of vision.

Xerostomia   Excessive mouth dryness.

THE LIVED EXPERIENCE

"I had to fly to Belfast last year. When I came to come back, I couldn't see my flight. I could see the actual board, I couldn't read so I had to ask one. I find that I have to ask people quite a bit, is that the right place or so I have to ask. As a rule, people don't mind, so I have to ask more about things."

"I've got very good friends who always know and they put—I don't have to ask them. They'll just read the menu to me to save me getting my phone, my torch out on my phone, which I did quite a lot in restaurants. But if I'm with my friends, they just read the menu to me."
AF1, older adult participant in study

From Taylor, D. J., Jones, L., Binns, A. M., et al. (2019). "You've got dry macular degeneration, end of story": A qualitative study into the experience of living with non-neovascular age-related macular degeneration. *Eye, 34,* 461–473. doi: 10.1038/s41433-019-0445-8.

L ater life is a time of opportunities and challenges. Among the challenges are those related to age-related physical changes. Some changes are considered a normal part of aging; others are the result of pathological conditions that are mistakenly considered to be an expected part of the aging process.

Aging consists of a series of complex changes and occurs in all living organisms. Most of these changes are intrinsic, coming from within; others are a result of extrinsic environmental factors, such as exposure to smoke or other pollutants. Exactly why the changes occur has been of interest to scientists for decades. It is known that the triggers of aging are influenced by genetics as well as by injury to the body earlier in life.

This chapter discusses the prominent biological theories of aging and some of the major physical changes that are a normal part of aging. This chapter also discusses some changes that indicate pathological conditions commonly seen in older adults. With this knowledge, the nurse can begin to differentiate normal age-related changes from health problems that require treatment and can help to facilitate prompt intervention to promote healthy aging.

BIOLOGICAL THEORIES OF AGING

A *theory* is an explanation that makes sense of some phenomenon. A theory remains a reasonable explanation until someone finds it to be incorrect. Most theories can be neither proved nor disproved, but they are useful as points of reference. Theories of aging provide clues to the aging process. However, many unanswered questions remain.

The biological theories of aging today evolved from the early study of changes over the lifespan of the organism. Two related viewpoints form the foundation of the biological theories. Stochastic theories include those theories describing changes that occur because of errors within cells or deoxyribonucleic acid (DNA), such as oxidative stress (i.e., free radicals). Nonstochastic theories describe changes that occur because of predetermined or preprogrammed processes. Both viewpoints agree that, in the end, the cells in the body become disorganized, the cells are no longer able to replicate, and cellular death occurs. When enough cells die, so does the organism. In recent years, research on the biological theories of aging has focused on cells, genes, and other cell components. A short description of emerging theories is provided in Box 6.1.

Error (Stochastic) Theories

Error theories explain aging as the result of an accumulation of errors in the synthesis of cellular DNA and ribonucleic acid (RNA), the basic building blocks of the cell (da Silva & Schumacher, 2019). With each replication, more errors occur, until the cell is no longer able to function. The visible signs of aging, such as grey hair, are thought to be the result of the accumulation of these cellular errors. Three of the most common theories of error are the wear-and-tear, cross-link, and oxidative stress theories.

Wear-and-Tear Theory

One of the earliest theories of aging is known as the wear-and-tear theory. According to this theory, cell

---

BOX 6.1
EMERGING BIOLOGICAL THEORIES OF AGING

NEUROENDOCRINE OR PACEMAKER THEORY

The neuroendocrine system regulates many essential activities related to an organism's growth and development. The neuroendocrine or pacemaker theory focuses on changes in the neuroendocrine system over time. Common neurons in the higher brain centres may act as pacemakers—regulators of the biological clock during development and aging—that slow down and eventually shut off at a predetermined time. Much of the current research in this area is on the influence of hormones (especially dehydroepiandrosterone and melatonin) on neuroendocrine functioning over time.

GENETIC RESEARCH

As the human genome is being mapped, scientists are examining the roles played by genetics (DNA and RNA) in both random and programmed aging. Among the findings are that telomeres (which cap the ends of chromosomes) shorten with each cellular reproduction until eventually the telomeres disappear and the cell can no longer reproduce and dies. Abnormal cells (such as cancer cells) produce an enzyme called *telomerase* that lengthens the telomeres, enabling the cells to continue to reproduce. The manipulation of telomerase may have implications for the control of both cellular reproduction and aging.

PROGERIN AND TELOMERES

Some of the latest research in this field has found an association between telomeres and a toxic protein called *progerin*. As long as a telomere is securely bound to the chromosome, the cell is able to replicate and essentially live forever. With aging, however, telomeres wear away at the same time the cell produces more and more progerin. Progerin, a mutated version of normal cell protein, interferes with the stability of the telomeres and ultimately the length of the cell's life (Cao et al., 2011).

Source: Cao, K., Blair, C. D., Faddah, D. A., et al. (2011). Progerin and telomere dysfunction collaborate to trigger cellular senescence in normal human fibroblasts. *The Journal of Clinical Investigation, 121*, 2833–2844. doi: 10.1172/JCI43578.

---

errors are the result of "wearing out" over time owing to trauma and continued use. Internal and external stressors (e.g., stressors in the shoulder joints of baseball pitchers or the knees of those who run frequently) increase the number of errors and the speed with which they occur. These errors cause a progressive decline in cellular function.

Cross-Link Theory

The cross-link theory explains aging in terms of the accumulation of errors by *cross-linking*, or the stiffening of proteins in the cell. Proteins link with glucose and other sugars in the presence of oxygen and become stiff and thick (Marin-Garcia, 2008). Cross-linking is most easily seen with collagens because they are the most plentiful proteins in the body. Skin that was once smooth, silky, firm, and soft becomes drier and less elastic with age. Collagen is also a key component of the lungs, the arteries, and the tendons, and similar changes can be seen in these body parts (e.g., stiffened joints).

Oxidative Stress (Free-Radical Theory)

The oxidative stress theory, also known as the free-radical theory of aging, is among the theories that are most accepted. *Free radicals* are natural byproducts of cellular activity and are always present to some extent. It is believed that cellular errors are the result of random damage from molecules (free radicals) in the cells. Exposure to environmental pollutants increases the production of free radicals, which in turn increases the rate of damage. Pollutants include smog and ozone, pesticides, and radiation (Manisalidis et al., 2020). Other environmental sources thought to cause increases in free radicals are gasoline, byproducts of the plastics industry, and drying linseed oil paints. In youth, naturally occurring vitamins, hormones, enzymes, and antioxidants neutralize the free radicals as needed (Valko et al., 2005). However, with aging, the damage caused by free radicals occurs faster than the rate at which cells can repair themselves, and cell death occurs (Vina et al., 2018).

Programmed Aging (Nonstochastic) Theories

The nonstochastic theories attribute aging to a process thought to be predetermined, or "programmed," at the cellular level; this means that each cell has a natural life expectancy. As more cells cease to replicate, the signs of aging appear, and ultimately the person dies at a "predetermined" age. These theories evolved from the groundbreaking work of Hayflick and Moorehead (1981), who referred to this process as the inner "biological clock." In other words, each cell is "born" with a limited number of replications and then stops replicating and dies.

Neuroendocrine–Immunological Theory

The neuroendocrine–immunological theory of aging attributes aging to changes in the integrated neuroendocrine and immune systems. The emphasis is on the programmed deaths of the immune cells due to damage caused by the increase in free radicals as aging progresses (Effros et al., 2005; Marin-Garcia, 2008). The immune system is a complex network of cells, tissues, and organs that function separately and together to protect the body from outside substances such as viruses and bacteria. The immune system is highly dependent on the release of hormones. In the simplest terms, the specialized B lymphocytes (humoral) and T lymphocytes (cellular) protect the body against infection or from other matter that is considered foreign, such as tissue or organ transplants. Animal studies have shown that the cells of the immune system become progressively more diversified with age and lose some of their ability to self-regulate. The reduced T cells are thought to be responsible for hastening the age-related changes caused by autoimmune reactions as the body battles itself; healthy cells are mistaken for foreign substances and are attacked.

In summary, it is important for the nurse to understand that the exact cause of aging is unknown. There is considerable variation in the aging process between persons and between the systems within any one person. Aging is a wholly unique and individual experience.

PHYSICAL CHANGES OF AGING

Integument

The skin is composed of the epidermis, the dermis, and the hypodermis. It is the largest and most visible organ of the body. The various layers of the skin meld and model the individual, providing much of their personal and sexual identity. The skin is important both in health and in illness; it provides clues to hereditary, racial, dietary, physical, and emotional conditions. Hair, also a part of the integument, provides recognizable characteristics.

Many age-related changes in the skin are functionally inconsequential. Others have implications for organs throughout the body and a more far-reaching impact. Changes in the skin are due to both genetic (intrinsic) factors and environmental (extrinsic) factors such as wind, sun, and pollution. Cigarette smoking causes coarse wrinkles, and photodamage from the sun is evidenced by a rough, leathery skin texture, itching, and mottled pigmentation, among other signs. Signs of skin changes that may be genetic, environmental, or both include dryness, thinning, decreased elasticity, and the development of prominent small blood vessels. Skin tears, purpura (large purple spots), and xerosis (excessive dryness) are common but not normal aspects of physical aging. Visible changes of the skin—colour, firmness, elasticity, and texture—affirm aging.

Epidermis

The *epidermis* is the tough outer layer of skin, composed primarily of *keratinocytes*, which are stratified, squamous, epithelial cells. With age, the epidermis thins, which makes blood vessels and bruises much more visible. T-cell function declines, and there may be a reactivation of a latent condition such as herpes zoster (shingles) or herpes simplex (see Chapter 11). The shingles vaccine, covered by some provincial and territorial health plans, is recommended for most people aged 60 years and older.

As one ages, there is an increase in skin renewal time and a 50% decrease in the turnover of epidermal replacement (Wounds Canada, 2018). This change significantly affects wound healing. If a younger adult's skin is injured (e.g., cut or scraped), the surrounding tissue becomes erythematous almost immediately. This inflammatory response is the first step in the natural healing process. For an older adult, this inflammatory first step may take 48 to 72 hours. A laceration that becomes pink several days after the event may be misinterpreted as being infected; in reality, the healing process will have only just started. Evidence of a true skin infection in older adults is no different from such evidence in younger adults—namely, increasing redness, pain, swelling, and purulent drainage.

Another change that occurs with aging is a reduction in the number of melanocytes in the epidermis. Melanocytes produce melanin, which gives the skin colour. Fewer melanocytes means a lightening of overall skin tone (regardless of the original skin colour) and a decrease in the amount of protection from ultraviolet (UV) rays. Thus, the importance of sunscreen use significantly increases with age (see Chapter 12). In some body areas, however, melanin synthesis is increased. Pigment spots (freckles and nevi) enlarge and become more numerous with increased exposure to light. Lentigines

(commonly referred to as "age spots" or "liver spots") appear; they are frequently found on the backs of the hands and the wrists and on the faces of light-skinned persons older than 50 years. Thick, brown, raised lesions with a "stuck-on" appearance (seborrheic keratoses) are more common in men; they are not clinically significant but can become cosmetically disfiguring if severe (see Chapter 11).

Dermis

The *dermis*, which lies beneath the epidermis, is a supportive layer of connective tissue. It is composed of a matrix of yellow elastic fibres, which provide stretch and recoil, and white fibrous collagen fibres, which provide tensile strength. The dermis supports hair follicles, sweat and sebaceous glands, nerve fibres, muscle cells, and blood vessels to provide nourishment to the epidermis. Sun exposure accelerates skin tissue changes by hastening collagen fibre alterations.

Many of the visible signs of skin aging are reflections of changes in the dermis. The dermis thins, causing older skin to look more transparent and fragile. Dermal blood vessels are reduced, resulting in skin pallor and cooler skin temperature. Collagen synthesis decreases, causing the skin to "give" less under stress and tear more easily. Elastin fibres thicken and fragment, leading to the loss of stretch and resilience and to a "sagging" appearance. Loss of elasticity accentuates jowls and elongated ears and contributes to the formation of a "double" chin. Breasts begin to sag and become pendulous. Melanocytes decrease, increasing the risk of UV damage from exposure to the sun.

Hypodermis

The *hypodermis* is the subcutaneous, innermost layer of the skin and contains connective tissues, blood vessels, and nerves. Its major component is subcutaneous fat, called adipose tissue. The primary purposes of adipose tissue are to store calories and provide thermal regulation. It also provides shape and form to the body and acts as a shock absorber against trauma. With age, some areas of the hypodermis atrophy. As the natural insulation of fat decreases, a person becomes more sensitive to cold.

Changes in the hypodermis also increase the chance for hyperthermia as a result of the reduced efficiency of the sweat (eccrine) glands. Sweat glands are located all over the body and respond to thermostimulation and neurostimulation in response to internal changes (e.g., fever, menopausal "hot flashes") or increases in environmental temperatures. The usual body response to heat is to produce moisture or sweat from these glands and thus cool the skin through evaporation. With aging, the glands become fibrotic, and the surrounding connective tissue becomes avascular, leading to a decline in the efficiency with which the body cools down. It is not uncommon for older adults to complain of being either too hot or too cold in environments that are comfortable to others. Older adults are at significant risk for both hyperthermia and hypothermia. Gerontological nurses can increase the comfort of frail, older adults by helping them avoid extremes of temperature, preventing drying of the skin, and preventing exposure to toxic products (see Chapter 11).

Sebaceous glands, which secrete sebum (oil), also atrophy. Sebum protects the skin by preventing the evaporation of water from the epidermis; it possesses bactericidal properties and contains a precursor of vitamin D. When the skin is exposed to sunlight, vitamin D is produced and absorbed into the skin. The production of vitamin D is especially important because it is essential for calcium absorption and the prevention of osteoporosis (see Chapters 12 and 18). Vitamin D deficiency is linked to higher risks for cancer, cardiovascular disease, diabetes, chronic pulmonary disease, kidney disease, and liver diseases (Meltzer et al., 2020). All people need sunshine or vitamin D supplementation every day (Osteoporosis Canada, 2017). In Canada, where direct sunlight is limited in the winter months, supplementation is recommended. Osteoporosis Canada (2017) recommends daily supplements of at least 800–2000 IU per day for people over 50 years of age.

Hair and Nails

As part of the integument, hair has biological, psychological, and cosmetic value. Hair is composed of tightly fused horny cells that arise from the dermal layer of the skin and obtain colouration from melanocytes. Genetics, race, sex, testosterone, and estrogen influence hair distribution in both men and women.

Race, sex, and hormones also determine the maximum amount of body and scalp hair and the changes that occur in the hair throughout life. Men and women of all races have less hair as they age. Hair loss in men is slightly more common than in women. By age 70,

approximately 75% of men will experience "male pattern baldness," characterized by a receding hairline and loss of hair at the top of the head (Canadian Dermatology Association, 2021). The hair in the ears, nose, and eyebrows of older men increases and stiffens. For women, female pattern baldness tends to involve thinning of the hair at the crown of the head (Canadian Dermatology Association, 2021). By age 50, approximately 40% of women will experience some type of thinning hair. Both genetics as well as hormonal changes play a role in both male and female pattern baldness (Canadian Dermatology Association, 2021). For some older adults, the accustomed hair colour remains; for most, however, there is a gradual loss of pigmentation (melanin), and the scalp hair becomes dryer and coarser. Older women develop chin and facial hair because of the decreased ratio of estrogen to testosterone. Leg, axillary, and pubic hair lessens and in some instances disappears in postmenopausal women. This normal absence of leg hair can be misinterpreted as a sign of peripheral vascular disease in older adults. People have distinctive hair characteristics that vary with race, which the nurse should keep in mind when caring for older adults.

The nails become harder and thicker, more brittle, dull, and opaque. They change shape, becoming flat or concave instead of convex. Vertical ridges appear because of decreasing water, calcium, and lipid content. The blood supply, as well as the rate of growth, decreases. The half-moon (lunule) of the fingernail may disappear, and the colour of the nails may vary from yellow to grey.

Fungal infection of the nails (onychomycosis) is not the result of aging but is quite common. Fungus invades the space between the layers of the nails, leaving a thick and unsightly appearance. The slowness of growth and the reduced circulation in the nails of older adults make treatment very difficult (see Chapter 11). Box 6.2 describes actions that older adults can take to keep skin healthy as they age.

Musculo-Skeletal System

A functioning musculo-skeletal system is necessary for movement, gross responses to environmental forces, and maintenance of posture. This complex system comprises bones, joints, tendons, ligaments, and muscles.

As seen with the skin, changes in the musculo-skeletal system are influenced by many factors, such as age, sex,

---

BOX 6.2
PROMOTING HEALTHY SKIN WHILE AGING

- Protect skin while outside, especially during the hours of 11:00 a.m. and 3:00 p.m., when the sun's UV rays are the strongest.
- Apply moisturizer to damp skin after bathing.
- Avoid the use of drying soaps; use low-pH cleansers.
- Always use sunscreens, paying special attention to the face, ears, neck, and hands.
- Wear a broad-brimmed hat when in sunshine.
- Keep well hydrated.

Sources: Canadian Dermatology Association. (2021). *Photoaging.* http://www.dermatology.ca/skin-hair-nails/skin/photoaging/#!/skin-hair-nails/skin/photoaging/what-is-photoaging/; Toronto Dermatology Centre. (2021). *How to get rid of dry skin.* https://torontodermatologycentre.com/news/how-to-get-rid-of-dry-skin/.

BOX 6.3
PROMOTING HEALTHY BONES AND MUSCLES

- Ensure regular intake of vitamin D and calcium (Osteoporosis Canada, 2017).
- Engage in regular weight-bearing exercise (e.g., tai chi).
- Engage in regular flexibility and balance exercises (e.g., yoga).
- Consider preventive pharmacotherapeutics if you are a woman.

---

race, and environment. Although none of the age-related changes to the musculo-skeletal system are life threatening, any of them could affect a person's ability to function and therefore affect their quality of life. Some of the changes are visible to others and have the potential to affect the individual's self-esteem.

The musculo-skeletal changes that have the most effect on function occur in the ligaments, tendons, and joints. Over time, these become dry, hardened, more rigid, and less flexible. In joints subjected to trauma earlier in life (e.g., from injuries or repetitive movement), these changes can be seen earlier and in more severe forms. If joint space is reduced, arthritis is diagnosed.

Bone mass decreases with age; the bones lose strength and become increasingly brittle. Bone loss is related to genetics, decreased hormone levels, decreased bone formation, deficiencies of vitamin D and calcium, and lifestyle (smoking and diet) (Karpouzos et al., 2017). Age-related changes to muscles are known as *sarcopenia* and are seen almost exclusively in skeletal muscle. Muscle mass can continue to build until a person is in their fifties. However, between 30% and 50% of the skeletal muscle mass may be lost by the time the person reaches their eighties or nineties (Crowther-Radulewicz, 2015; McCormick & Vasilaki, 2018). Disuse of the muscles accelerates the loss of strength. In key areas, muscle tissue mass decreases (atrophies), whereas adipose tissue increases. Replacement of lean muscle by adipose tissue is most noticeable in men in the area of the waist and in women between the umbilicus and the symphysis pubis. Nurses can encourage older adults to exercise, especially through weight-bearing exercises, to help maintain healthy bones and muscles as well as flexibility (Box 6.3). Chapter 10 discusses the importance of exercise.

Structure, Posture, and Body Composition

Changes in stature and posture, two of the more obvious signs of aging, are associated with factors that involve skeletal, muscular, subcutaneous, and fat tissue. Vertebral discs become thin as a result of dehydration, causing a shortening of the trunk. These changes may begin as early as one's forties (Cleveland Clinic, 2021). The trunk shortens as a result of gravity and dehydration of the vertebral discs. The person may have a stooped appearance from **kyphosis,** a curvature of the cervical vertebrae that results from reduced bone mineral density (BMD). Some loss of BMD in women is associated with the reduction of estrogen levels after menopause; with the shortened appearance, the bones of the arms and the legs may appear disproportionate in size. If a person's BMD is very low, osteoporosis is diagnosed; a loss of 5–8 cm (2–3 inches) in height is not uncommon (see Chapter 18).

Alteration in body shape and weight occurs as lean body mass declines and body water is lost. Fat tissue increases until 60 years of age. Therefore, body density is higher in youth because of the density of muscle compared to the lightness of fat. From 25 to 75 years of age, the fat content of the body increases by 16%. Changes in water distribution have significant implications for dramatically increased risk for dehydration (Fig. 6.1).

Proportion of Body Weight Represented by Water

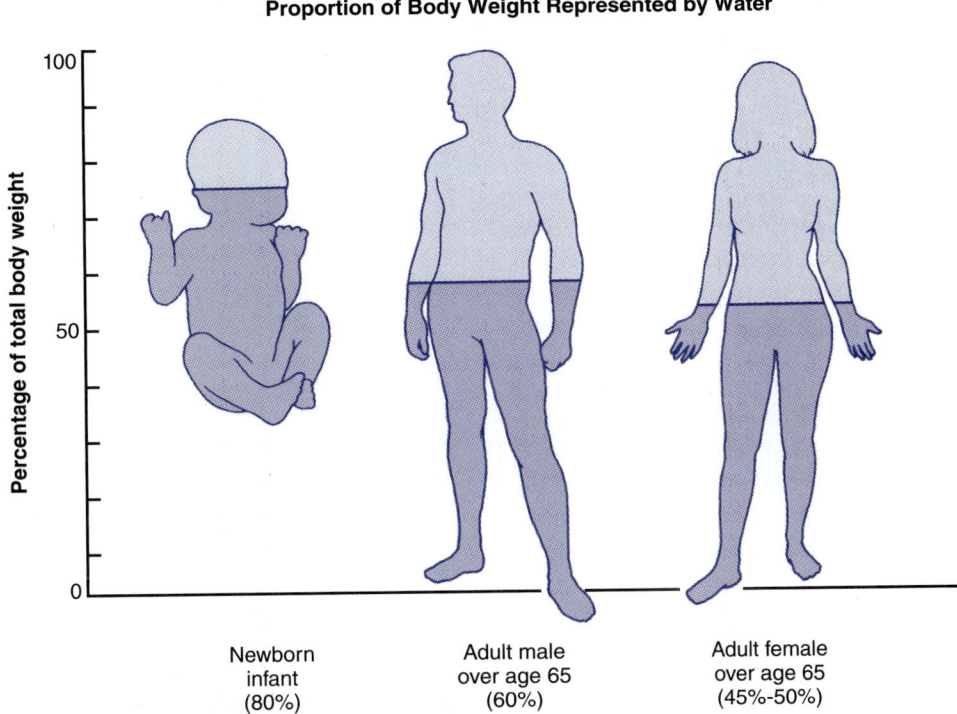

Fig. 6.1 ■ Changes in body water distribution. From Thibodeau, G. A., & Patton, K. T. (2004). *Structure and function of the body* (12th ed.). Mosby.

Cardiovascular System

The cardiovascular system is responsible for the transport of oxygen and nutrient-rich blood to the organs and the transport of metabolic waste products to the kidneys and bowels. The most relevant age-related changes are myocardial and blood vessel stiffening and a decreased responsiveness to sudden changes in oxygen demand (Gupta & Shea, 2019). Changes in the cardiovascular system are progressive and cumulative.

Cardiac Changes

The age-related changes of the heart (called *presbycardia*) are structural, electrical, and functional. The size of the heart remains relatively unchanged in healthy older adults. However, the left ventricle wall thickens by as much as 50% by 80 years of age, and the left atrium increases slightly in size—an adaptation that enhances ventricular filling. Maximum coronary-artery blood flow, stroke volumes, and cardiac output all decrease with age. The changes have little or no effect on the heart's ability to function in day-to-day life. The changes only become significant when there are environmental, physical, or psychological stresses. With sudden demands for more oxygen, the heart may not be able to respond adequately; it takes longer for the heart to accelerate and then return to a resting state. For the gerontological nurse, this means that the increased heart rate one might expect to see when a person is anxious, febrile, hemorrhaging, or in pain may not be present or will be delayed in an older adult. Similarly, the older heart may not be able to respond to other calls for increased cardiac demand, such as infection, anemia, pneumonia, cardiac dysrhythmias, surgery, diarrhea, hypoglycemia, and malnutrition. Instead, the nurse must depend on other signs of distress in the older adult and be alert to signs of rapid decompensation in both a previously well older adult and an adult who is frail.

Heart disease is the number one cause of nonaccidental death worldwide. Often, the changes associated with disease are thought to be a normal part of aging, but they are not. The gerontological nurse can promote healthy aging by making recommendations for heart-healthy life choices and supporting the older adult in obtaining excellent health care.

Blood Vessels

Several age-related changes in the skin and muscles affect the lining (*intima*) of the blood vessels, especially the arteries. As with the skin, the most significant change is decreased elasticity and recoil. The blood supply to various organs decreases, and peripheral resistance increases. Change in flow to the coronary arteries and the brain is minimal, but decreased perfusion of other organs, especially the liver and kidneys, has potentially serious implications for medication use (see Chapter 14). When a person already has or develops arteriosclerosis or hypertension, the age-related changes can have serious consequences.

Less dramatic changes are found in the veins, although the veins do become somewhat stretched and the valves less efficient. This means that lower-extremity edema develops more quickly and the older adult is at greater risk for deep vein thrombosis because of the increased sluggishness of the venous circulation. The normal changes, when combined with a longstanding but unknown weakness of the vessels, may become visible in marked varicosities and can lead to an increased rate of stroke and aneurysms. However, the promotion, and attainment, of a healthier heart is possible (Box 6.4).

Respiratory System

The respiratory system is the vehicle for ventilation and gas exchange, particularly the transfer of oxygen into and the release of carbon dioxide from the blood. The respiratory structures depend on the full functioning of the musculo-skeletal and nervous systems. The respiratory system matures by age 20 and then begins to decline. Subtle and mostly insignificant changes occur in the lungs, the thoracic cage, the respiratory muscles, and the respiratory centres in the central nervous system. The more specific changes include loss of elastic recoil, stiffening of the chest wall, inefficiency in gas exchange, and increased air flow resistance (Fig. 6.2). Respiratory problems are common but almost always result from exposure to environmental toxins (e.g., pollution) and not the aging process (Kim et al., 2018).

BOX 6.4
PROMOTING A HEALTHY HEART

- Do not smoke.
- Keep cholesterol, blood pressure, and blood sugar levels normal.
- Engage in at least 150 minutes of moderate to vigorous aerobic physical activity per week, in bouts of 10 minutes of more.
- Maintain a healthy weight.
- Eat a wide variety of foods, following *Canada's Food Guide*. Eat seven servings of vegetables and fruits each day.
- Learn how to cope with stress in a healthy way.
- Avoid trans fats and limit saturated fats.
- Limit sodium intake.

Sources: Adapted from Heart and Stroke Foundation of Canada. (2020). *How much physical activity do you need?* https://www.heartandstroke.ca/healthy-living/stay-active/how-much-physical-activity-do-you-need; Heart and Stroke Foundation of Canada. (2020). *Healthy eating basics.* https://www.heartandstroke.ca/healthy-living/healthy-eating/healthy-eating-basics; Heart and Stroke Foundation of Canada. (2020). *Lifestyle risk factors.* https://www.heartandstroke.ca/heart-disease/risk-and-prevention/lifestyle-risk-factors.

As with the cardiovascular system, the biggest change in respiration is in efficiency. Under normal conditions, this has little or no effect on the performance of customary life activities. However, when an individual is confronted with a sudden demand for increased oxygen, a respiratory deficit may become evident. Chemoreceptor function is altered or blunted at the peripheral and central chemoreceptor sites in the central nervous system, reducing the ability to respond to **hypoxia** or **hypercapnia.**

The changes that occur in the anatomical structures of the chest and the alterations in muscle strength can significantly affect one's ability to cough forcefully enough to quickly expel materials that accumulate in or obstruct airways. In addition, respiratory cilia are less effective. The reduced effectiveness of the cough response and cough reflex increases the risk of potentially life-threatening infections and aspiration, especially when the person has a swallowing or gastro-intestinal impairment such as dysphagia or decreased esophageal motility. The lack of basilar inflation, an ineffective cough response, and a less efficient immune system pose potential problems for older adults who are sedentary,

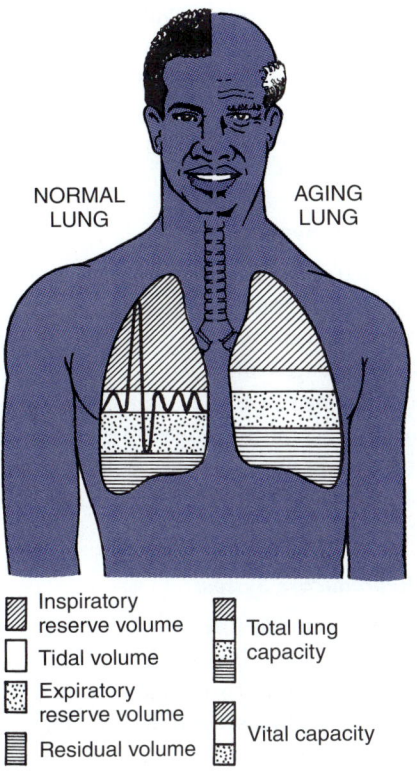

NORMAL
LUNG

AGING
LUNG

Inspiratory
reserve volume

Tidal volume

Expiratory
reserve volume

Residual volume

Total lung
capacity

Vital capacity

Fig. 6.2 ■ Changes in lung volumes with aging. From McCance, K. L., & Huether, S. E. (Eds.). (2006). *Pathophysiology: The biologic basis for disease in adults and children* (5th ed.). Mosby.

bedridden, or limited in activity. All these risks and conditions make the administration of annual influenza immunizations and a single pneumococcal vaccine of the highest importance. In promoting the appropriate immunizations, the nurse is promoting healthy aging (Box 6.5).

Renal System

The renal system is responsible for regulating water and salts in the body and for maintaining the acid–base balance in the blood. Blood passes through the nephrons in the kidneys for filtering. The glomerulus is the key structure that controls the rate of filtering (**glomerular filtration rate**). Kidney function is measured indirectly by means of the plasma creatinine by calculating the creatinine clearance rate.

Among the many changes to the kidneys are changes in blood flow and the ability to regulate body fluids.

Blood flow through the kidneys decreases by about 10% per decade (Xu et al., 2019), from about 1 200 mL/min in young adults to about 600 mL/min by the age of 80 years as a result of vascular and fixed anatomical and structural changes. The kidneys lose up to 50% of the nephrons, with little change in the body's ability to regulate body fluids. The age-related decrease in size and function occurs primarily in the kidney cortex and begins in a person's thirties or forties (Preminger, 2019). Renal reserve is lost, and the ability to respond to either a salt or water load or deficit is compromised.

Whereas plasma creatinine is constant throughout life, urine creatinine declines even in healthy aging because of reduced lean muscle mass. Creatinine clearance, a measurement of the glomerular filtration rate, decreases to 100 mL/min by the age of 80 years. Urine creatinine clearance is an important indicator for appropriate medication therapy, reflecting the ability to handle medications that are passing through and metabolized by the kidneys (see Chapter 14). Persons with a reduced creatinine clearance usually need lower doses of medications to prevent potential toxicity, and caution must be used in the administration of fluids (see Chapter 9).

Age-related changes in the renal system are significant because of the resultant heightened susceptibility to fluid and electrolyte imbalance, as well as structural damage from medications and from the contrast media used during diagnostic tests. Under normal circumstances, renal function is sufficient to meet the regulation and excretion demands of the body. However, with the stress of disease, surgery, or fever, the kidneys have a reduced capacity to respond and are therefore at greater risk for renal insufficiency and failure.

Endocrine System

The endocrine system, working in tandem with the neurological system, regulates and controls the integration of body activities by secreting hormones from glands throughout the body. As the body ages, most glands atrophy and decrease their rate of secretion. However, other than the decrease in estrogen, which causes menopause, the impact of the changes is not clear.

Pancreas Function

The endocrine pancreas secretes insulin, glucagon, somatostatin, and pancreatic polypeptides. The secretion of these substances does not appear to decrease to a level of any clinical significance in older adults. However, for unknown reasons, the tissues of the body often develop a decreased sensitivity to insulin. When combined with the increased need for insulin in the presence of obesity, the result is often the development of type 2 diabetes. Older adults have the highest rate of type 2 diabetes of any age group, with significant variation by ethnicity and region (see Chapter 17). When the pancreas is stressed with sudden concentrations of glucose, blood levels remain high for a longer duration. These temporary levels of increased blood glucose make the diagnosis of diabetes or glucose intolerance difficult.

Thyroid Function

With aging, slight changes occur in the structure and function of the thyroid gland, which may explain the increased incidence of hypothyroidism in older adults (Duntas, 2018). Some atrophy, fibrosis, and inflammation occur. Although other evidence of change is inconclusive at this time, diminished secretion of thyroid-stimulating hormone (TSH) and thyroxine (T_4) and decreased plasma triiodothyronine (T_3) appear to be age related. Serum T_3 decreases with age, perhaps as a result of decreased secretion of TSH by the pituitary gland. When thyroid hormone replacement therapy is needed, lower doses are necessary. The required dose of thyroxine may change over time,

and monitoring is required. Collective signs, such as a slowed basal metabolic rate, thinning hair, and dry skin, are characteristic of hypothyroidism in the young, but are normal manifestations in older adults who have no history of thyroid deficiencies, making the recognition of thyroid disturbances difficult.

Reproductive System

The reproductive systems in men and women serve the same physiological purpose—human procreation. Although aging men and women both undergo age-related changes, the changes affect women significantly more than men. Women lose the ability to procreate after menopause (cessation of ovulation), whereas men remain fertile their entire lives. Regardless of the physical changes, sexual needs remain. Chapter 26 discusses sexual health and well-being.

Female Reproductive System

As menopause signals the end of the reproductive phase in a woman's life, several other age-related changes occur, particularly in breast tissue and urogenital structures. The breasts of older women are smaller, pendulous, and less firm. The labia majora and minora become less prominent, and the pubic hair thins. The ovaries, cervix, and uterus slowly atrophy. The vagina shortens, narrows, and loses some of its elasticity. Vaginal walls lose their ability to lubricate quickly, especially if the woman is not sexually active, and more stimulation is needed to achieve orgasm. The vaginal epithelium changes considerably; the pH rises from 4.0 to 6.0 before menopause to 6.5 to 8.0 afterward (Tufts et al., 2015). The vaginal changes result in the potential for dyspareunia (painful intercourse), trauma during intercourse, and higher susceptibility to infection.

Hormone therapies can be used to treat hot flashes and other symptoms that accompany menopause such as vaginal dryness. For the treatment of hot flashes, hormones can be delivered orally, as a patch, through sprays, as gels, or as a vaginal ring; to treat vaginal dryness, hormones come in the form of a cream, pill, or vaginal ring (North American Menopause Society, 2021a). Estrogen therapy is typically indicated for women who have had a hysterectomy and do not require uterine protection to prevent uterine cancer (North American Menopause Society, 2021b). Progestogen therapy includes natural progesterone and synthetic progestins to treat symptoms such as hot flashes; it is typically indicated for women who cannot use estrogen (North American Menopause Society, 2021b). Progestogen therapy can also be used alongside estrogen therapy to protect against uterine cancer (estrogen–progestogen therapy) (North American Menopause Society, 2021b). Side effects of estrogen therapy include increased risk of stroke and blood clots. Estrogen therapy and estrogen–progestogen therapy can increase one's risk of breast cancer when used long term (more than 5 years) (North American Menopause Society, 2021b).

Male Reproductive System

Although men continue to have the ability to produce sperm in late life, changes in the functioning of the reproductive and urogenital organs occur. The changes are usually more subtle and are noticed only as they accumulate, beginning when men are in their fifties. The testes atrophy and soften, the seminiferous tubules thicken, and obstruction caused by sclerosis and fibrosis can occur. Although the sperm count does not decrease, fertility may be reduced because of sperm that lack motility or because of structural abnormalities. Erectile changes are also seen; more stimulation is needed to achieve a full erection, ejaculation is slower and less forceful, and refractory periods are longer (Tufts et al., 2015). As with women, alterations in hormone balance may play a part in the age-related changes in men. Testosterone level is reduced in all men but only rarely to a level that would be considered a true deficiency.

By the age of 50 years, up to 50% of men have some degree of prostatic enlargement, with prevalence increasing with age (Kim et al., 2016). The condition, known as *benign prostatic hypertrophy*, is so common that it is considered normal with aging. It is considered problematic only when the enlargement causes compression of the urethra. As a result, older men may experience urinary retention, leading to repeated urinary tract infections and overflow incontinence. Medications or surgical interventions are pursued only when the symptoms of benign prostatic hypertrophy interfere with quality of life (Kim et al., 2016). Medications may include alpha-blockers such as terazosin (Hytrin) or tamsulosin (Flomax) to relax the muscles around the prostate and relieve pressure on the urethra (Canadian Cancer Society, 2021). If surgery is indicated owing to urinary difficulties, then men typically undergo a transurethral resection of the prostate (TURP) to remove part of the prostate tissue through the urethra. Side effects may include bleeding, infection, and retrograde ejaculation (Canadian Cancer Society, 2021). Other surgeries include laser prostatectomy (using a laser to destroy prostate tissue) or transurethral incision of the prostate (TUIP) to make a small incision in the prostate and relieve pressure on the urethra (Canadian Cancer Society, 2021). Annual prostate examination by a primary health care provider is important.

Gastro-intestinal System

The digestive system includes the gastro-intestinal tract and the accessory organs that aid digestion. As with the endocrine system, few age-related changes affect function. However, a number of common health problems can have a great effect on the digestive system. Changes in other systems can also affect gastro-intestinal structure and function.

Mouth

Age-related changes affect both the teeth and the mouth. With the wear and tear of years of use, the teeth eventually lose enamel and dentin and become more vulnerable to decay and caries. The roots become more brittle and break more easily. For unknown reasons, the gums are also more susceptible to periodontal disease. Without good mouth care, teeth may be lost. Taste buds decline in number, reducing the sense of taste, and salivary secretion lessens. A very dry mouth (**xerostomia**) is common. When dentures are used, it is important to ensure their fit and cleanliness and the appropriate diet. A number of medications taken for common health problems can quickly exacerbate oral problems, especially xerostomia. When the gerontological nurse administers medications or teaches about medication, the older adult should be warned about this effect (see Chapter 14).

Esophagus

In youth, food passes quickly through the esophagus to the stomach because of the strong and coordinated contractions of associated muscle and peristalsis. In aging people, the contractions increase in frequency but are more disordered; thus, propulsion is less effective. This is called *presbyesophagus*. The sluggish emptying of the esophagus forces its lower end to dilate, creating greater stress in this area and possibly causing digestive discomfort. Pathological processes that are more common with advanced age include GERD and hiatal hernias.

Stomach

Decreased gastric motility and volume as well as reduced secretion of bicarbonate and gastric mucus are also associated with aging (Corey et al., 2020). These reductions are caused by gastric atrophy and result in hypochlorhydria (insufficient hydrochloric acid). Decreased production of intrinsic factor can lead to pernicious anemia if the stomach is not able to use ingested B_{12} vitamins. The protective alkaline viscous mucus of the stomach is lost because of the increase in stomach pH, which makes the stomach more susceptible to peptic ulcer disease, particularly if nonsteroidal anti-inflammatory drugs such as aspirin and ibuprofen are taken. The loss of smooth muscle in the stomach delays emptying time, which may lead to anorexia or weight loss (as a result of distension), meal-induced fullness, and a feeling of satiety (Landi et al., 2016).

Intestines

Age-related changes in the small intestine include those noted earlier that involve the villi, the anatomical structures in the intestinal walls that are essential for the absorption of nutrients. The villi become broader, shorter, and less functional. This affects nutrient absorption; proteins, fats, minerals (including calcium), vitamins (especially B_{12}), and carbohydrates (especially lactose) are absorbed more slowly and in lesser amounts (Doig & Huether, 2015). Changes in motility, epithelial membranes, vascular perfusion, and gastro-intestinal membrane transport may affect the absorption of lipids, amino acids, glucose, calcium, and iron.

Peristalsis slows with aging, and the response to rectal filling is blunted; the extent of the change should not be sufficient to cause problems with defecation. In other words, constipation, often thought of as a normal part of aging, is not normal. Constipation is often a side effect of medications, life habits, immobility, inadequate fluid intake, and lack of attention to the gastrocolic reflex and the postprandial urge to defecate (see Chapter 8). Suggestions for promoting healthy digestion are found in Box 6.6.

Accessory Organs

The accessory organs of the digestive system are the liver and the gallbladder. The liver continues to function

---

BOX 6.6
PROMOTING HEALTHY DIGESTION

- Practise good oral hygiene.
- Wear proper-fitting dentures.
- Seek prompt treatment of dental caries and periodontal disease.
- Eat meals in a relaxed atmosphere.
- Maintain adequate intake of fluids.
- Provide time for response to gastrocolic reflex.
- Respond promptly to the urge to defecate.
- Eat a balanced diet.
- Avoid prolonged periods of immobility.
- Avoid tobacco products.

---

throughout the lifespan despite a decrease in volume and weight (mass), a concomitant decrease in liver blood flow, and up to a 35% decrease in the liver's blood volume in those aged 65 years or older (Hunt et al., 2019). These decreases carry implications for impaired metabolism of medications and are associated with an increased half-life of fat-soluble medications (see Chapter 14). Liver regeneration, although slow, is not greatly impaired, and liver function test results remain unaltered with age.

There does not seem to be a specific change in the gallbladder with aging; however, the incidence of gallstones increases (Song et al., 2020), possibly owing to the increased lipogenic composition of bile from biliary cholesterol. The decrease in bile salt synthesis increases the incidence of cholelithiasis and cholecystitis (National Institute of Diabetes and Digestive and Kidney Diseases, 2017). In addition, the decrease in bile acid synthesis causes a reduction in hydroxylation of cholesterol. This change, in conjunction with a decrease in hepatic extraction of low-density lipoprotein cholesterol from the blood, increases the level of serum cholesterol in the older adult. In women, the increase in cholesterol begins to be seen after menopause.

Neurological System

Contrary to popular belief, the older adult's nervous system, including the brain, is remarkably resilient, and changes in cognitive functioning are not a normal part of aging. Neither the older adult nor the nurse should accept an assessment of "confusion" without making sure the cause is identified and treated if possible. Although many neurophysiological changes occur with aging, they do not occur in all older adults and do not affect everyone the same way. For example, neurofibrillary tangles are a classic sign of dementia and are present in the brains of all persons with Alzheimer's disease, but they are also found in the brains of persons without dementia. Although it is difficult to show the true causes and effects of age-related changes in the nervous system, some changes appear to be consistent.

Central Nervous System

The major changes in the aging nervous system are found in the central nervous system. With aging, the dendrites appear to "wear out," and the number of neurons decreases, along with a corresponding decrease in brain weight and size (Fig. 6.3). This change in size is primarily in the frontal lobe and appears as atrophy on computed tomography scans and magnetic resonance imaging; it is considered to be clinically insignificant. Decreased adherence of the dura mater to the skull, fibrosis, thickening of the meninges, narrowing of the gyri, widening of the sulcus, and increased subarachnoid space also occur (Sugarman, 2015).

Sleep changes resulting from changes in the reticular formation may also be a normal part of aging. The reticular formation is a set of neurons that extend from the spinal cord through the brainstem and into the cerebral cortex. With aging, there may be a loss of deep sleep (stages 3 and 4). Compared with younger people, older adults spend more time in bed to get the same amount of "sleep," because the time they spend in light sleep increases in proportion to the time they spend in deep sleep (National Institutes of Health, 2021). However, excessive daytime drowsiness is not typical and should lead to a thorough assessment of causative factors, especially depression and the side effects of medication (see Chapters 14 and 23).

Subtle changes in cognitive functioning (thinking) and motor functioning (movement) occur in very old people. Mild memory impairment and difficulties with balance may be seen as normal age-related changes in neurodegeneration and neurochemistry (see Chapters 7 and 22). Intellectual performance without brain dysfunction remains constant. However, the performance of tasks may take longer, an indication that central processing is slowed. There are also decreasing levels of the neurotransmitters acetylcholine, serotonin, dopamine, and catecholamine. Other enzymes, such as monoamine oxidase, increase. Redundancy of brain cells may

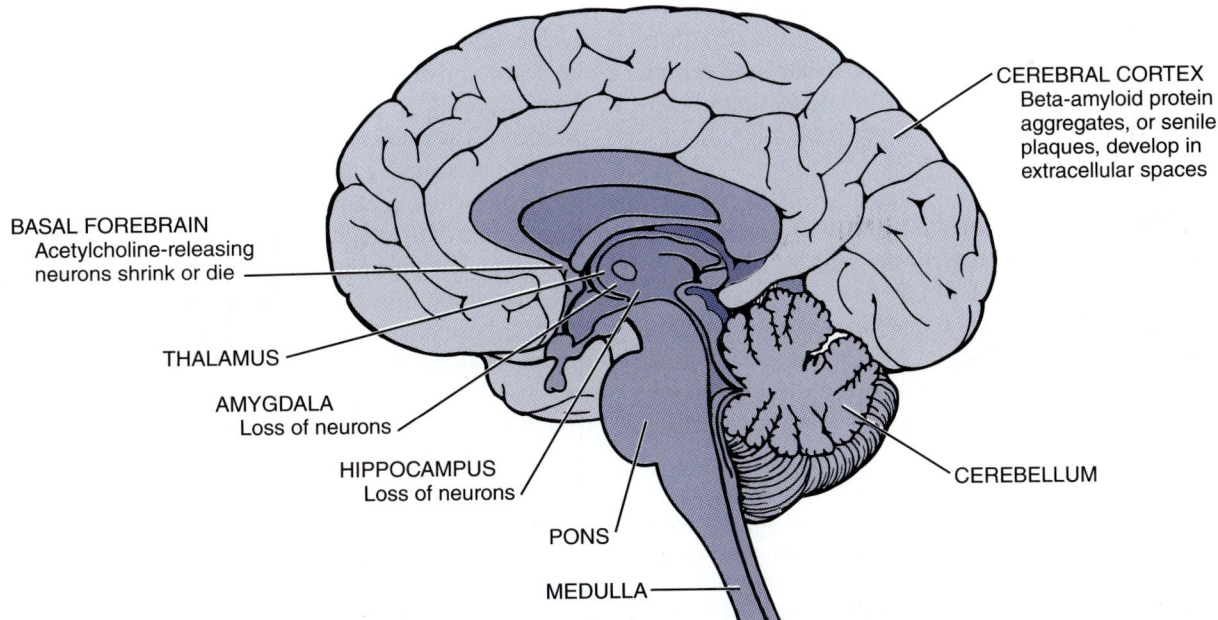

Fig. 6.3 ■ Changes in the brain with aging. Courtesy Carole Donner, Tucson, AZ, USA.

forestall the effects of these changes; the exact number of cells required for certain functions is unknown.

Peripheral Nervous System

The most important effect of normal changes in the aging peripheral nervous system is the increased risk for injury. Vibratory sense in the lower extremities may be nonexistent. Somesthesia, or tactile sensitivity, decreases in connection with the loss of nerve endings in the skin; this is most notable in the fingertips, the palms of the hands, and the lower extremities. This decreased sensitivity is translated into delayed reactions to things such as hot surfaces, significantly increasing the risk for burns and the extent of any burns. (The presence of a functioning smoke detector in the home is particularly important.)

Kinesthetic sense, or **proprioception,** is altered because of changes in both the peripheral and central nervous systems. If one is less aware of body position and has less tactile awareness, one's risk of falling is dramatically increased. With reduced proprioception, it takes a little longer to realize that the surface is uneven and a little longer still to realize that one has tripped (changed position in space). This slight delay can result in an older adult falling, whereas younger people are able to immediately balance themselves and prevent a fall. Conditions such as arthritis, stroke, some cardiac disorders, and damage to the structures of the inner ear may also affect peripheral and central mechanisms of mobility. A further discussion of sensory alterations appears in Chapter 19.

Sensory Changes

A number of changes (some loss of smell, sight, sound, and touch) occur in the sensory organs as a result of a combination of intrinsic and extrinsic factors. The gerontological nurse can make a significant difference in the quality of life for the person with sensory changes (Box 6.7). Chapter 3 discussed communication with older adults who have vision and/or hearing impairments.

Eyes and Vision. Changes in vision and the eyes begin very early and are both functional and structural. All changes affect visual acuity and accommodation (the ability of the eyes to adjust to changes in the environment).

BOX 6.7
PROMOTING HEALTHY EYES

- Have eyes examined regularly.
- Use bright lighting.
- Do not smoke.
- Reduce glare as much as possible.
- Wear sunglasses that provide 99% to 100% UV-A and UV-B protection.
- Protect eyes from accidents and injury (e.g., use grease shields, safety glasses).

Source: Government of Canada. (2017). *Seniors and aging—Vision care.* https://www.canada.ca/en/health-canada/services/healthy-living/your-health/lifestyles/seniors-aging-vision-care.html.

Presbyopia is an age-related decrease in near vision that typically becomes noticeable at the age of 40, where glasses are needed for close vision. Approximately 18% of older adults use a magnifying glass for reading and close work. Although presbyopia is first seen in people who are in their 40s, 80% of those older than 65 years have fair to adequate far vision past 90 years of age. Pathological conditions that are more common in aging include glaucoma, cataracts, and macular degeneration (see Chapter 19).

Extraocular Changes. Age-related changes affect both the form and function of the eyes. The eyelids lose elasticity, resulting in drooping (*senile ptosis*). In most cases, only the appearance is affected; in extreme cases, the lids sag enough to block vision. Spasms of the orbicular muscle may cause the lower lid to turn inward; the prolonged turning inward of the lower lid is called *entropion.* The lower lashes that curl inward irritate and scratch the cornea, and surgery may be needed to prevent permanent injury. Decreases in orbicular muscle strength may result in *ectropion,* the turning outward of the lower lid. Without the integrity of the trough of the lower lid, tears run down the cheek instead of bathing the cornea. Ectropion and an inability to close the lid completely leads to excessively dry eyes and the need for artificial tears. Exacerbating this problem is a decrease in the number of goblet cells that provide mucin, which is essential for eye lubrication and movement. A severe deficiency of lubrication is known as *dry eye syndrome.*

Ocular Changes. The cornea is the avascular transparent outer surface of the eye globe that refracts (bends) light rays entering the eye through the pupil. With aging, the cornea becomes flatter, less smooth, thicker, and duller in appearance. The result is increased far-sightedness (hyperopia). For a person who was nearsighted (myopic) earlier in life, this change may actually improve vision.

Arcus senilis, a ring or partial ring that is grey-white to silver in colour, may be observed 1–2 mm inside the limbus at the juncture of the iris and cornea. It is composed of deposits of calcium and cholesterol salts. It does not appear to have any clinical significance.

The anterior chamber is the space between the cornea and the lens. The edges of the chamber include canals that control the volume and movement of aqueous fluid within the space. With aging, the chamber decreases slightly in size and capacity because of thickening of the lens. Resorption of the intraocular fluid becomes less efficient with age; a significant decrease can lead to increased intraocular pressure and glaucoma (Huether et al., 2015). Any eye pain or acute changes in vision should be considered medical emergencies and be responded to accordingly.

The ability to adjust to changes in light and the need for higher levels of lighting are the result of reduced responsiveness of the pupils and changes in the lens. The lens—a small, flexible, biconvex, crystal-like structure just behind the iris—is most responsible for visual acuity; it adjusts the light entering the pupil and focuses it on the retina. Age-related changes in the lens begin in a person's forties. The origins of these changes are not fully understood, although the sun's UV rays contribute to the problem, and cross-linkage of collagen creates a more rigid and thickened lens structure.

With age, light scattering increases and colour perception decreases. As a result, glare is a problem not only when created by sunlight outdoors but also when created by the reflection of light from any shiny object, such as a polished floor or surface. Eventually, people require three times as much light to see things as they required when they were younger. It is more effective to place high-intensity light on the object or surface to be observed than to increase the intensity of the light in the entire room (for example, focusing a light directly on the newspaper a person is reading instead of adding more light sources to the room).

Intraocular Changes. The retina, which lines the inside of the eye, has less distinct margins and is duller in appearance in older adults than in younger adults. Colour clarity diminishes by 25% in the sixth decade and by 59% in the eighth decade, especially the clarity of blues, violets, and greens; light colours such as reds, oranges, and yellows are more easily seen. Some of this difficulty is linked to the yellowing of the lens and impaired transmission of light to the retina. Finally, the number of rods and associated nerves at the periphery of the retina is reduced, resulting in peripheral vision that is not as clear as before or is absent (Mehra & Le, 2020). Arteries in the back of the eye may show atherosclerosis and slight narrowing. If a person has a long history of hypertension, veins may show indentations (nicking) as they pass over the arteries. As long as these changes are not accompanied by distortion of objects or a significant decrease in vision, they are not clinically significant.

Ears and Hearing. Aging affects both the structure and the function of the ears. Hearing loss that affects the ability to hear normal speech is more common in older adults. Approximately 54% of Canadians aged 40 to 79 experience at least mild hearing loss (Ramage-Morin et al., 2019). This number increases to 93% of those aged 70 to 79 years (Ramage-Morin et al., 2019). The most common type of hearing loss in older adults is a high-frequency, sensorineural loss known as **presbycusis.** Hearing loss can lead to social withdrawal and increase the risk for depression and falls (Abrams, 2017).

Several age-related changes in the ear's appearance occur, especially in men. The auricle loses flexibility and becomes longer and wider as a result of diminished elasticity. The lobes sag, elongate, and wrinkle. Together, these changes make the ears appear larger. In addition, coarse, wiry, stiff hairs grow at the periphery of the auricle. In men, the tragus enlarges.

The auditory canal narrows through inward collapse, and stiffer and coarser hairs line the canal. Cerumen glands atrophy, producing a thicker and dryer wax that is more difficult to remove; this is a substantial cause for temporary, reversible obstructive hearing loss. The gerontological nurse should be sensitive to this possibility and be skilled at safe cerumen removal.

On otoscopic examination, the tympanic membrane appears dull and grey. Structurally, the ossicle joints between the malleus and the stapes become calcified, causing reduced vibration of these bones and a mechanical reduction in the amount of sound transmitted to the auditory nerve.

With presbycusis, there is a decrease in vestibular sensitivity as a result of optic nerve loss and the degeneration of the organ of Corti in the cochlea. The transmission of sound waves to the brain is thus impaired. Hearing loss develops slowly. Whereas obstructive causes are reversible, sensorineural ones are not.

Presbycusis is primarily the loss of the ability to hear high-frequency sounds, such as consonants, the chirping of birds, and the rustling of leaves. Although the person may be able to decipher what is said if it is in context, this processing takes longer than usual or language is processed incorrectly. With normal age-related hearing loss, the person can still hear but may not be able to make sense of the partially heard words. Inaccurate responses too often lead to the incorrect suspicion of cognitive impairment when in fact the problem is hearing loss.

Immune System

The immune system protects the host from invasions by foreign substances and organisms. To do so, it must be able to differentiate the self from the nonself (Delves, 2020). The immune system includes elements of many other systems, including white blood cells, bone marrow, the thymus, lymph nodes, and the spleen.

A number of age-related changes have been implicated in the increased risk for infection in the older adult. For example, the skin is thinner and therefore less resistant to bacterial invasion. The reduced number of cilia in the lungs leads to the increased risk for pneumonia. The friability of the urethra increases the risk for urinary tract infections, especially in women. But perhaps most important of all is the reduced immunity at the cellular level, which is now understood to have a significant genetic underpinning.

In late life, a decrease in innate immunity, adaptive immunity, and self-tolerance brings a decrease in T-cell function. The response to foreign antigens decreases, but immunoglobulins increase, creating an autoimmune response not associated with autoimmune diseases that may have developed earlier (Delves, 2020). Older adults are thus likely to experience infections in the absence of characteristic symptoms such as fever.

BOX 6.8
REDUCING RISK FOR FOODBORNE ILLNESS

- Follow Health Canada recommendations for safer choices among deli meats.
- Do not eat hot dogs straight from the package; heat to an internal temperature of 74°C.
- Avoid raw sprouts; refrigerated patés; raw or lightly cooked eggs; raw or undercooked meat; and unpasteurized dairy products, fruit juice, or cider.
- Take the following four steps for safe food handling, storage, and preparation:
  - Separate raw foods from cooked foods.
  - Wash your hands, kitchen surfaces, utensils, and reusable shopping bags with warm soapy water.
  - Promptly refrigerate food leftovers at 4°C or lower.
- Cook meat to recommended safe internal temperatures.

Source: Health Canada. (2015). *Food safety for adults ages 60 and older.* http://healthycanadians.gc.ca/eating-nutrition/healthy-eating-saine-alimentation/safety-salubrite/vulnerable-populations/older-adults-adultes-agees-eng.php.

For example, in older adults, urinary tract infections may present only with symptoms of changes in cognitive status (Public Health Ontario, 2019). Being alert for atypical signs and symptoms of infection is especially important to gerontological nursing, as is the responsibility to promote disease prevention and protection from infection. A pneumococcal vaccine is recommended for persons aged 65 years and older, and annual influenza vaccines are recommended for all adults. Older adults are also at increased risk for serious health effects from foodborne illnesses (Box 6.8).

The changes in immune function affect the older adult's response to illness. Early studies by Stengel (1983) found significantly lower oral temperature norms in healthy older adults. Thus, a febrile response suggestive of infection is not restricted to a temperature higher than 37°C. Instead, an older adult may have a core temperature elevation at much lower numbers. Very old persons may have an average normal temperature of 35.5°C and an average range of 35.0–36.1°C (Hogstel, 1994).

These findings emphasize the need to carefully evaluate the basal temperature of older adults and to recognize that even low-grade fevers (e.g., 37°C) may signify serious illness. When such temperature changes are combined with the age-related delay in the increases in white blood cell count seen in older adults as compared with that in younger adults, early detection of serious illness can be difficult. *A lack of fever (a temperature greater than 37°C) or a normal white blood cell count does not rule out infection.* Instead, the whole person must be considered, including mood, level of consciousness, and other factors, such as a recent fall or a change in cognitive abilities.

EVIDENCE-INFORMED PRACTICE: SMOKING CESSATION

Common health advice to older adults includes the recommendation to limit or quit smoking in order to promote oral health, heart health, and healthy eyes, lungs, digestion, and brain function. Cessation of smoking results in health benefits at any age, even in older age. The Registered Nurses' Association of Ontario (RNAO) has many resources (https://rnao.ca/category/topics/tobacco) that help nurses integrate smoking cessation into daily practice. The site includes a link to the relevant RNAO best practice guideline.

SUMMARY

Current biological theories of aging, supported by clinical evidence, indicate that complex functions of the body decline more than simple body processes do; that coordinated activity shows a greater decremental loss than that shown by single-system activity; and that a uniform and predictable loss of cell function occurs in all vital organs. Yet, the older adult is able to function effectively within the physical dictates of their body and often continues to live to a healthy and satisfactory old age while remaining capable of wisdom, judgement, and accomplishments.

The physical changes that accompany aging affect every body system, and the theories of why they occur are many. Although there are numerous ways and interventions by which nurses can promote healthy aging in the presence of these changes, the positive effect of these interventions is multiplied when nurses differentiate between normal changes and the signs and symptoms of potential health problems.

KEY CONCEPTS

- Many physical changes accompany aging; however, some of them are relatively insignificant in the absence of disease or unusual stress.
- Physiological aging begins at birth and is universal, progressive, and intrinsic.
- There are enormous individual variations in the rate of aging of body systems and functions.
- Many of the normal changes that occur with aging may be misinterpreted as pathological, and some pathological conditions may be mistaken for normal changes of aging.
- Careful assessment of lifestyle and individual age-related changes is fundamental to providing quality nursing care to older adults.

ACTIVITIES AND DISCUSSION QUESTIONS

1. Identify for each body system at least two normal changes that accompany aging.

2. Identify for each body system two abnormal physical, physiological, or both physical and physiological changes commonly seen in older adults.

3. Discuss the aging-related changes that you would find most difficult to accept.

4. Develop a nursing care plan for promoting the health of the older adult's cardiac system.

5. Describe some nursing interventions to maintain healthy skin for older adults.

6. Interview an older adult about their health practices and views on healthy aging. Discuss what you learned from the older adult with your classmates.

7. Search for images of healthy aging. Discuss how these images compare with the images of aging shown in popular media.

RESOURCES

Canadian Nurses Association. Aging and seniors care.
https://www.cna-aiic.ca/en/policy-advocacy/aging-and-seniors-care
Health Canada. Seniors.
*https://www.canada.ca/en/health-canada/services/healthy-living/
seniors.html*
Immunize Canada
https://www.immunize.ca/
Osteoporosis Canada
http://www.osteoporosis.ca/
Public Health Agency of Canada. Aging and seniors—Publications.
*https://www.canada.ca/en/public-health/services/health-promotion/
aging-seniors/aging-seniors-publications.html*
**Registered Nurses' Association of Ontario. Integrating tobacco
interventions into daily practice.**
*http://rnao.ca/bpg/guidelines/integrating-tobacco-interventions-
daily-practice*

For additional resources, please visit *http://evolve.elsevier.com/
Canada/Ebersole/gerontological/*

REFERENCES

Abrams, H. (2017). Hearing loss and associated comorbidities: What do we know. *Hearing Review, 24*(12), 32–35.

Canadian Cancer Society. (2021). *Benign prostatic hyperplasia (BPH).* https://www.cancer.ca/en/cancer-information/cancer-type/prostate/prostate-cancer/benign-prostatic-hyperplasia/?region=on.

Canadian Dermatology Association. (2021). *Alopecia.* https://dermatology.ca/public-patients/hair/alopecia/.

Cleveland Clinic. (2021). *Degenerative disc disease.* https://my.clevelandclinic.org/health/diseases/16912-degenerative-disc-disease.

Corey, B. L., Grams, J. M., Christein, J. D., et al. (2020). Benign disease of stomach and duodenum. In R. A. Rosenthal, M. E. Zenilman, & M. R. Katlic (Eds.), *Principles and practice of geriatric surgery* (pp. 1025–1049). Springer.

Crowther-Radulewicz, C. L. (2015). Structure and function of the musculoskeletal system. In K. L. McCance, S. E. Huether, V. L. Brashers, et al. (Eds.), *Pathophysiology: The biologic basis for disease in adults and children* (7th ed., pp. 1510–1539). Mosby.

da Silva, P. F. L., & Schumacher, B. (2019). DNA damage responses in ageing. *Open Biology, 9,* 190168. doi:10.1098/rsob.190168.

Delves, P. J. (2020). *Overview of the immune system.* https://www.merckmanuals.com/home/immune-disorders/biology-of-the-immune-system/overview-of-the-immune-system.

Doig, X. K., & Huether, S. E. (2015). Structure and function of the digestive system. In K. L. McCance, S. E. Huether, V. L. Brashers, et al. (Eds.), *Pathophysiology: The biologic basis for disease in adults and children* (7th ed., pp. 1393–1422). Mosby.

Duntas, L. H. (2018). Thyroid function in aging: A discerning approach. *Rejuvenation Research, 21*(1), 22–28. doi:10.1089/rej.2017.1991.

Effros, R. B., Dagarag, M., Spaulding, C., et al. (2005). The role of CD8+ T-cell replicative senescence in human aging. *Immunologic Review, 205,* 147–157. doi:10.1111/j.0105-2896.2005.00259.x.

Gupta, J. I., & Shea, M. J. (2019). *Effects on aging on the heart and blood vessels.* https://www.merckmanuals.com/home/heart-and-blood-vessel-disorders/biology-of-the-heart-and-blood-vessels/effects-of-aging-on-the-heart-and-the-blood-vessels.

Hayflick, L., & Moorehead, P. S. (1981). The serial cultivation of human diploid cell strains. *Experimental Cell Research, 25,* 585. doi:10.1016/0014-4827(61)90192-6.

Hogstel, M. O. (1994). Vital signs are really vital in the old-old. *Geriatric Nursing, 15*(5), 253. doi:10.1016/S0197-4572(09)90079-9.

Huether, S. E., Rodway, G., & DeFriez, C. B. (2015). Pain, temperature regulation, sleep, and sensory function. In K. L. McCance, S. E. Huether, V. L. Brashers, et al. (Eds.), *Pathophysiology: The biologic basis for disease in adults and children* (7th ed., pp. 484–526). Mosby.

Hunt, N. J., Kang, S. W. S., Lockwood, G. P., et al. (2019). Hallmarks of aging in the liver. *Computational and Structural Biotechnology Journal, 17,* 1151–1161. doi:10.1016/j.csbj.2019.07.021.

Karpouzos, A., Diamantis, E., Farmaki, P., et al. (2017). Nutritional aspects of bone health and fracture healing. *Journal of Osteoporosis, 2017,* 4218472. doi:10.1155/2017/4218472.

Kim, D., Chen, Z., Zhou, L., et al. (2018). Air pollutants and early origins of respiratory disease. *Chronic Diseases and Translational Medicine, 4*(2), 75–94. doi:10.1016/j.cdtm.2018.03.003.

Kim, E. H., Larson, J. A., & Andriole, G. L. (2016). Management of benign prostatic hyperplasia. *Annual Review of Medicine, 67,* 137–151. doi:10.1146/annurev-med-063014-123902.

Landi, F., Calvani, R., Tosato, M., et al. (2016). Anorexia of aging: Risk factors, consequences, and potential treatments. *Nutrients, 8*(2), 69. doi:10.3390/nu8020069.

Manisalidis, I., Stavropoulou, E., Stavropoulos, A., et al. (2020). Environmental and health impacts of air pollution: A review. *Frontiers in Public Health, 8,* 14. doi:10.3389/fpubh.2020.00014.

Marin-Garcia, J. (2008). *Aging and the heart: A post-genomic view.* Springer.

McCormack, R., & Vasilaki, A. (2018). Age-related changes in skeletal muscle changes to life-style as a therapy. *Biogerontology, 19,* 519–536. doi:10.1007/s10522-018-9775-3.

Mehra, D., & Le, P. H. (2020). *Physiology, night vision.* StatPearls. https://www.ncbi.nlm.nih.gov/books/NBK545246/.

Meltzer, D. O., Best, T. J., Vokes, T., et al. (2020). Association of vitamin D status and other clinical characteristics with COVID-19 test results. *JAMA Network Open, 3*(9), 32019722. doi:10.1001/jamanet-workopen.2020.19722.

National Institute of Diabetes and Digestive and Kidney Diseases. (2017). *Bile acids.* https://www.ncbi.nlm.nih.gov/books/NBK548626/.

National Institutes of Health. (2021). *Aging changes in sleep.* https://medlineplus.gov/ency/article/004018.htm.

North American Menopause Society. (2021a). *Hormone therapy & menopause FAQs.* http://www.menopause.org/for-women/expert-answers-to-frequently-asked-questions-about-menopause/hormone-therapy-menopause-faqs.

North American Menopause Society. (2021b). *Hormone help desk: ET, EPT, and more.* http://www.menopause.org/for-women/menopauseflashes/menopause-symptoms-and-treatments/hormone-help-desk-et-ept-and-more.

Osteoporosis Canada. (2017). *Vitamin D.* https://osteoporosis.ca/vitamin-d/.

Public Health Ontario. (2019). *Urinary tract infection (UTI) program. Causes of delirium and mental status changes.* https://www.publichealthontario.ca/-/media/documents/u/2016/uti-delirium-mental-status.pdf?la=en.

Preminger, G. M. (2019). *Effects of aging on the urinary tract.* https://www.merckmanuals.com/home/kidney-and-urinary-tract-disorders/biology-of-the-kidneys-and-urinary-tract/effects-of-aging-on-the-urinary-tract.

Ramage-Morin, P. L., Banks, R., Pineault, D., et al. (2019). *Unperceived hearing loss among Canadians aged 40 to 79.* https://www150.statcan.gc.ca/n1/pub/82-003-x/2019008/article/00002-eng.htm.

Song, S. T., Shi, J., Wang, X. H., et al. (2020). Prevalence and risk factors for gallstone disease: A population-based cross-sectional study. *Journal of Digestive Diseases, 21*(4), 237–245. doi:10.1111/1751-2980.12857.

Stengel, G. B. (1983). Oral temperature in the elderly. *Gerontologist, 23*(Special Issue), 306.

Sugarman, R. A. (2015). Structure and function of the neurologic system. In K. L. McCance, S. E. Huether, V. L. Brashers, et al. (Eds.), *Pathophysiology: The biologic basis for disease in adults and children* (7th ed., pp. 447–483). Mosby.

Tufts, G., Rodway, G., Heuther, S. E., et al. (2015). Structure and function of the reproductive systems. In K. L. McCance, S. E. Huether, V. L. Brashers, et al. (Eds.), *Pathophysiology: The biologic basis for disease in adults and children* (7th ed., pp. 768–799). Mosby.

Valko, M., Morris, H., & Cronin, M. (2005). Metals, toxicity and oxidative stress. *Current Medical Chemistry, 12*(10), 1161–1208.

Vina, J., Borras, C., & Gomez-Cabrera, M. C. (2018). A free radical theory of frailty. *Free Radical Biology and Medicine, 124*, 358–363.

Wounds Canada. (2018). *Skin: Anatomy, physiology and wound healing.* https://www.woundscanada.ca/docman/public/health-care-professional/bpr-workshop/166-wc-bpr-skin-physiology/file.

Xu, J., Yu, J., Xu, X., et al. (2019). Preoperative hidden renal dysfunction add an age dependent risk of progressive chronic kidney disease after cardiac surgery. *Journal of Cardiothoracic Surgery, 14*, 151. doi:10.1186/s13019-019-0977-9.

7

SOCIAL, PSYCHOLOGICAL, SPIRITUAL, AND COGNITIVE ASPECTS OF AGING

LEARNING OBJECTIVES

Upon completion of this chapter, the reader will be able to:

- Explain the major cognitive, psychological, and sociological theories of aging.
- Discuss the influence of culture and cohort on psychological and social adaptation.
- Discuss the importance of spirituality to healthy aging.
- Explain several normal cognitive changes of aging.
- Discuss factors influencing learning in late life and appropriate teaching and learning strategies.

GLOSSARY

Cognition   The mental process characterized by knowing, thinking, learning, and judging.

Cross-sectional   A study design in which data are collected at one time on several variables such as age, gender, education, and health status.

Face validity   "The extent to which a test appears to measure what it is intended to measure" (Johnson, 2013).

Geragogy   The application of the principles of adult learning theory to teaching older adults.

Health literacy   The ability to access, understand, and act on information concerning health.

Longitudinal research   A study that repeatedly and at predetermined intervals assesses the experiences, states, or situations of a group of research participants.

THE LIVED EXPERIENCE

Accounts of Aging Well

Carr and Weir (2017) explored factors that contribute to aging successfully. Participants shared the following:

"*Stay engaged with people, like not isolate yourself . . . I think you need to get out and talk to people.*" (J.W., 70 years of age)

"*[It] helps to have good genes.*" (M.T., 97 years of age)

"*Never look on the bad side of things . . . you've got to be positive.*" (A.N., 88 years of age)

"*Successful aging in my point of view is being able to maintain the ordinary things in your life in your own home, doing your own gardening, doing your own repairs, helping a neighbour, interacting with kids on the street, helping your wife.*" (B.G., 91 years of age)

"*You're retired now, if you're in good health, or in fairly good health, all the things you wanted to do in life, which you didn't do or couldn't do, now is the time to do them, while you got your health.*" (S.D., 82 years of age)

SOCIAL, PSYCHOLOGICAL, SPIRITUAL, AND COGNITIVE ASPECTS OF AGING

Each individual has unique life experiences. Thus, each person must be seen holistically, through the lens of their time, place, culture, gender, and personal history. The close relationship between biological, social, and psychological development that exists through childhood and adolescence varies more in adulthood because of the greater variations in life experiences and demands as one matures. This chapter discusses the psychological, social, cognitive, and spiritual aspects of aging. Also discussed are factors that influence learning later in life, as well as appropriate teaching and learning strategies for older adults.

LIFESPAN DEVELOPMENT AND LIFE-COURSE APPROACHES

Human development is a lifelong process of adaptation. *Lifespan development* is an individual's progress through time and the expected patterns of change, biologically, sociologically, and psychologically. The lifespan theory of development is a psychological theory. The key principles of this theory, which are based on the work of Baltes and colleagues (Baltes, 1987; Baltes et al., 1998), have been summarized by Papalia et al. (2002) as follows:

- Development is a lifelong process. Each part of the lifespan is influenced by the past and will affect the future. Each period of the lifespan has unique characteristics and value; no single period is more important than any other.
- Development depends on history and on social and cultural context. Each person develops under a certain set of circumstances and conditions that are defined by time and place.
- Development within each lifespan is multidimensional and multidirectional and involves a balance of growth and decline. Whereas children usually grow consistently in size and abilities, the balance gradually shifts in adulthood. Some abilities, such as acquiring a vocabulary, continue to increase, whereas others, such as speed of information retrieval, may decrease. New abilities, such as those involving wisdom and expertise, may emerge with age.
- Development is malleable and influenced by external conditions. With training and practice, a person's functioning and performance can improve throughout their lifespan. However, there are limits to how much performance can improve at any age.

Life-course theory is closely related to sociological theory; lifespan theory, social relations, age, and the timing of events in the course of life are integrated (Elder, 1998, as cited in Lerner, 2002). As explained by lifespan theory, historical times and places experienced during a lifetime affect the course of a person's life (Lerner, 2002). Furthermore, the impact of an event or transition depends on when it occurs during the life course. Social roles and interdependent social relationships are viewed as having an important influence on the life course. Finally, "individuals construct their own life course through the choices and actions they take within the constraints and opportunities of history and social circumstances" (Elder, 1998, as cited in Lerner, 2002, pp. 235–236).

TYPES OF AGING

People age in a number of ways. Aging can be viewed in terms of *chronological age, biological age, psychological age,* and *social age.* Chronological age is measured by the number of years lived. Biological age is predicted by the person's physical condition and by how well vital organ systems are functioning. Psychological age is indicated by the person's ability and control in regard to memory, learning capacity, skills, emotions, and judgement. Maturity and capacity direct the manner in which a person is able to adapt psychologically over time to the requirements of the environment. Social age is measured by age-graded behaviours that conform to an expected social status and social roles within a particular culture or society.

These different types of aging within a person do not necessarily match. A person may have a chronological age of 80 years but a biological age of 60 years because they have remained fit by maintaining a healthy lifestyle. Conversely, a person with a chronic illness may have a biological age of 70 years but a much younger psychological age owing to an active and involved lifestyle.

There are several psychological and sociological theories of aging. Not all theories acknowledge the importance of opportunity, ethnicity, gender, and social status. As current generations of older adults move through life, many of the current ideas and theories about this period of life development will continue to be redefined.

SOCIOLOGICAL THEORIES OF AGING

Sociological theories of aging attempt to explain and predict changes in roles and relationships in middle and late life, with an emphasis on adjustment. The basic theories were developed in the 1960s and 1970s and must be viewed within the context of the historical period from which they emerged. Some of the theories, such as modernization and social exchange theories, continue to generate interest and thought.

Activity Theory

Activity theory is based on the belief that remaining as active as possible contributes to successful aging (Maddox, 1963). Evidence from gerontological research connects continued physical activity, social engagement, and productive roles to better outcomes (Jakovljevic, 2018; Dause & Kirby, 2019). However, other research indicates that the meaning of an activity to the person may be more important than the activity per se (Rantanen et al., 2019). Many older adults judge successful aging partly in terms of physical, mental, and social activity (Mejía et al., 2017). Older adults tend to remain active in retirement and may do so through the "productive activity" of paid and unpaid work. A Canadian survey (Revera, 2019) found that more than one-third of older adults volunteer. Furthermore, older adults spend more time volunteering (an average of 223 hours per year) than younger Canadians do. Accessibility and opportunities to participate in society have an important influence on activity. The federal government's Age-Friendly Communities Initiative (Government of Canada, 2016), which is based on the World Health Organization's Global Age-Friendly Cities Project (World Health Organization, 2021), is an example of the application of this theory to policy. In age-friendly communities, "policies, services and structures related to the physical and social environment are designed to support and enable older adults to 'age actively' . . . to continue to participate fully in society" (Public Health Agency of Canada, 2016, p. 2). Older adults and their communities work together, for example, to reduce ageist attitudes in businesses, to lobby for accessible public transportation, or to make parks accessible and safe.

Continuity Theory

According to continuity theory, people use continuity strategies to adapt to the changes of normal aging; people are "motivated toward inner psychological continuity as well as outward continuity of social behaviour and circumstances" (Atchley, 2000, p. 47). Inner continuity is "a remembered inner structure such as ideas, temperament, affect, experiences, preferences, dispositions, and skills" (Atchley, 2000, p. 49). Inner continuity provides a foundation for decision making, is a means of meeting important needs, and supports a sense of self, identity, and self-esteem. External continuity, then, is "a remembered structure of physical and social environments, role relationships, and activities [that] result from being and doing in familiar environments, practicing familiar skills, and interacting with familiar people" (Atchley, 2000, p. 50). Too little or too much continuity feels uncomfortable to the person.

Continuity is a fluid concept and does not imply that people do not change; rather, there is coherence and consistency of patterns over time. For example, an older adult who enjoys decorating is more likely to take up a new activity in the same domain (such as painting) than a new activity in another domain (such as a sport). When people take on new volunteer roles after retirement, they tend to select volunteer roles in which they can work toward solutions on issues that are affecting the world, using their skills and knowledge to make a difference (Revera, 2019). Furthermore, research supports the continuity theory's prediction that retirement and the resultant relief from work pressure bring increased psychological well-being (Matthews & Nazroo, 2021).

Age-Stratification Theory

Age-stratification theory (Marshall, 1996) goes beyond the individual to the age structure of society. Social institutions such as workplaces or families are partly organized by age; within these institutions, older adults are segregated from younger people (Street, 2007). According to age-stratification theory, older adults can be understood as belonging to specific "birth cohorts" (e.g., "baby boomers") whose members have shared specific historical periods in their lives, and thus share the effect of having lived through similar conditions. They have been exposed to similar events and conditions; have lived under common global, environmental, and political circumstances (Street, 2007); and have had similar racial and cultural experiences (Hooks, 2000). Age norms are socially and culturally based ideas about what is appropriate at a certain age.

The cohort effect can be a powerful tool for understanding the life experiences of people from different cultures and different parts of the world. Structural lag, another concept of the age-stratification theory, "occurs when social structures (e.g., incentives for early retirement) are out of synch with population dynamics (fewer younger workers) and individual lives (increasing life expectancy, later onset of disabilities or frailty)" (Street, 2007, p. 156). Age-stratification theory may be particularly useful for examining aging in a global context.

Social Exchange Theory

Social exchange theory challenges the activity theory. It is based on the consideration of the cost–benefit model of social participation (Dowd, 1980). In social exchange theory, withdrawal or social isolation is the result of an imbalance in the social exchanges between older adults and younger members of society. The balance determines the older adult's personal satisfaction and social support at any point.

Older adults are often viewed as unequal partners in the exchange, and they may need to depend on metaphorical reserves of contributions to the pool of reciprocity. For example, this theory has been used to explain social support in families. In some cultures, there is an expectation that older adults should be cared for in return for their having provided care to others earlier in their lives (Mendez-Luck et al., 2017). It has been noted that "although older individuals may have fewer economic and material resources, they often have nonmaterial resources such as respect, approval, love, wisdom, and time for civic engagement and giving back to society" (Hooyman & Kiyak, 2008, p. 317). Some older adults care for their young grandchildren so that the parents can work; in return, they may receive other support (i.e., room, board, and income). Although this exchange may appear uneven, it can also be viewed from the more holistic perspective of a lifetime of exchanges and contributions. Intergenerational programs in which older and younger people interact, such as older adults volunteering in classrooms, are an example of the value of social exchange between generations.

Modernization Theory

Modernization theory focuses on the social changes that have resulted in the devaluation of the contributions of older adults as well as that of older adults themselves. According to this theory, before 1900, materials and political resources were controlled by the older members of society (Street, 2007). These resources included time, knowledge, skills, and experience. Modernization theory assumes "that there was a gold age of the aged: preindustrial societies where people were revered for their wisdom" (Street, 2007, p. 156). However, according to the modernization theory, the status and thus the value of older adults are lost to society when their labour is no longer considered useful. Kinship networks are dispersed, the information they hold is no longer useful to the society in which they live, and the culture to which they belong no longer reveres them. It has been proposed that these changes are the result of health technology, industrial technology, urbanization, and mass education.

The treatment of older adults in modern Japan was long considered evidence of the inaccuracy of the theory. Historically, older adults in Japan were given the highest status and held the greatest power. This did not seem to change with the industrial advances after World War II. Today, however, Japan is not only a highly modern country from an industrial standpoint; the country also shows signs of "modernization" in social relations with regard to older adults. Researchers have also found support for the modernization theory in other countries, such as India and Taiwan (Dandekar, 1996; Silverman et al., 2000).

Symbolic Interaction Theories

Symbolic interaction theories propose that the aging process a person experiences is a result of interactions between the environment, the person, and the meaning the person attributes to their activities (Gubrium, 1973; Hooyman & Kiyak, 2008). "Whether a new activity increases or decreases life satisfaction depends on an older individual's resources (health, socioeconomic status, and social support), along with the environmental norms for interpreting activities" (Hooyman & Kiyak, 2008, p. 313). With this perspective, one has to examine how the individual's resources and activities, as well as the environmental demands, can be altered to enhance satisfaction and self-concept. For example, if an older adult needs to move to a long-term care home, it is useful to determine how the new environment can be structured to support the person's resources and lifestyle so that they can continue to maintain a positive self-concept and experience life satisfaction and well-being.

IMPLICATIONS FOR GERONTOLOGICAL NURSING AND HEALTHY AGING

Sociological theories of aging give the gerontological nurse useful information and a background for enhancing healthy aging and adaptation (Box 7.1). The theories have been adapted and applied to contemporary approaches to aging in many ways, from the concept of seniors' centres (activity theory) to nursing assessments of social support (social exchange theory). Further research is needed to explore how culture, ethnicity, and gender influence aging and adaptation. Such research is particularly important in light of the growth of the diverse aging population in Canada.

PSYCHOLOGICAL THEORIES OF AGING

Psychological theories of aging presuppose that aging is one of many developmental processes experienced

---

between birth and death. Life, then, is a dynamic process. These theories are widely accepted because of their **face validity**. Like the sociological theories, however, they are not well suited to testing or measurement and do not always address the influence of culture, gender, and ethnicity.

Jung's Theories of Personality

Psychologist Carl Jung, a contemporary of Sigmund Freud, proposed a theory about the development of personality from childhood to old age (Jung, 1971). Jung was one of the first psychologists to regard the second half of life as having a purpose of its own. He noted that the second half of life is often a time of inner discovery, as opposed to the great amount of outward attention demanded by biological and social issues during the first half of life. Ideally, the second half of life is less intensely demanding and allows more time for inner growth, self-awareness, and reflection.

According to this theory, an individual's personality is either extroverted and thus oriented toward the external world or introverted and oriented toward the subjective inner world. Jung suggested that aging results in a movement from extraversion to introversion. Beginning perhaps in midlife, individuals begin to question their own dreams, values, and priorities. The potentially resulting crisis or emotional upheaval is a step in the process of personality development. Jung proposed that with chronological age and personality development, a person is able to move from a focus on outward achievement to an acceptance of the self and to an awareness that both the accomplishments and challenges of one's lifetime can be found within oneself. The development of the psyche and the inner person is accomplished by a search for personal meaning and the spiritual self. This personality of later life can easily be compared to Maslow's theory of self-actualization and Erikson's notion of ego integrity (Erikson, 1963; Maslow, 1968).

Maslow described self-actualization as "the [person's] desire for self-fulfillment, namely, to the tendency for him to become actualized in what he is potentially" (Maslow, 1943, pp. 382–383, in Koltko-Rivera, 2006). When one enters Maslow's hierarchy of self-actualization, they are seeking fulfillment of a personal potential (Gholamnejad et al., 2019). Pursuing spiritual enlightenment, being realistic, remaining autonomous, and maintaining interpersonal

---

BOX 7.1
AREAS OF NURSING ASSESSMENT AND EDUCATION CONSISTENT WITH SOCIOLOGICAL THEORIES OF AGING

- Currently held roles, role satisfaction, and emerging roles (*activity, continuity*).
- Individual's and family's expectations of age norms and the effects of these expectations on self-esteem (*age stratification*).
- Current level of activity and satisfaction with it (*activity*).
- Effect of changes in health on usual roles and activity (*activity, continuity*).
- Cultural beliefs and expectations related to roles and activity, and related engagement and disengagement (*activity, disengagement*).
- Usual life patterns and personality as they influence adaptation to change (*continuity*).
- Historical context of the individual and its potential influence on perception and responses (*age stratification*).
- Complexity of social support and network (*social exchange*).
- Opportunities to contribute knowledge to society (*modernization*).
- Sense of self and self-worth (*continuity, modernization*).

relationships are all examples of traits of someone who is self-actualizing (Gholamnejad et al., 2019).

Developmental Theories

The psychologist Erik Erikson is well known for articulating the developmental stages and tasks of life from early childhood to later "elderhood" (Erikson, 1963). Erikson theorized a predetermined order of development and specific tasks that were associated with specific periods in the course of life. He proposed that one needed to successfully accomplish one task before complete mastery of the next was possible, and he originally articulated these developmental tasks in "either–or" language. He proposed that all people would return again and again to a task that had been poorly resolved in the past. Erikson's task of middle age is generativity; contributing to the future and to future generations in meaningful ways. Failure to accomplish this task results in stagnation. Erikson saw the last stage of life as a vantage point from which one could look back with ego integrity or despair in one's life. *Ego integrity* implies a sense of the completeness and cohesion of the self. In achieving this final task, people can look back on their lives—at the joys, sorrows, mistakes, and successes— and feel satisfied with the way they lived.

In later years, as octogenarians, Erikson and his wife reconsidered his earlier work from the perspective of their own aging. They changed their "either–or" stance of the developmental tasks to the recognition of the balance of each of the tasks. Thus, ego integrity is tinged with some regrets, wisdom is balanced with frivolity, and letting go is balanced with hanging on (Erikson et al., 1986). Mrs. Erikson describes stated, "The more you know yourself, the more patience you have for what you see in others . . . You don't have to accept what people do, but understand what leads them to do it. The stance this leads to is to forgive even though you still oppose" (Goleman, 1988).

Peck (1968), expanding on the work of Erikson, identified the specific tasks of old age that must be addressed in order to establish ego integrity. Peck's tasks, which represent the process or movement toward Erikson's final stage, are as follows:

- *Ego differentiation* versus *work role preoccupation.* The individual is no longer defined by their work.
- *Body transcendence* versus *body preoccupation.* The body is cared for but does not consume the interest and attention of the individual.

- *Ego transcendence* versus *ego preoccupation.* The self becomes less central, and the person feels a part of the mass of humanity, sharing its struggles and its destiny.

Peck's theoretical model states that to achieve ego integrity, one must develop the ability to redefine the self, to let go of occupational identity in order to rise above bodily discomforts, and to establish meanings that go beyond the scope of self-centredness. Although these are admirable and idealistic goals, they place a considerable burden on the older adult. Not everyone may have the courage or the energy to laugh in the face of adversity or surmount all the challenges of old age. The wisdom of old age involves a crisis of understanding in which ordinary structures are shaken and the meaning of life is reexamined; it may or may not include the wisdom of questioning assumptions in the search for meaning in the last stage of life.

Havighurst (1971) is another developmental theorist who has proposed specific tasks to be accomplished in middle age and later maturity. Havighurst's developmental tasks are presented in Box 7.2.

BOX 7.2
HAVIGHURST'S DEVELOPMENTAL TASKS

MIDDLE AGE
- Assisting teenage children with becoming responsible and happy adults.
- Achieving adult social and civic responsibility.
- Reaching and maintaining satisfactory performance in one's occupational career.
- Developing adult leisure-time activities.
- Relating to one's spouse as a person.
- Accepting and adjusting to the physiological changes of middle age.
- Adjusting to aging parents.

LATER MATURITY
- Adjusting to decreasing physical strength and health.
- Adjusting to retirement and reduced income.
- Adjusting to the death of a spouse.
- Establishing an explicit affiliation with one's age group.
- Adopting and adapting social roles in a flexible way.
- Establishing satisfactory living arrangements.

Source: Havighurst, R. (1971). *Developmental tasks and education* (3rd ed.). Longman.

Theory of Gerotranscendence

Tornstam (1994, 1996, 2005) theorized that human aging brings about a general potential for *gerotranscendence*, a gradual and ongoing shift in perspective from the material world to the cosmic world, along with an increasing satisfaction with life. Gerotranscendence is generated by the normal processes of living, sometimes hastened by serious personal disruptions. Similar to Erikson's concept of integrity and Maslow's self-actualization, it is associated with wisdom and spiritual growth. The characteristics of gerotranscendence include the following:

- High degree of satisfaction with life
- Prime motivators other than midlife patterns and ideals
- Complex and active coping patterns
- Greater need for solitary philosophizing, meditation, and solitude
- Satisfaction with self-selected social activities
- Less concern with body image and material possessions
- Decreased fear of death
- Affinity with past and future generations, and
- Decreased self-centredness and increased altruism.

IMPLICATIONS FOR GERONTOLOGICAL NURSING AND HEALTHY AGING

Knowledge about lifespan development and the various ways in which people experience aging can help gerontological nurses understand the meaning of healthy aging for each person. Future generations of older adults will likely redefine what are now considered the norms for aging. People can expect to spend 30 or more years in "late life," and there are many important tasks to accomplish during this period.

SPIRITUALITY AND AGING

Spirituality is defined as "the intangible and immaterial and thus may be considered more of a general term, not associated with a particular group or organization. It can refer to feelings, thoughts, experiences, and behaviours related to the soul or to a search for the sacred" (Kaplan & Berkman, 2019). The spiritual aspect of people's lives transcends the physical and psychosocial

realms and reaches the deepest capacity for love, hope, and meaning.

Spirituality is a significant factor in understanding healthy aging. The model of successful aging proposed by Rowe and Kahn (1998) includes active engagement in life, minimal risk and disability, and high cognitive and physical function. Crowther et al. (2002) maintained that spirituality is the fourth integrated element of this model. Research has found that spirituality is associated with life satisfaction, over and above any other factors that influence healthy aging (Hosseini et al., 2019).

Spirituality and the religious practices of older adults are linked to positive health outcomes in regard to life expectancy, cardiovascular conditions, chronic conditions, disability, and mental health (Hosseini et al., 2019). The effects of religious practice on health outcomes may partly result from the social support obtained through religious communities. Canadian researchers who interviewed religious leaders and older churchgoers found that attending religious services has a direct effect on a person's mental health and also provides social connections, social activity, and social support (Hosseini et al., 2019).

Spirituality and religious practice may be particularly important to healthy aging (Kaplan & Berkman, 2019). Declining physical health, loss of loved ones, and a realization that life's end may be near often challenge older adults to reflect on the meaning of their lives, and spirituality may become more important (Harrington, 2016). Older Canadians are more likely than younger Canadians to report a religious affiliation (92% versus 76%, respectively) (Statistics Canada, 2016). Canadian researchers have found that spirituality and religion are important for older adults who are caring for a relative who has dementia (Hosseini et al., 2019).

IMPLICATIONS FOR GERONTOLOGICAL NURSING AND HEALTHY AGING

Gerontological nurses have many opportunities to help older adults reflect on the meaning and purpose of life and achieve spiritual well-being. Spiritual well-being can be considered the ability to experience and integrate meaning and purpose in life through connectedness with self, others, art, music, literature, nature, or a power greater than oneself.

Assessment

Older adults often welcome a discussion of spiritual matters, and some want health care providers to consider their spiritual needs. Some older adults may have a pressing need to talk about philosophy and spiritual development. Private time for prayer, meditation, and reflection may be needed. Nurses who neglect exploring this issue with older adults may do so because they perceive that religion and spirituality is not a priority. The older adult should be assured that religious longings and rituals are important and that opportunities to fulfill these longings or practice rituals can be made available as desired. Nurses must be knowledgeable about and respectful of various cultural beliefs, values, and religious rites and rituals; they must also understand age-related or generational differences in religious practices. It is important for the nurse to avoid imposing their own beliefs and to respect the older adult's privacy in matters of spirituality and religion (College of Nurses of Ontario, 2019).

The FICA spiritual assessment tool is a comprehensive, evidence-informed guideline to promote spirituality in the older adult (Puchalski, 1996–2021). The acronym "FICA" is used to recall what to ask during a spiritual history. The FICA tool is described in Box 7.3. Its use identifies older adults who may be at risk of spiritual distress (Box 7.4). Spiritual distress is "the impaired ability to experience and integrate meaning or purpose in life through connectedness with self, others, art, music, literature, nature, and/or a power greater than oneself" (Hall et al., 2019). The person experiencing spiritual distress is unable to experience hope, connectedness, and transcendence. Spiritual distress may manifest as anger, guilt, blame, hatred, expressions of alienation, turning away from others, an inability to enjoy, and an inability to participate in religious and spiritual activities and rituals that have provided comfort.

Interventions

Religious and spiritual resources, such as pastoral visits, should be available in all settings where older adults reside.

Caring relationships between the nurse and the older adult being cared for are at the heart of nursing that touches and supports the spirit. In one study by Desmet and colleagues (2020), four categories of spiritual needs were identified through an integrative literature review

---

BOX 7.3
FICA SPIRITUAL HISTORY TOOL

F—Faith, Belief, Meaning: Determine whether or not the patient identifies with a particular belief system or spirituality at all.
"Do you consider yourself to be spiritual?"
"Is spirituality something important to you?"
"What gives your life meaning?"
I—Importance and Influence: Understand the importance of spirituality in the patient's life and the influence on healthcare decisions.
"Has your spirituality influenced how you take care of yourself, particularly regarding your health?"
"Does your spirituality affect your healthcare decision making?"
C—Community: Find out if the patient is part of a spiritual community, or if they rely on their community for support.
"Are you part of a spiritual community?"
"Is your community of support to you and how?" (If they don't identify with a community, you can ask, "Is there a group of people you really love or who are important to you?")
A—Address/Action in Care: Learn how to address spiritual issues with regards to caring for the patient.
"How would you like me, as your healthcare provider, to address spiritual issues in your healthcare?"

Source: Adapted from Puchalski, C. (1996–2021). *The © FICA Spiritual History Tool: A guide for spiritual assessment in clinical settings.* https://smhs.gwu.edu/spirituality-health/sites/spirituality-health/files/FICA-PDF-Final-Nov2020.pdf.

BOX 7.4
INDICATIONS OF RISK OF SPIRITUAL DISTRESS

- Feelings of anger or hopelessness
- Difficulty sleeping
- Feelings of depression
- Feelings of anxiety
- Feeling abandoned by God
- Questioning the meaning of life or suffering
- Questioning beliefs or sudden doubt in spiritual or religious beliefs
- Asking why this situation occurred
- Seeking spiritual help or guidance

Source: Adapted from Crossroads Hospice & Palliative Care. (2018, October 10). *Signs and symptoms of spiritual distress.* https://www.crossroadshospice.com/hospice-palliative-care-blog/2018/october/10/signs-and-symptoms-of-spiritual-distress/.

of studies focusing on hospitalized older adults. The four categories include the following:

1. The need to be connected with others or with God/the transcendent/the divine
2. Religious needs
3. The need to find meaning in life, and
4. The need for maintaining identity.

Desmet and colleagues (2020) also highlighted the importance of assessing spiritual needs in order to provide the best comprehensive spiritual care. Knowing a person in their complexity, responding to that which matters most to the person, identifying and nurturing connections, listening, using presence and silence, and fostering connections to that which is sacred to the person are spiritual nursing responses that arise from a caring, connected relationship (Touhy, 2001). Suggestions for spiritual responses are presented in Box 7.5.

COGNITION AND AGING

Cognition is both a biological and a psychological factor that must be considered in caring for the older

---

BOX 7.5
SPIRITUAL RESPONSES

- Regard spirituality as a potentially important component of every patient's physical well-being and mental health.
- Address spirituality at each complete physical examination and continue addressing it at follow-up visits if appropriate. In patient care, spirituality is an ongoing issue.
- If a patient presents with distress, always assess for psycho-social and spiritual distress as well as physical.
- Respect a patient's privacy regarding spiritual beliefs; don't impose your beliefs on others.
- Make referrals to chaplains, spiritual directors, or community resources as appropriate.
- Be aware that your own spiritual beliefs will help you personally and will overflow in your encounters with those for whom you care to make the clinician–patient encounter a more humanistic one.

Source: Adapted from Puchalski, C. (1996–2021). *The © FICA Spiritual History Tool: A guide for spiritual assessment in clinical settings.* https://smhs.gwu.edu/spirituality-health/sites/spirituality-health/files/FICA-PDF-Final-Nov2020.pdf.

---

adult. This chapter discusses the processes of normal cognition and learning in late life. Care of older adults with impaired cognition is discussed in Chapter 21. Cognition is the "mental processes involved in acquiring and processing information that are necessary for everyday living" (Magni & Bilotta, 2016, p. 411).

Early studies about cognition and aging were based on **cross-sectional** rather than **longitudinal research** and were often conducted with older adults who were in an institution or who had coexisting illnesses. It has been generally believed that cognitive function declines in old age because of a shrinking hippocampus and the wearing down of the myelin sheath that surrounds and protects nerve fibers, which can slow the speed of communication between neurons. Some of the receptors on the surface of neurons that enable them to communicate with one another may not function as well as they once did. These changes can affect the person's ability to encode new information into the memory and retrieve information that is already in storage. On the other hand, researchers have found that in later life, the branching of dendrites can increase, and connections between distant brain areas can strengthen (Harvard University, 2017). These changes enable the aging brain to become better at detecting relationships between diverse sources of information, capturing the big picture, and understanding the global implications of specific issues; perhaps this is the foundation of wisdom. It is as if, with age, the brain becomes better at seeing the entire forest and worse at seeing the leaves (Harvard University, 2017).

The aging brain maintains resiliency (the ability to compensate for age-related changes). The old adage "use it or lose it" applies to cognitive as well as physical health. Stimulating the brain increases brain tissue formation, enhances the synaptic regulation of messages, and enhances the development of *cognitive reserve*. Cognitive reserve is based on the concept of neuroplasticity, which is the capacity of the brain to change in response to various stimuli, such as daily stressors and activities. Neuroplasticity was once thought to decrease with age, but current literature (National Institute on Aging, 2020) suggests that cognitive performance can be enhanced with mental stimulation. Maximizing the potential benefits of brain plasticity and cognitive reserve requires engaging in challenging cognitive, sensory, and motor activities, as well as meaningful social interactions, on a regular basis throughout life.

Many myths about aging and the brain may be believed by both health care providers and older adults. It is important to understand late-life cognition, memory, and learning, as well as to dispel myths that have a negative effect on wellness and that may in fact contribute to unnecessary cognitive decline.

Later life is no longer seen as a period when growth has ceased and cognitive development has halted; rather, it is seen as a life stage programmed for plasticity and the development of unique capacities. Older adults do maintain their ability to understand situations and learn from new experiences. These findings are significant to satisfaction in later life because the capacity for effective lifestyle management and one's cognitive resources contribute to adaptation and enjoyment. Brain function that becomes impaired in old age is a result of disease or illness, not aging.

Fluid and Crystallized Intelligence

Fluid intelligence (often called *native intelligence*) is biologically determined and independent of experiences or learning. It is associated with flexibility in thinking, inductive reasoning, abstract thinking, and integration; it helps people identify and draw conclusions about complex relationships. Fluid intelligence is related to learning and problem solving in novel situations. *Crystallized intelligence* comprises knowledge and abilities that a person acquires through education and life. Measures of crystallized intelligence include verbal meaning, word association, social judgement, and number skills. The performance of older adults declines on scales measuring fluid intelligence, but is stable on verbal scales (crystallized intelligence). This phenomenon is known as the *classic aging pattern* (Botwinick, 1977; Hooyman & Kiyak, 2008). The tendency to decline in performance tasks may be related to age-related changes in sensory and perceptual abilities as well as psychomotor skills. Lower cognitive processing speed and slower reaction time also affect performance.

Memory

Memory is the ability to retain or store information and retrieve it when needed. Memory is a complex set of processes and storage systems. Three components characterize memory: immediate recall, short-term memory (ranging from minutes to days), and remote or long-term memory (Family Practice Notebook,

2021). Biological, functional, environmental, and psychosocial influences affect memory development throughout adulthood. *Immediate recall* of newly encountered information seems to decrease with age, and declines in memory are noted in connection with complex tasks and strategies. Even though some older adults show decrements in reaction time, perception, the capacity for attentional tasks, and the ability to process information, most functioning remains intact and sufficient. *Recall of long-term events*, familiarity, previous learning, and life experience compensate for the minor loss of efficiency in the basic neurological processes. In unfamiliar, stressful, or demanding situations, however, these changes may be more marked.

Age-associated decline in memory is a major focus of research on aging and dementia. Healthy older adults may complain of memory problems, but their symptoms do not meet the criteria for mild cognitive impairment or dementia (see Chapter 21). *Age-associated memory impairment* is memory loss that is considered normal in light of a person's age and education level.

Many medical or psychiatric difficulties, such as depression and anxiety, also influence memory and concentration. Thus, it is important for older adults who have memory concerns to have a comprehensive geriatric assessment and evaluation. In some cases, memory impairment is related to reversible and treatable conditions such as delirium, thyroid disease, injury, infection, depression, untreated diabetes, vitamin B12 deficiency, and anxiety. The assessment of cognitive function is discussed in Chapter 21.

IMPLICATIONS FOR GERONTOLOGICAL NURSING AND HEALTHY AGING

Nurses can educate people of all ages about effective strategies to enhance cognitive health and vitality and how to promote cognitive reserve and brain plasticity. Suggested strategies include preventing and managing chronic conditions, maintaining a healthy weight, avoiding excess caloric intake, limiting sodium and fat intake, being physically active, participating in mentally stimulating activity, and engaging in social contact (National Institute on Aging, 2020).

Older adults should remain active and engaged in activities that stimulate the mind as well as the body.

Cognitive stimulation and memory training may be helpful for cognitively intact older adults, as well as for those with cognitive impairment (Djabelkhir et al., 2017). Cognitive stimulation and memory training techniques include mnemonics (strategies to enhance coding, storage, and recall), internal and external aids, reasoning and speed-of-processing training, cognitive games (e.g., Scrabble, chess, crossword puzzles), and spaced retrieval techniques (in which information is recalled over increasing lengths of time, such as 1 minute, 2 minutes, 4 minutes, and longer).

LEARNING IN LATE LIFE

Basic intelligence remains unchanged with increasing years, and older adults should be given opportunities for continued learning. **Geragogy** is the application of the principles of adult learning theory to teaching for older adults. Teaching for older adults should be relevant; new learning should be related to what is already known and should emphasize concrete and practical information. Box 7.6 presents additional strategies for enhancing the learning of older adults.

Opportunities for older adults to learn are available in many formal and informal modes: self-teaching, college and university classes, seminars and conferences, public broadcasting television programs, DVDs, web-based courses, and countless other modes. Older adults are able to learn and to reap the benefits of learning—improved health, life satisfaction, coping abilities, friendships, joy, and satisfaction from learning (Narushima et al., 2018) (Box 7.7). The benefits of engaging in lifelong learning are greater for vulnerable older adults (Narushima et al., 2018).

The Internet is one of the major vehicles of learning for older adults, and older adults make up the

---

BOX 7.6
STRATEGIES TO ENHANCE THE LEARNING OF OLDER ADULTS

- Make sure the person is ready to learn before trying to teach them. Watch for cues that may indicate that the person is preoccupied or too anxious to comprehend the material.
- Be sensitive to cultural, language, and other differences among the older adults you serve. Some suggestions may not be appropriate for everyone.
- Provide adequate time for learning, and use self-pacing techniques.
- Create a shame-free environment in which older adults feel free to ask questions and stay informed.
- Provide regular positive feedback.
- Avoid distractions, and present one idea at a time.
- Present pertinent, specific, practical, and individualized information. Emphasize concrete rather than abstract material.
- Use past experience; connect new learning to what has already been learned.
- Use written material to supplement verbal instruction. Use a list format; a vocabulary for low literacy levels; and large, readable font (e.g., 14- to 16-point Arial).

- Use high-contrast visual materials and handouts (e.g., black print on white paper).
- Consider using Braille and digitally recorded material whenever necessary.
- Pay attention to reading ability. Use tools other than printed material, such as drawings, pictures, and discussion.
- Use point form or lists to highlight pertinent information.
- Sit facing the person so they can watch your lip movements and facial expressions.
- Speak slowly.
- Keep the pitch of your voice low. Older adults hear low-frequency sounds better than they hear high-frequency sounds.
- Encourage the learner to develop various mediators or mnemonic devices (e.g., visual images, rhymes, acronyms, and self-designed coding schemes).
- Have shorter, more frequent sessions with appropriate breaks. Pay attention to fatigue and physical discomfort.

Source: Adapted from SPRY Foundation. (1999). *Bridging principles of older adult learning: Reconnaissance phase final report*; Hayes, K. (2005). Designing written medication instructions: Effective ways to help older adults self-medicate. *Journal of Gerontological Nursing, 32*(5), 5–10. doi:10.3928/0098-9134-20050501-04.

BOX 7.7

RESEARCH FOR EVIDENCE-INFORMED PRACTICE: LIFELONG LEARNING IN ACTIVE AGEING DISCOURSE: ITS LIFELONG EFFECT ON WELL-BEING, HEALTH, AND VULNERABILITY

Problem: It is important to understand the effect of older adults' participation in lifelong learning on their psychological well-being. Researchers also wanted to determine whether the duration of the program made a difference in psychological well-being.

Methods: The sample of the study included learners aged 60 years old or older who enrolled in a continuing education program. The program offered noncredit courses in four subject areas: (a) arts and crafts, (b) fitness and exercise, (c) music and dance, and (d) language, computer, and other practical skills. Questionnaires were completed that asked for information such as demographic, health-related information, and general psychological well-being questions. Psychological well-being, vulnerability level, self-rated health, and duration of learning were measured.

Findings: A total of 416 participants were included in the study. Most participants were female. Those who had a higher level of vulnerability were more likely to be distressed when compared to those with a lower level of vulnerability. There was an association between continuous participation in the courses and psychological well-being of older adults. Researchers found that the longer the participant pursued one course, the better the psychological well-being they reported.

Implications for Nursing Practice: The major benefits of learning identified in this study are all factors that promote psychosocial health. Researchers found that meaningful social participation enhanced psychological well-being and quality of life in older adults. Lifelong learning and continuing to pursue a course is associated with psychological well-being. Nurses can take these findings into consideration when discussing social activity options with older adults.

Source: Narushima, M., Liu, J., Diestelkamp, N. (2018). Lifelong learning in active ageing discourse: Its conserving effect on wellbeing, health and vulnerability. *Ageing and Society, 38*(4), 651–675. doi:10.1017/S0144686X16001136.

fastest-growing group using social networking sites such as Facebook. Internet use among older adults aged 65 years and older doubled from 2007 (32%) to 2016 (68%) (Davidson & Schimmele, 2019). Older adults are increasingly taking charge of their own learning and are scanning the Internet for information about health and lifestyles. There are many reliable Internet resources related to health and aging. Examples include the websites of Health Canada (https://www.canada.ca/en/health-canada/services/healthy-living/seniors.html), the Public Health Agency of Canada (https://www.canada.ca/en/public-health/services/health-promotion/aging-seniors.html), the Government of Canada's Programs and Services for Seniors (https://www.canada.ca/en/employment-social-development/campaigns/seniors.html) and the US National Institute on Aging (http://www.nia.nih.gov/health/).

Health Literacy

Health literacy is the ability to access, understand, and act on information concerning health. Health literacy is more than the ability to read and write. It includes listening skills, the ability to speak and communicate health needs, and the ability to act on written health information and instructions from health care providers. Factors influencing health literacy include the person's basic literacy skills and culture, the situations encountered in the health care system, and the cultural competence and communication skills of health care providers.

Six of ten adult Canadians do not have proficient health literacy. Literacy levels are lower for older adults (The University of British Columbia, 2016). Average health literacy varies among provinces and territories; the highest level is in Yukon and the lowest level is in Nunavut. Especially in the older population, lower literacy levels are found among those with less than a high school education. Chronic health conditions and vision and hearing impairments may further limit health literacy.

Limited literacy skills influence the learning and understanding of health-related information, such as prescription directions, consent documents, and health education materials. The consequences of limited literacy may include poorer health, poorer compliance with instructions, and increased hospitalizations. Agarwal and colleagues (2018) found an association between poor health literacy and pain and discomfort.

Health literacy experts recommend the "teach-back" method of health education, which results in better understanding and retention of information (Yen & Leasure, 2019). Using this method, the nurse breaks down the teaching into small chunks and then verifies the person's understanding by asking the person to explain what they need to do. It must be emphasized that it is the nurse's responsibility to explain the material clearly; the checking of the person's understanding is not a test. If needed, the nurse follows up by explaining again and checking understanding again. The 10 principles of the teach-back method are presented in Box 7.8. The Agency for Healthcare Research and Quality health literacy toolkit website has links to excellent online information about the teach-back method (https://www.ahrq.gov/professionals/quality-patient-safety/quality-resources/tools/literacy-toolkit/healthlittoolkit2-tool5.html).

IMPLICATIONS FOR GERONTOLOGICAL NURSING AND HEALTHY AGING

Caring for older adults means caring for body, mind, and spirit—holistic nursing at its finest. Understanding and appreciating the social, psychological, spiritual, and cognitive aspects of aging provides a foundation for nursing assessments and interventions that enhance lifelong growth, development, health, and well-being. A rich and stimulating environment should be available to all older adults in all care settings so that they can thrive, not merely survive, in old age.

BOX 7.8
TEN ELEMENTS OF THE TEACH-BACK METHOD OF HEALTH EDUCATION

1. Use a caring tone of voice and attitude.
2. Display comfortable body language and make eye contact.
3. Use plain language.
4. Ask the patient to explain back using their own words.
5. Use nonshaming, open-ended questions.
6. Avoid asking questions that can be answered with a simple "yes" or "no."
7. Emphasize that the responsibility to explain clearly is on you, the provider.
8. If the patient is not able to teach back correctly, explain again and re-check.
9. Use reader-friendly print materials to support learning.
10. Document use of and patient's response to teach-back.

Source: Adapted from Iowa Health System, Picker Institute, Des Moines University, and Health Literacy Iowa. (n.d.). *Always Use Teach-Back! Ten Elements of Competence for Using Teach-back Effectively.* http://www.teachbacktraining.org/assets/files/PDFS/Teach%20Back%20-%2010%20Elements%20of%20Competence.pdf.

KEY CONCEPTS

- Normal aging involves a gradual process of biopsychosocial change over time.
- Lifespan development theorists tend to study the total life course of cohort groups to determine the influence of major historical events on their development.
- The impact of gender, ethnicity, culture, and cohort must always be considered when discussing the validity of biopsychosocial theories.
- Spirituality is considered a significant factor in healthy aging.
- Late adulthood is seen as a life stage programmed for plasticity and the development of unique capacities.
- Cognitive stimulation and attention to brain health is just as important as attention to physical health.
- Learning in late life can be enhanced by using principles of geragogy and adapting teaching strategies to minimize barriers such as hearing and vision impairment and low literacy levels.

ACTIVITIES AND DISCUSSION QUESTIONS

1. Identify and discuss some flaws in the sociological theories of aging.

2. How well do the psychological and sociological theories of aging align with your own cultural perspective?

3. Discuss the variables that must constantly be considered when the psychosocial aspects of the aging experience are assessed. Identify and discuss those that seem most significant.

4. Discuss some of the problems of adequately testing cognitive function in an older adult.

5. How would you respond to the following myth of aging: "You can't teach an old dog new tricks."

6. Identify and discuss strategies you can use to dispel myths about older adults' adaptability, intelligence, activity, social relationships, and productivity.

7. Discuss some ways that nurses can respond to the spiritual needs and concerns of older adults.

8. Practice using the teach-back method with classmates.

RESOURCES

Agency for Healthcare Research and Quality. *Use the teach-back method.*
https://www.ahrq.gov/professionals/quality-patient-safety/quality-resources/tools/literacy-toolkit/healthlittoolkit2-tool5.html

Alzheimer Society of Canada. *Challenging your brain.*
https://alzheimer.ca/en/help-support/im-living-dementia/living-well-dementia/challenging-your-brain

Government of British Columbia. *Active aging.*
http://www2.gov.bc.ca/gov/content/family-social-supports/seniors/health-safety/active-aging

National Institute on Aging. *Health information (senior health: age pages and convenient one-page information sheets on health and aging).*
https://www.nia.nih.gov/health

Public Health Agency of Canada. *Age-Friendly Communities Initiative.*
https://www.canada.ca/en/public-health/services/health-promotion/aging-seniors/friendly-communities.html

The Hartford Institute for Geriatric Nursing. *FICA spiritual history tool.*
https://consultgeri.org/try-this/specialty-practice/issue-sp5

World Health Organization. *Age-friendly world.*
https://extranet.who.int/agefriendlyworld/

For additional resources, please visit *http://evolve.elsevier.com/Canada/Ebersole/gerontological/*

REFERENCES

Agarwal, G., Habing, K., Pirrie, M., et al. (2018). Assessing health literacy among older adults living in subsidized housing: A cross-sectional study. *Canadian Journal of Public Health*, 109, 401–409. doi:10.17269/s41997-018-0048-3.

Atchley, R. C. (2000). A continuity theory of normal aging. In J. F. Gubrium & J. A. Holstein (Eds.), *Aging and everyday life*. Blackwell Publishers.

Baltes, P. B. (1987). Theoretical propositions on life-span developmental theory: On the dynamics between growth and decline. *Developmental Psychology*, 23(5), 611–626. doi:10.1037/0012-1649.23.5.611.

Baltes, P. B., Lindenberger, U., & Staudinger, U. (1998). Life span theory in developmental psychology. In R. Lerner (Ed.), *Handbook of child psychology (Vol. 1): Theoretical models of human development* (pp. 569–664). John Wiley & Sons.

Botwinick, J. (1977). Intellectual abilities. In J. E. Birren & K. W. Schaie (Eds.), *Handbook of the psychology of aging* (pp. 580–605). Van Nostrand Reinhold.

Carr, K., & Weir, P. L. (2017). A qualitative description of successful aging through different decades of older adulthood. *Aging & Mental Health*, 21(12), 1317–1325. doi:10.1080/136077863.2016.1226764.

College of Nurses of Ontario. (2019). *Code of conduct.* https://www.cno.org/globalassets/docs/prac/49040_code-of-conduct.pdf.

Crowther, M., Parker, M., Achenbaum, W., et al. (2002). Rowe and Kahn's model of successful aging revisited: Positive spirituality—the forgotten factor. *Gerontologist*, 42(5), 613–620. doi:10.1093/geront/42.5.613.

Dandekar, K. (1996). *The elderly in India.* Sage.

Dause, T. J., & Kirby, E. D. (2019). Aging gracefully: Social engagement joins exercise and enrichment as a key lifestyle factor in resistance to age-related cognitive decline. *Neural Regeneration Research*, 14(1), 39. doi:10.4103/1673-5374.243698.

Davidson, J., & Schimmele, C. (2019). *Evolving Internet use among Canadian seniors.* https://www150.statcan.gc.ca/n1/pub/11f0019m/11f0019m2019015-eng.htm.

Desmet, L., Dezutter, J., Vandenhoeck, A., et al. (2020). Spiritual needs of older adults during hospitalization: An integrative review. *Religions*, 11, 529. doi:10.3390/rel11100529.

Djabelkhir, L., Wu, Y., Vidal, J. S., et al. (2017). Computerized cognitive stimulation and engagement programs in older adults with mild cognitive impairment: Comparing feasibility, acceptability, and cognitive psychosocial effects. *Clinical Interventions in Aging, 12,* 1967–1975. doi:10.2147/CIA.S145769.

Dowd, J. J. (1980). *Stratification among the aged.* Brooks Cole.

Erikson, E. H. (1963). *Childhood and society* (2nd ed.). W.W. Norton.

Erikson, E. H., Erikson, J. M., & Kivnick, H. Q. (1986). *Vital involvement in old age: The experience of old age in our time.* W.W. Norton.

Family Practice Notebook. (2021). *Memory evaluation.* https://fpnotebook.com/neuro/exam/MmryEvltn.htm.

Gholamnejad, H., Darvishpoor-Kakhki, A., Ahmadi, F., et al. (2019). Self-actualization: Self-care outcomes among elderly patients with hypertension. *Iranian Journal of Nursing and Midwifery Research, 24*(3), 206–212. doi:10.4103/ijnmr.IJNMK_95_18.

Goleman, D. (1988, June 14). Erikson, in his own old age, expands his view of life. *The New York Times.* https://www.nytimes.com/1988/06/14/science/erikson-in-his-own-old-age-expands-his-view-of-life.html.

Government of Canada. (2016). *Age-friendly communities.* https://www.canada.ca/en/public-health/services/health-promotion/aging-seniors/friendly-communities.html.

Gubrium, J. F. (1973). *The myth of the golden years.* Charles C. Thomas.

Harrington, A. (2016). The importance of spiritual assessment when caring for older adults. *Ageing & Society, 36,* 1–16. doi:10.1017/S0144688X14001007.

Hall, E., Hughes, B. P., & Handzo, G. (2019). Time to follow the evidence—Spiritual care in health care. *Ethics, Medicine and Public Health, 9,* 45–56. doi:10.1016/j.jemep.2019.04.011.

Harvard University. (2017, August 30). *How memory and thinking ability change with age.* https://www.health.harvard.edu/mind-and-mood/how-memory-and-thinking-ability-change-with-age.

Havighurst, R. (1971). *Developmental tasks and education* (3rd ed.). Longman.

Hooks, B. (2000). *Feminist theory: From margin to center.* South End Press.

Hooyman, N., & Kiyak, H. (2008). *Social gerontology* (8th ed.). Pearson.

Hosseini, S., Chaurasia, A., & Oremus, M. (2019). The effect of religion and spirituality on cognitive function: A systematic review. *Gerontologist, 59*(2), e76–e85.

Jakovljevic, D. G. (2018). Physical activity and cardiovascular aging: Physiological and molecular insights. *Experimental Gerontology, 109,* 67–74.

Johnson, E. (2013). Face validity. In F. R. Volkmar (Ed.), *Encyclopedia of autism spectrum disorders.* Springer. doi:10.1007/978-1-4419-1698-3.

Jung, C. (1971). The stages of life (R. F. C. Hull, Trans.). In J. Campbell (Ed.), *The portable Jung* (pp. 3–22). Viking Press. (Original work published 1928.)

Kaplan, D. B., & Berkman, B. J. (2019). *Religion and spirituality in older adults.* https://www.merckmanuals.com/professional/geriatrics/social-issues-in-older-adults/religion-and-spirituality-in-older-adults.

Koltko-Rivera, M. E. (2006). Rediscovering the later version of Maslow's hierarchy of needs: Self-transcendence and opportunities for theory, research and unification. *Review of General Psychology, 10*(4), 302–317. doi:10.1037/1089-2680.10.4.302.

Lerner, R. M. (2002). *Concepts and theories of human development* (3rd ed.). Lawrence Erlbaum Associates.

Maddox, G. (1963). Activity and morale: A longitudinal study of selected elderly subjects. *Social Forces, 42*(2), 195–204. doi:10.1093/sf/42.2.195.

Magni, G., & Bilotta, F. (2016). Chapter 41: Postoperative cognitive dysfunction. *Complications in Neuroanesthesia,* 411–427. doi:10.1016/B978-0-12-804075-1.00041-9.

Marshall, V. (1996). The state of theory in aging and the social sciences. In R. H. Binstock & L. K. Geroge (Eds.), *Handbook of aging and the social sciences* (4th ed., pp. 12–30). Academic Press.

Maslow, A. H. (1968). *Toward a psychology of being.* Van Nostrand.

Matthews, K., & Nazroo, J. (2021). The impact of volunteering and its characteristics on well-being after state pension age: Longitudinal evidence from the English Longitudinal Study of Ageing. *Journals of Gerontology: Series B, 76*(3), 632–641. doi:10.1093/geronb/gbaa146.

Mejía, S. T., Ryan, L. H., Gonzalez, R., et al. (2017). Successful aging as the intersection of individual resources, age, environment, and experiences of well-being in daily activities. *Journals of Gerontology: Series B, 72*(2), 279–289. doi:10.1093/geronb/gbw148.

Mendez-Luck, C. A., Amorim, C., Anthony, K. P., et al. (2017). Beliefs and expectations of family and nursing home care among Mexican-origin caregivers. *Journal of Women & Aging, 29*(5), 460–472.

Narushima, M., Liu, J., & Diestelkamp, N. (2018). Lifelong learning in active ageing discourse: Its conserving effect on wellbeing, health and vulnerability. *Ageing and Society, 38*(4), 651–675. doi:10.1017/S0144686X16001136.

National Institute on Aging. (2020). *Cognitive health and older adults.* https://www.nia.nih.gov/health/cognitive-health-and-older-adults.

Papalia, D., Sterns, H., Feldman, R., et al. (2002). *Adult development and aging.* McGraw-Hill.

Peck, R. (1968). Psychological developments in the second half of life. In B. Neugarten (Ed.), *Middle age and aging* (pp. 88–92). University of Chicago Press.

Public Health Agency of Canada. (2016). *Age-friendly communities initiative.* http://www.phac-aspc.gc.ca/seniors-aines/afc-caa-eng.php.

Puchalski, C. (1996–2021). *The © FICA spiritual history tool: A guide for spiritual assessment in clinical settings.* https://smhs.gwu.edu/spirituality-health/sites/spirituality-health/files/FICA-PDF-Final-Nov2020.pdf.

Rantanen, T., Pynnönen, K., Saajanaho, M., et al. (2019). Individualized counselling for active aging: Protocol of a single-blinded, randomized controlled trial among older people (the AGNES intervention study). *BMC Geriatrics, 19*(1), 5. doi:10.1186/s12877-018-1012-z.

Revera. (2019, June 20). *Living a life of purpose: New research shows Canadian seniors volunteer more time and money than any other age group.* https://cdn.reveraliving.com/-/media/files/news-releases/missing-files/2019/jun-20-2019reverareportonaginglivingalifeofpurpose.pdf.

Rowe, J. W., & Kahn, R. L. (1998). *Successful aging.* Pantheon Books.

Silverman, P., Hecht, L., & McMillin, J. (2000). Modeling life satisfaction among the aged: A comparison of Chinese and Americans. *Journal of Cross-Cultural Gerontology, 15*(4), 289. doi:10.1023/A:1006793304508.

Statistics Canada. (2016). *Religion (108), immigrant status and period of immigration (11), age groups (10) and sex (3) for the population in private households of Canada, provinces, territories, census metropolitan areas and census agglomerations, 2011 National Household Survey.* https://www12.statcan.gc.ca/nhs-enm/2011/dp-pd/dt-td/Rp-eng.cfm?LANG=E&APATH=3&DETAIL=0&DIM=0&FL=A&FREE=0&GC=0&GID=0&GK=0&GRP=0&PID=105399&PRID=0&PTYPE=105277&S=0&SHOWALL=0&SUB=0&Temporal=2013&THEME=95&VID=0.

Street, D. A. (2007). Sociological approaches to understanding age and aging. In J. A. Blackburn & C. N. Dulmus (Eds.), *Handbook of gerontology: Evidence based approaches to theory, practice, and policy* (pp. 143–168). John Wiley & Sons.

The University of British Columbia. (2016). *Health literacy in Canada.* https://wiki.ubc.ca/Health_Literacy_in_Canada.

Tornstam, L. (1994). Gerotranscendence: A theoretical and empirical exploration. In L. E. Thomas & S. A. Eisenhandler (Eds.), *Aging and the religious dimension* (pp. 203–225). Greenwood Publishing Group.

Tornstam, L. (1996). Gerotranscendence: A theory about maturing into old age. *Journal of Aging & Identity, 1*(1), 37–50.

Tornstam, L. (2005). *Gerotranscendence: A developmental theory of positive aging.* Springer.

Touhy, T. (2001). Nurturing hope and spirituality in the nursing home. *Holistic Nursing Practice, 15*(4), 45–56. doi:10.1097/00004650-200107000-00008.

World Health Organization. (2021). *Global Age-Friendly Cities Project: A guide.* https://www.who.int/ageing/publications/Global_age_friendly_cities_Guide_English.pdf.

Yen, P. H., & Leasure, A. R. (2019). Use and effectiveness of the teach-back method in patient education and health outcomes. *Federal Practitioner, 36*(6), 284–289.

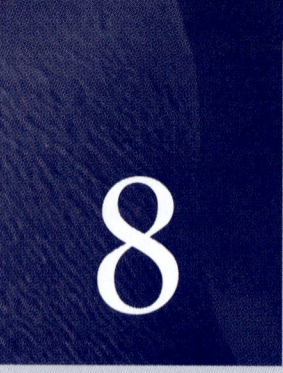

8

NUTRITIONAL NEEDS

LEARNING OBJECTIVES

Upon completion of this chapter, the reader will be able to:

- Assess nutritional requirements.
- Identify factors affecting nutrition.
- Discuss nursing interventions to promote nutrition.
- Discuss assessment and interventions for older adults with dysphagia.
- Identify strategies to promote adequate nutrition for older adults who are experiencing physical and cognitive impairments or are in an institution or hospital.
- Discuss nursing interventions that promote good oral hygiene.
- Discuss nursing interventions to promote healthy bowel function.
- Discuss assessments and interventions for older adults with malnutrition.

GLOSSARY

Dysphagia The sensation of impaired passage of food from the mouth to the esophagus and stomach; difficulty swallowing.

Gastro-esophageal reflux disease (GERD) The backward flow of stomach contents into the esophagus.

Xerostomia Excessive mouth dryness.

THE LIVED EXPERIENCE

"If I do reach the point when I can no longer feed myself, I hope that the hands holding my fork belong to someone who has a feeling for who I am. I hope

my helper will remember what she learns about me. If she would talk to me, if we could laugh together, I might even forget the chagrin of my useless hands. We could have a conversation rather than a feeding."

From Lustbader, W. (1999). Thoughts on the meaning of frailty. *Generations, 13*(4), 21–22.

HEALTHY AGING CARE PLAN

About D.M.

D.M. (pronouns he/him) is 82 and lives at home. You are a registered nurse who has come to visit D.M. in order to assess his needs for home care services. During your conversation with and observation of D.M., you notice that he is fairly independent. D.M. has well-managed osteoarthritis and is hard of hearing. He is not taking any medications except for acetaminophen for his osteoarthritis. You observe that his pants seem a bit loose on him. You also notice that he is mobile and does not need assistive devices to move around his home. When you ask about his dietary intake, D.M. says, "I can take care of myself for the most part, but ever since my wife passed away, I'm having trouble cooking for myself. Martha was always a wonderful cook and I miss the food she made."

QUESTIONS TO CONSIDER

1. Given your observations about D.M. and his home environment, what other questions should you ask him?
2. What key nursing interventions can you put in place to help D.M.?

NUTRITION

Nutrition is a leading indicator of the health status of Canadians (Statistics Canada, 2019a). Proper nutrition means that all the essential nutrients (carbohydrates, fat, protein, vitamins, minerals, and water) are adequately supplied and used to maintain optimal health and well-being. Adequate nutrition is critical to preserving the health of older adults and is an integral part of health, happiness, independence, quality of life, and physical, social, and mental functioning. This chapter discusses the dietary needs of older adults, risk factors that contribute to inadequate nutrition, bowel function, malnutrition, dental health concerns, the effects of disease and functional impairment on nutrition, age-related changes that affect nutrition, and special considerations for older adults who have cognitive and physical impairments.

Nutrition-Related Concerns for Older Adults

While the fulfillment of an older adult's nutritional needs can be affected by age-related changes, it is more often affected by numerous other factors, including lifelong eating habits, ethnicity, socialization, income, transportation, housing, food knowledge, health, and dentition.

Healthy Eating for Seniors, adapted from *Canada's Food Guide* (Government of Canada, 2019a), indicates the types and amounts of food that should be eaten to optimize nutrient intake (Fig. 8.1). The adapted food guide emphasizes increased servings of vegetables, fruits, and grain products. With proper instruction, this guide can be an easy and systematic way for a person to evaluate their own nutritional intake and independently make corrective adjustments. Health Canada also provides culturally relevant food guides for First Nations, Inuit, and Métis peoples (Health Canada, 2010). There is also a wide variety of recommended diets, such as diets for persons with diabetes and the Mediterranean diet for heart health (World Health Organization, 2017).

Age-Related Concerns

A number of age-related factors can contribute to poor nutrition for the older adult, including changes in taste, smell, the digestive system, and appetite.

Taste. The sense of taste primarily depends on receptor cells in the taste buds, which are scattered on the surface of the tongue, the cheek, the soft palate, the upper tip of the esophagus, and other parts of the mouth and throat. Individuals have varied levels of taste sensitivity that seem to be predetermined by genetics and constitution as well as by age. Research findings suggest that the number of taste buds decreases as a person ages and that the remaining taste cells shrink (Ogawa et al., 2017).

Age-related changes do not affect all taste sensations equally; with age, the ability to detect sweet taste seems to remain intact, whereas the ability to detect sour, salty, and bitter tastes declines. Many denture wearers say they lose some of their satisfaction with food, possibly because dentures cover the palate and because texture is a very important element in food enjoyment. The addition of flavour enhancers (e.g., bouillon cubes), concentrated flavours (e.g., jellies or sauces), and fresh herbs and spices can amplify both taste and smell and may increase enjoyment and interest in eating. The bland diets often found in hospitals and long-term care (LTC) homes contribute to decreased appetite.

Smell. Smell occurs when nerve receptors in the nose send messages to the brain. The oral and nasal senses interact to give the impression of a certain food, combining to heighten the sensory perceptions received. Smells also create positive or negative emotional responses to food, because the parts of the brain responsible for emotions and smell overlap.

Studies have shown that the sense of smell declines as a person ages. A decreased sense of smell may be related to many factors, including nasal sinus disease, repeated injury to olfactory receptors through viral infections, age-related changes in central nervous system functioning, cigarette smoking, medications, and periodontal disease or other dentition problems. Changes in the sense of smell are also associated with Parkinson's disease (Tarakad & Jancovic, 2017) and Alzheimer's disease (Cingi et al., 2020).

Many older adults, particularly those who are in LTC settings, no longer cook and never have the experience of smelling food as it is cooking, an important appetite stimulant. As a way of increasing residents' interest in and enjoyment of food, some LTC settings have adapted kitchens and dining rooms so that residents can smell the food cooking and even participate in the preparation of food.

My Food Guide

As a man aged 71 years or older, this is how many Food Guide Servings you need from each food group every day.

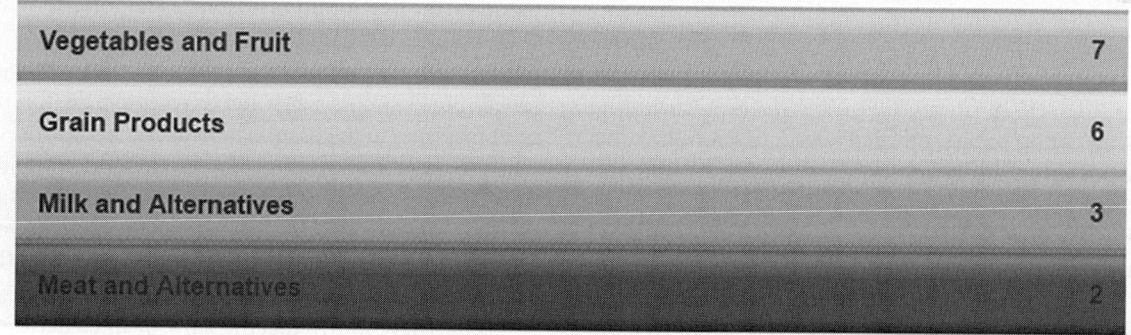

Vegetables and Fruit	7
Grain Products	7
Milk and Alternatives	3
Meat and Alternatives	3

My Food Guide

As a woman aged 71 years or older, this is how many Food Guide Servings you need from each food group every day.

Vegetables and Fruit	7
Grain Products	6
Milk and Alternatives	3
Meat and Alternatives	2

Fig. 8.1 ▓ Dietary Recommendations for Older Adults. Adapted from Health Canada. (2019). *Canada's Food Guide: Healthy eating for seniors*. https://food-guide.canada.ca/en/tips-for-healthy-eating/seniors/. Reproduced with permission of the Minister of Public Works and Government Services Canada, 2017.

Digestive System. Age-related changes in the oral cavity, esophagus, stomach, liver, pancreas, gallbladder, and small and large intestines may influence nutritional status. A study found that persons who have lost their teeth generally eat fewer servings of fruit and vegetables (Su et al., 2020).

Regulation of Appetite. Appetite in persons of all ages is regulated by a combination of a peripheral satiation system and a central feeding drive, and is influenced by physical activity, functional limitations, smell, taste, mood, socialization, and comfort. With aging, the physiological

basis for appetite regulation begins to differ from that of younger adults. Although the specifics await further research, changes in energy regulation mechanisms and neurotransmitter regulators of appetite have been implicated in impaired appetite and decreased intake associated with aging (Soenen & Chapman, 2017).

Disease states also increase cytokine levels as a result of diseased tissues being released, thereby decreasing appetite. There is some suggestion that alterations in endogenous opioid peptides are involved in food cravings, further contributing to decreased appetite (Bodnar, 2019). Valbrun and Zvonarev (2020) found that the blockade of opioid receptors diminishes patients' food intake, which could have implications for older adults who take opiates.

Nutritional Needs

Several considerations are important when nutrition for older adults is addressed. Box 8.1 discusses menu planning in LTC homes. Increased amounts of calcium and vitamins D and B12 are needed in later life. Total caloric intake should decline in response to corresponding changes in metabolic rate and a general decrease in physical activity. The Sodium Reduction Strategy for Canada has reduced the recommended daily value for sodium to 1 500 mg and even lower for older adults (https://www.canada.ca/en/health-canada/services/food-nutrition/healthy-eating/sodium.html). The intake of fluid is emphasized because thirst mechanisms may be less responsive in older adults.

BOX 8.1
NUTRITIONAL GOALS: KEY RECOMMENDATIONS FOR OLDER ADULTS IN LONG-TERM CARE

CANADA'S FOOD GUIDE RECOMMENDATION 1:

- Nutritious foods are the foundation for healthy eating.
- Promote regular intake of vegetables, fruits, and whole grains and protein-rich foods. Among protein foods, consume plant-based foods more often.
- Protein foods: legumes, nuts, seeds, tofu, fish, shellfish, eggs, poultry, lean red meats, lower-fat yogurts.
- Foods that contain mostly unsaturated fat should replace foods that contain mostly saturated fat.
- Water should be the beverage of choice.

DIETITIANS OF CANADA RECOMMENDED MODIFICATION:

- Owing to the high risk for malnutrition and increased need for protein, animal-based products that are nutrient dense and easy to consume (e.g., dairy) or increased use of soy-based fortified products are needed.
- Owing to challenges in eating, beverages (milk, soy beverage, vegetable and fruit juice) are important contributors to energy and nutrient intake.

CANADA'S FOOD GUIDE RECOMMENDATION 2:

- Processed or prepared foods and beverages that contribute to excess sodium, free sugars, or saturated fat undermine healthy eating and should not be consumed regularly.

DIETITIANS OF CANADA RECOMMENDED MODIFICATION:

- All menu items should be evaluated for nutrient density and contribution to resident satisfaction and preferences.
- Menu should include a range of foods and beverages to support nutrient needs and quality of life.
- Foods and beverages with higher sugar or fat content can support weight maintenance and may represent a high percentage of familiar foods for residents.

- Menus should emphasize high-quality protein and nutrients of concern for the resident population.
- Residents are offered choice to promote autonomy and quality of life; prepared or processed food options are commonly requested or are popular with residents, and inclusion on the menu should be based on resident input.
- Whether made in house or purchased ready prepared, menu items' nutrition profiles, taste, quality, and acceptance should be evaluated.

CANADA'S FOOD GUIDE RECOMMENDATION 3:

- Food skills are needed to navigate the complex food environment and support healthy eating.
- Cooking and food preparation using nutritious foods should be promoted as a practical way to support healthy eating.
- Food labels should be promoted as a tool to help Canadians make informed food choices.

DIETITIANS OF CANADA RECOMMENDATION MODIFICATION:

- Adequate numbers of qualified cooking staff are required to prepare high-quality nutrient-dense products.
- Adequate numbers of staff to service and assist residents at meals and snacks are required to optimize food and fluid intake.
- Standardized recipes for palatable and acceptable nutrient-dense foods with reasonable costs are needed.
- Ensure opportunities for residents to engage in menu planning and choose preferred foods and beverages at meals to increase satisfaction and intake.
- Review food labels for nutrition information and suitability of ingredients for specific diet types and allergies.

Source: Dietitians of Canada. (2019). *Menu planning in long term care and Canada's Food Guide.* https://www.dietitians.ca/DietitiansOfCanada/media/Documents/Resources/Menu-Planning-in-Long-Term-Care-with-Canada-s-Food-Guide-2020.pdf.

The major nutrition-related concerns with older adults are obesity and malnutrition. In 2018, approximately 75% of males and 70% of females over the age of 65 years were overweight or obese (Statistics Canada, 2019b). Obesity in later life can further exacerbate the seriousness of a number of age-related health problems, depending on weight gain patterns and the health history of the obese person. Obesity is also connected with hypertension, kidney disease, and cardiovascular disease. Intervention trials indicate clinically significant benefits of weight reduction with regard to lower blood pressure, cholesterol, and blood sugar (Centers for Disease Control and Prevention, 2020).

Malnutrition is the other major nutrition-related concern. Malnutrition often goes unrecognized and affects morbidity, mortality, and quality of life. Research into frailty has identified that two-thirds of malnourished older adults are frail and that being malnourished is associated with higher mortality risk (Rodriguez-Manas et al., 2020). Malnutrition emerged as a significant risk factor for developing frailty and death in a 3-year follow-up period (Rodriguez-Manas et al., 2020). Of note is that obese older adults are also at risk for malnutrition (Bell et al., 2021).

Lifelong Eating Habits

The nutritional state of a person often reflects their dietary history and present eating practices. Lifelong eating habits develop from tradition, ethnicity, religion, and societal influences (e.g., the availability of fast food), all of which can be collectively called "culture" and influence the food intake of older adults.

Members of a particular ethnic or religious group can have unique eating patterns, so individual assessment is important. Culturally and religiously appropriate diets should be available in any facility or congregate dining program.

For healthy older adults, essential nutrients should be obtained from food sources rather than dietary supplements. Recent studies have shown that diet can affect longevity and, when combined with lifestyle changes, reduce disease risk. A diet consisting of nutrient- and fibre-rich fruits, brightly coloured vegetables, whole grains, legumes, lean proteins, and healthy fats—as well as unrefined, unprocessed foods—is beneficial (Government of Canada, 2019a). By following the recommendations in *Eating Well With Canada's Food Guide*, older adults may lower their risk of chronic disease and ensure health-protective nutrition.

Socialization

The social aspect of eating involves sharing with others and a feeling of belonging. People use food as a means of giving and receiving love, friendship, or a sense of belonging. Often, older adults may be isolated from the mainstream of life because of chronic illness, depression, and other functional limitations. When the older adult has to prepare their own meals and eat alone, the outcome sometimes is either overindulgence or disinterest in eating. The presence of others during meals is a significant predictor of caloric intake (Keller et al., 2017a).

Disinterest in food may also result from the effects of medications or disease processes. Over-the-counter and prescribed medications have the potential to cause adverse effects that can affect dietary intake (Youdim, 2019). A number of medications also interact with food (in what are called drug–nutrient interactions), resulting in the reduced absorption of nutrients. Both of these problems can adversely affect nutritional status (Mohn et al., 2018).

The misuse of alcohol is prevalent among older adults and is a growing public health concern. Excessive consumption of alcohol interferes with nutrition; alcohol depletes the body of necessary nutrients and often replaces meals, thus making the person more susceptible to malnutrition (see Chapter 23).

Most cities and rural areas throughout Canada support a wide range of nutrition services for older adults, including home-delivered meals, congregate dining sites, and home visits by registered dietitians. Congregate dining programs and home-delivered meal services have been shown to improve or help maintain nutritional status in older adults, thereby enabling them to avoid or delay costly institutionalization and allowing them to stay in their homes and communities. Many of these programs are funded by municipal or provincial and territorial governments (sometimes by both), by charitable organizations such as the United Way, and by private donations.

Income

There is a strong relationship between poor nutrition and low income. In Canada, the most accepted measure of poverty is what is known as the low income cut-off

(LICO). Statistics Canada measures the number of families that are below the LICO—families that spend 20 percentage points or more of their gross income on food, shelter, and clothing. According to Statistics Canada, persons 65 years of age and older account for 3.5% of people below the LICO (Statistics Canada, 2020). Poverty rates among older Indigenous persons and recent immigrants are much higher, as these persons are more vulnerable to low income and unemployment than are other Canadians (Statistics Canada, 2019c; Statistics Canada, 2017).

Older adults with low incomes may need to choose among several essential needs, such as food, heat, telephone bills, medications, and health care visits, all of which affect overall health. Some older adults eat only once per day in an attempt to make their income last through the month. Free food programs and donated commodities are available at distribution centres (e.g., food banks) for those with limited incomes. Although this is a valuable option for older adults, the use of such programs is not always feasible. The types of food available any particular day or week can vary, and the quantities distributed are frequently too large for an older adult to use or even carry from the distribution site. Some food sources do not support the dietary recommendations to prevent or manage certain disease conditions (e.g., processed canned food is high in sodium and sugar). The distribution site may be too far away or difficult to reach, and the time of distribution may be inconvenient. Although some restaurants provide special meal prices for older adults, they often increase their prices as food costs rise.

Transportation

Available and easily accessible transportation to where food is sold or served is often limited for older adults. Many small, longstanding neighbourhood food stores have been closed in the wake of the expansion of larger supermarkets that are located in areas that serve a greater segment of the population. It may become difficult for an older adult to walk to the supermarket, reach it by public transportation, or carry a bag of groceries while using a cane or walker.

Functional impairments also make the use of public transportation difficult for some older adults. For a person whose income is limited, transportation by taxicab is often unrealistic, but sharing a taxicab with others who also need to shop may enable the older adult to purchase food. Organizations for older adults in many parts of Canada have been helpful in providing older adults with "van service" to shopping areas. In housing complexes, it may be possible to schedule group trips to the supermarket. Most communities have multiple sources of transportation available, but the older adult may be unaware of them. It is important for nurses to be knowledgeable about community resources that are available to older adults.

Many older adults, particularly widowed men, may never have learned how to shop for and prepare food. Older adults often have to rely on others to shop for them, and this may be a cause of concern, depending on the availability of support. The older adult may also be reluctant to be dependent on others, particularly family members. For older adults who own a computer, shopping on the Internet and having groceries delivered offers advantages, although prices may be higher than in-store prices. Another choice is home delivery of nutritious meals made without additives or preservatives. A newer option is to have fresh ingredients delivered to the door along with a recipe that the older adult can follow using those ingredients. Costs will vary, depending on ingredients and preferences.

Housing

The environments where older adults reside need to be functional and meet their changing needs (Government of Canada, 2019b). Some older adults who live in single rooms lack a stove for cooking, a means of refrigeration, and storage space for food. During the colder months, some single-room dwellers use window ledges and fire escapes to keep perishables cool for several days' use, which creates a high risk for food spoilage and hence food poisoning.

MALNUTRITION

Malnutrition among older adults has been documented in acute care, in LTC homes, and in the community. Protein-calorie malnutrition (PCM) is the most common form of malnutrition among older adults. It is characterized by clinical signs (muscle wasting, low body mass index) and biochemical signs (decreased albumin or other serum protein) indicative of insufficient intake. Many of the factors discussed previously contribute to malnutrition in older adults (Box 8.2).

BOX 8.2
RISK FACTORS FOR MALNUTRITION IN OLDER ADULTS

PSYCHOSOCIAL RISK FACTORS

Limited income
Misuse of alcohol and other central nervous system depressants
Bereavement, loneliness, isolation, or living alone
Removal from usual cultural patterns
Memory loss
Depression

MECHANICAL RISK FACTORS

Decreased or limited strength and mobility
Neurological deficits, arthritis, impairment of hand–arm coordination, loss of tongue strength, dysphagia
Blindness or decreased or diminished vision
Inability to shop, prepare food, or feed self, and lack of adequate assistance with these activities
Pressure ulcers
Loss of teeth, poor-fitting dentures, or chewing problems
Difficulty breathing
Polypharmacy
Surgery, nothing by mouth (NPO) orders for extended periods of time, and fluid restriction

The prevalence of PCM varies with the population observed and the definition of malnutrition. The prevalence of malnutrition in older adults depends on their health and functional capacity. As health and functional capacity deteriorate, the prevalence of malnutrition increases dramatically, reaching up to 60% in LTC homes or hospital settings (Sauer et al., 2016). Malnutrition has serious consequences, including infections, pressure ulcers, anemia, hypotension, impaired cognition, hip fractures, and increased mortality and morbidity. Most pathological causes of weight loss are considered to be reversible. A study by Julius and colleagues (2017) found that malnutrition is associated with an increased risk of falling and impaired activity in older adults who reside in LTC homes. Malnutrition can be assessed with standardized tools such as the Mini Nutritional Assessment or the Nutritional Risk Screening tool (Deer et al., 2017).

Depression, which frequently affects older adults, is a common and reversible cause of weight loss. Screening for depression with validated tools such as the Geriatric Depression Scale and the Cornell Scale for Depression in Dementia should be included in the assessment of older adults who are experiencing weight loss (see Chapter 23). A thorough medication review is important when nutritional concerns are assessed since many medications affect appetite and can affect nutritional status. Medications that are most frequently associated with malnutrition include digoxin, theophylline, nonsteroidal anti-inflammatory drugs, iron supplements, and psychoactive medications.

Oral Health

Dental health is a basic need for older adults that is increasingly neglected. Oral and dental health is integral to general health (Tabak et al., 2019). Poor oral health is recognized as a risk factor for dehydration as well as a number of systemic diseases (Kossioni, 2018). Furthermore, poor oral health—which leads to missing teeth, teeth in ill repair, and oral pain—contributes to chewing and swallowing problems that affect adequate nutritional intake (Kossioni, 2018). The Canadian Dental Association has written a report entitled the *State of Oral Health in Canada* (2017), which can be accessed on their website at https://www.cda-adc.ca/stateoforalhealth/_files/thestateoforalhealthincanada.pdf.

The percentage of people aged 60 to 79 years who are without natural teeth is 22.3% for men and 21.1% for women (Statistics Canada, 2015). The prevalence of periodontitis, which is the main cause of the loss of natural teeth, is decreasing as knowledge about it increases and more people use fluorides, improve their nutrition, engage in oral hygiene practices, and take advantage of improved dental health care. However, older adults may not have had the advantages of preventive treatment, and those with functional and cognitive limitations may be unable to perform oral hygiene. Access to dental care for older adults may be limited as well as cost prohibitive. Also, some Canadian cities, such as Calgary and Windsor, choose not to fluoridate the water (Government of Canada, 2018), which further affects residents' oral health.

The low priority of dental care in the existing health care system is reflected by the absence or inadequacy of third-party reimbursement for the type of dental care needed by older adults. The *Canada Health Act* has designated dental surgery in hospitals as a "medically necessary" health service, resulting in the coverage of this service by provincial health insurance. However, this health insurance does not cover regular dental services in a dentist's office. Canadians rely on their employers, individual private insurance, or their own financial resources to cover the cost of dental treatments. In some jurisdictions, public health units have been involved in providing targeted programs to address the needs of older adults or those who receive social assistance. The Canadian Association of Public Health Dentistry tracks those programs and has been advocating for the extension of coverage to persons who are currently unable to pay for dental care (Canadian Association of Public Health Dentistry, 2019).

Older adults make fewer visits to the dentist than members of any other age group. Older Canadians with the poorest oral health are those who are low income, lack insurance, and are members of racial and ethnic minorities. Furthermore, in hospitals and LTC homes, oral care is often overlooked (Keboa et al., 2019). Some of the age-related physiological changes and common problems associated with oral care are discussed later in this chapter.

Age-Related Changes to the Buccal Cavity

Aging teeth become worn and darker and tend to yellow over time (Government of Canada, 2019c). In addition to years of exposure of the teeth and related structures to microbial assault, the oral cavity shows evidence of wear and tear as a result of normal use (chewing and talking) and destructive oral habits such as bruxism (habitual grinding of the teeth). People who are edentulous and are using complete dentures continue to have oral health care needs. Ill-fitting dentures affect chewing and hence nutritional intake. Age-related changes in the buccal cavity also predispose older adults to oral and dental problems (Box 8.3).

Xerostomia

A common oral problem among older adults is dry mouth, or **xerostomia**. Prevalence of xerostomia increases with age and affects many older adults (Manlapaz, 2017). Reduced salivary flow is a side effect of more than 500 medications. A reduction in saliva and a dry mouth make eating, swallowing, and speaking difficult. It can also lead to significant problems of the teeth and their supporting structure. Artificial saliva preparations are available (those containing sorbitol should be avoided), and adequate fluid intake is also important when xerostomia occurs. Chewing gum with xylitol stimulates saliva

> **BOX 8.3**
> **AGE-RELATED CHANGES OF THE BUCCAL CAVITY**
>
> - Decrease in the cellular compartment
> - Loss of submucosal elastin in oral mucosa
> - Loss of connective tissue (collagen)
> - Increase in thickness of collagen fibres
> - Decrease in function of minor salivary glands
> - Decrease in number and quality of blood vessels and nerves
> - Attrition on occlusive contact surfaces
> - Decrease of enamel permeability (teeth more brittle)
> - Change of tooth colour
> - Formation of excessive secondary dentin
> - Decrease at the cement–enamel junction
> - Decrease in size of pulp chamber and root canals
> - Decrease in size and volume of tooth pulp
> - Increase in pulp stones and dystrophic mineralization

flow and promotes oral hygiene (Takeuchi et al., 2018). Medication review is also indicated in order to eliminate, if possible, the use of medications that contribute to xerostomia.

Oral Cancer

Oral cancers occur more frequently in late life, and men are affected twice as often as women. For all stages combined, the 5-year survival rate is 64%, while survival rates are higher for cervical cancer (72%), melanoma cancers (88%), and prostate cancer (93%) (Canadian Cancer Society, 2020). Oral examinations are important, as they can assist in the early detection and treatment of oral cancers and other oral and dental problems. Box 8.4 presents the common signs and symptoms of oral cancer.

Risk factors for oral cancer are tobacco use, alcohol use, and exposure to ultraviolet light (especially for cancer of the lips). Pipe, cigar, and cigarette smoking are all implicated. Other risk factors are age, sex, local tissue irritation, poor nutrition, use of mouthwash with a high alcohol content, human papillomavirus (HPV) infection, and immunosuppressant medications. Therapy options are based on diagnosis and staging and include surgery, radiation, and chemotherapy. If detected early, these cancers can often be treated successfully.

BOX 8.4

SIGNS AND SYMPTOMS OF ORAL AND THROAT CANCER

- Swelling or thickening, lumps or bumps, or rough spots or eroded areas on the lips, gums, or other areas inside the mouth
- Velvety white, red, or speckled patches in the mouth
- Persistent sores on the face, neck, or mouth that bleed easily
- Unexplained bleeding in the mouth
- Unexplained numbness, pain, or tenderness in any area of the face, mouth, neck, or tongue
- Soreness in the back of the throat; a persistent feeling that something is caught in the throat
- Difficulty chewing or swallowing, speaking, or moving the jaw or tongue
- Hoarseness, chronic sore throat, or changes in the voice
- Dramatic weight loss
- Lump or swelling in the neck
- Severe pain in one ear (with a normal eardrum)
- Pain around the teeth; loosening of the teeth
- Swelling or pain in the jaw; difficulty moving the jaw

IMPLICATIONS FOR GERONTOLOGICAL NURSING AND HEALTHY AGING

Assessment

Good oral hygiene and assessment of oral health are essentials of nursing care. In addition to identifying oral health problems, an examination of the mouth can lead to early diagnosis and treatment for some diseases. All persons, especially those over age 50, with or without dentures, should have oral examinations on a regular basis. Although an oral examination is best performed by a dentist, nurses can perform basic screening examinations. A list of instruments and signs and symptoms are also provided by the Registered Nurses' Association of Ontario as part of its Best Practice Guidelines (Registered Nurses' Association of Ontario [RNAO], 2020a) (Table 8.1). One example is the Oral Health Assessment Tool (OHAT) developed by Chalmers and colleagues (2005) (Fig 8.2).

Interventions

The prescribed oral hygiene regimen for a person with natural teeth consists of brushing and flossing twice a

TABLE 8.1		
Oral Signs and Symptoms Associated With Patient Stressors in the Critical Care Unit Setting		
Stressor	**Signs**	**Symptoms**
Mechanical Ventilation and Oxygen Therapy		
Dry mouth	■ Dry, red mucosa and depapillated, lobulated, or fissured tongue ■ Dry, cracked lips ■ Buildup of debris in mouth	■ Burning sensation ■ Dryness ■ Difficulty swallowing
Medication Therapy		
Immunosuppression, change in flora	■ White plaques and inflammation associated with *Candida albicans*, herpetic ulcers, and halitosis	■ Pain or discomfort ■ Halitosis
Xerostomia	■ Decreased salivary flow ■ Dry, red mucosa and depapillated, lobulated, or fissured tongue ■ Dry, cracked lips ■ Buildup of debris in mouth	■ Burning sensation ■ Dryness ■ Difficulty swallowing
Therapeutic Dehydration		
Xerostomia	■ See above	■ See above

Source: Registered Nurses' Association of Ontario. (2020). *Oral health: Supporting adults who require assistance* (2nd ed.). https://rnao.ca/sites/rnao-ca/files/bpg/RNAO_Oral_Health_Supporting_Adults_Who_Require_Assistance_Second_Edition_FINAL_WEB_Dec_2020.pdf.

Resident: _____	Date: ___/___/___
Completed by: _____	

<table>
<tr><td colspan="5">Scores - You can circle individual words as well as giving a score in each category
(* if 1 or 2 scored for any category please organize for a dentist to examine the resident)</td></tr>
<tr><th>Category</th><th>0 = healthy</th><th>1 = changes*</th><th>2 = unhealthy*</th><th>Category Scores</th></tr>
<tr><td>Lips</td><td>Smooth, pink, moist</td><td>Dry, chapped, or red at corners</td><td>Swelling or lump, white/red/ulcerated patch; bleeding/ulcerated at corners</td><td></td></tr>
<tr><td>Tongue</td><td>Normal, moist, roughness, pink</td><td>Patchy, fissured, red, coated</td><td>Patch that is red and/or white, ulcerated, swollen</td><td></td></tr>
<tr><td>Gums and tissues</td><td>Pink, moist, smooth, no bleeding</td><td>Dry, shiny, rough, red, swollen, one ulcer/sore spot under dentures</td><td>Swollen, bleeding, ulcers, white/red patches, generalized redness under dentures</td><td></td></tr>
<tr><td>Saliva</td><td>Moist tissues, watery and free flowing saliva</td><td>Dry, sticky tissues, little saliva present; resident thinks they have a dry mouth</td><td>Tissues parched and red, very little/no saliva present, saliva is thick, resident thinks they have a dry mouth</td><td></td></tr>
<tr><td>Natural teeth Yes/No</td><td>No decayed or broken teeth/roots</td><td>1–3 decayed or broken teeth/roots or very worn down teeth</td><td>4 + decayed or broken teeth/roots or very worn down teeth, or less than 4 teeth</td><td></td></tr>
<tr><td>Dentures Yes/No</td><td>No broken areas or teeth, dentures regularly worn, and named</td><td>1 broken areas/teeth or dentures only worn for 1–2 hrs daily, or dentures not named, or loose</td><td>More than 1 broken area/tooth, denture missing or not worn, loose and needs denture adhesive, or not named</td><td></td></tr>
<tr><td>Oral cleanliness</td><td>Clean and no food particles or tartar in mouth or dentures</td><td>Food particles/tartar/plaque in 1–2 areas of the mouth or on small area of dentures or halitosis (bad breath)</td><td>Food particles/tartar/plaque in most areas of the mouth or on most of dentures or severe halitosis (bad breath)</td><td></td></tr>
<tr><td>Dental pain</td><td>No behavioural, verbal, or physical signs of dental pain</td><td>Verbal and/or behavioural signs of pain such as pulling at face, chewing lips, not eating, aggression</td><td>Physical pain signs (swelling of cheek or gum, broken teeth, ulcers), as well as verbal and/or behavioural signs (pulling at face, not, eating, aggression)</td><td></td></tr>
</table>

☐ Organize for resident to have a dental examination by a dentist

☐ Resident and/or family/guardian refuses dental treatment

☐ Complete Oral Hygiene Care Plan and start oral hygiene care interventions for resident

☐ Review this resident's oral health again on Date: ___/___/___

TOTAL SCORE: ___ 16

Fig. 8.2 ■ Oral Health Assessment Tool (OHAT). Reprinted with permission of the Registered Nurses' Association of Ontario. *Sources:* Chalmers, J., King, P., Spencer, A., et al. (2005). The oral health assessment tool—Validity and reliability. *Australian Dental Journal, 50*(3), 191–199; Registered Nurses' Association of Ontario. (2020). *Oral health: Nursing assessment and interventions.* https://rnao.ca/sites/rnao-ca/files/bpg/RNAO_Oral_Health_Supporting_Adults_Who_Require_Assistance_Second_Edition_FINAL_WEB_Dec_2020.pdf.

day and using a fluoride dentifrice and nonalcoholic mouthwash. There is evidence that cleaning the teeth with a toothbrush after meals lowers the risk for aspiration pneumonia (Longo et al., 2019).

Impaired manual dexterity may make it difficult for older adults to adequately maintain their dental routine and remove plaque adequately. The handgrip of a manual toothbrush is often too small to grasp and manipulate easily. Using a child's toothbrush or enlarging the handle of an adult-sized toothbrush by adding a foam grip or wrapping it with gauze has been effective in facilitating grasp. The ultrasonic toothbrush is an effective tool that older adults or their caregivers can use. Occupational therapists can be helpful in the assessment of functional impairments and the provision of adaptive equipment for oral care.

Therapeutic rinses contain an agent that is beneficial to the surface of the teeth and to the oral environment. Some therapeutic rinses (such as chlorhexidine [Peridex], which contains alcohol but is also a broad-spectrum antimicrobial agent that helps control plaque) require a prescription. Original-formula Listerine, a commercial over-the-counter product, should not be used by persons who have severe oral mucositis, because it contains a high quantity of alcohol (26.9% by volume). Listerine and generic equivalents that contain alcohol may be mixed with water but should always be used in conjunction with, not instead of, brushing.

Enteral feeding of older adults is associated with significant pathological colonization of the mouth, greater than that observed in people who receive oral feeding. Therefore, oral care should be undertaken every 4 hours for people who have gastrostomy tubes, and teeth should be brushed after each feeding to decrease the risk for aspiration pneumonia (Li et al., 2016). The oral mucosa of unconscious or severely cognitively impaired patients should be hydrated by using gauze soaked in physiological saline, and the lips should be coated with petroleum jelly or lip balm (Kobayashi et al., 2017).

When the person is unable to carry out their own dental or oral regimen, it is the responsibility of the caregiver to provide oral care (Box 8.5). Oral care is an often neglected part of daily nursing care. Poor oral health and a lack of attention to oral hygiene are major concerns in residential settings and contribute significantly to poor nutrition and other negative outcomes

---

BOX 8.5

INSTRUCTIONS FOR CAREGIVERS PROVIDING DENTAL CARE

1. If the person is in bed, elevate their head by raising the bed or propping up the patient's head and neck with pillows, and have the person turn their head to face you. Place a clean towel across the chest and under the chin, and place a basin under the chin.
2. If the person is sitting in a chair or a wheelchair, stand behind the person and stabilize the head by placing one hand under the chin and resting the head against your body. Place a towel across the chest and over the shoulders. The basin can be kept handy in the person's lap or on a table placed at the front or side. A wheelchair may be positioned in front of the sink.
3. Brush and floss the person's teeth (use an electric toothbrush if possible). It may be helpful to retract the person's lips and cheek with a tongue blade or with the fingers in order to see the area that is being cleaned. Use a mouth prop as needed. If manual flossing is too difficult, use a floss holder or interproximal brush to clean the proximal surfaces between the teeth.
4. If the person's lips are dry or cracked, apply a light coating of petroleum jelly or lip balm.
5. Provide a conscious person with fluoride rinses or other rinses as indicated.

---

such as aspiration pneumonia. There are many reasons for this deficit, including inadequate knowledge of how to assess and provide care, difficulty in providing oral care to dependent and cognitively impaired older adults, inadequate training and staffing, and the lack of appropriate supplies.

Many LTC homes have implemented specific programs, such as staff training or dental care teams, mobile dentistry units, or oral screening and teeth cleaning done by dental students. Evidence-informed protocols combined with educational training sessions have been shown to have a positive impact on the oral health status of older adults (RNAO, 2020a).

Dentures

Older adults who have dentures should be taught the proper care of their dentures and oral tissue to prevent odour, staining, plaque buildup, and oral infections. Care should include the removal of debris under dentures in order to prevent pressure and shrinkage of underlying support structures. Dentures and other dental appliances, such as bridges, should be rinsed after each meal and brushed thoroughly once a day, preferably at night (Box 8.6). To allow relief from compression on the gums, dentures should not be worn at night.

Dentures are very personal and expensive possessions; in LTC homes, hospitals, and other care centres, patients' dentures are often misplaced or mixed up with those of others. The utmost care should be taken when handling, cleaning, and storing dentures. Dentures should incorporate some means of identifying the patient who owns them. Broken or damaged dentures and dentures that no longer fit because of the wearer's weight loss are a common problem for

older adults. Relining (adding material to the acrylic surface of the denture) can be used to improve the fit of dentures. Ill-fitting dentures or dentures that are not cleaned contribute to oral problems as well as to poor nutrition and reduced enjoyment of food. Daily removal and cleaning of dentures and brushing of teeth should be a part of the care routines in every facility.

All staff need to be knowledgeable about oral hygiene and techniques for the care of teeth and dentures. Oral hygiene protocols and appropriate oral care equipment should be available. Older adults and families also need to be educated about the importance of oral health and taught the techniques of adequate oral care.

HEALTH CONDITIONS AFFECTING NUTRITION

Chronic Diseases

Chronic diseases and their sequelae that pose nutritional challenges to older adults include osteoporosis, gastro-intestinal disorders, obesity, diabetes, cardiovascular and respiratory diseases, cancer, **dysphagia**, and dementia. Functional impairments associated with chronic disease interfere with the person's ability to shop, cook, and eat independently. For example, heart failure and chronic obstructive pulmonary disease are associated with fatigue, increased energy expenditure, and decreased appetite. Alzheimer's disease and other dementias affect adequate nutritional intake. Depression can cause changes in appetite (resulting in weight loss or gain), and the side effects of antidepressant medications affect appetite and nutrition (see Chapters 14 and 23). A number of prevalent disorders of the gastrointestinal tract—including **gastro-esophageal reflux disease (GERD)**, ulcers, constipation, diverticulosis, and colon cancer—are associated with nutritional problems.

The following section discusses nutritional concerns and nursing interventions related to dementia, dysphagia, constipation, and fecal impaction. (For more detailed information on health conditions and chronic diseases in older adults, see Chapters 15, 17, 18, 20, and 22.)

Dementia

Dementia affects adequate nutritional intake, and weight loss and malnutrition become considerable concerns in late dementia. Weight loss may be the result of physiological changes, cognitive deficits, lack of awareness of the need to eat, loss of independence for self-feeding, ill-fitting dentures, depression, or increased energy output caused by pacing or wandering (Lopez & Molony, 2018).

One of the best strategies for managing poor food intake for a person with dementia is to find foods that the person enjoys. Nutrient-dense foods are preferred. Attention to mealtime ambience is important, and the person should be able to take as much time as needed to eat. Food should be available 24 hours a day, and the person should be allowed to follow their accustomed eating schedule (e.g., late breakfast, early dinner). Finger foods may be a good choice when utensils are too difficult to manage. Serving one dish and using only one utensil at a time may assist in promoting adequate intake. Demonstrate eating motions that the person can imitate; use verbal cueing and prompting (e.g., take a bite, chew, swallow) and the hand-over-hand guiding technique to support self-feeding. Offer small amounts of fluid between bites of food and throughout the day. Refreshment stations with easy access to juices, water, and healthy snacks also promote adequate food intake.

Dysphagia

Dysphagia is difficulty swallowing. Dysphagia may occur as a result of neurological conditions such as stroke, Parkinson's disease, multiple sclerosis, and dementia. Dysphagia can be classified as oropharyngeal or esophageal. *Oropharyngeal dysphagia* refers to difficulty in the passage of food from the mouth to the esophagus. *Esophageal dysphagia* refers to disordered passage of food through the esophagus. The two types can be distinguished on the basis of the person's medical history, specific signs and symptoms on physical examination, and diagnostic tests.

Dysphagia is a serious problem; its consequences include malnutrition, dehydration aspiration, and pneumonia (Namasivayam-MacDonald et al., 2017). For the older adult, dysphagia is superimposed on the slowed swallowing rate associated with normal aging, creating an even greater risk for complications.

The exact prevalence of dysphagia is unknown, but one study by Andrade and colleagues (2018) indicates that the risk of dysphasia amongst older adults is about 10.5%.

IMPLICATIONS FOR GERONTOLOGICAL NURSING AND HEALTHY AGING

Assessment

A careful history of the older adult's response to dysphagia and observation of the person during mealtimes are important. Box 8.7 lists symptoms that will alert the nurse to possible swallowing problems and aspiration. When any of these symptoms are present, it is important to contact a speech-language pathologist (SLP), who will conduct specific tests to identify the cause of the person's swallowing problem and restore swallowing function to as normal a level as possible.

Interventions

The most profound and dangerous problem for older adults experiencing dysphagia is aspiration, in which oral or gastric contents (food, saliva, or nasal secretions) enter the bronchial tree. Aspiration during swallowing is best detected by procedures such as videofluoroscopy or fibre-optic endoscopy, but clinical observations and evaluation by an SLP are important as well.

BOX 8.7

SYMPTOMS OF DYSPHAGIA OR POSSIBLE ASPIRATION

- Difficult, laboured swallowing
- Drooling
- Copious oral secretions
- Coughing or choking while eating
- Holding or pocketing food in the mouth
- Difficulty moving food or liquid from mouth to throat
- Difficulty chewing
- Nasal voice or hoarseness
- Wet or gurgling voice
- Excessive throat clearing
- Sensation of something stuck in the throat during swallowing
- Reflux of food or liquid into the throat, mouth, or nose
- Heartburn
- Chest pain
- Hiccups
- Weight loss
- Frequent respiratory infections, pneumonia

Aspiration pneumonia (i.e., bronchopneumonia as a result of aspiration) is underdiagnosed in older adults, and its signs and symptoms manifest themselves differently in members of this age group as compared to other age groups. Small-volume aspirations, or microaspirations, that produce few overt symptoms are common and may not be discovered until the condition has progressed to a more serious state, such as aspiration pneumonia (Canadian Patient Safety Institute, 2020). An elevated respiratory rate and alterations in mental status may be early symptoms of aspiration pneumonia.

It is important to have suctioning equipment available at the bedside or in the dining room in institutional settings. In the home setting, a call for emergency help should be immediate if the person is having trouble breathing, is choking, or has stopped breathing. Perform first aid and cardiopulmonary resuscitation (CPR) if consented to and necessary. People with dysphagia should have supervision at all mealtimes, and observation of persons who are at high risk for aspiration pneumonia should be ongoing.

The gerontological nurse must work closely with other members of the interprofessional team, such as the SLP, in implementing suggested interventions to prevent aspiration. Research on the appropriate management of swallowing disorders in older adults, particularly during acute illness and in LTC, is limited. A comprehensive protocol for preventing aspiration in older adults with dysphagia is available from https://hign.org/sites/default/files/2020-06/Try_This_General_Assessment_20.pdf. Interventions that are helpful in preventing aspiration during hand feeding are presented in Box 8.8.

Constipation

Bowel function in the older adult, although normally only slightly altered by physiological changes of age, can be a source of concern and a potentially serious problem, especially for the older adult who is functionally impaired. Normal elimination is the easy passage of feces without undue straining or a feeling of incomplete evacuation or defecation. Constipation is a common gastro-intestinal complaint; laxative use is common among older adults (RNAO, 2020b).

Constipation is a symptom that nurses should know how to recognize. It is often a reflection of poor habits, postponed passage of stool, and many chronic physical and psychological illnesses. It is also a common side effect

BOX 8.8
PREVENTING ASPIRATION IN OLDER ADULTS WITH DYSPHAGIA

- Provide a 30-minute rest period before feeding; a rested person will likely have less difficulty swallowing.
- The person should sit at 90° during all oral (PO) intake.
- Maintain the 90° positioning for at least 1 hour after PO intake.
- Avoid mixed-consistency food items (e.g., fruit cups, soup).
- Adjust the rate of feeding and the size of bites to the person's tolerance; avoid rushed or forced feeding.
- Alternate solid and liquid boluses.
- Follow the speech-language pathologist's recommendation for safe swallowing techniques and modified food consistency (thickened liquids, pureed foods).
- Place food on the unimpaired side of the mouth.
- Avoid sedatives and hypnotics that may impair the cough reflex and swallowing ability.
- Keep suction equipment ready at all times.
- Supervise all meals.
- Visually check the mouth for pocketing of food in cheeks.

Source: Adapted from Metheny, N. A. (2018). Preventing aspiration in older adults with dysphagia. *ConsultGeri: Try this: Series. The Hartford Institute for Geriatric Nursing, 20.* https://hign.org/consultgeri/try-this-series/preventing-aspiration-older-adults-dysphagia.

of medication. Constipation can also signal more serious underlying problems, such as colonic dysmotility or mass lesions. Poor diet and lack of activity play significant roles in constipation. Numerous precipitating factors or conditions can cause or worsen constipation.

Fecal Impaction. Fecal impaction is a major complication of unrecognized or unattended constipation. Fecal impaction, which is especially common in older adults who are cognitively impaired and living in institutions, is a serious and often dangerous problem. The symptoms of fecal impaction include malaise; urinary retention; elevated temperature; incontinence of bladder, bowel, or both; alterations in cognitive status; fissures; hemorrhoids; and intestinal obstruction. Leakage of liquid stool from around the impaction can be seen. Continued obstruction by a fecal mass may eventually impair sensation, leading to the need for larger stool volume to stimulate the urge to defecate, which contributes to megacolon (Zhang & Ding, 2019). Valsalva's manoeuvre with straining during stool defecation can cause transient ischemic attacks and syncope, especially in frail older adults.

Removal of a fecal impaction is at times worse than the misery of the condition. The management of fecal impaction requires the digital removal of the hard, compacted stool from the rectum with the use of a lubricant containing lidocaine jelly. Generally, this is preceded by an oil-retention enema to soften the feces in preparation for manual removal. Suppositories are not effective, because their action is blocked by the amount and size of the stool in the rectum.

Several sessions or days may be necessary to totally clear the sigmoid colon and rectum of impacted feces. Once this is achieved, attention should be directed to planning a regimen that includes adequate fluid intake, increased dietary fibre, administration of stool softeners if needed, and many of the suggestions presented here for the prevention of constipation. For persons who are in hospital or residing in LTC settings, accurate bowel records are essential; unfortunately, they are often overlooked or inaccurately completed. All direct care providers should be educated about the importance of bowel function and the accurate reporting of the size and consistency of stools and the frequency of bowel movements.

IMPLICATIONS FOR GERONTOLOGICAL NURSING AND HEALTHY AGING

Assessment

The precipitants and causes of constipation must be included in the evaluation of the older adult. A review of these factors will also determine whether the person is at risk for altered bowel function. Older adults at high risk for constipation and subsequent fecal impaction are those who have hypotonic colon function, who are immobilized and cognitively impaired, or who have central nervous system lesions. Incontinence, increased temperature, poor appetite, unexplained falls, or altered cognitive status may be the only clinical symptom of constipation in a cognitively impaired or frail older adult.

Recognizing constipation can be a challenge because there may be a significant difference between a patient's definition of constipation and that of the clinician. Assessment begins with the clarification of what the older adult means by "constipation." A bowel history should also be obtained that includes the person's usual patterns of elimination; the frequency, size, and consistency of bowel movements; and any changes that have occurred. Many clinicians think of bowel movement infrequency as the main indicator of constipation, but people with chronic constipation are more likely to report straining, a sense of incomplete or ineffective defecation, and hard or lumpy stools (RNAO, 2020b).

A physical examination is needed to rule out systemic causes of constipation such as neurological, endocrine, or metabolic disorders. Symptoms that may indicate an underlying gastro-intestinal disorder are abdominal pain, nausea, cramping, vomiting, weight loss, melena, rectal bleeding, rectal pain, and fever. A review of food and fluid intake may be necessary to determine the amount of fibre and fluid ingested. The nurse should ask questions about the level of physical activity and the use of medications. A psychosocial history with attention to depression, anxiety, and stress management is also indicated.

The abdomen should be examined for masses, distension, tenderness, and high-pitched or absent bowel sounds. A rectal examination is important for revealing painful anal disorders such as hemorrhoids or fissures, which impede the evacuation of stool, and for evaluating sphincter tone, stool presence, and anal reflex, as well as the presence of an enlarged prostate, rectal prolapse, strictures, and masses. Biochemical tests should include a complete blood count, fasting glucose, chemistry panel, and thyroid studies. Other diagnostic studies such as flexible sigmoidoscopy, colonoscopy, a computed tomography scan of the abdomen, or an abdominal X-ray study may also be indicated.

Interventions

The first steps in treating constipation are to examine the medications the person is taking, eliminate any that cause constipation, and change the regimen to medications that do not cause constipation. Medications that affect the central nervous system, nerve conduction, and smooth muscle function are associated with the highest frequency of constipation. Anticholinergics, opiates, and many psychoactive medications can be especially problematic.

Nonpharmacological interventions for constipation include (1) fluid- and fibre-related interventions,

(2) exercise, or (3) a combination of these. Adequate hydration, mainly with water, is the cornerstone of constipation therapy (RNAO, 2020b).

A low-fibre diet and insufficient fluid intake contribute to constipation. Fibre is an important dietary component that many older adults do not consume in sufficient quantities. Fibre is abundant in raw fruits and vegetables and in unrefined grains and cereals. It facilitates the absorption of water, increases bulk, and improves intestinal motility. Fibre helps prevent or reduce the incidence of constipation by increasing the weight of the stool and shortening transit time.

Individuals who can chew foods well can benefit from eating increased amounts of fresh fruits and vegetables daily or combining unsweetened bran with other types of food. People who have difficulty chewing can sprinkle bran on cereals or use it in soups and casseroles. The quantity of bran depends on the individual, but generally 1 to 2 tablespoons (15–30 mL) daily is sufficient. Individuals who have not used bran previously should begin with 1 teaspoon (5 mL) and progressively increase the amount until the quantity of fibre intake is enough to accomplish its purpose. Adequate fluid intake is also important. If megacolon or colonic dilation from bowel obstruction is suspected, fibre supplements are not advised.

Exercise

Exercise is important as an intervention to stimulate colon motility and bowel evacuation. Daily walking for 20 to 30 minutes is helpful, especially after a meal. Pelvic-tilt and range-of-motion exercises (passive or active) are beneficial for those who are less mobile or who are bedridden (see Chapter 10).

Positioning

A squatting or sitting position, if the person is able to assume it, facilitates bowel function. A similar position may be obtained by leaning forward and applying firm pressure to the lower abdomen or placing the feet on a stool. Massaging the abdomen may help stimulate the bowel.

Regularity

Establishing a toileting routine promotes or normalizes (retrains) bowel function. The gastrocolic reflex occurs after breakfast or supper and may be enhanced by a warm drink. Given privacy and sufficient time (a minimum of 10 minutes), many people will have a daily bowel movement. Any urge to defecate should be followed by a trip to the toilet. Older adults who depend on others to meet toileting needs should be assisted in maintaining normal routines and be provided with opportunities for routine toilet use. (Additional information on bowel management programs can be found in Chapter 9.)

Laxatives

When changes in diet and lifestyle are not effective in treating constipation, the use of laxatives can be considered. Older adults receiving opiates need to have a constipation prevention program in place, because these medications delay gastric emptying and decrease peristalsis. The correction of constipation associated with opiate use calls for a senna or osmotic laxative to overcome the strong opioid effect; stool softeners and bulking agents alone are inadequate. Commonly used laxatives for chronic constipation include the following:

- Bulking agents (e.g., psyllium, methylcellulose)
- Stool softeners (e.g., docusate sodium)
- Osmotic laxatives (e.g., lactulose, sorbitol)
- Stimulant laxatives (e.g., senna, bisacodyl)
- Saline laxatives (e.g., milk of magnesia)

Because of their safety, bulk laxatives are often the first laxatives prescribed. Bulk laxatives absorb water from the intestinal lumen and increase stool mass; adequate fluid intake is essential. The use of these laxatives is contraindicated in the presence of obstruction or compromised peristaltic activity. A saline or osmotic laxative can be added if the bulk laxative is not effective, but saline laxatives should be avoided in people with poor renal function or heart failure, because they may cause electrolyte imbalances. Stimulant laxatives should be used when other laxatives are ineffective. An emollient laxative, such as mineral oil, should be avoided because of the risk for lipoid aspiration pneumonia. Stool softeners have shown little effect when given to older adults with limited mobility, and their use should be limited to people who experience excessive straining or painful defecation or to people who are at a high risk for developing constipation (Emmanuel et al., 2017).

Combinations of natural fibre, fruit juices, and natural laxative mixtures (raisins, pitted prunes, figs, dates, currants, and prune concentrate) are often recommended in clinical practice. Some studies have found an increase in bowel frequency and a decrease in laxative use when these mixtures are used (Emmanuel et al., 2017) (Box 8.9).

Enemas

An enema is a procedure for introducing liquids into the rectum and colon via the anus. Enemas should not be used on a regular basis and should be used only when other methods produce no response or when there is an impaction. A normal saline or tap-water enema (500 to 1 000 mL) at 40.5°C is the best choice. Soap suds (a mixture of mild soap and warm water)

BOX 8.9

RESEARCH FOR EVIDENCE-INFORMED PRACTICE: CONSTIPATION IN OLDER ADULTS: A CONSENSUS STATEMENT

Purpose: The aim of the study was to evaluate the existing guidance and best clinical practice to improve the care of older adults with constipation.

Study Design: Six health care experts attended a face-to-face meeting. The panel consisted of experts from five European countries who came from various backgrounds (gastroenterology, nursing, geriatrics, pharmacology, and clinical research). Participants discussed their understanding of constipation and how it is addressed in their own country, as well as their own experience treating constipation.

Results: All panel experts believed that constipation is a serious problem for older adults. Increasing dietary fibre is recommended, but health care providers must take caution because it can also make constipation worse or cause additional discomfort. Reduced physical activity may also play a role in constipation, but reduced physical activity in older adults may be the result of poor mobility and frailty. Increased fluid intake has been promoted. Experts from Germany, Italy, and the Netherlands recommend use of medicinal treatments such as macrogol, biacodyl, and sodium picosulfate as a first-line treatment. In France, the first line of treatment is to maintain regular toilet habits. Many older adults may choose to self-medicate and therefore do not benefit from the expertise of health care providers.

Implications for Nursing Practice: It is important to understand the different treatment options available to promote healthy bowel habits in older adults.

Source: Emmanuel, A., Mattace-Raso, F., Neri, M. C., et al. (2017). Constipation in older people: A consensus statement. *The International Journal of Clinical Practice, 71*(1). doi:10.1111/ijcp.12920.

---

and phosphate enemas irritate the rectal mucosa and should not be used. Oil-retention enemas such as bisacodyl (Dulcolax) are used to increase the motility of the bowel (Mitchell, 2019).

A constipation prevention and treatment program that includes a high-fibre diet, liberal fluid intake, daily exercise, and environmental modifications that promote a regular pattern of bowel elimination must be developed for each older adult.

Older Adults in Hospitals and Institutions

Older adults in hospitals and LTC settings are more likely to experience a number of problems that contribute to inadequate nutrition. In addition to the risk factors already mentioned, isolation, severely restricted diets, long periods of nothing-by-mouth (NPO) status, and insufficient time and support staff for meals contribute to inadequate nutrition. Malnutrition can cause prolonged hospital stays, increased risk of poor health status, institutionalization, and mortality (Allard et al., 2016). Assessing the patient's nutritional status to identify malnutrition and the risk factors for malnutrition is important. Sufficient time, care, and attention should be given to helping dependent older adults with meals.

About 86% of residents of LTC homes require some assistance with activities such as eating (Ontario Long Term Care Association, 2019). Inadequate staffing in LTC homes is associated with inadequate organizational support, which may lead to poor nutrition in residents (Smith et al., 2019). Keller and colleagues found that residents significantly increased their oral food and fluid intake when they received one-on-one eating assistance (Keller et al., 2017b).

Family members (and volunteers in some settings) are often able to assist at mealtimes and provide a familiar social context for the older person. Nurses need to support and provide guidance to families around meal assistance and nutritional intake.

The use of restrictive therapeutic diets (e.g., low cholesterol, low salt, no concentrated sweets) for frail older adults in LTC homes often reduces their food intake without significantly helping their clinical status (Farrer et al., 2017). If caloric supplements are used (e.g., Ensure, Boost, Sustacal), they should be administered at least 1 hour before meals or else they will interfere with food intake. These products are widely used, can be expensive, and are often not dispensed or consumed as ordered. More research related to their effectiveness is needed.

Dispensing a small amount (2 calories/mL) of calorically dense oral nutritional supplement during the routine medication pass may have a greater effect on weight gain than a traditional supplement (1.06 calories/mL) with or between meals. Small volumes of nutrient-dense supplements may also have less of an effect on appetite and will increase food intake during meals and snacks. This method of dispensing supplements allows nurses to observe and document consumption.

Attention to the environment in which meals are served is also important. Assisting older adults who have difficulty eating independently can become mechanical and devoid of feeling. The assistance process becomes a task; even if the older adult requires additional time, the meal may be ended abruptly, depending on the time the caregiver has allotted for assistance. Any pleasure derived through socialization and eating and any dignity that could be maintained are often lost. Older adults who are accustomed to certain table manners may feel ashamed about their inability to behave in a way that they feel is appropriate.

In addition to having competent and adequate staff, LTC homes can use innovative and evidence-informed strategies to improve their residents' nutritional intake. The many suggestions in the literature include the following:

- Restorative dining programs
- Home-like dining rooms
- Individualized menu choices that include ethnic foods
- Cafeteria-style service
- Kitchens on the units or wards
- Availability of food around the clock
- Choice of mealtimes
- Liberal diets
- Finger foods
- Visually appealing puréed foods (with texture and shape)
- Music
- Touch
- Verbal cueing
- Hand-over-hand guiding
- The nurse's sitting (instead of standing) while assisting the person to eat

Other suggestions can be found in Box 8.10.

BOX 8.10

SUGGESTIONS FOR IMPROVING OLDER ADULTS' NUTRITIONAL INTAKE

- Serve meals to the person while they sit in a chair rather than in bed when possible.
- Provide analgesics and antiemetics on a schedule that provides comfort at mealtime.
- Determine the person's food preferences; include culturally appropriate food.
- Have food available 24 hours per day; provide snacks between meals and at night.
- Do not interrupt meals to administer medication if possible.
- Walk around the dining area or the rooms at mealtime to determine whether food is being eaten or assistance is needed.
- Encourage family members to be present during mealtimes to provide an enhanced social situation.
- Offer caloric supplements, if used, between meals or with the medication pass.
- Recommend an exercise program that may increase appetite.
- Ensure proper fit of dentures and proper denture use.
- Provide oral hygiene, and allow the person to wash their hands.
- Offer the person their eyeglasses if the person is vision impaired.
- Sit while assisting the person with the meal, use touch, and carry on a social conversation.
- Provide soft music during the meal.
- Use small round tables seating six to eight people; consider using tablecloths and centrepieces.
- Seat people with similar interests and abilities together, and encourage socialization.
- Use restorative dining programs and adaptive equipment.
- Make diets as liberal as possible, especially for frail older adults who are not consuming adequate amounts.
- Consider a referral to a speech-language pathologist for a person experiencing difficulties with eating, a referral to an occupational therapist for adaptive equipment, or a referral to both.

In light of current population projections, the number of older adults requiring hospital care, rehabilitative care, and LTC will dramatically increase, leading to increased hospital stays, increased costs, and considerable mortality. Since the risk for malnutrition rises as soon as a person is put under one of these three types of care, malnutrition is a serious challenge for health care providers in all settings.

IMPLICATIONS FOR GERONTOLOGICAL NURSING AND HEALTHY AGING

Assessment

Older adults are less likely than younger people to show the signs of malnutrition and nutrient malabsorption. Although the evaluation of nutritional health can be difficult in the absence of severe malnutrition, a comprehensive assessment and physical examination can reveal deficits (Reber et al., 2019). The nurse needs to ensure holistic care while assessing the patient, taking into consideration both subjective and objective information.

A nutritional assessment that provides the most conclusive data about a person's actual nutritional state consists of the following steps: interview, physical examination, anthropometric measurements, and biochemical analysis. The collective result can provide the gerontological nurse with the data needed to identify immediate and potential nutritional problems. The nurse can then begin to establish plans for supervising, assisting, and educating the person, with the goal being adequate nutrition.

The Mini Nutritional Assessment, developed by Nestlé of Geneva, Switzerland, is intended for use by health care providers who are screening patients for malnutrition (https://www.mna-elderly.com). More information on nutrition and older adults can be found at https://uwaterloo.ca/nutrition-and-aging-lab/.

The minimum data set (MDS) includes assessment information that can be used to identify potential nutritional problems, risk factors, and potential for improved function. The nutrition and dehydration resident assessment protocols (RAPs) guide staff in the assessment of nutritionally related problems. Triggers for more thorough investigation include weight loss, alterations in taste, medical therapies, prescription medications, hunger, parenteral or intravenous feedings, mechanically altered or therapeutic diets, percentage of food left uneaten, pressure ulcers, and edema. Chapters 5 and 13 provide further information on the MDS and RAPs. An evidence-informed guideline on nutritional management in LTC is available at https://ltctoolkit.rnao.ca/clinical-topics/all.

Interview

The interview provides background information and clues to the older adult's nutritional state and to the actual and potential challenges facing the older adult. The nurse should ask questions about state of health, social activities, normal patterns, and changes that have occurred. The nurse should also explore the person's needs, how the person obtains food, and the person's ability to prepare food.

Information about the relationship of food to daily events will provide clues to the meaning and significance of food. The older adult who eats alone is considered a candidate for malnutrition. Information about occupation and daily activities will suggest the degree of energy expenditure and caloric intake most appropriate for the overall activity. A person's economic status will have a direct bearing on nutrition. It is therefore important to explore the person's financial resources to determine how much income is available for purchasing food.

The nutrition history should include data on the medications being taken. Additional medical information about visual difficulty, bowel and bladder function, and the presence or absence of mouth pain or discomfort should be obtained, as well as a history of illness.

Diet Histories. A 24-hour diet recall compared with the age- and gender-specific recommendations in *Eating Well With Canada's Food Guide* can provide an estimate of nutritional adequacy. When the older adult cannot supply all the information requested, it may be possible to obtain it from a family member or another source. There will be times, however, when the information is not as complete as one would like or when the older adult, too proud to admit that they are not eating well, furnishes erroneous information. Even so, the nurse will be able to obtain additional data from other areas of the nutritional assessment, as discussed later in this chapter.

Keeping a dietary record for 3 days is another assessment tool. What food was eaten, when it was eaten, and the amount eaten must be carefully recorded. Analysis of the dietary records provides information on energy, vitamin, and mineral intake. The accuracy of dietary records in hospitals and LTC homes can be problematic, as intake may be either underestimated or overestimated. Standardized observational protocols can improve the accuracy of oral intake documentation as well as the quality of feeding assistance. Nurses should ensure that direct caregivers are educated on the proper observation and documentation of intake.

Physical Examination

The physical examination furnishes clinically observable evidence of the existing state of nutrition. Data such as height and weight; vital signs; condition of the tongue, lips, and gums; skin turgor, texture, and colour; and functional ability are assessed, and the overall general appearance is scrutinized for evidence of wasting. Height should be measured and not estimated or self-reported. If the person cannot stand, an alternative way of measuring standing height is to use knee-height calipers (Cirillo et al., 2018). The body mass index (BMI) should be calculated to determine whether weight for height is within the normal range of 18.5 to 24.9. A BMI below 18.5 is a sign of undernutrition (Health Canada, 2019a).

A detailed weight history should be taken along with a measurement of current weight. This history should include information about the person's history of weight loss, the period during which the weight loss occurred, and whether the weight loss was intentional or unintentional. How to determine the appropriate weight charts for an older adult is still under debate. Although weight alone does not indicate the adequacy of diet, unplanned fluctuations in weight are significant and should be evaluated.

Weight changes may be the result of fluid retention, edema, or ascites and thus merit investigation. An unintentional weight loss of more than 5% of body weight in 1 month, more than 7.5% in 3 months, or more than 10% in 6 months is considered a significant indicator of poor nutrition as well as an MDS trigger.

Anthropometric Measurements

Obtained with simple procedures, anthropometric measurements include measurements of height, weight, midarm circumference, and triceps skinfold thickness. These measurements offer information about the status of the older adult's muscle mass and body fat in relation to height and weight. Muscle mass is found by measuring the circumference of the nondominant upper arm. Body fat and lean muscle mass are assessed by measuring specific skinfolds with Lange or Harpenden calipers at the midpoint of the upper arm. If there is a neuropathological condition or hemiplegia following a stroke, the unaffected arm should be used for measurements.

Biochemical Examination

The final step in a nutritional assessment is the biochemical examination. Suggested biochemical parameters include serum albumin, cholesterol, and serum transferrin. Although these parameters may also be abnormal in several conditions not associated with malnutrition, they

are useful as guides to interventions (Zhang et al., 2017). Serum albumin of more than 40 g/L (4 g/dL) is desirable; less than 35 g/L (3.5 g/dL) is an indicator of a poor nutritional state. Prealbumin level may be a better indicator of protein loss, because it changes rapidly in the presence of malnutrition. Transferrin, an iron transport protein, is diminished in protein malnutrition. However, it increases in iron deficiency anemia, which is common in older adults, so it is not a sensitive indicator of protein-caloric malnutrition. Laboratory test results, although not definitive for malnutrition, provide important clues to nutritional status but should be evaluated in relation to the person's overall health status.

Interventions

Interventions are often formulated around the identified nutritional problem. Nursing interventions are centred on techniques to increase food intake and enhance and manage the environment to promote increased food intake (Palese et al., 2018). Collaboration with the interprofessional team (which may include a dietitian, pharmacist, social worker, occupational therapist, or SLP) is important in planning interventions. For the community-dwelling older adult, intervention involves nutrition education and working together with the person and their family members on how to best resolve the potential or actual nutritional deficit.

The causes of poor nutrition are complex. It is important to assess all the factors emphasized in this chapter when individualized interventions to ensure adequate nutrition are being planned.

Pharmacological Therapy

Medications that stimulate the appetite (*orexigenic medications*) should be considered for reversing resistant anorexia after all other interventions have been attempted. Older adults taking these medications must be monitored closely for side effects, as these medications have not been evaluated well in frail older adults. Their benefits are restricted to small weight gains without indication of decreased morbidity, mortality, or improved quality of life or functional ability. Megestrol acetate (Megace) may be effective at a dosage of 800 mg daily for 3 months as prescribed by provider. Older adults should be monitored closely for adrenocortical insufficiency, and megestrol should not be given to bedridden older adults because of the risk for deep venous thrombosis. Dronabinol (Marinol), although not adequately tested with older adults, has shown some potential benefits because it stimulates appetite, has antinausea properties, decreases pain, and enhances general well-being. More research is needed to further understand the specific functions of Megace and Marinol in promoting weight gain for older adults (Levitt & O'Neil, 2018).

For older adults who are depressed and have weight loss or a poor appetite, mirtazapine (Remeron), an antidepressant, has been shown to increase appetite and weight gain as well as improve depressed mood (Levitt & O'Neil, 2018).

Patient and Family Education

Patients and families need to be educated about how to read nutritional information on labels. In 2016, the Food and Drug Regulations were modified to mandate nutritional labelling on most food labels (Government of Canada, 2020). The choice of nutrients was based on evidence that eating too much or too little of these substances has the greatest impact on health. Health Canada defines a "good source" as a food that contains 5% to 15% of the recommended daily value per serving (Health Canada, 2019b). Balance is the key to a healthy diet.

Enteral Feeding

When all the aforementioned interventions fail and challenges with nutritional intake in older adults persist, the decision is sometimes made to insert a feeding tube into the patient to provide an enteral feeding route. A comprehensive assessment of swallowing problems and other factors that influence intake must be conducted before initiating severely restricted diet modifications or considering the use of feeding tubes, particularly for older adults with advanced dementia. The use of enteral feeding routes for people with advanced dementia to prevent aspiration, pneumonia, malnutrition, and infections provides few long-term benefits and may in fact contribute to further decline. Enteral feeding has never been shown to reduce a person's risk of regurgitating gastric contents and cannot be expected to prevent the aspiration of oral secretions (Adeyinka et al., 2020).

The use of percutaneous endoscopic gastrostomy (PEG) feeding tubes in older adults has increased at an astonishing rate in recent years. Few complications occur with the insertion of a PEG tube; however, numerous complications occur from having one (Hucl & Spicak, 2016). Aspiration pneumonia, diarrhea, metabolic problems, and cellulitis are just a few of these complications.

Persons who aspirate oral feedings are also likely to aspirate enteral feedings, be they by way of either nasogastric tubes or gastrostomy tubes (Adeyinka et al., 2020).

As discussed earlier, food and eating are closely tied to socialization, comfort, pleasure, love, and basic biological needs. Decisions about enteral feeding are some of the most challenging of the many decisions that face families, health care providers, and facilities that care for older adults with dementia. Decisions to provide or not provide enteral feeding must be made carefully. Health care providers must take the time to listen to the wishes and concerns of the person and their family.

Individuals have the right to refuse or accept enteral feeding but should be given accurate information about its risks and benefits (Jones, 2018). Discussion about advance directives and feeding support should begin early in the course of the illness rather than being delayed until a crisis develops. The best advice is to allow individuals to state their preferences regarding enteral feeding in a written advance directive. Surrogate decision makers should use advance directives and previously expressed wishes to decide what a person with advanced dementia who is not eating would want in the particular circumstance.

Hospitals, LTC homes, and other care settings must promote choice and honour patient preferences in regard to enteral feeding and should not exert pressure on patients or on medical care providers to institute artificial feeding. LTC homes should have policies in place to ensure that patients with remediable causes of weight loss are appropriately evaluated and treated and that enteral feeding is not regarded as the only treatment of choice (Hanson et al., 2016).

Everyone involved in the care of the older adult must be informed about the potential benefits and risks of enteral feeding. Whether enteral feeding provides any benefit to the person is uncertain. However, the question should never be whether enteral feeding is or is not to be used. No family members should be made to feel that they are starving their loved one to death if it is decided not to institute enteral feeding. Comprehensive attempts to continue to provide nutrition should always be made. Excellent information about enteral feeding, both for patients and their families, can be found at http://www.chcr.brown.edu/dying/consumerfeedingtube.htm.

Short-term enteral feeding may be indicated for some conditions (e.g., after a hip fracture when serum albumin is low), but evidence supporting the effectiveness of enteral feeding for older adults with dementia is scant. When enteral feeding is indicated, the nurse and dietitian must work closely together to determine the appropriate formula and rate of administration, as well as the patient's tolerance, weight, and hydration status. The head of the bed should be elevated at least 30° for patients receiving continuous enteral feedings. When patients receive nutrition by bolus, the head of the bed should be elevated at least 30° during feeding and for 1 hour after feeding.

SUMMARY

The maintenance of adequate nutritional health as a person ages is extremely complex. A knowledge of normal nutrition in later years and the many factors contributing to inadequate nutrition is essential for the gerontological nurse, and the consideration of these matters should be a part of every assessment of the older adult. Whether in a community, hospital, or LTC setting, nurses must work with members of the interprofessional team to conduct appropriate assessments and develop therapeutic interventions. The use of evidence-informed practice protocols is important for determining nursing interventions to support and enhance nutritional status and promote adequate bowel function. The prevention of undernutrition and malnutrition and the maintenance of dietary needs and food enjoyment until the end of the patient's life are also ethical responsibilities of gerontological nurses. No older adult should be hungry or thirsty because they cannot shop, cook, or buy food, nor should any older adult have to suffer because of a lack of assistance with these activities, regardless of the setting in which they reside.

KEY CONCEPTS

- Recommended dietary patterns for the older adult are similar to those for younger persons but incorporate some reduction in caloric intake, based on decreased caloric requirements.
- Many factors affect adequate nutrition in later life, including income, chronic illness, dentition, mood disorders, capacity for food preparation, functional limitations, and lifetime eating habits.
- Protein-caloric malnutrition is the most common form of malnutrition in older adults. Estimates are that 50% of residents of LTC homes, 50% of patients in hospital, and 44% of home care patients over the age of 65 years are malnourished.
- A comprehensive nutritional assessment is an essential component of the assessment of older adults.
- Making mealtime pleasant and attractive for the older adult who is unable to eat unassisted is a nursing priority, and adequate assistance must be provided.
- Dental health is a basic need of older adults that is increasingly neglected. Poor oral health is a risk factor for dehydration, malnutrition, and aspiration pneumonia.
- Bowel function in older adults is minimally affected by the physiological changes of aging. Constipation is a common complaint, and non-pharmacological interventions, such as exercise and increased fluid and fibre intake, are important to maintain normal bowel function.

ACTIVITIES AND DISCUSSION QUESTIONS

1. What factors affect nutrition in the older adult?

2. How can the nurse intervene to provide better nutrition for older adults in the community, in acute care, and in LTC settings?

3. What are the causes of malnutrition?

4. What is included in the nutritional assessment of an older adult?

5. What factors contribute to changes in bowel function as a person ages?

6. What proactive measures can the nurse take to promote adequate bowel function for older adults in the community, in acute care, and in LTC settings?

7. How is dysphagia assessed, and what interventions may be helpful in preventing aspiration?

8. Develop a nursing care plan for an older adult at risk for malnutrition.

HEALTHY AGING CARE PLAN

Caring for D.M.

Recall the *Lived Experience* testimonial and D.M.'s case presented at the beginning of the chapter.

1. You continue your conversation with D.M. You ask D.M. how many meals he has in a day, to which he responds, "I always make two eggs in the morning and eat that with white toast and butter. I don't eat much the rest of the day. At night I might have a slice of white toast with an apple." You say to D.M., "I've noticed your pants seem a bit loose on you. Have you lost weight since your wife passed away?" D.M. describes how all his clothes have become loose, so he needed to buy a smaller belt to help secure them.

2. With D.M.'s approval, you put him in touch with Meals on Wheels, which will deliver nutritious meals to help increase his dietary intake. As a home care nurse, you also put in a referral to a dietitian with your agency to help D.M. ensure he is meeting his nutritional needs.

RESOURCES

Nutrition

Alzheimer Society of Canada. *Mealtimes.*
https://alzheimer.ca/en/Home/Living-with-dementia/Day-to-day-living/Meal-time

American Geriatrics Society's Health in Aging Foundation
https://www.healthinaging.org/

An approach to the management of unintentional weight loss in elderly people
https://www.cmaj.ca/content/cmaj/172/6/773.full.pdf

Assessing nutrition in older adults
https://hign.org/consultgeri/try-this-series/assessing-nutrition-older-adults

Eating and feeding issues in older adults with dementia: Part I: Assessment
https://hign.org/consultgeri/try-this-series/eating-and-feeding-issues-older-adults-dementia-part-i-assessment

Eating and feeding issues in older adults with dementia: Part II: Interventions
https://hign.org/consultgeri/try-this-series/eating-and-feeding-issues-older-adults-dementia-part-ii-interventions

EatRightOntario. *Older adults eating well.*
https://www.eatrightontario.ca/en/Articles/Seniors-nutrition/Older-adults-eating-well

Government of British Columbia. *Healthy Eating for Seniors Handbook.*
https://www2.gov.bc.ca/gov/content/family-social-supports/seniors/health-safety/active-aging/healthy-eating/healthy-eating-for-seniors-handbook

Government of Canada. *Canada's Food Guide.*
https://www.canada.ca/en/health-canada/services/canada-food-guides.html

Preventing aspiration in older adults with dysphagia
https://hign.org/consultgeri/try-this-series/preventing-aspiration-older-adults-dysphagia

Oral Health

Registered Nurses' Association of Ontario. *Oral Health: Supporting Adults Who Require Assistance* (2nd ed.).
https://rnao.ca/bpg/guidelines/oral-health-supporting-adults-who-require-assistance-second-edition

Constipation

Registered Nurses' Association of Ontario. *A Proactive Approach to Bladder and Bowel Management in Adults* (4th ed.)
https://rnao.ca/sites/rnao-ca/files/bpg/Bladder_and_Bowel_Management_FINAL_WEB.pdf

For additional resources, please visit *http://evolve.elsevier.com/Canada/Ebersole/gerontological/*

REFERENCES

Adeyinka, A., Rouster, A. S., & Valentine M. (2020). *Enteric feedings.* StatPearls. https://pubmed.ncbi.nlm.nih.gov/30422471/.

Allard, J. P., Keller, H., Jeejeebhoy, K. N., et al. (2016). Malnutrition at hospital admission—Contributors and effect on length of stay: A prospective cohort study from the Canadian Malnutrition Task Force. *Journal of Parenteral and Enteral Nutrition, 40*(4), 487–497. doi:10.1177/0148607114567902.

Andrade, P. A., dos Santos, C. A., Firmino, H. H., et al. (2018). The importance of dysphasia screening and nutritional assessment in hospitalized patients. *Einstein, 16*(2), eAO4189. doi:10.1590/S1679-45082018AO4189.

Bell, J. J., Pulle, R. C., Lee, H. B., et al. (2021). Diagnosis of overweight or obese malnutrition spells DOOM for hip fracture patients: A prospective audit. *Clinical Nutrition, 40*(4), 1905–1910. doi:10.1016/j.clnu.2020.09.003.

Bodnar, R. J. (2019). Endogenous opioid modulation of food intake and body weight: Implications for opioid influences upon motivation and addiction. *Peptides, 116*, 42–62. doi:10.1016/j.peptides.2019.04.008.

Canadian Association of Public Health Dentistry. (2019). *NEEDED: A Made-in-Canada solution to deliver dental care for all.* http://www.caphd.ca/sites/default/files/Federal%20Dental%20Care%20Ask%202019%20-%20For%20Members.pdf.

Canadian Cancer Society. (2020). *Oral cancer.* https://www.cancer.ca/en/cancer-information/cancer-type/oral/prognosis-and-survival/survival-statistics/.

Canadian Patient Safety Institute. (2020). *Aspiration pneumonia: Introduction.* https://www.patientsafetyinstitute.ca/en/toolsResources/Hospital-Harm-Measure/Improvement-Resources/Aspiration-Pneumonia/Pages/default.aspx.

Centers for Disease Control and Prevention. (2020). *The health effects of overweight and obesity.* https://www.cdc.gov/healthyweight/effects/index.html.

Chalmers, J., King, P., Spencer, A., et al. (2005). The oral health assessment tool—Validity and reliability. *Australian Dental Journal, 50*(3), 191–199. doi:10.1111/j.1834-7819.2005.tb00360.x.

Cingi, C. C., Eroglu, E., & Kreps, G. (2020). Role of anosmia on personal communication. In C. Cemal & N. Bayar Muluk (Eds.), *All around the nose: Basic science, diseases and surgical management* (pp. 247–251). Springer.

Cirillo, D. M., Hart, S. K., Reich, R. R., et al. (2018). Height measures: Evaluating alternatives to standing height in the ambulatory setting. *Clinical Journal of Oncology Nursing, 22*(5), 529–533. doi:10.1188/18.CJON.529-533.

Deer, R. R., Goodlett, S., & Volpi, E. (2017). Comparison of four malnutrition screening tools to the Subjective Global Assessment (SGA) in a cohort of acutely ill older adults. *The FASEB Journal, 31*(Suppl. 1), 151–154. doi:10.1096/fasebj.31.1_supplement.151.4.

Emmanuel, A., Mattace-Raso, F., Neri, M. C., et al. (2017). Constipation in older people: A consensus statement. *International Journal of Clinical Practice, 71*(1), e12920. doi:10.1111/ijcp.12920.

Farrer, O., Yaxley, A., Walton, K., et al. (2017). The 'diabetic diet': A web based survey for determining the incidence, rationale, composition and implications in Australian residential aged care facilities. *Journal of Nursing Home Research, 3*, 50–53. doi:10.14283/jnhrs.2017.8.

Government of Canada. (2018). *The state of community water fluoridation in Canada.* https://www.canada.ca/en/services/health/publications/healthy-living/community-water-fluoridation-across-canada-2017.html.

Government of Canada. (2019a). *Canada's Food Guide: Healthy eating for seniors.* https://food-guide.canada.ca/en/tips-for-healthy-eating/seniors/.

Government of Canada. (2019b). *Report on housing needs of seniors.* https://www.canada.ca/en/employment-social-development/corporate/seniors/forum/report-seniors-housing-needs.html.

Government of Canada. (2019c). *Oral health for seniors.* https://www.canada.ca/en/public-health/topics/oral-health/caring-your-teeth-mouth/senior.html.

Government of Canada. (2020). *Food labelling changes.* http://www.healthycanadians.gc.ca/eating-nutrition/label-etiquetage/changes-modifications-eng.php.

Hanson, E., Hellström, A., Sandvide, Å., et al. (2016). The extended palliative phase of dementia—An integrative literature review. *Dementia, 18*, 108–134. doi:10.1177/1471301216659797.

Health Canada. (2010). *Eating well with Canada's Food Guide—First Nations, Inuit and Métis.* https://www.canada.ca/en/health-canada/services/food-nutrition/canada-food-guide/eating-well-with-canada-food-guide-first-nations-inuit-metis.html.

Health Canada. (2019a). *Canadian guidelines for body weight classification in adults.* https://www.canada.ca/en/health-canada/services/food-nutrition/healthy-eating/healthy-weights/canadian-guidelines-body-weight-classification-adults/questions-answers-public.html.

Health Canada. (2019b). *How do you use the % DV?* https://www.canada.ca/en/health-canada/services/food-nutrition/food-labelling/nutrition-labelling/educators.html.

Hucl, T., & Spicak, J. (2016). Complications of percutaneous endoscopic gastrostomy. *Best Practice & Research Clinical Gastroenterology, 30*(5), 769–781. doi:10.1016/j.bpg.2016.10.002.

Jones, A. L. (2018). Refusal of PEG feeding following a carotid endarterectomy. *Cureus, 10*(7), e3046. doi:10.7759/cureus.3046.

Julius, M., Kresevic, D., Turcoliveri, M., et al. (2017). Malnutrition as a fall risk factor. *Federal Practitioner, 34*(2), 27.

Keboa, M., Beaudin, A., Cyr, J., et al. (2019). Dentistry and nursing working together to improve oral health care in a long-term care facility. *Geriatric Nursing, 40*(2), 197–204. doi:10.1016/j.gerinurse.2018.10.002.

Keller, H. H., Carrier, N., Slaughter, S., et al. (2017a). Making the Most of Mealtimes (M3): Protocol of a multi-centre cross-sectional study of food intake and its determinants in older adults living in long term care homes. *BMC Geriatrics, 17*(15). doi:10.1186/s12877-016-0401-4.

Keller, H. H., Carrier, N., Slaughter, S. E., et al. (2017b). Prevalence and determinants of poor food intake of residents living in long-term care. *Journal of the American Medical Directors Association, 18*(11), 941–947. doi:10.1016/j.jamda.2017.05.003.

Kobayashi, K., Ryu, M., Izumi, S., et al. (2017). Effect of oral cleaning using mouthwash and a mouth moisturizing gel on bacterial number and moisture level of the tongue surface of older adults requiring nursing care. *Geriatrics & Gerontology International, 17*, 116–121. doi:10.1111/ggi.12684.

Kossioni, A. E. (2018). The association of poor oral health parameters with malnutrition in older adults: A review considering the potential implications for cognitive impairment. *Nutrients, 10*(11), 1709: doi:10.3390/nu10111709.

Levitt, A., & O'Neil, J. (2018). Older adults with unintended weight loss: The role of appetite stimulants. *Home Healthcare Now, 26*(5), 312–318. doi:10.1097/NHH.0000000000000692.

Li, C., Zhang, Q., Ng, L., et al. (2016). Oral care measures for preventing nursing home-acquired pneumonia. *Cochrane Oral Health Group, 27*, CD012416. doi:10.1002/14651858.CD012416.

Longo, D. L., Mandell, L. A., & Niederman, M. S. (2019). Aspiration pneumonia. *New England Journal of Medicine, 380*, 651–663. doi:10.1056/NEJMra1714562.

Lopez, R. P., & Molony, S. L. (2018). Dementia: Weight loss and mealtime challenges. *Journal for Nurse Practitioners, 14*(3), 153–159.

Manlapaz, H. J. (2017). Implications of xerostomia and caries in community-dwelling older adults. *Canadian Journal of Dental Hygiene, 51*(3): 126–131.

Mitchell, A. (2019). Administering an enema: Indications, types, equipment and procedure. *British Journal of Nursing, 28*(3), 154–156. doi:10.12968/bjon.2019.28.3.154.

Mohn, E. S., Kern, H. J., Saltzman, E., et al. (2018). Evidence of drug–nutrient interactions with chronic use of commonly prescribed medications: An update. *Pharmaceutics*, *10*(1), 36. doi:10.3390/pharmaceutics10010036.

Namasivayam-MacDonald, A. M., Morrison, J. M., Steele, C. M., et al. (2017). How swallow pressures and dysphagia affect malnutrition and mealtime outcomes in long-term care. *Dysphagia*, *32*(6), 785–796.

Ogawa, T., Annear, M. J., Ikebe, K., et al. (2017). Taste-related sensations in old age. *Journal of Oral Rehabilitation*, *44*(8), 626–635.

Ontario Long Term Care Association. (2019). *This is long-term care 2019*. https://www.oltca.com/OLTCA/Documents/Reports/TILTC2019web.pdf.

Palese, A., Bressan, V., Kasa, T., et al. (2018). Interventions maintaining eating independence in nursing home residents: A multicenter qualitative study. *BMC Geriatrics*, *18*, 292. doi:10.1186/s12877-018-0985-y.

Reber, E., Gomes, F., Vasiloglou, M. F., et al. (2019). Nutritional risk screening and assessment. *Journal of Clinical Medicine*, *8*(7), 1065. doi:10.3390/jcm8071065.

Registered Nurses' Association of Ontario (RNAO). (2020a). *Oral health: Supporting adults who require assistance* (2nd ed.). https://rnao.ca/bpg/guidelines/oral-health-supporting-adults-who-require-assistance-second-edition.

Registered Nurses' Association of Ontario (RNAO). (2020b). *A proactive approach to bladder and bowel management in adults* (4th ed.) https://rnao.ca/sites/rnao-ca/files/bpg/Bladder_and_Bowel_Management_FINAL_WEB.pdf.

Rodriguez-Manas, L., Rodriguez-Sanchez, B., Carnicero, J. A., et al. (2020). Impact of nutritional status according to GLIM criteria on the risk of incident frailty and mortality in community-dwelling older adults. *Clinical Nutrition*, *40*(3), 1192–1198. doi:10.1016/j.clnu.2020.07.032.

Sauer, A. C., Alish, C. J., Strausbaugh, K., et al. (2016). Nurses needed: Identifying malnutrition in hospitalized older adults. *NursingPlus Open*, *2*, 21–25. doi:10.1016/j.npls.2016.05.001.

Smith, K. M., Thomas, K. S., Johnson, S., et al. (2019). Dietary service staffing impact nutritional quality in nursing homes. *Journal of Applied Gerontology*, *38*(5), 639–655.

Soenen, S., & Chapman, I. (2017). Appetite regulation in healthy aging. In R. R. Watson (Ed.), *Nutrition and functional foods for healthy aging* (pp. 35–42). Academic Press.

Statistics Canada. (2015). *Oral health: Edentulous people in 2007 to 2009*. http://www.statcan.gc.ca/pub/82-625-x/2010001/article/11087-eng.htm.

Statistics Canada. (2017). *Chronic low income among immigrants in Canada and its communities*. https://www150.statcan.gc.ca/n1/pub/11f0019m/11f0019m2017397-eng.htm.

Statistics Canada. (2019a). *Health indicators: Non-medical determinants of health*. https://www150.statcan.gc.ca/n1/pub/82-221-x/2017003/ndh-dns-eng.htm.

Statistics Canada. (2019b). *Overweight and obese adults*. Catalogue No. 82-625-X. https://www150.statcan.gc.ca/n1/en/pub/82-625-x/2019001/article/00005-eng.pdf%3Fst%3DOBRuwojR.

Statistics Canada. (2019c). *Results from the 2016 Census: Housing, income and residential dissimilarity among Indigenous people in Canadian cities*. https://www150.statcan.gc.ca/n1/pub/75-006-x/2019001/article/00018-eng.htm.

Statistics Canada. (2020). *Low income statistics by age, sex and economic family type*. https://www150.statcan.gc.ca/t1/tbl1/en/tv.action?pid=1110013501.

Su, Y., Yuki, M., Hirayama, K., et al. (2020). Denture wearing and malnutrition risk among community-dwelling older adults. *Nutrients*, *12*(1), 151. doi:10.3390/nu12010151.

Tabak, L., Green, E., Devaney, S., et al. (2019). Precision health: Bringing oral health into the context of overall health. *Advances in Dental Research*, *30*(2), 31–33. doi:10.1177/0022034519877392.

Takeuchi, K., Asakawa, M., Hashiba, T., et al. (2018). Effects of xylitol-containing chewing gum on the oral microbiota. *Journal of Oral Science*, *60*(4), 588–594. doi:10.2334/josnusd.17-0446.

Tarakad, A., & Jankovic, J. (2017). Anosmia and ageusia in Parkinson's disease. *International Review of Neurobiology*, *133*, 541–556. doi:10.1016/bs.irn.2017.05.028.

Valbrun, L. P., & Zvonarev, V. (2020). The opioid system and food intake: Use of opiate antagonists in treatment of binge eating disorder and abnormal eating behavior. *Journal of Clinical Medicine Research*, *12*(2), 41. doi:10.14740/jocmr4066.

World Health Organization. (2017). *Diet, nutrition and the prevention of chronic diseases: Report of the joint WHO/FAO expert consultation*. WHO Technical Report Series 916. https://www.who.int/publications/i/item/924120916X.

Youdim, A. (2019). *Nutrient–drug interactions*. https://www.merckmanuals.com/professional/nutritional-disorders/nutrition-general-considerations/nutrient-drug-interactions.

Zhang, M., & Ding, K. (2019). Adult congenital megacolon with acute fecal obstruction and diabetic nephropathy: A case report. *Experimental and Therapeutic Medicine*, *18*(4), 2726–2730. doi:10.3892/etm.2019.7852.

Zhang, Z., Pereira, S. L., Luo, M., et al. (2017). Evaluation of blood biomarkers associated with risk of malnutrition in older adults: A systematic review and meta-analysis. *Nutrients*, *9*(8), 829. doi:10.3390/nu9080829.

9

HYDRATION AND CONTINENCE

LEARNING OBJECTIVES

Upon completion of this chapter, the reader will be able to:

- Identify risk factors for dehydration.
- Discuss interventions to prevent or treat dehydration.
- Define *urinary* and *fecal incontinence*.
- List factors contributing to urinary and fecal incontinence.
- Explain the types of urinary incontinence and their causes.
- Discuss nursing interventions for urinary and fecal incontinence.

GLOSSARY

Dehydration   A harmful reduction in the amount of water in the body.

Detrusor   A body part that pushes down, such as the bladder muscle.

Incontinence   The inability to control excretory function.

Micturition   Urination.

Transient   Temporary.

THE LIVED EXPERIENCE

"I knew this problem could happen to me. I think it's related to miscarriages, childbirth, the muscles, etc., and these are the consequences."

"In the morning, when I cough a bit more and I sit on the toilet, like women do, sitting down, I go until I think I'm done . . . and I don't use pads because that would make me more feminine."

"I talk to my friends, who have the same problem as me, who have already gone through this. Talking to my friends helps me let off some steam, because they know what it's like to have urinary incontinence."

"When I'm around my children, I feel embarrassed because sometimes you leak very often and the truth is, I really feel embarrassed."

Comments from participants in a study of living with urinary incontinence (Esparza et al., 2018).

HYDRATION

Hydration Management

Hydration management is the maintenance of an adequate fluid balance, which prevents complications resulting from abnormal or undesirable fluid levels (Mentes & Gaspar, 2020). Water, a commodity that is accessible and available to almost all people, is often overlooked as an essential part of nutrition. Water's functions in the body include thermoregulation, dilution of water-soluble medications, facilitation of renal and bowel function, and creation of requisite conditions for and maintenance of metabolic processes.

Daily needs for water can usually be met through the intake of fluids with meals and by social drinks. However, a significant number of older adults (up to 85% of those aged 85 and older) drink less than 1 L of fluid per day. Older adults, with the exception of those requiring fluid restrictions, should consume at least 3.7 L (men) or 2.7 L (women) of fluid per day (Mentes & Gaspar, 2020). Maintenance of the balance between fluid intake and fluid output (when fluid intake equals fluid output) is

HEALTHY AGING CARE PLAN
About P.D.

P.D. (pronouns she/her), 83 years old, has been living in a long-term care (LTC) facility in Ottawa, Ontario, for the last 6 months. She came to the home after an admission to the hospital for a fall. P.D. and her family decided it was unsafe for her to stay at home any longer. P.D. likes being in the LTC home. Her care consists of support with activities of daily living, medication management, and fall prevention. When entering P.D.'s room one morning to help her get ready for breakfast, you notice that the room smells like urine. You observe that her bedsheets and nightgown are wet. P.D. tells you, "I could not get out of bed in time to use the bathroom and I could not hold it in. I really had to go." She hides her face in her hands and starts to cry.

QUESTIONS TO CONSIDER

1. What immediate steps do you take to care for P.D.?
2. What type of incontinence could P.D. be experiencing?
3. What key nursing interventions can you put in place to help P.D.?

---

essential to health, regardless of a person's age (Bak et al., 2017). Age-related changes, medication use, functional impairments, and comorbid medical illness place some older adults at risk for changes in fluid balance and especially dehydration (Picetti et al., 2017). A comprehensive hydration management guideline as well as intervention strategies can be found on the ConsultGeri website (https://hign.org/consultgeri/resources/protocols/hydration-management). Detailed recommendations for care planning to reduce the risk of dehydration and to maintain hydration are available on the Registered Nurses' Association of Ontario (RNAO) *Long-Term Care Best Practices Toolkit* website (http://ltctoolkit.rnao.ca/).

Dehydration

Dehydration results from insufficient fluid intake, is indicated by elevated directly measured serum osmolality, and undermines the health of older adults (Lešnik et al., 2017). Dehydration is a geriatric syndrome frequently associated with common diseases (e.g., diabetes, respiratory illness, and heart failure) and with frailty (Lešnik et al., 2017).

Dehydration is a problem among older adults in all settings. Not only is dehydration a significant risk factor for delirium, thromboembolic complications, infections, and kidney stones, but it also contributes to constipation and obstipation, falls, medication toxicity, renal failure, seizure, electrolyte imbalance, hyperthermia, and delayed wound healing (Bak et al., 2017; Picetti et al., 2017). Due to a lack of understanding of the pathogenesis and consequences of dehydration in older adults, dehydration in these persons is often attributed to poor care by LTC home staff, physicians, or both. However, for most older adults, dehydration is the result of increased fluid loss combined with decreased fluid intake due to decreased thirst.

Risk Factors for Dehydration

Most healthy older adults maintain adequate hydration. However, physical or emotional illness, surgery, trauma, or conditions with higher physiological demands increase the risk of dehydration. At that time, the limited capacity of the body's homeostatic mechanisms to maintain fluid balance can put an older adult's fluid balance at risk (Williams et al., 2017).

Age-related changes in the thirst mechanism, a decrease in total body water (TBW), and decreased kidney function increase the risk for dehydration. TBW decreases with age. In young adults, TBW is about 60% of body weight in men and 52% of that in women. In older adults, TBW decreases to about 52% of body weight in men and 46% of that in women. The loss of muscle mass with age increases the proportion of fat cells. This loss is greater in women because they have a higher percentage of body fat and less muscle mass than men have. Because fat cells contain less water than muscle cells, older adults have a lower volume of intracellular fluid. Furthermore, thirst sensation diminishes, resulting in the loss of an important defence against dehydration. Creatinine clearance also declines with age, and the kidneys are less able to concentrate urine. These changes are more pronounced among persons with illnesses that affect kidney function (see Chapter 6).

Risk factors for dehydration include the use of medications that directly affect renal function and fluid balance (e.g., diuretics, laxatives, and angiotensin-converting enzyme inhibitors) and the use of psychoactive medications that have anticholinergic effects (dry mouth, urinary retention, and constipation). The concurrent use of four or more medications is also a risk factor (Paulis et al., 2018).

Functional deficits, communication and comprehension problems, oral problems, dysphagia, depression, dementia, hospitalization, low body weight, diagnostic procedures that necessitate fasting, inadequate assistance with fluid intake, diarrhea, fever, vomiting, infections, bleeding, draining wounds, artificial ventilation, fluid restrictions, high environmental temperature, and multiple comorbidities have all been noted as risk factors for dehydration in older adults (Paulis et al., 2018). Nothing-by-mouth (NPO) periods for diagnostic tests and surgical procedures should be avoided or made as short as possible for older adults, and adequate fluids should be given once procedures have been completed. Research has determined that consuming clear liquids (e.g., water, apple juice, black tea, black coffee) 2 to 3 hours before surgery does not increase gastric residual volume or the risk for aspiration (Schmidt et al., 2018). Box 9.1 presents a simple screen for dehydration.

Hyponatremia is a decrease in sodium plasma concentration (<135 mmol/L) caused by an excess of water relative to solute. Differential diagnosis includes the syndrome of inappropriate antidiuretic hormone (SIADH) (Leonard & Lee, 2017). Selective serotonin reuptake inhibitors (SSRIs) increase the risk for hyponatremia, with risk being greatest in the first 2 weeks of treatment. Monitoring the sodium level and fluid intake of individuals taking recently prescribed SSRIs is important. Changes in mental status, including lethargy or acute confusion, should be investigated immediately (see Chapter 21). Other risk factors include certain medications, such as thiazide and loop diuretics, and comorbidities such as renal and hepatic insufficiencies, congestive heart failure,

---

BOX 9.1
SIMPLE SCREEN FOR DEHYDRATION

Drugs
End of life
High fever
Yellow urine turns dark
Dizziness (orthostasis)
Reduced oral intake
Axillae dry
Tachycardia
Incontinence (fear of)
Oral problems
Neurological impairment (confusion)
Sunken eyes

Source: Thomas, D., Cote, T., Lawhorne, L., et al. (2008). Understanding clinical dehydration and its treatment. *Journal of the American Medical Directors Association, 9*(5), 292–301.

---

and respiratory infections. Hyponatremia is especially common in older adults (Boyer et al., 2019).

IMPLICATIONS FOR GERONTOLOGICAL NURSING AND HEALTHY AGING

Assessment

Prevention of dehydration is essential, but the assessment of dehydration in older is complex; clinical signs may not appear until dehydration is advanced. Attention to risk factors is very important for identifying possible dehydration and intervening early. In addition, the minimum data set has 12 triggers for dehydration-fluid maintenance and seven additional risk factors. Older adults and their caregivers should be taught about the need for fluids and about the signs and symptoms of dehydration. Acute episodes of vomiting, diarrhea, or fever should be quickly recognized and treated. Older adults over the age of 85 years who have experienced volume deficits, weight loss, malnutrition, or infections are at a high risk for dehydration, as are older adults with dementia, delirium, and functional impairments.

Older adults may not always show the typical signs of dehydration (Brandstrup & Moller, 2019). Skin turgor, assessed at the sternum and commonly included in the assessment of dehydration, is an unreliable marker in older adults because of the loss of subcutaneous tissue that occurs with aging. Dry mucous membranes in the mouth and nose, longitudinal furrows on the tongue, orthostasis, speech incoherence, weakness of extremities, dry axillae, and sunken eyes may indicate dehydration.

Laboratory tests for suspected dehydration include blood urea nitrogen (BUN) and tests for sodium, creatinine, glucose, and bicarbonate. Osmolarity should be either directly measured or calculated. While most cases of dehydration involve elevated BUN, there are many other causes of elevated BUN (Ren et al., 2018). Changes in body weight should also be assessed, as they indicate changes in hydration.

Interventions

Interventions for dehydration are derived from a comprehensive assessment that consists of risk identification and hydration management (Mentes & Gaspar, 2020). Hydration management involves both acute and ongoing management of oral intake. Oral hydration is the first treatment approach for dehydration. Individuals with mild to moderate dehydration who can drink and do not have significant mental or physical compromise due to fluid loss may be able to replenish fluids orally. Water is considered the best fluid for this purpose, but other clear fluids may also be offered, depending on the person's preference.

Rehydration methods depend on the severity and type of dehydration and may include either intravenous administration or hypodermoclysis, an infusion of isotonic fluids into the subcutaneous space. A general rule is to replace 50% of the loss within the first 12 hours (1 L per day in afebrile older adults) or a sufficient quantity to relieve tachycardia and hypotension. Further fluid replacement can be administered over a longer period.

Hypodermoclysis is safe, easy to administer, and a useful alternative to intravenous administration for persons with mild to moderate dehydration, particularly those with altered mental status. Normal saline (0.9%), half-normal saline (0.45%), a 5% dextrose in water infusion (D5W), or Ringer's solution can be used (Epstein & Waseem, 2020). Because hypodermoclysis can be administered in almost any setting, hospital admission may be avoided.

Ongoing management of oral hydration includes the following five steps: (1) calculate a daily fluid goal; (2) compare the person's current intake to the amount

---

BOX 9.2

FLUID INTAKE CALCULATION AND ONGOING MANAGEMENT OF HYDRATION

FLUID INTAKE CALCULATION:

- Recommended intake of 3.7 L per day for men and 2.7 L per day for women aged 70 and older who are active and not frail.
- For those in a LTC home and who may be sedentary, the following daily fluid intake is recommended:
  - 100 mL/kg for the first 10 kg of body weight
  - 50 mL/kg for the remaining kilograms of body weight

ONGOING MANAGEMENT OF HYDRATION:

1. Provide fluids consistently throughout the day:
   - Offer a variety of fluids
   - Integrate fluid rounds mid-morning and late afternoon
   - If taking thickened liquids, encourage intake, as intake has been reported as lower than if taking thin liquids
2. Make drinking opportunity a pleasurable and social experience:
   - Offer "happy hours" or "teatime" in the afternoon where residents can gather together for additional fluids and socialization
3. Ensure utensils are resident centered:
   - Use modified fluid containers based on resident intake behaviours
   - Use high-contrast tableware during meals for those with dementia

Source: Adapted from Mentes, J. C., & Gaspar, P. M. (2020). Hydration management. *Journal of Gerontological Nursing,* 46(2), 20–30.

---

calculated, to evaluate the person's hydration status; (3) provide fluids consistently throughout the day; (4) plan for at-risk individuals; and (5) perform fluid regulation and documentation (Mentes & Gaspar, 2020). Box 9.2 further discusses fluid intake calculation and ongoing management of hydration.

URINARY CONTINENCE

Bladder Function

Normal bladder function requires an intact brain and spinal cord, competent lower urinary tract function, motivation to maintain continence, functional ability to recognize voiding signals and use a toilet, and an environment that facilitates the process. A full bladder increases pressure and alerts the spinal cord and the brainstem centre to the need to micturate. Social training then dictates whether **micturition** should be attended to or postponed (e.g., until there is an opportunity to access toilet facilities). However, when bladder contents reach 500 mL or more, the pressure is such that the urge to void becomes more difficult to control. As volume increases, emptying the bladder becomes an uncontrollable act.

Age-Related Changes in Bladder Function

Bladder changes that occur with aging include decreased capacity, increased irritability, contractions during filling, and incomplete emptying. These changes may lead to frequency, nocturia, urgency, and vulnerability to infection. The warning period between the desire to void and actual micturition is shortened. This shorter warning period—combined with illness, cognitive impairments, challenges in manipulating clothing, or difficulty in walking to the toilet or handling a bedpan or urinal—can affect an older adult's ability to maintain continence.

Urinary Incontinence

Urinary **incontinence** (UI) is the involuntary loss of urine (Trad et al., 2019) and an important yet neglected geriatric syndrome. Because of its high prevalence and chronic but preventable nature, UI is considered a public health issue—a stigmatized, underreported, underdiagnosed, and undertreated condition that is thought to be part of normal aging (Biswas et al., 2017).

Individuals may not seek treatment for UI, because they are embarrassed by the dysfunction or because they do not know that successful treatments are available. In one study by Waetjen and colleagues, (2018), 61% of women who experienced UI chose not to seek treatment. Most of these women did not believe that the UI was "bad enough" (73%), believed that UI was a normal part of aging (53%), or stated that they did not bring it up because their health care provider did not ask (55%) (Waetjen et al., 2018). Men may be unlikely to report UI to their primary care providers because they feel that UI is a woman's condition. Nurses caring for older adults in all practice settings should be prepared to assess the person for urine control and

implement nursing interventions that promote continence (Trad et al., 2019). *Incontinence: Breaking the Silence*, a fact sheet for public education, is available from the RNAO (http://rnao.ca/bpg/fact-sheets/incontinence-breaking-silence).

Epidemiology of Urinary Incontinence

Millions of adults worldwide are affected by UI. In Canada, 50% of adults report symptoms of urge incontinence. Women are more likely than men to have UI (14% versus 9%). In addition, UI is more common among older adults: at age 85 years or older, 11% of men and between 10% and 58% of women experience UI (Registered Nurses' Association of Ontario [RNAO], 2020). An estimated 79% of LTC home residents are incontinent (Ontario Long Term Care Association, 2019).

Urinary incontinence is more prevalent than diabetes, Alzheimer's disease, and many other chronic conditions that receive more attention and treatment. Incontinence also costs Canadians approximately $8.5 billion annually (RNAO, 2020). A recent study of UI in LTC homes reported that staff education and staff perceptions of the effectiveness of UI treatment influenced care intervention. Enabling factors included teamwork and the experience of success (French et al., 2017).

Consequences of Urinary Incontinence

UI affects quality of life and has physical, psychosocial, and economic consequences. It is associated with falls, skin irritations and infections, urinary tract infections (UTIs), and pressure ulcers. It also affects self-esteem and increases the risk for depression, anxiety, social isolation, and avoidance of sexual activity. Older adults with UI experience a loss of dignity, loss of independence, and loss of self-confidence, as well as feelings of shame and embarrassment (Trad et al., 2019). The psychosocial impact of UI affects both the person and family caregivers. Three instruments are available to assess the psychological effects of UI: the Incontinence Impact Questionnaire (Uebersax et al., 1995), the International Consultation on Incontinence Questionnaire (ICIQ) (Volz-Sidiropoulou et al., 2018), and the Male Urinary Symptom Impact Questionnaire (Robinson & Shea, 2002).

Risk Factors for Urinary Incontinence

Cognitive impairment, limitations in daily activities, and institutionalization are associated with higher risk for UI. Stroke and diabetes are also associated with UI (Northwood et al., 2020). Pregnancy, childbirth, menopause, and hysterectomy are other factors that contribute to UI. It can also be exacerbated by medications that increase urinary output and by sedative–hypnotic medications, which produce drowsiness, confusion, or limited mobility, thus dulling the desire to urinate.

In a study of LTC home residents with dementia, 48% had UI upon admission, and 81% had UI 6 months after admission. Dementia does not cause UI but affects the ability of the person to recognize the urge to void and to find a washroom in which to do so. Mobility problems and dependency in transfers are better predictors of continence status than is dementia, which suggests that persons with dementia may be able to remain continent as long as they are mobile. Making toilets easily visible, helping persons go to the washroom at regular intervals, and implementing prompted voiding protocols can help promote continence for people with dementia.

Box 9.3 presents risk factors for UI.

Types of Urinary Incontinence

Incontinence is classified as either **transient** (acute) or established (chronic). Transient incontinence has a sudden onset, is present for 6 months or less, and is usually caused by treatable factors, such as UTIs, delirium, constipation and stool impaction, and increased urine production caused by metabolic conditions such as hyperglycemia and hypercalcemia. *Iatrogenic* (treatment-induced) incontinence is a type of transient UI that results from the use of restraints, limited fluid intake, bedrest, or intravenous fluid administration. The use of anticholinergics, calcium channel blockers, and alpha-adrenergic agonists and blockers can also lead to transient UI (Boockvar et al., 2020; Nerli & Hiremath, 2017).

Established UI may have either a sudden or a gradual onset and is categorized into the following types:

- *Urge incontinence* (overactive bladder) is defined as involuntary urine loss that occurs soon after feeling an urgent need to void. The bladder muscles are overactive and cause a sudden urge to void—the "gotta go right now" syndrome (Aoki et al., 2017). The defining characteristics of urge

> **BOX 9.3**
> **RISK FACTORS FOR**
> **URINARY INCONTINENCE**
>
> - Age
> - Immobility, functional limitations
> - Diminished cognitive capacity (dementia, delirium)
> - Medications (anticholinergics, sedatives, diuretics)
> - Smoking
> - High caffeine intake
> - Obesity
> - Constipation, fecal impaction
> - Pregnancy, vaginal delivery, episiotomy
> - Low fluid intake
> - Environmental barriers
> - High-impact physical exercise
> - Diabetes
> - Stroke
> - Parkinson's disease
> - Hysterectomy
> - Pelvic muscle weakness
> - Childhood nocturnal enuresis
> - Prostate surgery
> - Estrogen deficiency
> - Arthritis
> - Hearing and vision impairments
>
> *Source:* Adapted from Dowling-Castronovo, A., & Bradway, C. (2012). Urinary incontinence. In M. Boltz, E. Capezuti, T. T. Fulmer, & D. Zwicker (Eds.), *Evidence-based geriatric nursing protocols for best practice* (4th ed., pp. 363–387). Springer.

incontinence include the loss of moderate to large amounts of urine before reaching a toilet and an inability to suppress the need to urinate. Urinary frequency and nocturia may also be present. Postvoid residual urine reveals a small amount of urine left in the bladder after voiding. Urge incontinence is the most common type of UI in older adults (Nerli & Hiremath, 2017).

- *Stress incontinence* (outlet incompetence) is defined as an involuntary loss of less than 50 mL of urine during actions that increase intra-abdominal pressure (e.g., coughing, sneezing, exercising, lifting, and bending). Stress incontinence is more common in women because of their short urethras and poor pelvic-muscle tone (as a result of pregnancies); it also occurs in men who have undergone prostatectomy and radiation treatment. Postvoid residual urine is low (Nerli & Hiremath, 2017).

- *Urge* or *stress UI with high postvoid residual incontinence* (formerly called "overflow incontinence") is what occurs when the bladder does not empty normally and becomes overdistended (beyond regular distention when filled with a normal amount of urine). This condition is accompanied by frequent or nearly constant urine loss (dribbling). Its symptoms include hesitancy in starting urination, slow urine stream, infrequent urination or small volumes of urine, a feeling of incomplete bladder emptying, and large volumes of postvoid residual urine. Persons with diabetes and men with enlarged prostates are at risk for this type of UI. The use of calcium channel blockers, anticholinergics, and adrenergics also contributes to symptoms.
- *Functional incontinence* is defined as a situation in which the lower urinary tract is intact but the individual is unable to reach a toilet because of environmental barriers, physical limitations, or severe cognitive impairment. The person may be dependent on others for assistance in reaching a toilet but have no genitourinary problems other than incontinence. Older adults in institutions have higher rates of functional incontinence (Jachan et al., 2019). Functional incontinence may also occur in the presence of other types of UI.
- *Mixed incontinence* is defined as a combination of more than one type of UI, usually stress and urge. Mixed incontinence is the most prevalent type of incontinence in older women; with increasing age, older women with stress incontinence begin to experience urge incontinence.

IMPLICATIONS FOR GERONTOLOGICAL NURSING AND HEALTHY AGING

Nurses in all practice settings with older adults should be prepared to assess continence and implement nursing interventions that promote continence.

Assessment

Continence must be routinely addressed in the initial assessment of every older adult, yet many people do not bring up their concerns about incontinence, and many health care providers do not ask. Health care providers must begin to change their thinking about incontinence and acknowledge that it can be cured or treated to minimize its detrimental effects. Nurses are often the ones to identify UI, but neither nurses nor physicians have been particularly aggressive in its management.

Assessment is multidimensional: it includes a health history, targeted physical examination, urinalysis, and a determination of postvoid residual urine. More extensive examinations are considered after the initial findings are assessed. A thorough health history should focus on the medical, neurological, and genitourinary history; functional assessment; cognitive assessment; psychosocial effects; strategies currently used to control UI; medication review of both prescribed and over-the-counter medications; detailed exploration of the symptoms of the UI; and associated symptoms and other factors. In care facilities, an environmental assessment, including the accessibility of bathrooms, room lighting, and the use of aids such as raised toilet seats or commodes, is also important.

In an LTC home, the completed minimum data set may trigger the resident assessment protocol for incontinence. Several tools can be used for comprehensive continence assessment, treatment, and evaluation for LTC home residents. The ICIQ-Urinary Incontinence-Short Form (ICIQ-UI-SF) is another instrument that can be used to evaluate UI (Timmermans et al., 2016).

One of the best ways to establish the presence of incontinence problems and to describe them is with a voiding diary, the "gold standard" for obtaining objective information about voiding patterns and the frequency and severity of UI episodes (Elmer et al., 2017). Older adults living in the community can usually keep a voiding diary without much difficulty. In LTC homes, voiding diaries are usually maintained by the staff. The voiding diary should record the character of the urine (colour, odour, sediment, clearness) and any difficulty the person has starting or stopping the urinary stream. The person's ability to accomplish activities of daily living (such as reaching and using a toilet) and their finger dexterity for manipulating clothing should also be documented.

Interventions

Behavioural

Continence can be improved when appropriate care is provided. A number of behavioural interventions have a good basis in research and can be implemented by nurses without extensive and expensive evaluation. These treatments are viewed as healthy bladder behaviour skills (French et al., 2017). These interventions will do no harm; if they bring no improvement, further evaluation can be sought. Behavioural techniques such as scheduled voiding, prompted voiding, bladder training, biofeedback, vaginal weight training, and pelvic floor muscle exercises (PFMEs) are recommended as first-line treatment for UI. The selection of a modality and interventions will depend on a comprehensive assessment, the type of incontinence and its underlying cause, and whether the goal is to cure or to minimize the extent of the incontinence. Interventions and treatment planning for UI should involve the interprofessional team and everyone involved with the person's care. Physiotherapy and occupational therapy, restorative programs, or all should be part of the treatment plan for persons with impaired mobility. For example, there are physiotherapists who specialize in incontinence care and management, such as pelvic floor physiotherapy. Occupational therapists are able to assist with environmental modifications to help prevent incontinence. Box 9.4 lists nursing interventions in the treatment of UI that focus on supportive measures and restorative therapeutic modalities.

■ *Scheduled (timed) voiding* is used to treat urge and functional UI in both cognitively intact and

cognitively impaired older adults. The scheduling or timing of voiding is based on the voiding patterns shown in the person's bladder diary or on common voiding patterns (i.e., voiding upon arising, before and after meals, and at midmorning, midafternoon, and bedtime). Generally, regular toileting is scheduled at 2- to 4-hour intervals. People can be taught to do this routinely, or they can be helped to the bathroom at the scheduled intervals.

■ *Prompted voiding* combines scheduled voiding with monitoring, prompting, and verbal reinforcement. With a cognitively intact person, the objective is to increase self-initiated voiding and decrease the episodes of UI. With a cognitively impaired person, caregivers should regularly ask whether they need assistance in using the toilet. The person is assisted to the toilet if they request. Positive feedback is provided after successful voiding. Newman (2019) describes how prompted voiding reduces the severity of UI, prevents complications associated with UI, and increases the resident's self-initiated requests to use the toilet in LTC homes.

Newly admitted LTC home residents should be thoroughly assessed for continence. Those who are incontinent yet able to use the toilet should undergo a 3- to 5-day trial of prompted voiding. The trial can help demonstrate a person's response to toileting and determine patterns of and symptoms associated with the incontinence. Residents who are unresponsive to toileting programs or are unable or unwilling to participate in toileting can be provided with supportive management, including the use of absorbent pads and briefs, with attention to the prevention of skin breakdown (Brennan et al., 2017; Rice et al., 2018).

Continence programs in LTC homes are required by regulations in some provinces and territories. Monitoring and the documentation of continence status in relation to implemented continence care should be a quality-of-care indicator for LTC homes (RNAO, 2020).

■ *Bladder training* aims to increase the interval between the urge to void and voiding. This method is appropriate for people with urge UI who are cognitively intact and independent in toileting. The person follows an established voiding schedule

---

BOX 9.4

NURSING INTERVENTIONS AND SUPPORT MEASURES IN THE TREATMENT OF URINARY INCONTINENCE

- Appropriate attitude
- Accessible toilets and toilet substitutes (bedpan, urinal, commode)
- Avoidance of iatrogenic conditions (UTIs, constipation or impaction, excessive sedation, medications adversely affecting the bladder or urethral function)
- Protective undergarments
- Absorbent bed pads
- Behavioural techniques: bladder training, scheduled (timed) voiding, prompted voiding, biofeedback, PFMEs, vaginal weight training
- Good skin care

until UI episodes cease. The interval between voidings is then extended, and techniques (e.g., PFMEs) for overcoming the urge to urinate and for postponing urination are taught.

- PFMEs, also called *Kegel exercises*, involve repeated voluntary pelvic floor muscle contraction. The targeted muscle is the pubococcygeal muscle; this muscle forms the support for the pelvis and surrounds the urethra and rectum in men and the urethra, rectum, and vagina in women. The goal of the repetitive contractions is to strengthen the muscle and decrease UI episodes. PFMEs are recommended for stress, urge, and mixed UI in older women and have also been shown to be helpful for men who have undergone prostatectomy. Contractions should be repeated 30 to 100 times a day; the contraction is held for 10 seconds and is followed by 10 seconds of relaxation.

Correct identification of the pelvic floor muscles and compliance with the exercise regimen are key to success. Improvement may not be noted until 2 to 4 weeks of exercising have been successfully completed. To help the person identify the correct muscle groups, the caregiver can tell the person to try to tighten the anal sphincter, as if controlling the passage of flatus or feces, and then to tighten the urethral muscles, vaginal muscles, or both, as if stopping the flow of urine. The stomach, thigh, or buttock muscles should not be contracted, since this increases intra-abdominal pressure. This exercise may be taught during a vaginal or rectal examination, when the clinician helps the patient identify the pelvic muscles by having them "squeeze" the clinician's gloved examination finger (Healy et al., 2013).

- *Biofeedback* may be helpful in identifying the correct muscles and visualizing the strength and time of the contraction (Perez et al., 2018).
- *Vaginal weight training* is an alternative for women who have difficulty identifying the pelvic floor muscles. The woman wears graded-weight vaginal balls or cones for two 15-minute periods each day or uses them in addition to doing PFMEs. When the weighted ball or cone is placed in the vagina, the pelvic floor muscle contractions keep it from slipping out. Although this technique involves less time and is more easily taught than PFMEs, discomfort and difficulties inserting the objects have been noted as deterrents to this approach.

Lifestyle Modifications

Several lifestyle factors are associated with either the development or exacerbation of UI. Lifestyle modifications that can diminish UI include modification of dietary factors, weight reduction, smoking cessation, bowel management, and physical activity. The University Health Network in Toronto, Ontario, has recommended limiting the consumption of caffeinated foods and drinks such as coffee, tea, and chocolate, and increasing noncaffeinated and nonalcoholic fluid intake (Samuel et al., 2021). Box 9.5 presents other recommendations to community-dwelling older adults for controlling or eliminating UI.

BOX 9.5

HELPFUL RECOMMENDATIONS TO COMMUNITY-DWELLING OLDER ADULTS FOR CONTROLLING OR ELIMINATING URINARY INCONTINENCE

- Empty the bladder completely before and after meals and at bedtime.
- Urinate whenever the urge arises; never ignore it.
- Try a schedule of urinating every 2 hours during the day and every 4 hours at night, which is often helpful in retraining the bladder. The use of an alarm clock may be necessary.
- Drink 1.5–2.0 L of fluid before 2000 hours each day to help the kidneys function properly. Limit fluids after supper to 125–250 mL, except in very hot weather.
- Eliminate or reduce the consumption of coffee, tea, brown cola, and alcohol, since they have a diuretic effect.
- Take prescription diuretics in the morning upon rising.
- Limit the use of sleeping pills, sedatives, and alcohol; they decrease the sensation of urinating and can increase incontinence, especially at night.
- Lose weight if overweight.
- Try doing PFMEs, which are often helpful for women with stress, urge, and mixed UI. They may also be helpful for men after prostatectomy.
- Make sure the toilet is nearby, has a clear path to it, and has good lighting, especially at night. Grab bars or a raised toilet seat may be needed.
- Dress protectively with cotton underwear and protective pants or incontinent pads if necessary.

Absorbent Products

A variety of protective undergarments and adult briefs are available for the older adult who is incontinent. Disposable types come in several sizes, as determined by hip and waist measurements, or as a one-size-fits-all garment. Many of these undergarments look like regular underwear and contribute to greater dignity. Some individuals may prefer to use absorbent products in addition to toileting interventions to maintain "social continence."

Urinary Catheters

External catheters (condom catheters) are used in male patients who are incontinent and cannot be toileted. Long-term use of external catheters can lead to fungal skin infection, penile skin maceration, edema, fissures, contact burns from urea, phimosis, UTIs, and septicemia. The catheter should be removed and replaced daily, the meatal area washed with soap and water, and the penis washed, dried, and aired to prevent irritation, maceration, pressure ulcers, and skin breakdown. If the catheter is not sized appropriately and is not applied and monitored correctly, strangulation of the penile shaft can occur.

Intermittent catheterization may be used in persons with urinary retention related to a weak **detrusor** muscle (e.g., diabetic neuropathy), a blockage of the urethra (e.g., benign prostatic hypertrophy), or reflex incontinence related to a spinal cord injury. The goal is to maintain a urine volume of 300 mL or less in the bladder. Most of the research on intermittent catheterization has been conducted with children or young adults with spinal cord injuries, but the procedure may be useful for older adults who are able to self-catheterize. Intermittent catheterization is an important alternative to indwelling catheterization.

Long-term indwelling urinary catheters have been used to manage urinary retention and UI, but this must be justified on the basis of medical conditions and failure of other efforts to maintain continence.

The use of indwelling catheters in hospitals is often unjustified, and they are used inappropriately (for example, for the convenience of staff) or left in place too long. The misuse of catheterization should be considered a medical error. About one in four indwelling catheters in hospitalized patients aged 70 years or older and one in three patients aged 85 years or older turn

out to be unnecessary (Griebling, 2017). Urinary catheterization is a risk factor for delirium (see Chapter 21), and catheterization without a specific medical indication is associated with a greater risk of death and longer hospital stays (Griebling, 2017).

If nurses must insert an indwelling catheter or leave it in place, daily assessment is key in preventing infections, sepsis, and delirium (Canadian Nurses Association, 2019). Policies, procedures, and clarity on long-term indwelling catheter management is lacking (Canadian Agency for Drugs and Technologies in Health [CADTH], 2019), and more information is needed on the proper indication for long-term indwelling catheter use.

Long-term catheter use increases the risk of recurrent urinary tract infections, leading to urosepsis, urethral damage in men secondary to urethral erosion, urethritis or fistula formation, and bladder stones or cancer. UTIs are the most common infections among residents of LTC homes. Asymptomatic bacteria in the urine are considered benign in older adults and should not be treated with antibiotics. Screening of urine cultures should not be performed for asymptomatic patients. Symptomatic UTIs necessitate antibiotic treatment, but it is important to pay attention to the range of symptoms that older adults may present (fever, dysuria, flank pain, abdominal pain, new-onset incontinence, decreased appetite, changes in mental status, or even respiratory distress). It is important to continue providing appropriate perineal care owing to the increased risk for infection.

Pharmacological

Typically, nonpharmacological therapies are more effective in treating UI and should be implemented before pharmacological treatment is considered. Pharmacological treatment, including anticholinergic–antimuscarinic (antispasmodic) agents—toterodine, darifenacin, and solifenacin succinate—may be indicated for urge UI and overactive bladder (Tadrous et al., 2018). Undesirable side effects of anticholinergic medications (such as dry mouth and eyes, constipation, confusion, and the precipitation of glaucoma) are sometimes problematic in older adults.

Nonsurgical Devices

Stress incontinence can be treated with intravaginal support devices, pessaries, and urethral plugs. Primarily used to prevent uterine prolapse, a pessary is a device that is fitted into the vagina and exerts pressure to ele-vate the urethro-vesical junction of the pelvic floor. The patient is taught to insert and remove the pessary, much like a diaphragm used for contraception is inserted and removed. The pessary is removed weekly or monthly for cleaning with soap and water and then reinserted. Adverse effects include vaginal infection, low back pain, and vaginal mucosal erosion. Another concern is the danger of forgetting to remove the pessary.

Surgical

Surgical intervention is appropriate for some condi-tions of incontinence. Surgical suspension of the bladder neck (sling procedure) is effective in 80% to 95% of women who elect to have this surgical correc-tive procedure. In men, outflow obstruction inconti-nence secondary to prostatic hypertrophy is generally corrected by prostatectomy. Sphincter dysfunction resulting from nerve damage following surgical trauma or radical perineal procedures is 70% to 90% repair-able through sphincter implantation. Periurethral bulking—the injection of collagen or polytetrafluoro-ethylene into the periurethral area to increase pressure on the urethra—has been added to the list of surgical procedures that address UI. This procedure adds bulk to the internal sphincter and closes the gap that allowed leakage to occur.

FECAL AND BOWEL INCONTINENCE

Fecal incontinence (FI) is defined as the continuous or recurrent uncontrolled passage of fecal material for at least 1 month in a mature person. Its prevalence is dif-ficult to determine with accuracy because many peo-ple are reluctant to discuss this disorder and many health care providers do not ask about it. Prevalence varies with the study population. In one study, 16.1% of participants reported FI, but when researchers used an assessment called the Rome IV Criteria, this preva-lence dropped to 3.3% (Whitehead et al., 2019). Other estimated prevalence rates are 2% to 17% in commu-nity-dwelling older persons, 50% to 65% in older adults living in LTC homes, and 33% in older adults in hospital. Higher prevalence rates are found among patients with diabetes, irritable bowel syndrome, stroke, multiple sclerosis, and spinal cord injury (Frank et al., 2020).

Often, FI is associated with UI, and as many as 50% to 70% of patients with UI also have FI. It can be transient (in episodes of diarrhea, acute illness, or fecal impaction) or persistent. Like UI, FI has devastating social ramifications for individuals and their families. Both UI and FI have similar contributing factors, including damage to the pel-vic floor as a result of surgery or trauma, neurological dis-orders, functional impairment, immobility, and dementia.

IMPLICATIONS FOR GERONTOLOGICAL NURSING AND HEALTHY AGING

Assessment

For most older adults, FI can be improved or resolved. In many cases, multiple factors interact to cause FI. Assessment should include a complete history (as is done in UI assessment, described earlier in this chapter) and investigation of the following: diet, stool consis-tency and frequency, use of laxatives or enemas, surgi-cal and obstetrical history, use of medications that could exacerbate FI, and the effect of FI on the person's quality of life. A focused physical examination (with attention to the gastro-intestinal system) and a bowel record are also necessary. A digital rectal examination should be performed to identify the presence of any mass, impaction, or occult blood.

Because FI is often associated with fecal impaction, reports of diarrhea in older adults must be thoroughly assessed before using antidiarrheal medications, as these may further complicate the problem of fecal im-paction. Digital rectal examination for impacted stool and an abdominal plain film will confirm the presence of impacted stool. Stool analysis for *Clostridium difficile* toxin should be ordered for patients who develop new-onset diarrhea with incontinence (Nelson et al., 2017). Additional tests may be indicated by assessment find-ings. Comprehensive assessment seeks to identify un-derlying and potentially treatable causes of FI, such as fecal loading, infection, inflammatory bowel disease, lower gastro-intestinal cancer, and rectal prolapse. Maintenance of healthy bowel function and prevention of constipation are discussed in Chapter 8.

Interventions

Interventions depend on the underlying cause of FI. Condition-specific interventions for treatable causes of FI should be implemented first. Nursing interventions are aimed at managing bowel continence, restoring bowel continence, or both, and for persons with intractable FI, preserving health and dignity. Therapies similar to those used to treat UI, such as environmental manipulation (for toilet access), diet alterations, habit-training schedules, improvement in transfer and ambulation ability, sphincter-training exercises, biofeedback, medications, or surgery to correct underlying defects, are effective in the treatment of FI.

Keeping accurate bowel records and identifying triggers that initiate incontinence are important. For example, eating a meal stimulates defecation 30 minutes following the completion of the meal, or defecation is stimulated after a morning cup of coffee. If its patterns are identified, FI can be controlled with preparation. Placing the person on the toilet or commode or having a bedpan available at a given time following the trigger event facilitates defecation. The judicious use of nonirritant laxatives can help to promote complete rectal emptying. Box 9.6 describes a bowel training program.

As in the treatment of UI, goals must be realistic. It cannot be stated too often or too strongly that the nurse must always provide immaculate skin care to incontinent persons, because the person's self-esteem and skin integrity depend on it. When FI is intractable, interventions are aimed at preserving the person's dignity and independence and providing psychological and emotional support. Patients may require advice about skin care, talking to friends and family, and

---

BOX 9.6
BOWEL TRAINING PROGRAM

Obtain a bowel history, complete a bowel record, and establish a schedule for the bowel training program that is comfortable and conforms to the patient's lifestyle.

Ensure adequate fibre intake (to normalize stool consistency):
1. Recommendations for adequate fibre intake:
   a. Add high-fibre foods (dried fruit and beans, vegetables, whole-grain products) to the person's diet.
   b. Add 15–45 mL of bran to the person's diet one or two times per day, or administer a bulk laxative (e.g., Metamucil, Benefibre, Prodiem). Titrate the dosage, based on the person's response.
   c. Use the following recipe for a natural laxative: 250 mL wheat bran, 250 mL applesauce, and 250 mL prune juice. Mix and store in refrigerator. Start with 15 mL per day and increase slowly until the desired effect is achieved (see Chapter 8).

Ensure adequate fluid intake (to normalize stool consistency):
1. Recommendations for adequate fluid intake:
   a. The person should drink 2–3 L daily (unless contraindicated).
   b. The person should consume 4 oz of prune, fig, or pear juice (or a warm fluid) daily as a stimulus (e.g., 30 to 60 minutes before established time for defecation).

Encourage exercise:
1. Pelvic tilt and modified sit-ups for abdominal strength.
2. Walking for general muscle tone and cardiovascular system.
3. A more vigorous program if appropriate.

Facilitate bowel movements:
1. Establish a regular routine and time for bowel movements, depending on person's schedule. The best times are 20 to 40 minutes after regularly scheduled meals, when the gastrocolic reflex is active.
2. Attempts at evacuation should be made daily within 15 minutes of the established time and whenever the person senses rectal distension.
3. Promote normal posture for defecation (i.e., sitting on the toilet or commode; for persons who are unable to get out of bed, a left-side lying position).
4. Instruct the person to contract the abdominal muscles and "bear down."
5. Have the person lean forward to increase intra-abdominal pressure by using compression against the thighs.
6. Stimulate the anorectal reflex and rectal emptying if necessary by one of the following actions:
   a. Administer an enema or insert a rectal suppository into the rectum 15 to 30 minutes before the planned bowel movement. (The suppository should be placed against the bowel wall.)
   b. Insert a gloved, lubricated finger into the anal canal, and gently dilate the anal sphincter.

obtaining and using continence products. Problems with toilet access can be addressed by clearly indicating location and through environmental modifications. Patients can be referred to support groups.

SUMMARY

Gerontological nurses play a pivotal role in continence care. It is important that nurses and other health care providers understand the risk factors for incontinence, the causes of incontinence, and evidence-informed protocols for interventions. Health promotion, public education, comprehensive assessments of incontinence, education of informal and formal caregivers, and evidence-informed interventions should be part of individualized care for all older adults experiencing symptoms of incontinence.

KEY CONCEPTS

- Age-related changes in the thirst mechanism, a decrease in total body weight, and decreased kidney function increase the risk for dehydration in older adults.
- Most healthy older adults maintain adequate hydration, but physical or emotional illness, surgery, trauma, or conditions with physiological demands increase the risk for dehydration.
- Urinary incontinence is not a normal part of aging; it is a symptom of underlying dysfunction and calls for thorough assessment.
- Urinary incontinence can be minimized or cured, and many therapeutic modalities for its treatment are available for nurses to implement.
- Health promotion teaching, identification of risk factors, comprehensive assessments, education of informal and formal caregivers, and use of evidence-informed interventions are basic continence competencies for nurses.
- A number of interventions for urinary incontinence are applicable to the management of fecal incontinence.

ACTIVITIES AND DISCUSSION QUESTIONS

1. Explain the problems associated with dehydration in the older adult.

2. Identify the signs and symptoms of dehydration.

3. Discuss interventions to prevent and treat dehydration.

4. Discuss risk factors for urinary incontinence in older adults.

5. Conduct a urinary incontinence history with a partner or with an older adult.

6. Explain what measures can be taken to cure or decrease the incidence or impact of urinary or fecal incontinence in the community and in long-term care settings.

7. Devise a nursing care plan for an older adult with urinary or fecal incontinence.

HEALTHY AGING CARE PLAN

Caring for P.D.

Recall the *Lived Experience* testimonials and P D.'s case presented at the beginning of the chapter.

1. As P.D.'s nurse, you listen to P.D. and reassure her. You inform her that you will help her and begin by assisting her with hygienic care and getting dressed for breakfast. You remove the soiled bed linens and nightgown and replace these with fresh ones. You document the care.

2. P.D. has experienced an incontinent episode, possibly due to an overactive bladder (urge incontinence). Urge incontinence is the most common type of urinary incontinence in older adults.

3. Nursing interventions should include ensuring that P.D. has assistance to use the toilet as soon as she wakes up in the morning and before breakfast (scheduled/timed voiding). Consultation with other members of the interprofessional health care team can help determine whether further assessment and treatment is needed.

RESOURCES

Agency for Healthcare Research and Quality. Prevention of urinary and fecal incontinence in adults.
https://archive.ahrq.gov/downloads/pub/evidence/pdf/fuiad/fuiad.pdf

Canadian Society of Intestinal Research. Research summaries and patient information.
http://www.badgut.com

Hartford Institute for Geriatric Nursing. Urinary incontinence in older adults admitted to acute care.
https://www.guidelinecentral.com/summaries/urinary-incontinence-in-older-adults-admitted-to-acute-care-in-evidence-based-geriatric-nursing-protocols-for-best-practice/

Hydration Management
https://hign.org/consultgeri/resources/protocols/hydration-management

Regional Geriatric Program Central. Professional and patient education resources for hydration and continence.
http://www.rgpc.ca/resources/

Registered Nurses' Association of Ontario. Best practice guideline for continence care and bowel management.
http://ltctoolkit.rnao.ca/resources/continence-and-constipation-assessment-and-management

The Canadian Continence Foundation
http://www.canadiancontinence.ca/EN/?index.html

The Canadian Nurse Continence Advisors. Standards of practice, continuing education, and pamphlets and video clips for patient education.
http://www.cnca.ca

For additional resources, please visit *http://evolve.elsevier.com/Canada/Ebersole/gerontological/*

REFERENCES

Aoki, Y., Brown, H. W., Brubaker, L., et al. (2017). Urinary incontinence in women. *Nature Reviews. Disease Primers, 3,* 17042. doi:10.1038/nrdp.2017.42.

Bak, A., Tsiami, A., & Greene, C. (2017). Methods of assessment of hydration status and their usefulness in detecting dehydration in the elderly. *Current Research in Nutrition and Food Science, 5*(2), 43–54. doi:10.12944/crnfsj.5.2.01.

Biswas, B., Bhattacharyya, A., Dasgupta, A., et al. (2017). Urinary incontinence, its risk factors, and quality of life: A study among women aged 50 years and above in a rural health facility of West Bengal. *Journal of Mid-life Health, 8*(3), 130–136. doi:10.4103/jmh.JMH_62_17.

Boockvar, K. S., Song, W., Lee, S., et al. (2020). Comparing outcomes between thiazide diuretics and other first-line hypertensive drugs in long-term nursing home residents. *Clinical Therapeutics, 42*(3), 583–591. doi:10.1016/j.clinthera.2020.02.016.

Boyer, S., Gayot, C., Bimou, C., et al. (2019). Prevalence of mild hyponatremia and its association with falls in older adults admitted to an emergency geriatric medicine unit (the MUPA unit). *BMC Geriatrics, 19*(265), 2–6. doi:10.1186/s12877-019-1282-0.

Brandstrup, B., & Moller, A. M. (2019). The challenge of perioperative fluid management in elderly patients. *Geriatric Anesthesia, 9,* 406–413. doi:10.1007/240140-019-0034906.

Brennan, M., Milne, C., Agrell-Kann, M., et al. (2017). Clinical evaluation of a skin protectant for the management of incontinence-associated dermatitis. *Journal of Wound, Ostomy, and Continence Nursing, 44*(2), 172–180. doi:10.1097/WON.0000000000000307.

Canadian Agency for Drugs and Technologies in Health (CADTH). (2019). *Management of patients with long-term indwelling urinary catheters: A review of guidelines.* https://cadth.ca/sites/default/files/pdf/htis/2019/RC1112%20Indwelling%20Urinary%20Catheters%20Final.pdf.

Canadian Nurses Association. (2019). *Nine things nurses and patients should question.* https://www.cna-aiic.ca/~/media/cna/page-content/pdf-en/nine-things-nurses-and-patients-should-question.pdf?la=en.

Elmer, C., Murphy, A., Elliot, J., et al. (2017). Twenty-four-hour voiding diaries versus 3-day voiding diaries: A clinical comparison. *Female Pelvic Medicine & Reconstructive Surgery, 23*(6), 429–432. doi:10.1097/SPV.0000000000000412.

Epstein, E. M., & Waseem, M. (2020). *Crystalloid fluids.* StatPearls. https://www.ncbi.nlm.nih.gov/books/NBK537326/.

Esparza, A. O., Tomás, C., & Pina-Roche, F. (2018). Experiences of women and men living with urinary incontinence: A phenomenological study. *Applied Nursing Research, 40,* 68–75. doi:10.1016/j.apnr.2017.12.007.

Frank, C., Molnar, F., & Spencer, M. (2020). Fecal incontinence in older adults. *Canadian Family Physician, 66,* 264.

French, B., Thomas, L. H., Harrison, J., et al. (2017). Client and clinical staff perceptions of barriers to and enables of the uptake and delivery of behavioural interventions for urinary incontinence: Qualitative evidence synthesis. *Journal of Advanced Nursing, 73*(1), 21–38. doi:10.1111/jan.13083.

Griebling, T. L. (2017). Re: Inappropriate use of urinary catheters among hospitalized elderly patients: Clinician awareness is key. *Journal of Urology, 197*(3 Part 1), 707–709.

Healy, F., Barry, E., & O'Sullivan, S. (2013). Physiotherapy service provision and its effectiveness after obstetric anal sphincter injuries. *Journal of the Association of Chartered Physiotherapists in Women's Health, 113,* 30–41.

Jachan, D., Müller-Werdan, U., & Lahmann, N. (2019). Impaired mobility and urinary incontinence in nursing home residents: A multicenter study. *Journal of Wound, Ostomy, and Continence Nursing, 46*(6), 524–529. doi:10.1097/WON.0000000000000580.

Leonard, S. D., & Lee, J. F. (2017). Hyponatremia and syndrome of inappropriate antidiuretic hormone after orthopedic surgery. *Proceedings of UCLA Healthcare, 21.*

Lešnik, A., Piko, N., Železnik, D., et al. (2017). Dehydration of older patients in institutional care and the home environment. *Research in Gerontological Nursing, 10*(6), 260–266. doi:10.3928/19404921-20171013-03.

Mentes, J. C., & Gaspar, P. M. (2020). Hydration management. *Journal of Gerontological Nursing, 46*(2), 19–30. doi:10.3928/00989134-20200108-03.

Nelson, R., Suda, K., & Evans, C. (2017). Antibiotic treatment for *Clostridium difficile*-associated diarrhoea in adults. *Cochrane Database of Systematic Reviews, 3,* CD004610. doi:10.1002/1451858. CD004610.pub5.

Nerli, R., & Hiremath, M. (2017). Urinary incontinence in the elderly. *RGUHS Journal of Medical Sciences, 7*(3), 90–93. doi:10.26463/rjms/2017/v7/i3/116933.

Newman, D. K. (2019). Prompted voiding for individuals with urinary incontinence. *Journal of Gerontological Nursing, 45*(2), 14–26. doi:10.3928/00989134-20190111-03.

Northwood, M., Markle-Reid, M., Sherifali, D., et al. (2020). Cross-sectional study of prevalence and correlates of urinary incontinence in older home-care clients with type 2 diabetes in Ontario, Canada. *Canadian Journal of Diabetes, 45*(1), 47–54. e4. doi:10.1016/j.jcjd.2020.05.005.

Ontario Long Term Care Association. (2019). *This is long-term care 2019.* https://www.oltca.com/OLTCA/Documents/Reports/TILTC2019web.pdf.

Paulis, S. J., Everink, I. H., Halfens, R. J., et al. (2018). Prevalence and risk factors of dehydration among nursing home residents: A systematic review. *Journal of the American Medical Directors Association, 19*(8), 646–657. doi:10.1016/j.jamda.2018.05.009.

Perez, F. S. B., Rosa, N. C., da Rocha, A. F., et al. (2018). Effects of biofeedback on preventing urinary incontinence and erectile dysfunction after radial prostatectomy. *Frontiers in Oncology, 8*, 20. doi:10.3389/fonc.2018.00020.

Picetti, D., Foster, S., Pangle, A. K., et al. (2017). Hydration health literacy in the elderly. *Nutrition and Healthy Aging, 4*(3), 227–237. doi:10.3233/NHA-170026.

Registered Nurses' Association of Ontario (RNAO). (2020). *A proactive approach to bladder and bowel management in adults* (4th ed.). Author.

Ren, X., Qu, W., Zhang, L., et al. (2018). Role of blood urea nitrogen in predicting the post-discharge prognosis in elderly patients with acute decompensated heart failure. *Scientific Reports, 8*(1), 1–7. doi:10.1038/s41598-018-31059-4.

Rice, S., Pendrill, L., Petersson, N., et al. (2018). Rationale and design of a novel method to assess the usability of body-worn absorbent incontinence care products by caregivers. *Journal of Wound, Ostomy, and Continence Nursing, 45*(5), 456–464. doi:10.1097/WON.0000000000000462.

Robinson, J. P., & Shea, J. A. (2002). Development and testing of a measure of health-related quality of life for men with urinary incontinence. *Journal of the American Geriatric Society, 50*(5), 935–945. doi:10.1046/j.1532-5415.2002.50223.x.

Samuel, S. E., Suresh, B. V., & Sushmitha, A. S. (2021). Influence of lower urinary tract dysfunction on functional status among ambulant stroke survivors: A pilot study. *Indian Journal of Physiotherapy and Occupational Therapy, 15*(4). doi:10.37506/ijpot.v15i4.16514.

Schmidt, A., Buehler, K., Both, C., et al. (2018). Liberal fluid fasting: Impact on gastric pH and residual volume in healthy children undergoing general anesthesia for elective surgery. *British Journal of Anesthesia, 121*(3), 647–655. doi:10.1016/j.bja.2018.02.065.

Tadrous, M., Elterman, D., Khu, W., et al. (2018). Publicly funded overactive bladder drug treatment patterns in Ontario over 15 years: An ecological study. *Canadian Urological Association Journal, 12*(3), E142–E145. doi:10.5489/cuaj.4541.

Timmermans, L., Falez, F., Melot, C., et al. (2016). Use of the International Consultation on Incontinence Questionnaire-Urinary Incontinence-Short Form (ICIQ-UI-SF) for an objective assessment of disability determination according to the Modified Katz Scale: A prospective longitudinal study. *Italian Journal of Urology and Nephrology, 68*(4), 317–323.

Trad, W., Flowers, K., Caldwell, J., et al. (2019). Nursing assessment and management of incontinence among medical and surgical adult patients in a tertiary hospital: A best practice implementation project. *JBI Database of Systematic Reviews and Implementation Reports, 17*(12), 2578–2590.

Uebersax, J. S., Wyman, J. F., Shumaker, S. A., et al. (1995). Short forms to assess life quality and symptom distress for urinary incontinence in women: The Incontinence Impact Questionnaire and the Urogenital Distress Inventory. Continence Program for Women Research Group. *Neurology & Urodynamics, 14*(2), 131–139.

Waetjen, L. E., Xing, G., Johnson, W. O., et al. (2018). Factors associated with reasons incontinent mid-life women report for not seeking urinary incontinence treatment over 9 years across the menopausal transition. *Menopause, 25*(1), 29–39. doi:10.1097/GME.0000000000000943.

Volz-Sidiropoulou, E., Rings, R., Wagg, A. S., et al. (2018). Development and initial psychometric properties of the 'ICIQ-Cog': A new assessment tool to measure the disease-related impact and care effort associated with incontinence in cognitively impaired adults. *BJU International, 122*(2), 309–3016. doi:10.1111/bju.14186.

Whitehead, W. E., Simren, M., Busby-Whitehead, J., et al. (2019). Fecal incontinence diagnosed by the Rome IV Criteria in the United States, Canada, and the United Kingdom. *Clinical Gastroenterology and Hepatology, 18*(2), 385–391. doi:10.1016/j.cgh.2019.05.040.

Williams, D., Sandler, A., Koepke, E., et al. (2017). Fluid management in the elderly. *Current Anesthesiology Reports, 7*(4), 357–363. doi:10.1007/s40140-017-0243-4.

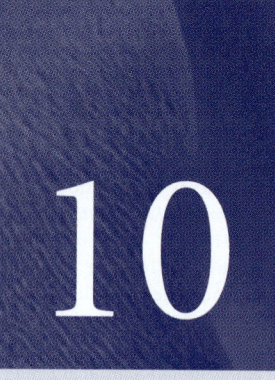

10 REST, SLEEP, AND ACTIVITY

Upon completion of this chapter, the reader will be able to:

- Identify age-related changes that affect rest, sleep, and activity.
- Discuss the importance of sleep and activity to the health and well-being of older adults.
- Describe nursing assessment relevant to rest, sleep, and activity.
- Explain nursing interventions useful in the promotion of rest, sleep, and activity.

GLOSSARY

Circadian rhythm   The regular recurrence of certain phenomena in cycles of approximately 24 hours.

Insomnia   Disturbed sleep pattern (difficulty falling asleep, staying asleep, or feeling restored following sleep) in the presence of adequate opportunity and circumstances for sleep.

Nocturia   Excessive urination at night.

Non–rapid eye movement (NREM) sleep   The first four stages of sleep.

Obstructive sleep apnea (OSA)   Repetitive cessation (>10 seconds) of respiration during sleep.

Rapid eye movement (REM) sleep   Wakeful and active form of sleep, during which dreaming occurs or tension is discharged.

THE LIVED EXPERIENCE

"You know, I never get a decent night's sleep. I wake up at least four times every night, and I just know I won't get back to sleep. I really don't want to keep taking pills for sleep, but when I lie there awake, I just think of all the difficult times and situations I can't manage. After a while, I'm really in a stew about everything."

Richard, a 67-year-old recent retiree

"This is really beginning to tire me out. Richard keeps waking me at night because he can't sleep. I try to tell him to get up and read or something. I really need my sleep if I'm going to get to work on time. I wonder if Richard needs to see a doctor. Maybe he is depressed about being retired and alone while I'm at work. I'll talk to him about it."

Clara, Richard's wife

Rest, sleep, and activity depend on one another. Inadequacy of rest and sleep affects any activity, be it an activity requiring strenuous exertion or an activity of daily living. Activity, in turn, is necessary to maintain physical and physiological integrity (such as that of cardiopulmonary endurance and function and that of musculo-skeletal strength, agility, and structure). Activity also helps people obtain adequate sleep. Together, rest, sleep, and activity contribute greatly to overall physical and mental well-being.

REST AND SLEEP

The human organism needs rest and sleep to conserve energy, prevent fatigue, provide organ respite, and relieve tension. Rest occurs with sleep in sustained, unbroken periods, whereas sleep is an extension of rest. Both are physiological and mental necessities for the preservation of life. Our lives proceed in a series of rhythms that influence and regulate physiological function, chemical concentrations, performance, behavioural responses, moods, and the ability to adapt.

Gerontologists are now studying the relevance of age-related changes in **circadian rhythm** to health, illness, and the process of aging. It is clear that body temperature, pulse, blood pressure, neurotransmitter excretion, and hormonal levels change significantly and predictably in a circadian rhythm. With aging, there is a reduction in the amplitude of all these circadian endogenous responses. The most important and obvious biorhythm is the circadian sleep–wake rhythm. Abnormalities of this endogenous cycle may be responsible for some of the sleep difficulties of old age. Complaints of sleep difficulty are common, since aging is associated with changes in the amount of sleep, sleep quality, and specific sleep disorders, such as **insomnia**, sleep apnea, restless legs syndrome (RLS), and circadian rhythm disturbances (Miner & Kryger, 2017).

The predictable pattern of normal sleep is called *sleep architecture* (Palinkas et al., 2017). The body progresses through five stages in the normal sleep pattern, which consists of **rapid eye movement (REM) sleep** and **non–rapid eye movement (NREM) sleep** (Box 10.1). The amount of deep sleep (stages 3 and 4) contributes to how rested and refreshed a person feels the next day. Sleep architecture changes in aging; less time is spent in stages 3 and 4, and more time is spent in stage 1. These declines start between 20 and 30 years of age, going against the stereotype that sleep disturbances occur only in older adults. Time spent in REM sleep also declines with age, and transitions between stages 1 and 2 are more common.

As a result, older adults' sleep is lighter, more fragmented, and characterized by frequent awakenings (Miner & Kryger, 2017). Older adults report more time in bed, reduced total sleep time, prolonged sleep latency (i.e., the amount of time it takes to fall asleep), more frequent awakenings, increased wakefulness after the onset of sleep, and increased frequency of daytime naps (Koščec Bjelajac et al., 2020) (Box 10.2). Sleep deprivation and fragmentation of sleep in older adults may promote the experience of pain and adversely affect cognitive functioning, respiratory function, and general health status (Chen et al., 2019). These concerns are greater when older adults are in hospital or reside in long-term care (LTC) homes (FitzGerald et al., 2017; Hjetland et al., 2020).

BOX 10.1
SLEEP STRUCTURE

FOUR STAGES OF NON–RAPID EYE MOVEMENT SLEEP

Stage 1
Lightest level
Between being awake and falling asleep
Light sleep

Stage 2
Onset of sleep
Disengagement from surroundings
Regular breathing and heart rate
Lowering of body temperature

Stages 3 and 4
Sleep is at deepest and most restorative level
Blood pressure drops
Breathing becomes slower
Muscles are relaxed
Blood supply to muscles increases
Tissue growth and repair occurs
Energy is restored
Hormones (such as growth hormone, essential for growth and development [including muscle development]) are released

Rapid Eye Movement Sleep
Takes up 25% of sleep
First occurs about 90 minutes after falling asleep
Recurs about every 90 minutes, getting longer throughout the night
Provides energy to brain and body
Supports daytime performance
Brain is active and dreams occur
Eyes dart back and forth
Muscles relax and body becomes immobile

Source: Adapted from National Sleep Foundation. (2017). *What happens when you sleep?* https://sleepfoundation.org/how-sleep-works/what-happens-when-you-sleep.

Older adults may not be exposed to adequate amounts of bright outdoor light, particularly in certain climates or in LTC homes. Bright-light therapy (exposure to bright outdoor light or to an indoor light box later in the afternoon) may assist in resetting the circadian rhythm (Schotland, 2019).

Older adults who are in good general health, have positive moods, and engage in active lifestyles and meaningful activities report better sleep and express fewer sleep complaints. Poor sleep is not an inevitable

BOX 10.2
AGE-RELATED SLEEP CHANGES

- Total sleep time and sleep efficiency are reduced.
- Deep sleep (slow-wave sleep) decreases with age.
- Daytime napping increases with age. Rapid eye movement sleep is shorter and less intense.
- Poorer subjective sleep quality is seen in older adults when compared to younger adults.
- Circadian rhythm changes.

Source: Adapted from Li, J., Vitiello, M. V., & Gooneratne, N. (2018). Sleep in normal aging. *Sleep Medicine Clinics,* 13(1), 1–11. doi:1016/j.jsmc.2017.09.001.

BOX 10.3
FACTORS CONTRIBUTING TO SLEEP PROBLEMS IN OLDER ADULTS

- Comorbidities (cardiovascular disease, diabetes), central nervous system disorders (Parkinson's disease, dementia), gastro-intestinal disturbances
- Depression, anxiety
- Medications
- Environmental noises, room sharing, health care organizational routines
- Poor sleep hygiene
- Lack of exercise
- Excessive napping
- Sleep apnea
- Restless legs syndrome/Willis–Ekbom disease
- Periodic limb movement
- Rapid eye movement sleep behaviour disorder
- Alcohol consumption

Source: Adapted from Lavoie, C. J., Zeidler, M. R., & Martin, J. L. (2018). Sleep and aging. *Sleep Science and Practice,* 2(3). doi:10.1186/s41606-018-0021-3.

consequence of aging; poor sleep is an indicator of health status and calls for further investigation.

Sleep Disorders

Sleep disorders include insomnia, sleep apnea, RLS, and rapid eye movement sleep behaviour disorder (RBD).

Insomnia

Insomnia is a subjective perception of insufficient or non-restorative sleep (Castelnovo et al., 2019). Insomnia can be classified as sleep-onset insomnia, sleep-maintenance insomnia, or nonrestorative sleep (awakening without feeling refreshed or rested). Insomnia has a high prevalence in older adults and results from numerous factors (Box 10.3).

Comorbid medical and psychiatric conditions contribute to insomnia in older adults. The most common reason for interrupted sleep is **nocturia** (Vaughan et al., 2016). Gastro-esophageal reflux disease (GERD) is also a common cause of sleeplessness. During REM sleep, more acid is produced. Because the esophageal sphincter at the gastric inlet is more relaxed in older adults, acid refluxes into the esophagus, which does not have the same protective lining that the stomach has. Over time, the lining of the esophagus becomes scarred, and protective secretions emerge into the back of the throat, resulting in frequent coughing during sleep. Treatment includes elevating the head of the bed (not just the mattress) 18–20 cm (7–8 inches) so that gravity keeps the secretions in the lower part of the esophagus. Other treatments for GERD include the use of proton pump inhibitor (PPI) medications and education on the avoidance of caffeine and alcohol. Although PPI therapy

is highly effective for the treatment of GERD, its long-term use has been associated with an increased risk of hip fractures (Torvinen-Kiiskinen et al., 2018).

Sleep problems among older adults with dementia can include sleeping too much or too little, wandering during the night, or rising earlier than usual (Lo et al., 2016). According to the Alzheimer Society of Canada, someone with dementia who sleeps during the day may eventually have difficulty sleeping at night because sleeping during the day tends to increase. In extreme situations, sleep patterns may reverse, as the person may sleep mostly during the day and stay awake most of the night (Alzheimer Society of Canada, 2020). Anxiety and depression also contribute to insomnia (see Chapter 23). There is some evidence that nonpharmacological complementary therapies (such as light therapy) and daytime activities help people with dementia sleep better, and bedtime music and reduced ambient noise at night may also be helpful for those with dementia (van Maanen et al., 2016; Gibson et al., 2017).

The side effects of many common medications used by older adults could also include sleep disturbances and insomnia (Box 10.4). A medication review is always indicated when sleep complaints are investigated.

BOX 10.4
MEDICATIONS THAT MAY CAUSE FRAGMENTED SLEEP, NIGHTMARES, NOCTURIA, OR STIMULATION

ANTIDEPRESSANTS

- Selective serotonin reuptake inhibitors
- Monoamine oxidase inhibitors
- Bupropion
- Venlafaxine

CARDIOVASCULAR

- Alpha-blockers (tamsulosin)
- Beta-blockers (propranolol, metoprolol)
- Diuretics (furosemide)
- Statins

OPIOIDS

- In combination with caffeine (acetaminophen)

RESPIRATORY

- Beta-agonists (salbutamol, formoterol, terbutaline)

STIMULANTS

- Amphetamine
- Caffeine
- Cocaine
- Ephedrine

OTHERS

- Alcohol
- Corticosteroids (prednisone)
- Dopamine receptor agonists (levodopa)
- Nicotine
- Phenytoin
- Thyroid supplements

Source: Adapted from Centre for Effective Practice. (2017). *Management of chronic insomnia.* https://cep.health/media/uploaded/CEP_Management_of_Chronic_Insomnia_2017.pdf.

BOX 10.5
RISK FACTORS FOR SLEEP APNEA

- Increasing age
- Increased alcohol and tobacco use
- Increased neck circumference
- Male sex
- Family history
- Excess weight

Source: Adapted from National Heart, Lung, and Blood Institute. (2020). *Sleep apnea.* https://www.nhlbi.nih.gov/health-topics/sleep-apnea.

Sleep Apnea

Sleep apnea is a condition in which people stop breathing while asleep. Apnea (complete cessation of respiration) and hypopnea (partial decrease in respiration) result in hypoxemia and changes in autonomic nervous system activity. The result is increased systemic and pulmonary arterial pressure and changes in cerebral blood flow. The episodes are generally terminated by an arousal (a brief awakening), which results in fragmented sleep and excessive daytime sleepiness. Other symptoms of sleep apnea include loud periodic snoring, gasping and choking on awakening, unusual nighttime activity (such as sitting upright or falling out of bed), morning headache, poor memory and intellectual functioning, and irritability and personality change. If the person has a sleeping partner, it is often the partner who reports the nighttime symptoms.

The two types of sleep apnea are **obstructive sleep apnea (OSA)** and central sleep apnea (CSA). OSA, caused by obstruction of the upper airway, is the most common; CSA is due to central nervous system or cardiac dysfunction. In Canada, older adults are three times as likely to report being diagnosed with sleep apnea (Statistics Canada, 2018).

In LTC homes, OSA is often underdiagnosed. The age-related decline in the activity of the upper-airway muscles, which results in compromised pharyngeal patency, predisposes older adults to OSA. Older adults with sleep apnea show a significant cognitive decline as compared with younger people with the same disease severity. Sleep apnea is most likely underdiagnosed, though the prevalence of symptoms related to sleep apnea is high (Laratta et al., 2017). Additional risk factors for sleep apnea are listed in Box 10.5.

The assessment of sleep apnea includes a sleep study and information collected from the sleeping partner if possible. Physical assessment often reveals that the person is obese, the neck is often short and thick, the uvula is large, and the soft palate hangs low. Tonsils may be enlarged, adenoids are enlarged, and the chin may be small or receded. It is important to look for upper-airway tumours or cysts. Therapy will depend on the severity of the sleep apnea. Specific treatment may involve weight loss, avoidance of alcohol and sedatives, cessation of smoking, and avoidance of supine sleep positions. There should also be risk counselling about impaired judgement from sleeplessness and the possibility of accidents when driving. Continuous positive airway pressure (CPAP) is the most effective treatment and the treatment of choice for older adults. A CPAP device delivers pressurized air through tubing to a nasal mask or nasal pillows that are fitted around the head. The pressurized air acts as an airway splint and gently opens the person's throat and breathing passages, allowing the person to breathe normally but only through the nose. CPAP has been shown to be well tolerated by older adults and effective for OSA in older adults with dementia (Owen et al., 2018). Another therapy, for mild cases of OSA, is the use of a dental appliance that moves the jaw forward, preventing the throat from closing (Haviv et al., 2018).

Restless Legs Syndrome

RLS is a sensorimotor neurological disorder characterized by the uncontrollable need to move the legs, often accompanied by discomfort in the legs. The estimated prevalence of RLS among the adult population is 5% to 10%, and it most commonly occurs in women older than 35 years of age (Rizek & Kumar, 2017).

Primary RLS starts at a younger age, has no predisposing factors, and probably has a genetic basis. Secondary RLS can result from a variety of medical conditions that involve iron deficiency, the most common of which are iron deficiency anemia, end-stage renal disease, and pregnancy. Impairment in dopamine transport in the substantia nigra owing to reduced intracellular iron seems to play a critical role in the disease.

Other symptoms of RLS include paresthesias; creeping sensations; crawling sensations; tingling, cramping, and burning sensations; pain; or even indescribable sensations. The syndrome has a circadian rhythm, and the intensity of the symptoms becomes worse at night and improves toward the morning. It may be temporarily relieved by movement.

Other sleep disorders, periodic limb movements of sleep, and periodic limb movement disorder are often associated with RLS. These movement disorders of sleep are sometimes called nocturnal myoclonus or periodic leg movements and involve repeated rhythmical extensions of the big toe and dorsiflexion of the ankle. Disrupted sleep is why people with these disorders seek help.

Antidepressants and neuroleptic medications can aggravate RLS symptoms. Increased body mass index, caffeine use, tobacco use, and a sedentary lifestyle are also contributing factors. Diagnosis of RLS includes ruling out or treating any medical condition as indicated. Oral iron supplements should be prescribed for patients with serum iron levels lower than 45 mcg/L (Harvard Health Publishing, 2020). Dopamine receptor agonists (e.g., pramipexole, ropinirole) are the medications of choice for RLS. Gabapentin may also be effective for people with comorbid RLS and peripheral neuropathy (Wijemanne & Ondo, 2017). Nonpharmacological therapy includes stretching of the lower extremities, mild to moderate physical activity, hot baths, relaxation techniques, and avoidance of alcohol.

Rapid Eye Movement Sleep Behaviour Disorder

RBD is a sleep disorder common in older adults. It is characterized by the loss of normal voluntary muscle atonia during REM sleep and is associated with complex behaviour while dreaming (Iranzo et al., 2016). Individuals report elaborate enactment of their dreams (the contents of which are often violent) during sleep. This may include violent actions such as punching and kicking, which can potentially injure both the affected person and any bed partner.

The mean age of a person at the emergence of RBD is 60 years, and the disorder is more common in males than in females. It may be primary or secondary to neuro-degenerative diseases such as Parkinson's disease, diffuse Lewy body disease, and Alzheimer's disease (Pham & Slowik, 2020). Up to 80% of people diagnosed with RBD will develop Parkinson's disease (Kahn et al., 2019).

Caffeine and some medications (selective serotonin reuptake inhibitors [SSRIs] and tricyclic antidepressants) may contribute to RBD. Interventions include neurological examination, removal of aggravating medications, and counselling related to safety measures in the sleep environment. Clonazepam, melatonin, or both may be effective in treating RBD, although melatonin is more favourable since it is less likely to pose any adverse reactions (Pham & Slowik, 2020). However, clonazepam should be used cautiously in older adults, and close monitoring is required because older adults are at greater risk for adverse central nervous system effects.

IMPLICATIONS FOR GERONTOLOGICAL NURSING AND HEALTHY AGING

Sleep Assessment

Older adults' sleep habits should be reviewed in all settings. Many people do not seek treatment for insomnia and may blame poor sleep on the aging process. Nurses are in an excellent position to assess sleep and to improve the quality of the older adult's sleep. Night-shift nursing staff in health care settings have the opportunity to assess sleep patterns and implement appropriate interventions to enhance sleep (Kikhia et al., 2018). A thorough assessment includes exploring how well the person sleeps at home, how many times the person wakes up at night, what time the person retires to bed, and what rituals occur at bedtime. Bedtime rituals include any activities that are crucial to the individual's ability to fall asleep (e.g., eating snacks, watching television, listening to music, and reading). Other assessment data should include the amount and type of daily exercise, favourite position in bed, room environment (including temperature, ventilation, and illumination), activities that are engaged in several hours before bedtime, and all medications. Additional assessment includes gathering information about the individual's satisfaction with life, perception of health status, and involvement in hobbies. The person should also be assessed for depression. The person's bed partner, caregivers, and family members can also provide valuable information about the person's sleep habits and lifestyle.

Subjective methods for assessing sleep include visual analog scales, subjective rating scales (e.g., 0 to 10, or 0 to 100), questionnaires, interviews, and daily sleep charts. A self-rating scale, the Pittsburgh Sleep Quality Index (PSQI), can be used to measure the quality and patterns of sleep in the older adult (https://www.sleep.pitt.edu/instruments/). An online video demonstrating the assessment of sleep with the PSQI can be found at http://journals.lww.com/ajnonline/Pages/videogallery.aspx?videoId=17&autoPlay=true. A sleep diary or log is an important part of the assessment, as it provides an accurate account of the person's sleep problem. Usually, a family member or caregiver records specific behaviours on a flow sheet. A period of 2 to 4 weeks is needed to obtain a clear picture of the sleep problem (Box 10.6). Objective measures include direct observation and polysomnography (including electro-encephalography and electro-myography) conducted in a sleep laboratory.

Some recently developed technology (i.e., cameras, sensors, and Fitbit-type activity trackers) can be used to assess sleep patterns.

Interventions

Nonpharmacological Interventions

Attention to sleep hygiene principles is important to promote good sleep habits (Box 10.7). Cognitive behavioural therapy, stimulus control, sleep restriction therapy, and relaxation therapy are all effective and produce sustained positive effects. These behavioural treatments have been reported to be effective and practical treatments for chronic insomnia in older adults. Tai chi also improves an older adult's sleep quality (Chan et al., 2017). Box 10.8 presents other nonpharmacological therapies for sleep disorders.

In all health care settings, the promotion of a good sleep environment is important. A sleep improvement protocol (including do-not-disturb periods; provision of usual bedtime routines; and soft music, relaxation techniques, massage, and aromatherapy) may improve sleep. An interprofessional approach to identifying sources of noise and light, such as equipment and staff interactions, can result in modification without compromising the older adult's safety and quality of care (Grossman et al., 2017). Because a full sleep cycle of 90 minutes can have a positive influence on sleep effectiveness, any effort to allow sufficient time for a

---

BOX 10.6
SLEEP DIARY

INSTRUCTIONS

Record the following for 2 to 4 weeks:
1. The number of times a call for assistance is made (e.g., concerning the bathroom, pain medication, and subjective symptoms of inability to sleep).
2. Whether the person appears to be asleep or awake when checked during the night.
3. Time and dosage of sleep medication.
4. Time the person awakens in the morning.
5. Where the person falls asleep in the evening.
6. Duration of daytime naps.

BOX 10.7
SLEEP HYGIENE RULES

1. Limit daytime naps to 30 minutes.
2. Avoid stimulants (caffeine and nicotine) before sleeping.
3. Engage in daily exercise.
4. Avoid consuming spicy foods, fried meals, and carbonated drinks before bedtime.
5. Ensure adequate exposure to natural light during the day and darkness at night, as this will help maintain a healthy sleep–wake cycle.
6. Establish a regular bedtime routine, including the use of relaxation techniques such as having a warm bath, reading a book, or doing light stretches.
7. Ensure the sleep environment is pleasant; for optimal sleep, have the bedroom at a cool temperature (between 15.5 and 19.4°C); turn off TVs, and avoid light from computer and cell phone screens.

Source: Adapted from National Sleep Foundation. (2017). *How can I improve my sleep hygiene?* https://sleepfoundation.org/sleep-topics/sleep-hygiene.

BOX 10.8
NONPHARMACOLOGICAL THERAPIES FOR SLEEP DISORDERS

TRANSCUTANEOUS ELECTRICAL NERVE STIMULATION (TENS)

TENS is a noninvasive treatment that uses low-voltage electric currents to treat chronic pain. Because it helps to relieve pain, it can help with improving sleep.

COGNITIVE BEHAVIOURAL THERAPY FOR INSOMNIA

Behavioural therapy is stimulus control therapy that connects the way we think, the things we do, and how we sleep. The bedroom should be used only for sleep and for sexual activity. The goal is to strengthen the person's emotional perception of the bedroom as a place for sleeping instead of a place for experiencing insomnia.

RELAXATION TECHNIQUES

Relaxation techniques include progressive relaxation exercises, guided imagery, meditation, and electro-myographic biofeedback. The goal is to minimize the physical and emotional stressors that affect sleep.

EXERCISE

Regular exercise during the day enhances the ability to sleep. Exercise should be avoided in the 4 hours before bedtime.

LIGHT THERAPY

Light therapy consists of exposure to natural light, the use of a light box, and the elimination of nighttime light (especially in health care settings).

Sources: O'Caoimh, R., Mannion, H., Sezgin, D., et al. (2019). Non-pharmacological treatments for sleep disturbance in mild cognitive impairment and dementia: A systematic review and meta-analysis. *Maturitas, 127,* 82–94. doi:10.1016/j.maturitas.2019.06.007; Gozani, S. N., Ferree, T. C., Moynihan, M., et al. (2019). Impact of transcutaneous electrical nerve stimulation on sleep chronic low back pain: A real-world retrospective cohort study. *Journal of Pain Research, 12,* 743–752. doi:10.2147/JPR.S196129; Sleep Foundation (2020). *How does CBT-I work?* https://www.sleepfoundation.org/insomnia/treatment/cognitive-behavioral-therapy-insomnia.

full sleep cycle is important (Wai & Yu, 2019). Box 10.9 provides suggestions for promoting sleep for older adults who live in LTC homes.

Aromatherapy, such as the use of essential oils, has been mentioned as beneficial in sleep promotion (Takeda et al., 2017). Outdoor physical activities for LTC residents can promote well-being, activity, and sleep. An example of such an activity program for older adults is that offered at Oliver Woods Wellness Park in British Columbia.

Pharmacological Interventions

Medications may be used in combination with behavioural interventions, but they must be chosen carefully, started at the lowest possible dosage, and monitored closely to avoid untoward effects in older adults. Older adults should be educated on the proper use of medications and on their side effects. Sedatives and hypnotics, including benzodiazepines and barbiturates, should be avoided. Over-the-counter medications such as diphenhydramine (Benadryl) and Tylenol PM (containing diphenhydramine), often thought to be relatively harmless, should be avoided because of their antihistaminic and anticholinergic side effects.

Benzodiazepine receptor agonists (such as zolpidem, eszopiclone, and zaleplon) have shorter half-lives for older adults than other insomnia prescription medications (Patel et al., 2018). However, they also have undesirable effects and a narrow safety margin and should be used in the short term only. Because of the rapid action of these medications, they should be taken immediately before bedtime. Recent research has reported that hospitalized patients who took zolpidem had a fall rate that was more than four times higher than that of patients who did not take that medication. Precautions against falls should be taken for people who take sleeping medications (Musich et al., 2018). Ramelteon, a melatonin receptor agonist that promotes sleep via action on the circadian system, can be used for individuals who have difficulty falling asleep.

ACTIVITY

Activity is a direct use of energy—in voluntary, involuntary, physical, and mental ways—that alters a person's microenvironment and macroenvironment. Few factors contribute as much to health in aging as physical activity. One of the goals of promoting healthy aging is having more people participate in regular physical activity to improve functional fitness and overall physical and mental health (Sanchez-Lopez et al., 2018). Regular physical activity throughout life is likely to enhance health and functional status as a person ages. It also decreases the number of persistent or chronic illnesses and the mobility and functional limitations that are often assumed to be part of aging.

Physical activity is important for all older adults, not just those who are active and healthy. Studies have found that increasing physical activity improves health outcomes for persons with persistent illnesses (regardless of severity) and for those with functional impairment (Sanchez-Lopez et al., 2018). Exercise has also been shown to be beneficial for frail LTC residents diagnosed with illnesses ranging from arthritis to lung disease and dementia (Gallaway et al., 2017).

Despite a large body of evidence about the importance of physical activity for maintaining and improving function, it was found that only 13% of older adults aged 60 to 79 years old were accumulating at least 150 minutes per week of moderate to vigorous physical activity, as per public health guidelines (Statistics Canada, 2017). The levels of physical activity among older adults in Canada have not improved significantly over the past 5 years (Statistics Canada, 2017). Inactivity poses serious health hazards to young and old alike. It can lead to hypertension, coronary artery disease, osteoporosis, obesity, tension, chronic fatigue, premature aging, depression, poor musculature, inadequate flexibility, and decreased cognitive function (González et al., 2017). Many older adults mistakenly believe that they are too old to begin an active fitness program. Even a small amount of time (e.g., 30 minutes of moderate activity several days a week) can improve health.

IMPLICATIONS FOR GERONTOLOGICAL NURSING AND HEALTHY AGING

Assessment

When promoting a healthy lifestyle for older adults, it is important for the nurse to understand the individual needs, circumstances, and situations of the person. Exercise counselling and an assessment of functional abilities should be part of the health assessment of all older adults. The purpose of screening is to (1) identify medical problems while allowing the individual to achieve the maximal benefit from physical activity; (2) identify functional limitations that will be addressed in the exercise program; and (3) minimize injury and other serious harmful effects. The Physical Activity Readiness Questionnaire for Everyone (PAR-Q+) (http://eparmedx.com/wp-content/uploads/2013/03/PARQPlus2019ImageVersion2.pdf) can be used to screen the older adult before they are started on a moderate program of physical activity. Depending on the results of the initial screening, older adults may need to be evaluated by their primary care provider. Frail or vulnerable older adults will also need close monitoring to ensure benefit without a compromise to their safety.

Interventions

Suggestions for exercise programs are based on the person's preference and medical history. Exercise programs often include the following components:

- *Endurance exercises* are composed of continuous movement involving large muscle groups for a minimum of 10 minutes. These exercises increase breathing and heart rates and improve the health of the heart, lungs, and circulatory system. Examples of endurance exercises are swimming, cycling, brisk walking, tennis, dancing, and gardening. Endurance exercises should initially be of short duration and gradually increased.
- *Strength (resistance) exercises* build muscles and increase muscle strength by the moving or lifting of objects that provide resistance, such as hand or ankle weights or resistance bands. The exercises should be performed at least twice a week.
- *Balance exercises* improve standing and gait and help prevent falls. Tai chi has been shown to be of benefit for older adults (Box 10.10).
- *Flexibility exercises* keep the body limber and increase range of motion. These exercises should be performed at least 3 days a week. Yoga is a form of exercise that can be practised regardless of one's condition.

Nonambulatory older adults can also engage in physical activity and may benefit the most from an exercise program in terms of function and quality of life. Both muscle weakness and atrophy are functionally relevant and are reversible through exercise in nonambulatory older adults. Upper-extremity cycling, marching in place, stretching, range-of-motion exercise, water-based activities, and chair yoga are examples of exercises for nonambulatory older adults. For older adults who reside in LTC homes, participation in self-care activities improves functioning and also contributes to greater staff, family, and resident satisfaction. The restorative care (Res-Care) intervention, a self-efficacy–based approach to restoring or maintaining one's physical function, can be used as a model for restorative care in LTC homes, and can help

---

BOX 10.10

RESEARCH FOR EVIDENCE-INFORMED PRACTICE: TAI CHI EXERCISE FOR IMPROVING SLEEP QUALITY: A SYSTEMATIC REVIEW AND META-ANALYSIS

Problem: Sleep plays an important role in the health of the human body. Currently, there is a lack of nonpharmacological treatments. This study looked at tai chi and its effect on patients with sleep complaints.

Method: A systematic review was completed by the researchers. English-language databases were searched, with searches conducted in both English and Chinese. The researchers were looking specifically for randomized controlled studies.

Findings: A total of 20 randomized controlled studies from five different countries were included in this meta-analysis. Those who practised tai chi found that their sleep quality improved, when compared both to those who did not use any intervention and to those who used different interventions (such as health education or another exercise regimen).

Source: Li, H., Chen, J., Xu, G.,et al. (2020). The effect of Tai Chi for improving sleep quality: A systematic review and meta-analysis. *Journal of Affective Disorders, 274*(1), 1102–1112. doi:10.1016/j.jad.2020.05.076.

---

improve or maintain residents' physical and mental function (Wang et al., 2019).

The older adult may be able to integrate activity into daily life rather than doing specific exercises. An example is walking to the store instead of driving there. Older adults limited to LTC homes should also be encouraged to increase their amount of walking. First they might walk only from the bed to the bathroom; with time, they can walk down the hall; and eventually they can walk around the entire facility or even outside. Restorative walking programs and other exercise programs should be integral activity in all LTC homes.

When especially low-intensity exercise is needed, the person can exercise for 2 to 3 minutes, rest for 2 to 3 minutes, and continue this pattern for 15 to 20 minutes. The Public Health Agency of Canada (2015) provides an excellent resource and also offers educational materials on exercise at https://www.canada.ca/en/public-health/services/being-active.html.

Exercise Prescription

As noted earlier, most older adults do not exercise regularly. Motivational interventions are important when encouraging older adults to begin an exercise program, and such interventions should be continued to ensure that the person stays with the program. Emphasis on the immediate benefits of regular exercise (i.e., improvement of current health and quality of life) can be an important motivator for the patient. A list of safety tips for exercise should also be provided. Exercise tips for older adults are presented in Box 10.11.

SUMMARY

This chapter has discussed the older adult's need for rest, sleep, and activity. It is apparent that each area influences the function of the other. The quality and the overall perception of life can be augmented when nurses monitor these specific functions and provide support or assistance according to the identified problems. Gerontological nurses must be knowledgeable about age-related changes in sleep and activity and about the effect of lifestyle on these changes. Many older adults may have misconceptions about sleep and exercise; the nurse can assess persons' beliefs and understanding and provide education to enhance their optimal well-being.

The assessment of sleep, the chosen level of activity, and the design of interventions must be grounded in evidence-informed knowledge and applied to meet the needs of each person. Common practices (such as the use of hypnotics for sleep) without thorough assessment, or a person's confinement to a wheelchair because there is no one to help maintain their walking skills, lead to disabling and preventable problems for older adults. Improvement of function is possible for even the frailest older adult, and gerontological nurses must incorporate the health promotion activities discussed here into any plan of care for an older adult.

BOX 10.11
12 TIPS TO GET ACTIVE

1. Take part in at least 2.5 hours of moderate to vigorous intensity aerobic activity each week.
2. Spread out the activities into sessions of 10 minutes or more.
3. Add muscle- and bone-strengthening activities using major muscle groups at least twice a week. This will help your posture and balance.
4. Find an activity you like such as swimming or cycling.
5. Minutes count—increase your activity level 10 minutes at a time. Every little bit helps.
6. Active time can be social time—look for group activities or classes in your community, or get your family or friends to be active with you.
7. Walk wherever and whenever you can.
8. Take the stairs instead of the elevator, when possible.
9. Carry your groceries home.
10. Start slowly.
11. Listen to your body.
12. Every step counts!

Source: Adapted from: Government of Canada. (2019). *Physical activity tips for older adults (65 years and older).* https://www.canada.ca/en/public-health/services/publications/healthy-living/physical-activity-tips-older-adults-65-years-older.html.

KEY CONCEPTS

- Rest and sleep are restorative, recuperative, and necessary for the preservation of life. Many persistent and chronic conditions can interfere with the quality and quantity of sleep.
- Complaints of sleep difficulties should be thoroughly investigated and not attributed to age. Nonpharmacological interventions should always be considered in any plan of care to improve sleep.
- Activity is an indication of an individual's health and wellness; the inability to exercise, do physical work, or perform activities of daily living is one of the first indicators of decline.
- Lack of physical activity increases the risk for many medical conditions experienced by older adults. Exercise can be done by individuals who are ambulatory, chairbound, or bedridden and should include endurance exercises, strength training, balance exercises, and flexibility exercises.
- The benefits of exercise include maintenance of functional ability, enhanced self-confidence and self-sufficiency, decreased depression, improvement in general lifestyle, maintenance of mental functional capacity, and decreased risk for medical problems.
- Exercise counselling and an exercise prescription should be taken into consideration for all older adults.

ACTIVITIES AND DISCUSSION QUESTIONS

1. Discuss the age-related changes that affect rest, sleep, and activity in older adults.

2. Describe the assessment of an older adult for adequacy or inadequacy of rest, sleep, and activity.

3. Develop an exercise prescription for an older adult who resides in the outside community.

4. Discuss nursing interventions for promoting rest, sleep, and activity.

5. Devise a nursing care plan for an older adult who has insomnia.

RESOURCES

Canadian Society for Exercise Physiology. *Canadian 24-Hour Movement Guidelines.*
https://csepguidelines.ca/

Canadian Society for Exercise Physiology. *Canadian 24-Hour Movement Guidelines for Adults Ages 65 Years and Older: An Integration of Physical Activity, Sedentary Behaviour, and Sleep.*
https://csepguidelines.ca/adults-65/

Government of Canada. *Physical activity tips for older adults (65 years and older).*
https://www.canada.ca/en/public-health/services/publications/healthy-living/physical-activity-tips-older-adults-65-years-older.html

Physical Activity Readiness Questionnaire for Everyone (PAR-Q+)
http://eparmedx.com/wp-content/uploads/2013/03/PARQPlus2019 ImageVersion2.pdf

Public Health Agency of Canada. *Educational materials on exercise.*
https://www.canada.ca/en/public-health/services/being-active.html

For additional resources, please visit *http://evolve.elsevier.com/ Canada/Ebersole/gerontological/*

REFERENCES

Alzheimer Society of Canada. (2020). *Sleep.* https://alzheimer.ca/en/Home/Living-with-dementia/Day-to-day-living/Sleep.

Castelnovo, A., Ferri, R., Punjabi, N. M., et al. (2019). The paradox of paradoxical insomnia: A theoretical review towards a unifying evidence-based definition. *Sleep Medicine Reviews, 44,* 70–82. doi:10.1016/j.smrv.2018.12.007.

Chan, A. W., Yu, D. S., & Choi, K. C. (2017). Effects of tai chi qigong on psychosocial well-being among hidden elderly, using elderly neighborhood volunteer approach: A pilot randomized controlled trial. *Clinical Interventions in Aging, 12,* 85. doi:10.2147/CIA.S124604.

Chen, T., Lee, S., Schade, M. M., et al. (2019). Longitudinal relationship between sleep deficiency and pain symptoms among community-dwelling older adults in Japan and Singapore. *SLEEP, 42*(2). doi:10.1093/sleep/zsy219.

FitzGerald, J. M., O'Regan, N., Adamis, D., et al. (2017). Sleep–wake cycle disturbances in elderly acute general medical inpatients: Longitudinal relationship to delirium and dementia. *Alzheimer's & dementia (Amsterdam, Netherlands), 7,* 61–68. doi:10.1016/j.dadm.2016.12.013.

Gallaway, P. J., Miyake, H., Buchowski, M. S., et al. (2017). Physical activity: A viable way to reduce the risks of mild cognitive impairment, Alzheimer's Disease, and vascular dementia in older adults. *Brain Sciences, 7*(2), 22. doi:10.3390/brainsci7020022.

Gibson, R., Gander, P., Dowell, A., et al. (2017). Non-pharmacological interventions for managing dementia-related sleep problems within community dwelling pairs: A mixed-method approach. *Dementia, 16*(8), 967–984. doi:10.1177/1471301215625821.

González, K., Fuentes, J., & Márquez, J. L. (2017). Physical inactivity, sedentary behavior and chronic diseases. *Korean Journal of Family Medicine, 38*(3), 111. doi:10.4082/kjfm.2017.38.3.111.

Grossman, M. N., Anderson, S. L., Worku, A., et al. (2017). Awakenings? Patient and hospital staff perceptions of nighttime disruptions and their effect on patient sleep. *Journal of Clinical Sleep Medicine, 13*(2), 301–306. doi:10.5664/jcsm.6468.

Harvard Health Publishing. (2020). *Are you missing this simple treatment for restless legs?* https://www.health.harvard.edu/diseases-and-conditions/are-you-missing-this-simple-treatment-for-restless-legs.

Haviv, Y., Kamer, L., Sheinfeld, R., et al. (2018). Successful treatment of extremely severe obstructive sleep apnea with a dental appliance. *The Israel Medical Association Journal, 20*(7), 429–432.

Hjetland, G. J., Pallesen, S., Thun, E., Kolberg, E., Nordhus, I. H., & Flo, E. (2020). Light interventions and sleep, circadian, behavioral, and psychological disturbances in dementia: A systematic review of methods and outcomes. *Sleep Medicine Reviews, 52,* 101310. https://doi.org/10.1016/j.smrv.2020.101310.

Iranzo, A., Santamaria, J., & Tolosa, E. (2016). Idiopathic rapid eye movement sleep behaviour disorder: Diagnosis, management, and the need for neuroprotective interventions. *Lancet Neurology, 15*(4), 405–419. doi:10.1016/S1474-4422(16)00057-0.

Kahn, L., Abosch, A., Kern, D. S., et al. (2019). Chapter 49—Rapid eye movement sleep behavior disorder: Pathological neural circuits and association with Parkinson's disease. *Handbook of Behavioral Neuroscience, 30,* 723–730. doi:10.1016/B978-0-12-813743-7.00049-9.

Kikhia, B., Stavropoulos, T. G., Meditskos, G., et al. (2018). Utilizing ambient and wearable sensors to monitor sleep and stress for people with BPSD in nursing homes. *Journal of Ambient Intelligence and Humanized Computing, 9*(2), 261–273.

Košćec Bjelajac, A., Holzinger, B., Despot Lučanin, J., et al. (2020). Sleep quality and daytime functioning in older European adults. *European Psychologist, 25*(3), 186–199. doi:10.1027/1016-9040/a000406.

Laratta, C. R., Ayas, N. T., Povitz, M., et al. (2017). Diagnosis and treatment of obstructive sleep apnea in adults. *Canadian Medical Association Journal, 189*(48), E1481–E1488. doi:10.1503/cmaj.170296.

Lo, J. C., Groeger, J. A., Cheng, G. H., et al. (2016). Self-reported sleep duration and cognitive performance in older adults: A systematic review and meta-analysis. *Sleep Medicine, 17*, 87–98. doi:10.1016/j.sleep.2015.08.021.

Miner, B., & Kryger, M. H. (2017). Sleep in the aging population. *Sleep Medicine Clinics, 12*(1), 31–38.

Musich, S., Wang, S. S., Slindee, L. B., et al. (2018). Characteristics of new-onset and chronic sleep medication users among older adults: A retrospective study of a US medigap plan population using propensity score matching. *Drugs & Aging, 35*(5), 467–476. doi:10.1007/s40266-018-0543-5.

Owen, J., Gislasson, T., Benediktsdottir, B., et al. (2018). Continuous positive airway pressure use is associated with a lower burden of Alzheimer's disease neuropathology in obstructive sleep apnea patients compared to non-use. *Sleep, 41*, A114. doi:10.1093/sleep/zsy061.295.

Palinkas, M., Semprini, M., Filo, J. E., et al. (2017). Nocturnal sleep architecture is altered by sleep bruxism. *Archives of Oral Biology, 81*, 56–60. doi:10.1016/j.archoalbio.2017.04.025.

Patel, D., Steinberg, J., & Patel, P. (2018). Insomnia in the elderly: A review. *Journal of Clinical Sleep Medicine, 14*(6), 1017–1024. doi:10.5664/jcsm.7172.

Pham, C. K., & Slowik, J. M. (2020). *Rapid eye movement sleep behavior disorder*. StatPearls. https://www.ncbi.nlm.nih.gov/books/NBK534239/.

Public Health Agency of Canada. (2015). *Physical activity guide for older adults*. https://www.canada.ca/en/public-health/services/health-promotion/healthy-living/physical-activity.html.

Rizek, P., & Kumar, N. (2017). Restless legs syndrome. *Canadian Medical Association Journal, 189*(6), E245. doi:10.1503/cmaj.160527.

Sanchez-Lopez, J., Silva-Pereyra, J., Fernández, T., et al. (2018). High levels of incidental physical activity are positively associated with cognition and EEG activity in aging. *PLOS One, 13*(1), e0191561. doi:10.1371/journal.pone.0191561.

Schotland, H. (2019). Artificial bright light therapy for circadian rhythm sleep–wake disorders. *American Journal of Respiratory and Critical Care Medicine, 200*(6), 11–12.

Statistics Canada. (2017). *Canadian Health Measures Survey: Activity monitor data*. https://www150.statcan.gc.ca/n1/daily-quotidien/170419/dq170419e-eng.htm.

Statistics Canada. (2018). *Sleep apnea in Canada, 2016 and 2017*. https://www150.statcan.gc.ca/n1/pub/82-625-x/2018001/article/54979-eng.htm.

Takeda, A., Watanuki, E., & Koyama, S. (2017). Effects of inhalation aromatherapy on symptoms of sleep disturbance in the elderly with dementia. *Evidence-Based Complementary and Alternative Medicine, 2017*, 1902807. doi:10.1155/2017/1902807.

Torvinen-Kiiskinen, S., Tolppanen, A., Koponen, M., et al. (2018). Proton pump inhibitor use and risk of hip fractures among community-dwelling persons with Alzheimer's disease—A nested case-control study. *Alimentary Pharmacology & Therapeutics, 47*(8), 1135–1142. doi:10.1111/apt.14589.

van Maanen, A., Meijer, A., van der Heijden, K., et al. (2016). The effect of light therapy on sleep problems: A systematic review and meta-analysis. *Sleep Medicine Reviews, 29*, 52–62. doi:10.1016/j.smrv.2015.08.009.

Vaughan, C. P., Fung, C. H., Huang, A. J., et al. (2016). Differences in the association of nocturia and functional outcomes of sleep by age and gender: A cross-sectional, population-based study. *Clinical Therapeutics, 38*(11), 2386–2393. doi:10.1016/j.clinthera.2016.09.009.

Wai, J. L. T., & Yu, D.S.F. (2019). The relationship between sleep–wake disturbances and frailty among older adults: A systematic review. *Journal of Advanced Nursing, 76*, 96–108. doi:10.1111/jan.14231.

Wang, Y., Liu, L., Chang, L., et al. (2019). The implementation of restorative care and factors associated with resident outcomes in long-term care facilities in Taiwan. *International Journal of Environmental Research and Public Health, 16*(20), 3860. doi:10.3390/ijerph16203860.

Wijemanne, S., & Ondo, W. (2017). Restless legs syndrome: Clinical features, diagnosis and a practical approach to management. *Practical Neurology, 17*, 444–452. doi:10.1136/practneurol-2017-001762.

11

PROMOTING HEALTHY SKIN AND FEET

LEARNING OBJECTIVES

Upon completion of this chapter, the reader will be able to:

- Identify normal age-related changes of the integument and feet.
- Identify skin and foot problems commonly found in later life.
- Use standardized tools to assess the skin and feet of older adults.
- Identify preventive, maintenance, and restorative measures for skin and foot health.

GLOSSARY

Debride   To remove dead or infected tissue, usually from a wound.

Emollient   A medication that softens and smooths the skin.

Eschar   Black, dry, dead tissue.

Hyperemia   Redness caused by increased blood flow, such as in an area of infection.

Maceration   Tissue that is overhydrated and subject to breakdown.

Slough   Dead tissue that has become wet, appearing as yellow to white and fibrous.

Tissue tolerance   The amount of pressure a tissue (i.e., skin) can endure before it breaks down, as in a pressure injury.

Xerosis   Very dry skin.

THE LIVED EXPERIENCE

"I talk a lot with my nurse, he's nice and I have a very good relationship. I told him when it hurt the most and when I was better, he saw how I was improving or worsening, as at times I got worse."
J.B., 90 years old

From García-Sánchez, F.J., Martínez-Vizcaíno, V., & Rodríguez-Martín, B. (2019). Patients' and caregivers' conceptualisations of pressure ulcers and the process of decision-making in the context of home care. *International Journal of Environmental Research and Public Health, 16*(15), 2719. doi:10.3390/ijerph16152719.

HEALTHY AGING CARE PLAN
About J.B.

J.B. (pronouns she/her) is 90 years old and has just moved into a long-term care home after recovering from a fall and hip fracture surgery. While in the hospital, she developed a stage 2 pressure injury. She also has been diagnosed with moderate Alzheimer's Disease and heart failure. She is frail, nonambulatory, and not eating well. As the nurse caring for her, you understand that she is at high risk for worsening and developing additional pressure injuries.

QUESTIONS TO CONSIDER

1. What are some steps you can take to help heal J.B.'s existing pressure injury?
2. What are some priority nursing interventions you would need to put in place to prevent J.B. from developing additional pressure injuries?
3. Which members of the interprofessional team should be involved in J.B.'s care?

Gerontological nurses play an instrumental role in promoting the health of the skin and the feet of the persons who seek their care. These areas of function may often be overlooked when the focus is on management of disease or acute problems. However, preservation of the integrity of the skin and the functioning of the feet is essential to well-being. To promote healthy aging, the nurse needs information about common problems encountered by the older adult and skill in developing effective interventions for both acute and chronic conditions.

INTEGUMENT

Integument is defined as the natural covering of an organism or organ. The skin, an example of integument, is the largest organ of the body and performs several physiological functions, including maintaining a homeostatic environment and protecting the body from exposure to heat, cold, water, trauma, friction, and pressure (Box 11.1). Healthy skin is durable, pliable, and strong enough to protect the body by absorbing, reflecting, cushioning, and restricting various substances and forces that might enter and alter its function, yet it is sensitive enough to relay subtle messages to the brain. When the integument malfunctions or is overwhelmed, discomfort, disfigurement, or death may ensue. Nurses can recognize and prevent many of the sources of danger to an older adult's skin in the promotion of the best possible health.

Many skin problems are seen as people age, both when people are in health and when they are compromised by illness or limited mobility. Skin problems seen in older adults are influenced by the environment and by age-related changes (see Chapter 6). The most common skin problems for older adults are xerosis, pruritus, seborrheic keratosis, herpes zoster, and cancer. People who are immobilized or medically fragile, such as residents in long-term care (LTC) or residential homes, are at a higher risk for fungal infections and pressure injuries, both of which are major threats to wellness.

Common Skin Problems

Xerosis

Xerosis is extremely dry, cracked, and itchy skin. Xerosis is the most common skin problem experienced by older adults. The thinner epidermis of older skin makes it less efficient, thus allowing more moisture to escape. Inadequate fluid intake worsens xerosis, as the body will pull moisture from the skin in an attempt to combat systemic dehydration. Xerosis occurs primarily in the extremities, especially the legs, but can affect the face and trunk as well.

Exposure to environmental elements such as artificial heat, decreased humidity, harsh soaps, and frequent hot baths or hot tub use contributes to skin dryness. Nutritional deficiencies and smoking can also lead to dehydration of the outer layer of the epidermis.

Hospitals and LTC homes accelerate the development of xerosis in older adults through routine baths, the use of drying soap, prolonged bed rest, and the action of bed linen on the person's skin (Hahnel et al., 2017). For persons with incontinence, the skin must be protected from both the burning of urine or feces and from the excess dryness that arises from frequent washing and drying.

Pruritus

One of the consequences of xerosis is *pruritus*, or itchy skin. It is a symptom, not a diagnosis or disease, and is a threat to skin integrity because of the person's attempts to relieve it by scratching. Pruritus is aggravated by perfumed detergents, fabric softeners, heat, sudden temperature changes, pressure, vibration, electrical stimuli, sweating, restrictive clothing, fatigue, exercise, and anxiety. If rehydration of the stratum corneum is not sufficient to control itching, cool compresses or oatmeal or Epsom salt baths may be helpful. Failure to control the itching increases the risk for eczema, excoriations, cracks in the skin, inflammation, and infection. Pruritus also may accompany systemic disorders such as chronic renal failure, biliary or hepatic disease, and iron deficiency anemia. The nurse should be alert for signs of infection.

BOX 11.1
PHYSIOLOGICAL FUNCTIONS OF THE SKIN

- Protects underlying structures
- Regulates body temperature
- Serves as a vehicle for sensation
- Stores fat
- Is a component of the metabolism of salt and water
- Is a site for two-way gas exchange
- Is the site for the production of vitamin D, when exposed to sunlight

Herpes Zoster

Herpes zoster (HZ), or shingles, is a viral infection frequently seen in older adults. Immunosuppressed older adults and those with a history of chicken pox are at greatest risk for the reactivation of dormant varicella-zoster virus within the sensory ganglia. However, HZ can occur in healthy people as well. It always occurs along a nerve pathway, or *dermatome*. The more dermatomes involved, the more serious the infection, especially if it involves the head. Involvement with the eye is always a medical emergency owing to the possibility of scarring and blindness (Meyers et al., 2018). In most cases, the severity of the infection increases with age.

The onset of HZ may be preceded by chills, fever, gastro-intestinal disturbance, malaise, and pain or paresthesia. Before diagnosis, the person may complain of pain, tingling, and a painful rash (Shiraki et al., 2017). The area where the eruption *will* occur is burning, painful, or tender, and this is often a predictive sign.

During the healing process, clusters of papulovesicles develop along a nerve pathway. The lesions themselves eventually rupture, crust over, and resolve. Scarring may result, especially if scratching or poor hygiene leads to a secondary bacterial infection. Shingles is infectious until it becomes crusty. The condition may be very painful and pruritic, and as many as 20% of older adults may have postherpetic neuralgia (PHN) lasting weeks or months after the acute infection resolves. The pain of PHN is difficult to control and can significantly affect the person's quality of life (see Chapter 16). In Ontario, as of January 2017, the shingles vaccine has been free for adults aged 65 to 70 years (Government of Ontario, 2016). The more common vaccine, Shingrix, is administered intramuscularly in two doses. The interval between the doses is 2 to 6 months (Government of Canada, 2020).

IMPLICATIONS FOR GERONTOLOGICAL NURSING AND HEALTHY AGING

Gerontological nurses are in a perfect position to promote healthy skin in older adults. In embracing this position, they can significantly improve older adults' quality of life and comfort.

Xerosis

Because age-related changes are one of the major causes of xerosis, nurses need to pay attention to the environment and provide preventative treatment to help older adults maintain healthy skin. Maintaining the environment's humidity at about 60% is a start. The challenge is to find ways to rehydrate the epidermis (Box 11.2).

Skin can be hydrated only with water. Topical skin products can help retain natural moisture in the skin. Most lubricants such as creams, lotions, and **emollients** work by trapping moisture and are most effective when applied to towel-patted, damp skin immediately after a shower or bath. Bath oils and other hydrophobic preparations may also be used to hold in moisture. Oils can be directly applied to moist skin; water-laden emulsions without perfumes or alcohol are best.

To prevent excessive loss of moisture and natural oil during bathing, only tepid water temperatures and superfatted soaps or skin cleansers without hexachlorophene or alcohol should be used. Soap products or bath washes that have low potential for irritation, are fragrance-free or unscented, do not contain common allergens, and are noncomedogenic help prevent the loss of the protective lipid film from the skin surface.

BOX 11.2
SKINCARE TIPS FOR OLDER ADULTS

- Watch for any break in the skin, and initiate treatment as soon as possible.
- Use a humidifier to keep the room humid.
- Use only tepid water for bathing, and limit time in the water.
- Use only mild skin cleansers without perfume or lanolin.
- Pat dry; do not rub.
- Do not add bath oil to water in order to minimize risk of slipping.
- Apply moisturizers as often as necessary to maintain continuous coverage.
- Choose clothing made of soft cotton or other non-abrasive materials.
- Maintain systemic hydration (a balance between fluid intake and hydration status).
- Protect skin from exposure to cold temperatures.

Some examples can be found on the Canadian Dermatology Association's website (https://dermatology.ca/recognized-products/skincare/). The use of deodorant soaps and detergents containing alcohol as a drying agent should be avoided, except in the axilla and groin.

In cases of extreme dryness, petroleum jelly can be applied to the affected areas before bed, and the skin will be smoother and have more moisture in the morning. Oils and ointments with zinc oxide are designed to coat the skin and replace the skin's natural oil barrier. These products are often used to prevent excoriations from feces or urine; however, they can be applied only to skin that is clean and intact.

Pruritus

When xerosis leads to pruritus, the goal of treatment is to reduce and alleviate the itching. If rehydration of the epidermis is not sufficient to control itching, then cool compresses or baths with oatmeal or Epsom salts may be helpful. Nurses should educate patients on the importance of hydration and skin protection to prevent scratching. Failure to control the itching increases the risk for eczema, excoriations, cracks in the skin, inflammation, and infection. Nurses should be alert to signs of infection and rough, scaly, or flaky skin. Pharmacological treatment can be used if necessary.

Herpes Zoster

Most care and treatment for herpes zoster is medical, involving the prompt initiation of antiviral medications and optimal pain management. Nursing care includes providing both emotional support during the outbreak and education in regard to reducing secondary infections and cross-contamination. Weeping and ruptured vesicles should be covered with an absorbent yet nonadherent product, such as gauze. If the gauze adheres to the skin, warm normal saline applied to it will help release it. Hands, bedding, towels, and clothing should be washed before and after contact.

PHN requires optimal pain management. The pain may persist for many months or even years; it may be severe and interfere with sleep and activities of daily living, resulting in weight loss, fatigue, and depression. Tricyclic antidepressants, tramadol (Ultram), long-acting opioids, or anticonvulsants (i.e., gabapentin [Neurontin] or pregabalin [Lyrica]) can decrease the pain of PHN. If topical therapy is indicated, capsaicin cream (Zostrix) or a lidocaine patch (Lidoderm) may lessen the pain (Mallick-Searle et al., 2016).

Given the frequent occurrence of herpes zoster in older adults and its associated morbidity, prevention should be considered. The zoster vaccine significantly boosts immunity to the varicella-zoster virus in older adults (Schwarz et al., 2018). Additionally, the zoster vaccine can significantly reduce the burden of illness and the incidence of PHN (Saguil & Lauters, 2017).

PREMALIGNANT CONDITIONS OF THE SKIN

Older adults can have premalignant conditions of the skin, some of which lead to skin cancer. The most common of these conditions are keratoses and photodamage to the skin.

Keratoses

A *keratosis* is a thick, scaly, or crusty patch of skin associated with frequent exposure to the sun. There are two types of keratoses: seborrheic and actinic.

Seborrheic keratosis is a benign growth that appears mainly on the trunk, face, neck, and scalp as single or multiple lesions. One or more lesions are present on nearly all adults older than 65 years of age, and the lesions are more common in men. A person may have dozens of these benign lesions. A seborrheic keratosis is a waxy, raised, verrucous lesion that is flesh-coloured or pigmented in various sizes (Fig. 11.1). The lesions have a "stuck on" appearance, as if they could be scraped off. If there are cosmetic concerns, seborrheic keratoses may be removed by a dermatologist. A variant seen in darkly pigmented persons occurs mostly on the face and appears as numerous small, dark, and possibly tag-like lesions (see http://www.dermweb.com/photo_atlas/).

An *actinic keratosis* is a precancerous lesion that may become a squamous cell carcinoma. It is characterized by rough, scaly, sandpaper-like patches that are pink to reddish-brown on an erythematous base (Stockfleth, 2017). Lesions may be single or multiple and may be painless or mildly tender. Actinic keratosis is found on the face, lips, hands, and forearms—areas of sun exposure in everyday life. Risk factors are age and fair complexion. A person with actinic keratoses should be monitored by a dermatologist every 6 to 12 months for any change in the appearance of the lesions. Early

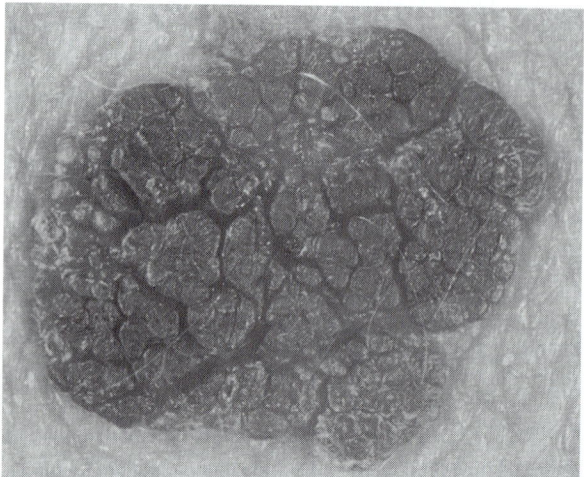

Fig. 11.1 ■ Seborrheic keratosis in an older adult. ***Source:*** Habif, T. P. (2004). *Clinical dermatology: A color guide to diagnosis and therapy* (4th ed.). Mosby.

recognition, treatment, and removal of the lesion are easy yet very important.

Photodamage to the Skin

Although exposure to sunlight is necessary for the production of vitamin D, the sun is also the most common cause of skin damage and skin cancer. With accumulating years of sun exposure, the risk of damage to the skin is significantly increased for older adults. The damage results from prolonged exposure to ultraviolet light (photo or solar) from the environment or from tanning booths. Although the amount of sun-induced damage varies with skin type and genetics, much of the associated damage is preventable. Ideally, preventive measures begin in childhood, but clinical evidence has shown that by limiting a person's sun exposure and having the person regularly use sunscreen, some measures can be effective at any time.

SKIN CANCERS

Worldwide, one of every three diagnosed cancers are skin cancers (*neoplasms*), which are growths on the skin (World Health Organization, 2017). The three most common skin cancers are basal cell cancer, squamous cell cancer, and melanoma; each is named for the type of skin cell from which it arises.

Skin cancer generally develops in the epidermis (the outermost layer of skin), and a tumour is therefore usually clearly visible, making most skin cancers detectable in the early stages. Nonmelanoma skin cancer represents approximately 30% of all new cancer cases in Canada (Government of Canada, 2019a). It is difficult to retrieve statistics for nonmelanoma skin cancer because it is typically treated with success at the doctor's office and does not require any further treatment or hospitalization (Government of Canada, 2019a).

Most of these skin cancers are curable; the type with the greatest potential to cause death is melanoma (Government of Canada, 2019b). Persons with a history of sunburn, tanning bed use, skin cancer, exposure to carcinogenic materials, sun sensitivity, or a depressed immune system are at particular risk. Treatment depends on the type of cancer, the stage of the cancer, and the thickness and location of the lesion (Canadian Cancer Society, 2021a).

Basal Cell Carcinoma

Basal cell carcinoma and squamous cell carcinoma are the most common types of skin cancer in Canada, making up to 80% of all cases of nonmelanoma skin cancers in the country (Canadian Cancer Society, 2021b). A basal cell lesion can be triggered by extensive sun exposure (especially that leading to sunburn), chronic irritation, and chronic ulceration of the skin. Basal cell carcinoma usually begins as a pearly papule with prominent telangiectasis (pattern or widened tiny blood vessels) or as a scar-like area with no history of trauma. It may be indistinguishable from squamous cell carcinoma and is diagnosed by biopsy. Basal cell carcinoma grows slowly, and metastasis is rare. Early detection and treatment are necessary to minimize disfigurement.

Squamous Cell Carcinoma

Squamous cell carcinoma is the second most common skin cancer; however, it is aggressive and has a high incidence of metastasis if not identified and treated promptly. Squamous cell cancer is more prevalent in fair-skinned older men who live in sunny climates and is usually found on the head, neck, or hands. Individuals in their mid-sixties who have been or are chronically exposed to the sun (e.g., persons who work outdoors, athletes) are at high risk for this type of cancer. Less common causes include persistent stasis ulcers, scars from injury, and exposure to chemical carcinogens. The lesion begins as a firm, irregular, fleshy, pink nodule that becomes reddened and scaly, much like actinic keratosis, but it may increase rapidly in size. The lesions may also be hard and wart-like, with a grey top and a horny texture, or they may be ulcerated and indurated, with raised, defined borders. Because the lesions can vary so much in appearance, they are often overlooked or thought to be insignificant. The best advice to give older adults, especially those who live in sunny climates, is to be regularly screened by a nurse practitioner, family physician, or dermatologist.

Melanoma

Melanoma, a neoplasm of melanocytes, is the least common skin cancer, but it has a high mortality rate because of its ability to metastasize quickly. Blistering sunburns before the age of 18 years are thought to damage Langerhans cells, which affects the skin's immune response and increases the risk for a later melanoma. The legs and backs of women and the backs of men are the most common sites. Two-thirds of melanomas develop from preexisting moles; only one-third arise alone. A melanoma lesion has a multi-coloured, raised appearance with an asymmetrical, irregular border. It may appear to be of any size, but, much like an iceberg, its surface

diameter does not necessarily reflect its size beneath the surface. It is treatable if caught very early, before it has a chance to invade surrounding tissue. If a nurse finds any questionable lesions upon assessment, the person should be referred to a dermatologist immediately. A common approach to assessing potential lesions is the ABCDE method (Box 11.3).

IMPLICATIONS FOR GERONTOLOGICAL NURSING AND HEALTHY AGING

Gerontological nurses have an active role to play in the prevention and early recognition of skin cancers. This role may include working within community awareness and education programs, working in screening clinics, and providing direct care. In promoting skin health, nurses should be vigilant in observing the skin for any changes that require further evaluation. Several applications for electronic devices—Spot Check, Skin of Mine, Skin Prevention, Mole Detective 2, and Skin Scan—can be helpful in the detection of skin cancer (Kassianos et al., 2015).

By far the most important preventive nursing intervention is educating the older adult about the risks caused by photodamage and smoke damage. Preventive

---

BOX 11.3

ABCDE RULES OF MELANOMA DIAGNOSIS

Asymmetry: One half does not match the other half.
Border irregularity: The edges are ragged, notched, or blurred.
Colour: The pigment is not uniform in colour, having shades of tan, brown, or black, or a mottled appearance with red, white, or blue areas.

Diameter: The diameter is greater than the size of a pencil eraser or is increasing in size.
Evolution: There is a change or evolution in size, shape, symptoms, surface, and/or shades of colour.

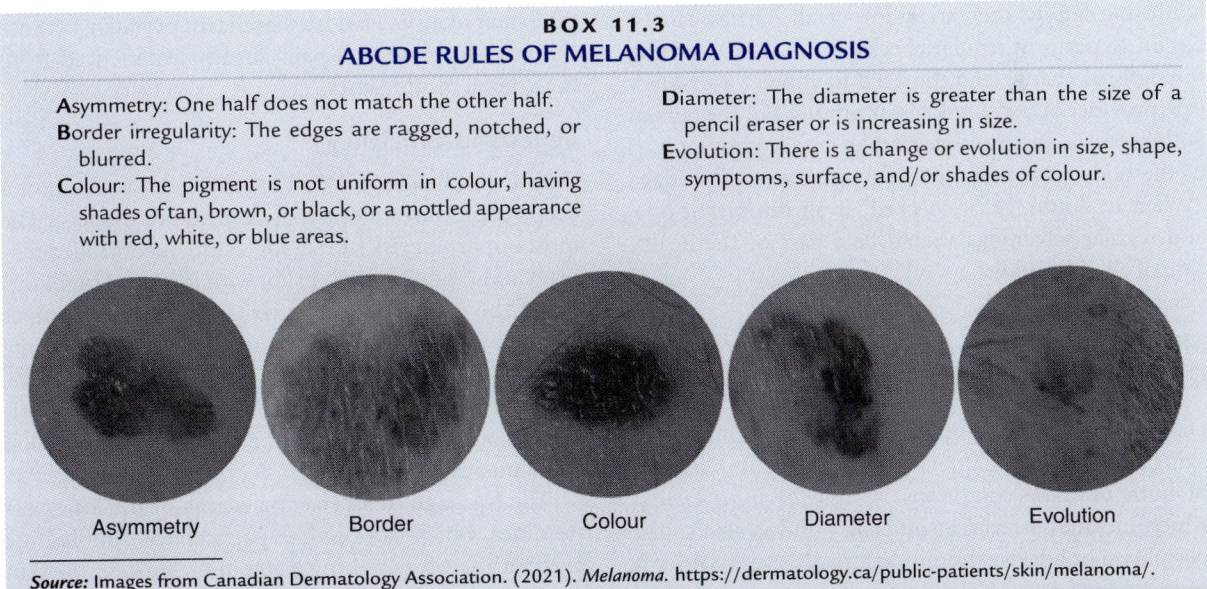

| Asymmetry | Border | Colour | Diameter | Evolution |

Source: Images from Canadian Dermatology Association. (2021). *Melanoma.* https://dermatology.ca/public-patients/skin/melanoma/.

BOX 11.4
SUN PROTECTION RECOMMENDATIONS

- Avoid midday sun (1000 to 1500 hours), when ultraviolet radiation is most intense.
- Use sunscreen daily if going outdoors in sunny or potentially sunny regions, regardless of the weather.
- Wear clothing that covers the normally exposed areas of the skin, and wear a broad-brimmed hat to protect the face and top of the head, especially when working outdoors in sunny regions.
- Use a sunscreen with a sun protection factor (SPF) of 15 or higher; apply before sun exposure, and reapply periodically after perspiring heavily or swimming.
- Avoid getting sunburned, and limit sun exposure at all times.
- Be aware of reflections from sand, snow, and water; these will intensify the radiation.
- Avoid sun if taking photosensitizing medications such as tetracyclines.
- Avoid sunscreens with para-aminobenzoic acid if allergic to procaine, sulphonamides, or hair dyes (because of cross-sensitization).
- Avoid tanning beds and sun lamps.

strategies include using sunscreen, wearing protective clothing, and limiting sun exposure (Box 11.4).

Secondary prevention of skin cancer is early diagnosis. Following a thorough clinical screening, the older adult, the family, the care aides, or all parties can be taught to perform regular checks of the skin, watching for signs of change and the need to contact a primary care provider or dermatologist promptly. For the person with keratosis and multiple freckles (*nevi*), photographs of the body parts may be useful references. The adage "When in doubt, get it checked" is an important one, and regular screenings should be a part of the health care of all older adults.

SKIN PROBLEMS ASSOCIATED WITH CARDIOVASCULAR PROBLEMS

Diabetes and hypertension are common problems for aging persons (see Chapters 17 and 20). A complication of both of these conditions is *vascular insufficiency*, which includes arterial insufficiency and is also called peripheral or lower-extremity artery disease; another is *venous insufficiency*. Vascular insufficiency may lead to

serious skin infections and lesions, from mild stasis dermatitis to ulceration and gangrene. In promoting healthy aging, nurses need to be aware of the signs of vascular insufficiency and protect the person's limb and skin from further injury.

Arterial Insufficiency

Peripheral artery disease (PAD) affects more than 200 million people worldwide (Shu & Santulli, 2018). The disease is often caused by increased atherosclerotic plaques, which lead to ischemia of the limb and can result in severe infections and limb loss. Many persons with PAD, whether diagnosed or not, complain of pain or muscle fatigue when they exercise. In more severe cases, the lower extremity can be extremely painful when the person is walking or when the legs are elevated (a condition called *intermittent claudication*). The person's pain is relieved only when the legs are returned to a dependent position (because of increased arterial flow downward) or when the person stops walking and rests, thus eliminating the extra circulatory demands made by exercise. Risk factors for PAD include obesity, coronary artery disease, smoking, dyslipidemia, hypertension, and diabetes.

As a result of PAD, the slightest trauma to a lower extremity, such as that caused by bumping the side of a wheelchair, can result in an arterial ulcer, which is very difficult and sometimes impossible to heal without surgical intervention. Pain is a significant problem, because the ulcer increases the pain already experienced from the arterial insufficiency.

Venous Insufficiency

Venous insufficiency (VI) is usually a consequence of a deep venous thrombosis that occurred in the past. The most important risk factors for VI are uncontrolled diabetes and venous hypertension with impaired functioning of the valves within the veins. Skin tissue becomes vulnerable to insignificant trauma, such as an insect bite or the pressure from snug elastic-topped ankle socks. These insignificant traumatic events may also precipitate venous ulcer formation, or ulceration can develop spontaneously.

The first sign of VI may be edema of the lower extremities, which can become particularly troublesome and can affect functioning. Later in the process, the skin on the lower half of the extremity develops a brownish

TABLE 11.1
Comparison of Arterial and Venous Insufficiency of the Lower Extremities

Characteristics	Arterial Insufficiency	Venous Insufficiency
Location	Between toes or on tips of toes Over phalangeal heads and on heels Lateral malleolus or pretibial area (in diabetic patients), over metatarsal heads, on sides or soles of feet	Lower calf and ankle (especially medial malleolus)
Appearance	Well-defined edges Black or necrotic tissue Deep, pale base Nonbleeding	Uneven edges Ruddy granulation tissue Superficial Bleeding
Pain	Extreme pain with elevation of leg (relieved by dependent position) Persistent pain Constant severe pain with complete occlusion of blood supply	Deep muscle pain if deep vein thrombosis develops Relieved by elevation
Pulses	Absent or weak	Normal
Associated changes in leg and foot	Thin, shiny, dry skin Thickened toenails Absence of hair growth Temperature variations (cooler if there is no cellulitis) Elevational pallor Dependent rubor	Firm edema Reddish-brown discolouration of skin Evidence of healed ulcers Dilated and tortuous superficial veins

discolouration caused by the leakage of iron from red blood cells. In people with dark-pigmented skin, the discoloured skin is darker than the surrounding skin.

Venous ulcerations are painful and difficult to heal (Gohel et al., 2018). Although they are most often found over the outer malleolus, they can become quite extensive. The characteristics of venous ulcers are summarized in Table 11.1.

IMPLICATIONS FOR GERONTOLOGICAL NURSING AND HEALTHY AGING

The most important aspect of caring for the person with VI and PAD is to ensure that a proper and timely diagnosis is made and that treatment is consistent. To promote the health of the person's lower extremities, nurses must stay alert for signs of potential problems and take prompt action to minimize tissue damage. If ulcers develop, treatment must be consistent with evidence-informed practice. Nurses can also help older adults reduce risk factors whenever possible;

for example, nurses can encourage smoking cessation and careful control of hypertension. Nurses can help reduce the incidence of ulcerations by protecting an affected limb from accidental injury.

A complaint of lower-extremity pain at rest necessitates a prompt referral to a vascular surgeon. Since the symptoms and problems associated with PAD are the result of ischemia of the extremity, interventions that promote circulation, such as finding ways for the older adult to dangle their feet, are helpful. In the LTC setting, caregivers must recognize that a resident may be refusing to elevate the lower extremities because doing so causes sudden and severe pain.

A person may be more comfortable sleeping in a recliner, where the feet can dangle. If an ulcer develops, then the emphasis should be on preventing it from worsening. The wound should be kept warm and covered, but compression is contraindicated. The goals of care are to maximize function, relieve edema and pain, and treat the ulcer as needed. Treatment usually consists of a combination of therapies, such as leg elevation whenever the person is sitting and support stockings worn during waking hours. Although the stockings are usually considered uncomfortable, wearing them should nonetheless be encouraged. Support stockings are now available in an assortment of colours, including skin tones that are more acceptable than the traditional white. For maximal effect, support stockings should be put on before the person gets out of bed. They should extend to the top of the leg and be prevented from "rolling," since constriction is increased at the roll. Treatment of the venous ulcer includes managing the exudate and preventing worsening.

SKIN PROBLEMS OF PARTICULAR CONCERN FOR PERSONS WITH LIMITED MOBILITY

Persons with limited mobility, compromised immunity, or both are at particular risk for fungal skin infections and pressure injuries.

Candidiasis

The fungus *Candida albicans* (referred to as yeast) is present on the skin of any healthy person. However, under certain circumstances and in the right environment, a fungal infection can develop. Persons who are obese, are malnourished, are receiving antibiotic or steroid therapy, or have diabetes are at increased risk. *Candida* grows especially well in areas that are moist, warm, and dark, such as in skinfolds, in the axilla and groin, under pendulous breasts, at the corners of the mouth, and in the vagina.

When it occurs inside the mouth, a *Candida* infection is referred to as *thrush* and is associated with those who have poor hygiene and are immunocompromised, such as that seen in persons engaged with long-term steroid use (e.g., because of chronic obstructive pulmonary disease), people who are receiving chemotherapy, or people who are infected with human immunodeficiency virus (HIV) or have developed acquired immunodeficiency syndrome (AIDS). In the mouth, candidiasis appears as irregular, white, and flat to slightly raised patches on an erythematous base that cannot be scraped off. The infection can extend down into the throat and cause painful swallowing. In severely immunocompromised persons, the infection can extend down the entire gastro-intestinal tract.

On the skin, a *Candida* infection usually manifests as maculopapular and glazed; it is dark pink on persons with less pigmentation and greyish on persons with more pigmentation. If the infection is advanced, the central area may be completely red or dark (or both) and weeping, with characteristic bright red, dark, or bright red and dark satellite lesions (distinct lesions a short distance from the centre). At that point, the skin may be edematous, itching, and burning.

The best approach to managing fungal infections is to prevent them. The key to prevention is limiting the conditions that encourage fungal growth. People who are at risk are those who are bedridden, incontinent, obese, or diaphoretic. It is important to pay attention to the adequate drying of target areas of the body after bathing, prompt management of incontinent episodes (see Chapter 9), the use of loose-fitting cotton clothing and underwear, and the avoidance of incontinence products that are tight or have plastic that touches the skin.

One of the best ways to dry hard-to-reach, vulnerable areas is with a hair dryer set on low. A folded dry washcloth or a cotton sanitary pad can be placed under the breasts or between skinfolds to allow exposure to air and light. Cornstarch should never be used because it promotes the growth of *Candida* organisms. Optimizing nutrition and glycemic control are also important.

The goal of treatment is to eradicate the infection. Eradication requires not only the use of prescribed antifungal medication but also the active involvement of nurses or caregivers in reducing or eliminating the conditions that created the problem. The affected area of the skin must be cleansed carefully with a mild soap or cleansing agent (such as Cetaphil) and dried thoroughly before antifungal preparations are applied. Antifungal preparations are available as powders, creams, and lotions. Because creams and lotions trap moisture, powder is recommended. These preparations are usually needed for 7 to 14 days, or until the infection has completely cleared. Antifungal medications include miconazole (Micatin), clotrimazole (Canesten, Clotrimaderm, Lotriderm), nystatin (Mycostatin), and econazole (Ecostatin).

Pressure Injuries

According to the Registered Nurses' Association of Ontario (RNAO), a pressure injury is "any lesion caused by unrelieved pressure that results in damage to underlying tissue. Pressure injuries usually occur over a bony prominence and are staged to classify the degree of tissue damage observed" (Registered Nurses' Association of Ontario [RNAO], 2016). As tissue is compressed, blood is diverted, and blood vessels are forcibly constricted by the persistent pressure on the skin and underlying structures; thus, cellular respiration is impaired, and cells die from ischemia and anoxia. Intervention at any point in this development can stop the advancement of the pressure injury. Just how much pressure can be endured by tissue, known as **tissue tolerance**, is highly variable between body locations and persons. Tissue tolerance is inversely affected by moisture, friction, shearing, amount of pressure, and age, and is directly related to malnutrition, anemia, and low arterial pressure.

The prevalence of pressure injuries is quite high in later life. Data from the Canadian Institute for Health Information indicates that between 2011 and 2012, 2.4%, 14.1%, and 6.7% of patients experienced a pressure injury in home care, complex continuing care, and LTC settings, respectively (Denny et al., 2014). Pressure injuries are highly preventable; however, they remain prevalent, particularly in LTC settings (Jorgensen et al., 2018). According to some researchers, pressure injuries are associated with adverse effects on health, social well-being, quality of life, and high treatment cost (RNAO, 2017). The cost of treating pressure injuries range from $26,800 to $231,000 per injury (RNAO, 2017).

Risk Factors

Persons who are frail, nonambulatory, or neurologically impaired are at the greatest risk for the development of a pressure injury. The most important predictors of pressure injuries are severity of illness and involuntary weight loss owing to problems of poor nutrition, especially dehydration, hypoproteinemia, and vitamin deficiencies. Other important indicators of increased risk are impaired sensory feedback systems (which prevent discomfort from being noticed) and impaired mobility or immobilization by sedation. Nevertheless, most pressure injuries are considered preventable.

Pressure injuries can develop anywhere on the body but are most frequently seen on posterior aspects, especially the sacrum, coccyx, knees, heels, and toes (RNAO, 2016). Secondary areas of breakdown include the lateral condyles of the knees and ankles. The pinna of the ears is also subject to breakdown, as are the elbows and

---

BOX 11.5

EXAMPLES OF COMPLICATIONS OF PRESSURE INJURIES

- Local infection of wound or surrounding tissue
- Loss of function
- Tetanus
- Extension of the infection to the bone: osteomyelitis
- Systemic infection: septicemia
- Extended period of acute and continuous medical and nursing care

---

the scapulae. If a person is lying prone, the knees, shins, and pelvis sustain undue pressure. In some circumstances, pressure injuries develop as a result of a fall at home, when the person stays in the same position and is unable to move for a prolonged period of time.

Heels are particularly apt to develop pressure injuries, since heels are small surfaces that receive a high degree of pressure. People who have peripheral vascular insufficiency and are immobile are at high risk for heel ulcers. In the acute care setting, patients who are supine for prolonged periods during surgical procedures may leave the operating room with newly acquired pressure injuries.

For many older adults, an ulcer will prolong recovery and lengthen rehabilitation. Complications include sepsis, the need for grafting, and the need for amputation; even death can occur (Box 11.5).

The development of pressure injuries is a dynamic process that makes constant vigilance and reassessment necessary, and nurses play an extremely important role in preventing them and in assessing the skin. The Braden Scale (Fig. 11.2) and the Norton Scale are risk assessment tools frequently used in the clinical setting to identify persons who are at high risk for pressure injuries (Bergstrom et al., 1994; Norton, 1996).

IMPLICATIONS FOR GERONTOLOGICAL NURSING AND HEALTHY AGING

Of all health care providers, nurses are the most responsible for the prevention and treatment of pressure injuries and other interruptions in skin integrity. Nurses are in an ideal position to implement preventive measures, identify early signs, and implement appropriate interventions to

Braden Scale for Predicting Pressure Sore Risk

Resident's Name _____   Evaluator's Name _____

				Date of assessment				
SENSORY PERCEPTION Ability to respond meaningfully to pressure-related discomfort	**1. Completely Limited** Unresponsive (does not moan, flinch or grasp) to painful stimuli, due to diminished level of consciousness or sedation. OR limited ability to feel pain over most of body.	**2. Very Limited** Responds only to painful stimuli. Cannot communicate discomfort except by moaning or restlessness. OR has a sensory impairment that limits the ability to feel pain or discomfort over ½ of body.	**3. Slightly Limited** Responds to verbal commands, but cannot always communicate discomfort or the need to be turned. OR has some sensory impairment which limits ability to feel pain or discomfort in 1 or 2 extremities.	**4. No Impairment** Responds to verbal commands. Has no sensory deficit which would limit ability to feel or voice pain or discomfort.				
MOISTURE Degree to which skin is exposed to moisture	**1. Constantly Moist** Skin is kept moist almost constantly by perspiration, urine, etc. Dampness is detected every time patient is moved or turned.	**2. Very Moist** Skin is often, but not always, moist. Linen must be changed at least once a shift.	**3. Occasionally Moist** Skin is occasionally moist, requiring an extra linen change approximately once a day.	**4. Rarely Moist** Skin is usually dry. Linen only requires changing at routine intervals.				
ACTIVITY Degree of physical activity	**1. Bedfast** Confined to bed.	**2. Chairfast** Ability to walk severely limited or non-existent. Cannot bear own weight and/or must be assisted into chair or wheelchair.	**3. Walks Occasionally** Walks occasionally during day, but for very short distances with or without assistance. Spends majority of each shift in bed or chair.	**4. Walks Frequently** Walks outside the room at least twice a day and inside room at least every 2 hours during waking hours.				
MOBILITY Ability to change and control body position	**1. Completely Immobile** Does not make even slight changes in body or extremity position without assistance.	**2. Very Limited** Makes occasional slight changes in body or extremity position, but unable to make frequent or significant changes independently.	**3. Slightly Limited** Makes frequent though slight changes in body or extremity position independently.	**4. No Limitation** Makes major and frequent changes in position without assistance.				

Fig. 11.2 ▓ Braden Scale for Predicting Pressure Sore Risk. **Source:** Regional Geriatric Program of Toronto. (n.d.). *Braden Scale for Predicting Pressure Sore Risk.* © Barbara Braden and Nancy Bergstrom, 1988. Reprinted with permission. All rights reserved. https://bpgmobile.rnao.ca/sites/default/files/Braden%20Scale%20for%20Predicting%20Pressure%20Sore%20Risk.pdf.

	1. Very Poor	2. Probably Inadequate	3. Adequate	4. Excellent	
NUTRITION Usual food intake pattern	Never eats a complete meal. Rarely eats more than 1/3 of any food offered. Eats 2 servings or less of protein (meat or dairy products) per day. Takes fluids poorly. Does not take a liquid dietary supplement. OR is NPO and/or maintained on clear liquids or IVs for more than 5 days.	Rarely eats a complete meal and generally eats only about ½ of any food offered. Protein intake includes only 3 servings of meat or dairy products per day. Occasionally will take a dietary supplement. OR receives less than optimum amount of liquid diet or tube feeding.	Eats over half of most meals. Eats a total of 4 servings of protein (meat or dairy products) each day. Occasionally will refuse a meal, but will usually take a supplement if offered. OR is on tube feeding or TPN regimen, which meets most of nutritional needs.	**4. Excellent** Eats most of every meal. Never refuses a meal. Usually eats a total of 4 or more servings of meat and dairy products. Occasionally eats between meals. Does not require supplementation.	
FRICTION AND SHEAR	**1. Problem** Requires moderate to maximum assistance in moving. Complete lifting without sliding against sheets is impossible. Frequently slides down in bed or chair, requiring frequent repositioning with maximum assistance. Spasticity, contractures or agitation lead to almost constant friction.	**2. Potential Problems** Moves feebly or requires minimum assistance. During a move skin probably slides to some extent against sheets, chair restraints, or other devices. Maintains relatively good position in chair or bed most of the time but occasionally slides down.	**3. No Apparent Problem** Moves in bed and chair independently and has sufficient muscle strength to lift up completely during move. Maintains good position in bed or chair.		**Total Score**

© Copyright Barbara Braden and Nancy Bergstrom, 1988.

Note: (Braden, 2001)
15 to 18 = At Risk
13 to 14 = Moderate Risk
10 to 12 = High Risk
≤ 9 = Very High Risk

Assessment Schedule:
Very High to High Risk = minimum monthly
Moderate Risk = q3months
Low/No Risk = q6months

Consider other resident factors that will also increase risks, e.g., advanced age, uncontrolled pain, underlying disease conditions, low albumin and HGB.

Fig. 11.2, cont'd

prevent skin breakdown and promote healing. Failure to take these actions jeopardizes the health and life of the person receiving care. The nurse can inform other health care providers of the need for prevention, recommended treatments, evaluation of the status of the wound or wounds, and the adequacy of interventions. A detailed best practice guideline can be found at https://ltctoolkit.rnao.ca/clinical-topics/pressure-ulcer/pressure-ulcers.

Assessment

Assessment begins with a detailed head-to-toe skin examination and an analysis of laboratory test findings (Box 11.6). Laboratory values that have been correlated with risk for the development and poor healing of pressure injuries include those that indicate anemia and poor nutritional status. Visual and tactile inspection of the entire skin surface, with special attention to bony prominences, is essential. Special attention must be paid to affected areas when an individual uses orthotic devices such as corsets, braces, prostheses, postural supports, splints, slings, or casts.

The nurse will look for any interruption in skin integrity or other changes, including **hyperemia** (redness). Any pressure should be relieved and the area reassessed in 1 hour. Redness may be less noticeable on darkly pigmented persons than on lightly pigmented persons; it may be necessary to look for induration, darkening, or a shadowed appearance. Pressure areas should be palpated for changes in temperature and tissue resilience. Blisters or pimples (with or without hyperemia) and scabs over weight-bearing areas in the absence of trauma should be considered suspect.

Existing pressure injuries are assessed with each dressing change, and detailed assessment is repeated as needed (Box 11.7). The purpose of the assessment is to carefully evaluate the effectiveness of treatment. If there are no signs of healing from week to week or if worsening is seen, then either the treatment is insufficient or the wound has become infected; in either case, treatment must be changed.

Pressure Injury Classification

Pressure injuries are classified according to the scale developed and updated by the National Pressure Ulcer Advisory Panel (2016). The scale encompasses suspected injury, pressure injury stages 1 through 4, and "unstageable" pressure injury (Fig. 11.3). An ulcer is always classified by the highest stage; this means that the wound is documented at the stage that represents the maximum damage that has occurred. As the wound heals, it fills with granulation tissue composed of endothelial cells, fibroblasts, collagen, and an extracellular

---

BOX 11.6
RISK ASSESSMENT AND PREVENTION OF PRESSURE INJURIES

- Carry out a daily head-to-toe assessment of persons who are at risk for skin breakdown; pay particular attention to bony prominences.
- Assess risk for pressure injury development with a valid and reliable tool, such as the Braden Scale for Predicting Pressure Sore Risk (Fig. 11.2).
- Assess persons who have restricted mobility for pressure, friction, and shearing forces, in all positions and during lifting, turning, and repositioning.
- Develop a collaborative, individualized plan of care based on assessment data, identified risk factors, and the patient's goals.
- Use proper positioning, transferring, and turning techniques.
- Avoid massaging over bony prominences.
- Protect and promote skin integrity through hydrating the skin, minimizing force and shear during cleansing, using protective barriers to reduce friction, and so on.

Source: Adapted from Registered Nurses' Association of Ontario. (2016). *Assessment and management of pressure injuries for the interprofessional team* (3rd ed.). https://rnao.ca/sites/rnao-ca/files/Pressure_Injuries_BPG.pdf.

BOX 11.7
KEY ASPECTS OF ASSESSMENT OF A PRESSURE INJURY

1. Stage and size (width, depth, length)
2. Location
3. Surface area (length × width) (mm², cm²)
4. Odour
5. Sinus tracts, undermining, tunnelling
6. Exudate
7. Condition of surrounding tissue
8. Condition of wound edges (e.g., smooth and white or irregular and pink)
9. Wound bed (warmth, moisture, odour, amount, and colour of exudates)

DEFINITION	SCHEMATIC DRAWING	EXAMPLE

STAGE 1 PRESSURE INJURY

Non-blanchable erythema of intact skin

Intact skin with a localized area of non-blanchable erythema, which may appear differently in darkly pigmented skin. Presence of blanchable erythema or changes in sensation, temperature, or firmness may precede visual changes. Colour changes do not include purple or maroon discoloration; these may indicate deep tissue pressure injury.

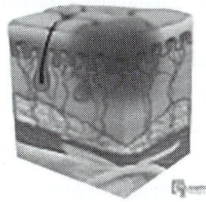 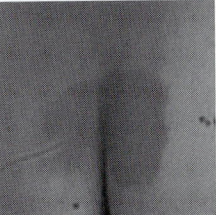

STAGE 2 PRESSURE INJURY

Partial-thickness skin loss with exposed dermis

Partial-thickness loss of skin with exposed dermis. The wound bed is viable, pink or red, moist, and may also present as an intact or ruptured serum-filled blister. Adipose (fat) is not visible and deeper tissues are not visible. Granulation tissue, slough and eschar are not present. These injuries commonly result from adverse microclimate and shear in the skin over the pelvis and shear in the heel. This stage should not be used to describe moisture associated skin damage (MASD) including incontinence associated dermatitis (IAD), intertriginous dermatitis (ITD), medical adhesive related skin injury (MARSI), or traumatic wounds (skin tears, burns, abrasions).

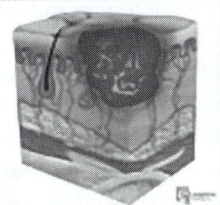 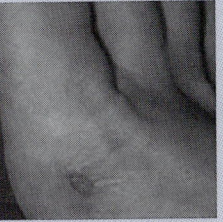

STAGE 3 PRESSURE INJURY

Full-thickness skin loss

Full-thickness loss of skin, in which adipose (fat) is visible in the ulcer and granulation tissue and epibole (rolled wound edges) are often present. Slough and/or eschar may be visible. The depth of tissue damage varies by anatomical location; areas of significant adiposity can develop deep wounds. Undermining and tunneling may occur. Fascia, muscle, tendon, ligament, cartilage or bone are not exposed. If slough or eschar obscures the extent of tissue loss this is an Unstageable Pressure Injury.

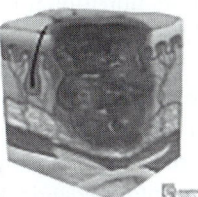 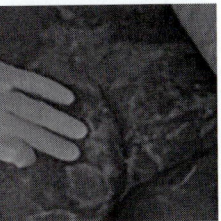

STAGE 4 PRESSURE INJURY

Full-thickness loss of skin and tissue

Full-thickness skin and tissue loss with exposed or directly palpable fascia, muscle, tendon, ligament, cartilage or bone in the ulcer. Slough and/or eschar may be visible. Epibole (rolled edges), undermining and/or tunneling often occur. Depth varies by anatomical location. If slough or eschar obscures the extent of tissue loss this is an Unstageable Pressure Injury.

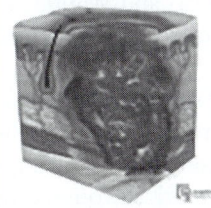 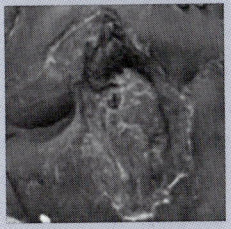

Fig. 11.3 ▪ Pressure sore development. ***Source:*** National Pressure Injury Advisory Panel. (2016). *Pressure injury and stages.* © 2016 National Pressure Injury Advisory Panel. https://npiap.com/, https://cdn.ymaws.com/npiap.com/resource/resmgr/NPIAP-Staging-Poster.pdf.

matrix. Muscle, subcutaneous fat, and dermis are not replaced. The staging of a pressure injury cannot be reversed; that is, a stage IV pressure injury that is healing is not reclassified as stage III and then stage II; it remains defined as a (healing) stage IV pressure injury. Wounds that are covered in black (**eschar**) or yellow fibrous (**slough**) necrosis cannot be staged, because it is not possible to determine the condition of the underlying wound bed. These wounds are documented as unstageable. Once the dead tissue has been removed (**debrided**), the wound can be staged.

Careful and detailed documentation of the condition of the skin is required at the onset of the problem and at intervals during its treatment.

Interventions

The goal of nurses is to help maintain skin integrity against the various environmental, mechanical, and chemical assaults that are potential causes of breakdown. In promoting the healthy aging of all persons, nurses focus on prevention by taking action to eliminate friction and irritation to the skin (such as that caused by shearing); to reduce moisture so that tissues do not **macerate**; and to displace body weight from prominent areas in order to facilitate circulation to the skin. Nurses should assess the frequency of position changes, add pillows so that skin surfaces do not touch, and establish a turning schedule if needed. They should also be familiar with the various types of supportive surfaces and dressings so that the most effective products are used.

Nutritional intake should be monitored, as well as serum albumin, hematocrit, and hemoglobin levels. Diets high in protein, carbohydrates, and vitamins are necessary to maintain and promote tissue growth. If the patient lacks appetite, appetite stimulants may be prescribed. Nurses can promote nutritional health by ensuring that dining is a pleasant experience for the person (see Chapter 8).

It is not always possible to prevent interruptions in skin integrity that are caused by overwhelming conditions. Fortunately, the state of the science of wound care is well developed, and evidence-informed guidelines are available. Sources of information include the websites of the RNAO (http://www.rnao.ca) and Wounds Canada (Canadian Association of Wound Care) (https://www.woundscanada.ca).

Consultation with a nurse specialized in wound care is advisable for wounds that are extensive or nonhealing. Specialized nurses such as enterostomal therapists or nurse practitioners, who may work at wound centres or with surgeons, provide consultation in hospitals, LTC homes, offices, and clinics (see Chapter 2). In 2003, the province of Quebec introduced Bill 90 (Fédération Interprofessionnelle de la Santé du Quebec [FIQ], 2009). Bill 90 brought a revision of the fields of practice of the 11 professional orders and introduced activities reserved for each profession. These activities refer to a group of operations or interventions that can be carried out within the framework of the professional field of practice. One example is wound care. For the nurse, caring for wounds is considered a "reserved activity" according to Bill 90: "determine the treatment plan for wounds and alterations of the skin and teguments and provide the required care and treatment" (FIQ, 2009).

HEALTHY FEET

Feet influence the older adult's physical, psychological, and social well-being. Feet carry the body's weight, hold the body erect, coordinate and maintain balance in walking, and must be adaptable enough to conform to changing walking surfaces. Little attention is given to a person's feet until they interfere with moving and ultimately the ability to remain independent. Promoting healthy feet and good care of the feet can alleviate disability and pain and lessen the risk of falling.

Common Foot Problems

The human foot is a complex structure with many bones, joints, tendons, muscles, and ligaments. Some foot irregularities and problems are inherited; however, many problems occur because of wear and tear, the shoes the person wears, or misuse of the feet.

Older feet, subjected to a lifetime of stress, may not be able to continue to adapt, and inflammatory changes in bone and soft tissue can occur. Foot health and function may reflect systemic disease or give early clues to physical illness. Changes in the nails or skin of the feet or the recurrence of infections may be precursors of more serious health problems.

Major abnormalities occur gradually. Rheumatological disorders (such as the various forms of arthritis) usually affect other joints but can also affect the feet. Gout is a systemic disease that occurs most often in the joint of the great toe (see Chapter 18). Both diabetes and VI commonly cause lower-extremity problems that can quickly become life threatening.

Without proper care and treatment, these conditions become disabling and threaten the person's mobility and independence. Care of the feet requires a team approach that includes the older adult, the nurse, the podiatrist, and the person's primary health care provider. Nurses have the opportunity to promote healthy aging by applying their knowledge of the common problems of the feet and their skills in foot care.

Corns and Calluses

Corns and *calluses* are both growths of compacted skin that occur as a result of prolonged pressure, usually from ill-fitting, tight shoes. Corns are cone shaped and develop on the top of the toe joints as the result of the rubbing of the shoe on the joint. Calluses are parts of the skin that become thickened and hardened as a result of repeated friction or pressure. Soft corns form between opposing surfaces of the toes from prolonged squeezing. Corns and calluses can interfere with the ability to walk and to wear shoes comfortably. Once a corn forms, continued pressure on it will cause pain. Unless the friction and pressure are relieved, the corn will continue to enlarge and cause increasing pain.

Many older adults self-treat corns and calluses with over-the-counter preparations to remove the corn temporarily. However, chemical burns and ulcerations from these products can result in the loss of toes or a leg for a person with diabetes, neurological impairment, or poor circulation in the lower extremities. Some people use razor blades and scissors to remove the affected tissue; this is very dangerous and is never recommended. Oval corn pads, moleskin, or lambswool, with a hole cut in the centre for the corn, can be used for more proper treatment. Irritation from soft corns between the toes can be eased by loosely wrapping a small amount of lambswool around the involved toe, or cotton balls can be placed between the toes. Gel pads are also useful in protecting the toes from friction and pressure. For persons who are prone to developing calluses, daily lubrication of the feet is important. For persons with VI and diabetes, foot care should be performed only by a trained nurse, a physician, or a podiatrist.

Mild corns may resolve themselves when pressure is removed and tight shoes are replaced by larger shoes with a better fit. Bigger or resistant corns may need to be surgically removed by a podiatrist. For persons at high risk, such as those with diabetes or VI, corns are not usually removed because of the risk of poor wound healing at the surgical site.

Bunions

Bunions are bony deformities that develop from the longstanding squeezing together of the first (great or big) and second toes. Bony prominences develop over the medial aspect of the joint of the great toe and, at times, at the lateral aspect of the fifth metatarsal head (*tailor's bunion* or *bunionette*). Heredity may be a factor in their development. Walking can be markedly compromised by any of these deformities. Bunions may be treated with corticosteroid injections, anti-inflammatory pain medications, or surgery if necessary. Shoes that provide forefoot space (e.g., running shoes) and sandals work well, or a custom-made shoe could be considered. Nurses can promote comfort by helping the person find shoes that properly support and protect the foot.

Hammer Toes

A *hammer toe* is a toe that is permanently flexed, giving it a claw-like appearance. The condition is a result of muscle imbalance and pressure from the great toe slanting toward the second toe. The toe then contracts, leaving a bulge on top of the joint. It is aggravated by poor-fitting shoes and is often seen in conjunction with bunions. This condition limits the ability to walk and restricts balance and comfort. As with bunions, treatment includes professional orthotics or specially designed protective devices; properly fitting, nonconstricting shoes; or surgical intervention.

Fungal Infections

Fungal infections are very common on the aging foot, and the incidence increases with age. These infections may affect the skin of the foot as well as the nails. Nail fungus, or *onychomycosis*, is characterized by degeneration of the nail plate, change in the colour of the nail (to yellow or an opaque brown), and brittleness and thickening of the nail (Fig. 11.4). A fine, powdery collection of fungus forms under the centre of the nail, separating

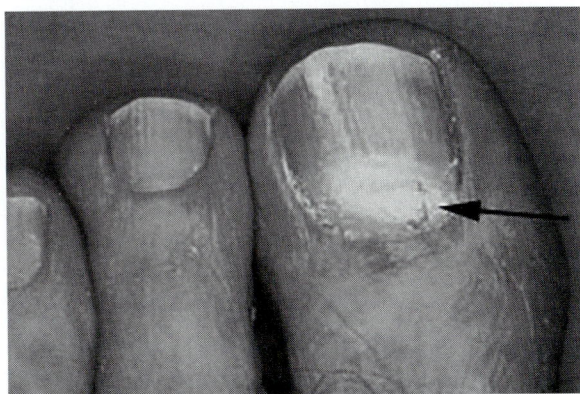

Fig. 11.4 ■ Onychomycosis: Yellowing, crumbling, and thickening of the toenails (arrow). ***Source:*** From Rodgers, P., & Bassler, M. (2001). Treating onychomycosis. *American Family Physician, 63*(4), 663–673. (Figure 5: Proximal subungual onychomycosis.)

the layers and pushing the nail up, causing the sides of the nail to dig into the skin like an ingrown toenail. Culturing is the only definitive way to diagnose onychomycosis. Several oral medications are available but are expensive and of limited effectiveness, need to be taken for 3 to 12 months, and are potentially toxic to the liver and heart. When nails are involved, a cure is difficult to impossible because of limited circulation.

Another common fungal infection is *tinea pedis* (athlete's foot). Many of the causes of candidiasis are also causes of this infection. Tinea pedis is treated as any other fungal infection is treated. Feet, especially the area between the toes, should be kept dry and clean and regularly exposed to sun and air. Topical application of antifungal powders, in addition to the hygiene measures already noted, is the usual treatment.

IMPLICATIONS FOR GERONTOLOGICAL NURSING AND HEALTHY AGING

Gerontological nurses should advocate the best foot health possible. Foot care is a prime factor in the maintenance of mobility and independence. Nursing care of the older adult with foot problems should be directed toward maintaining optimal comfort and function, removing possible mechanical irritants, and decreasing the likelihood of infection. The nurse has to assess the feet for clues of functional ability and their owner's well-being (Box 11.8). Nurses can identify potential and actual problems and make referrals or seek assistance from the primary care provider or podiatrist as needed.

Gerontological nursing care includes the observation of gait, postural deformities, physical limitations, the position of the foot with the heel strike, and the type of shoe worn and its condition, including sole wear. Assessment also includes an inspection of the feet for irritation, abrasions, and other lesions; hazards to the maintenance of adequate circulation to the lower extremities and the existing circulatory status; and the individual's general mobility. Periodic assessment of the feet is especially important for persons with diabetes, heart disease, VI, thyroid or renal conditions, and any neurological impairment, such as reduced or absent sensations resulting from a stroke.

Care of Toenails

Poor close vision, difficulty bending, obesity, or increased thickness of the nails makes self-care of the

---

BOX 11.8
ESSENTIAL ASPECTS OF FOOT ASSESSMENT

OBSERVATION OF MOBILITY
- Gait
- Use of assistive devices
- Footwear type and pattern of wear

PAST MEDICAL HISTORY
- Neuropathies
- Musculo-skeletal limitations
- Vascular insufficiency
- Vision problems
- Falls
- Pain affecting movement

BILATERAL ASSESSMENT
- Colour
- Circulation and warmth
- Pulses
- Structural deformities
- Skin lesions
- Lower extremity edema
- Evidence of scratching
- Rash or excessive dryness
- Condition and colour of toenails

---

toenails difficult. Care of the feet and toenails of persons in LTC is the nurse's responsibility. Nails that become too long will begin to interfere with stockings, hose, or shoes. Ideally, toenails should be trimmed after the bath or shower when they are soft, but if this is not possible, soaking the feet for 20 to 30 minutes before care is sufficient. Nails should be clipped straight across and even with the top of the toe, with the edges filed slightly (to remove sharpness) but not to the point of rounding (Fig. 11.5). The foot care of persons with diabetes should be done only by a podiatrist or a trained registered nurse, and special care must be taken to prevent accidental damage or trauma to the skin (RNAO, 2015). Persons with diabetes or peripheral neuropathy should never have pedicures from commercial establishments.

Nails that are neglected become long and curved. Hard, thickened nails indicate inadequate nutrition to the nail matrix because of trauma or poor circulation. Once the nail becomes thickened, it will remain so. Thick, hard nails split easily, causing trauma, pain, and possibly infection. Any attempt by the nurse or other caregiver to cut these nails may result in further damage

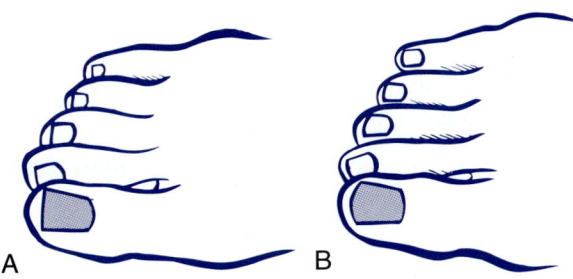

Fig. 11.5 ■ Cutting toenails. (A) Correct angle and shape. (B) Incorrect angle and shape.

to the matrix or precipitate an infection. These conditions should be brought to the attention of a podiatrist.

An ingrown toenail is a fragment of nail that pierces the skin at the edge of the nail. This problem is often a consequence of the hypertrophy of the nail with onychomycosis, improper cutting of the nail, or pressure exerted on the toes by tight hosiery or shoes. Ingrown toenails should be referred to a podiatrist because of the risk of infection. Temporary relief can be provided by inserting a small piece of cotton under the affected nail corner.

Nursing interventions include helping the older adult understand the necessity of appropriate footwear and helping the person obtain such footwear. For persons with diabetes or other neurological impairments, the shoes should cover and protect the foot entirely without pressure areas. For persons with arthritis, firm soles are more comfortable than soft soles and may decrease pain associated with walking (Frecklington et al., 2018).

Shoes should be functional; that is, they should cover, protect, and stabilize the foot and provide maximum toe space to prevent bunions, corns, and calluses. One foot is usually larger than the other. Feet lengthen slightly with age; one foot is usually larger than the other, and the feet are largest in the afternoon. Thus, shoes should be fitted to the largest foot, and afternoon purchases are advised. Fabric shoes are not recommended for persons with diabetes or VI because they do not provide enough support. Low-heeled shoes place less stress on the legs and back than completely flat shoes do.

Slip-on shoes are helpful for those who are unable to bend or lace shoes, but care must be taken that the person's feet will not accidentally slip out of the shoes, which can lead to a fall. Velcro closures are useful for those who have limited finger dexterity. Custom-made shoes, although expensive, may be necessary for persons with bunions or any other deformity.

SUMMARY

Gerontological nurses have an instrumental role in promoting the health of the skin and feet of the older adult, but this is sometimes overlooked when dealing with other, more immediately life-threatening problems. However, preservation of the integrity of the skin and the functioning of the feet is essential to mobility, well-being, and quality of life. To promote healthy aging, the nurse needs to be able to assess common skin and foot problems encountered by older adults and to develop effective interventions both for acute and for persistent conditions.

KEY CONCEPTS

- The skin is the largest and most visible organ of the body and has multiple roles in maintaining health.
- Maintaining adequate moisture and skin lubrication will reduce the incidence of xerosis and other skin problems.
- The best way to minimize the risk for skin cancer is to avoid prolonged sun and smoke exposure.
- Prompt treatment of persons with herpes zoster infection is needed to lessen the risk of postherpetic neuralgia.
- Problems of the skin and feet may reflect systemic disease.
- Mobility is fundamental to independence; therefore, care of the feet and toenails is an important concern for the gerontological nurse.
- A pressure injury is documented by stage, which indicates the degree of tissue damage; a healing ulcer retains its original staging.
- A pressure injury that is covered in dead tissue (eschar or slough) cannot be staged until it has been debrided.
- Persons with darkly pigmented skin will not display the "typical" erythema of a stage I pressure injury or early stage VI; therefore, closer vigilance is necessary for these persons.
- Persons with VI, diabetes, or peripheral neuropathy are at special risk for serious skin problems.
- Foot care for older adults with diabetes should always be performed by a podiatrist or a trained registered nurse.

ACTIVITIES AND DISCUSSION QUESTIONS

1. Describe the common skin and foot problems an older adult is likely to experience.

2. Describe the nurse's responsibility in maintaining the patient's skin integrity.

3. List several interventions that apply to skin and foot care.

4. Develop a nursing care plan for an older adult experiencing xerosis and pruritus.

HEALTHY AGING CARE PLAN

Caring for J.B.

Recall the *Lived Experience* testimonial and J.B.'s case presented at the beginning of the chapter.

1. You understand that new pressure injuries are preventable and that the stage 2 pressure injury needs to be treated. To promote healthy skin, you should focus on eliminating friction and irritation of the skin. You should also attempt to reduce moisture, make sure that J.B. receives assistance to use the toilet, and ensure that her bedsheets are changed often.

2. You would help J.B. change her position frequently during the day, including getting her up out of bed.

3. You would consult with other members of the interprofessional team, including a dietitian to optimize J.B.'s nutritional intake and a physiotherapist to work with J.B. to promote as much physical activity as possible.

RESOURCES

Hartford Institute for Geriatric Nursing
https://hign.org/
National Pressure Ulcer Advisory Panel
https://npiap.com/
Registered Nurses' Association of Ontario. *Evidence Booster: Best Practice Guideline Implementation to Reduce Diabetic Foot Ulcers.*
https://rnao.ca/sites/rnao-ca/files/Evidence_Boosters_Winter-2018Assessment_foot_ulcers_homecare_FINAL_March2018.pdf
Registered Nurses' Association of Ontario. *Assessment and Management of Pressure Injuries for the Interprofessional Team* (**3rd ed.**).
https://rnao.ca/sites/rnao-ca/files/Pressure_Injuries_BPG.pdf
Wound Assessment and Treatment Flowsheet
https://www.clwk.ca/buddydrive/file/watfs-portrait/
Wounds Canada (Canadian Association of Wound Care)
http://www.woundscanada.ca

For additional resources, please visit *http://evolve.elsevier.com/Canada/Ebersole/gerontological/*

REFERENCES

Bergstrom, N., Allman, R., Alvarez, O. M., et al. (1994). *Treatment of pressure ulcers.* Clinical Practice Guideline No. 15, AHCPR Publication No. 95-0652. US Department of Health and Human Services, Public Health Service, Agency for Health Care Policy and Research.

Canadian Cancer Society. (2021a). Treatments for melanoma skin cancers. https://cancer.ca/en/cancer-information/cancer-types/skin-melanoma/treatment.

Canadian Cancer Society. (2021b). Types of non-melanoma skin cancer. https://cancer.ca/en/cancer-information/cancer-types/skin-non-melanoma/what-is-non-melanoma-skin-cancer/types-of-non-melanoma.

Denny, K., Lawand, C., & Perry, S. D. (2014). *Compromised wounds in Canada. Healthcare Quarterly, 17*(1), 7–10. doi:10.12927/hcq.2014.23787.

Fédération Interprofessionnelle de la Santé du Quebec (FIQ). (2009). *Revision of the professional system. Impacts of Bill 90.* http:// www.fiqsante.qc.ca.

Frecklington, M., Dalbeth, N., McNair, P., et al. (2018). Footwear interventions for foot pain, function, impairment and disability for people with foot and ankle arthritis: A literature review. *Seminars in Arthritis and Rheumatism, 47*(6), 814–824. doi:10.1016/j.semarthrit.2017.10.017.

Gohel, M. S., Heatley, F., Liu, X., et al. (2018). A randomized trial of early endovenous ablation in venous ulceration. *New England Journal of Medicine, 378*(22), 2105–2114.

Government of Ontario. (2016, December 29). *Shingles vaccine free for Ontario seniors.* https://news.ontario.ca/mohltc/en/2016/12/shingles-vaccine-free-for-ontario-seniors.html.

Government of Canada. (2019a). *Non melanoma skin cancer.* https://www.canada.ca/en/public-health/services/chronic-diseases/cancer/non-melanoma-skin-cancer.html.

Government of Canada. (2019b). Melanoma skin cancer. https://www.canada.ca/en/public-health/services/chronic-diseases/cancer/melanoma-skin-cancer.html.

Government of Canada. (2020). *Herpes zoster (shingles) vaccine: Canadian immunization guide.* https://www.canada.ca/en/public-health/services/publications/healthy-living/canadian-immunization-guide-part-4-active-vaccines/page-8-herpes-zoster-(shingles)-vaccine.html.

Hahnel, E., Blume-Peytavi, U., Trojahn, C., et al. (2017). Associations between skin barrier characteristics, skin conditions and health of aged nursing home residents: A multi-center prevalence and correlational study. *BMC Geriatrics, 17*(1), 263. doi:10.1186/s12877-017-0655-5.

Jorgensen, M., Siette, J., Georgiou, A., et al. (2018). Longitudinal variation in pressure injury incidence among long-term aged care facilities. *International Journal of Quality Health Care, 30*(9), 684–691. doi:10.1093/intqhc/mzy087.

Kassianos, A., Emery, J., Merchie, P., et al. (2015). Smartphone applications for melanoma detection by community, patient and generalist clinician users: A review. *British Journal of Dermatology, 172*(6), 1507–1518. doi:10.1111/bjd.13665.

Mallick-Searle, T., Snodgrass, B., & Brant, J. M. (2016). Postherpetic neuralgia: Epidemiology, pathophysiology, and pain management pharmacology. *Journal of Multidisciplinary Healthcare, 9,* 447. doi:10.2147/JMDH.S106340.

Meyers, J. L., Candrilli, S. D., Rausch, D. A., et al. (2018). Cost of herpes zoster and herpes zoster-related complications among immunocompromised individuals. *Vaccine, 36*(45), 6810–6818. doi:10.1016/j.vaccine.2018.08.080.

National Pressure Ulcer Advisory Panel. (2016). *Pressure injury and stages.* https://cdn.ymaws.com/npiap.com/resource/resmgr/NPIAP-Staging-Poster.pdf.

Norton, D. (1996). Calculating the risk: Reflections on the Norton Scale. *Advances in Wound Care, 9*(6), 38–43. https://www.ncbi.nlm.nih.gov/pubmed/9069755.

Registered Nurses' Association of Ontario (RNAO). (2015). *RNAO submission to the Health Professions Regulatory Advisory Council: Regulation of chiropody and podiatry in Ontario.* https://rnao.ca/sites/rnao-ca/files/RNAO_Submission_to_HPRAC_re_The_College_of_Chiropodists.pdf.

Registered Nurses' Association of Ontario (RNAO). (2016). *Assessment and management of pressure injuries for the interprofessional team* (3rd ed.). https://rnao.ca/sites/rnao-ca/files/Pressure_Injuries_BPG.pdf.

Registered Nurses' Association of Ontario (RNAO). (2017). *Best practice guideline implementation to reduce hospital-acquired pressure injuries.* https://rnao.ca/sites/rnao-ca/files/FINAL_Evidence_Boosters_-_Spring_2017_HAPU_May_25_17_FINAL.pdf.

Saguil, A., & Lauters, R. (2017). Herpes zoster and postherpetic neuralgia: Prevention and management. *American Family Physician, 96*(10), 656–663.

Schwarz, T. F., Volpe, S., Catteau, G., et al. (2018). Persistence of immune response to an adjuvanted varicella-zoster virus subunit vaccine for up to year nine in older adults. *Human Vaccines & Immunotherapeutics, 14*(6). doi:10.1080/21645515.2018.1442162.

Shiraki, K., Toyama, N., Daikoku, T., et al. (2017). Herpes zoster and recurrent herpes zoster. *Open Forum Infectious Diseases, 4*(1), ofx007. doi:10.1093/ofid/ofx007.

Shu, J., & Santulli, G. (2018). Update on peripheral artery disease: Epidemiology and evidence-based facts. *Atherosclerosis, 275,* 379–381. doi:10.1016/j.atherosclerosis.2018.05.033.

Stockfleth, E. (2017). The importance of treating the field in actinic keratosis. *Journal of the European Academy of Dermatology and Venereology, 31,* 8–11. doi:10.1111/jdv.14092.

World Health Organization. (2017). *Radiation: Ultraviolet (UV) radiation and skin cancer.* https://www.who.int/news-room/q-a-detail/radiation-ultraviolet-(uv)-radiation-and-skin-cancer.

12

MAINTAINING MOBILITY AND ENVIRONMENTAL SAFETY

LEARNING OBJECTIVES

Upon completion of this chapter, the reader will be able to:

- Discuss the effects of impaired mobility on general function and quality of life.
- Specify risk factors for impaired mobility.
- Identify older adults at risk for falls, and list several interventions to reduce fall risk.
- Understand the negative effects of restraints, and discuss appropriate alternatives for safety promotion and fall risk reduction.
- Identify factors in the environment that contribute to the safety and security of the older adult.
- Relate strategies for protecting the older adult from injury and accidents.
- Develop a nursing care plan appropriate for an older adult at risk of falling.

GLOSSARY

Agility   The ability to change the body's position efficiently.

Orthostatic (postural) hypotension   A drop in blood pressure that occurs when a person assumes an upright position from sitting or lying down.

Sarcopenia   The loss of skeletal muscle mass, strength, and function.

Syncope   A brief lapse in consciousness caused by transient cerebral hypoxia.

THE LIVED EXPERIENCE

"After that fall last year when I slipped in the bathroom, I feel so insecure. I find myself taking small, shuffling steps to avoid falling again, but it makes me feel awkward and clumsy. When I was younger, I never worried about falling, but now I'm so afraid I will break a bone or something."
Betty, 75 years old

MOBILITY

Mobility is the capacity for movement within the immediate and larger-scale environment. Older adults move more slowly and purposefully, sometimes with more forethought and caution. This chapter focuses on the maintenance of maximal mobility, both in health and in the presence of various disorders; the assessment of gait and mobility status; the negative consequences of restraints; measures to achieve safety without using restraints; causes and consequences of falls in older adults; reduction of the risk of falling; and aids and interventions that are useful when mobility is impaired. Specific information is provided to promote a safe environment for older adults in all health care settings and in the community. Challenges related to transportation and driving as essential aspects of environmental mobility are also included. Chapter 10 provides a further discussion about activity and exercise, and bone and joint problems affecting mobility are addressed in Chapter 18.

Age-Related Changes in Mobility and Agility

Mobility and **agility** are affected by the strength of the muscles, flexibility, postural stability, vibratory sensation, cognition, and perceived stability. With aging, changes occur in muscles and joints, particularly those of the back and the legs. Strength and flexibility of muscles and endurance decrease, especially if there is a decrease in activity. Movements and range of motion become more limited and are less fluid, and joints change as the regeneration of tissue slows and muscle wasting occurs. Normal wear and tear reduces the smooth cartilage of joints. Proper management of persistent illnesses and maintenance of healthy lifestyles can forestall the onset of mobility limitations for older adults.

Sarcopenia, a loss of skeletal muscle mass, strength, and function, is thought to be related to aging and contributes to mobility impairments and disability. Sarcopenia is therefore a marker of frailty (D. Wilson et al., 2017). Some of the gait changes that are thought to be associated with aging include a narrower standing base, wider side-to-side swaying when walking, slower responses, a greater reliance on proprioception, diminished arm swing, and increased care in gait. Steps are slower, and there is a decrease in step height (lifting of the foot when taking a step). These changes are less pronounced in people who remain active and at a desirable weight. A sedentary lifestyle, excess weight, and smoking are all associated with mobility problems (Agahi et al., 2018; DiPietro et al., 2019; Kim & Lee, 2019). Health promotion programs to address these factors contribute to improving the mobility and functional status of older adults. Even for frail older adults, exercise and strength training will improve mobility and function (see Chapter 10).

Because of aging and a variety of comorbidities, older adults are vulnerable to becoming immobilized. Various degrees of immobility are often temporary or the permanent consequences of illnesses, falls, and fractures. Immobility, a common problem for older adults in hospital or residing in institutions, can have severe consequences (Box 12.1).

Older adults frequently have limited environmental mobility because of a lack of transportation or the loss of their driver's licence. Impairment of mobility is highly associated with poor outcomes and quality of

---

BOX 12.1
CONSEQUENCES OF IMMOBILITY

- Dehydration
- Bronchial pneumonia
- Contractures
- Deep vein thrombosis
- Constipation
- Pressure ulcers
- Incontinence
- Hypothermia
- Iatrogenic complications
- Disability
- Institutionalization
- Loss of independence
- Isolation and depression

---

life for older adults (Kim & Lee, 2019). Therefore, the maintenance of mobility and safety for older adults is one of the most important components of gerontological nursing.

Disorders Affecting Mobility

To prevent the problems associated with immobility, nurses need to pay special attention to common conditions that accompany the normal changes of aging, as well as to disorders that occur more frequently in older adults. Osteoporosis, gait disorders, Parkinson's disease, stroke, and arthritic conditions markedly affect movement and functional capacities (see Chapter 18). Mobility may also be limited by paresthesias, amputations, neuromotor disturbances, fractures, joint problems, and illnesses that deplete the person's energy.

FALLS

A fall is "an event which results in a person coming to rest inadvertently on the ground or floor or other lower level" (World Health Organization, 2021). Unfortunately, falls are a common and often devastating problem for older adults, causing a tremendous amount of morbidity and mortality (Berková & Berka, 2018). This section discusses the significance of falls for the older adult, the risk factors of falling, and different nursing assessments.

Falls: A Significant Geriatric Syndrome

Among older adults, falls are the leading cause of death by injury and the most common cause of nonfatal injuries and hospital admissions for trauma (Registered Nurses' Association of Ontario [RNAO], 2017). Approximately 20% to 30% of older adults fall each year (Public Health Agency of Canada [PHAC], 2016). The number of falls among older adults that result in serious injury are increasing dramatically, and falls are a serious public health concern (PHAC, 2016). In Canada, 81% of injury hospitalizations in older adults were due to falls (Canadian Institute for Health Information, 2019). In addition, 95% of all hip fractures are directly caused by falls (PHAC, 2016).

In response to rising fall-related sentinel events in health care organizations, several national and international professional organizations and governments have established fall-prevention guidelines based on systematic reviews of research evidence on best practices for working with older adults. The Public Health Agency of Canada has engaged community organizations in fall prevention for older adults (PHAC, 2016). The Registered Nurses' Association of Ontario (RNAO) has developed a best practice guideline, *Preventing Falls and Reducing Injury from Falls* (RNAO, 2017), which includes practices for addressing education and post-fall prevention. Internationally, one of the most widely adopted guidelines is the American Geriatrics Society's *Guideline for the Prevention of Falls in Older Adults*, prepared in collaboration with the British Geriatrics Society (Panel on Prevention of Falls in Older Persons, American Geriatrics Society and British Geriatrics Society, 2010). In addition, most provinces and territories have implemented mandatory reporting of falls that occur in long-term care (LTC) settings.

Factors Contributing to Falls

Falls are a geriatric syndrome and a symptom of a problem or underlying issue, but they become the core of the problem when they occur. The etiology of falls is multifactorial; falls may indicate neurological, sensory, cognitive, medication-related, osteoporotic, or musculoskeletal problems, or they may indicate impending physical illness. The cause of a fall is usually an interaction between an environmental factor, such as a wet floor, and an intrinsic factor, such as limited vision, cognitive impairment, or a gait problem. In health care settings, iatrogenic factors (such as limited staffing), a lack of toileting programs, and the use of restraints and side rails can also interact to increase the risk of falls.

TABLE 12.1	
Fall Risk Factors for Older Adults	
Intrinsic Factors	**Extrinsic Factors**
Advanced age	Lack of handrails on stairs
History of previous falls	Poor design of stairs
Gait and balance problems	Lack of grab bars in bathroom
Poor vision	Dim lighting
Postural hypotension	Obstacles or tripping hazards
Chronic conditions: arthritis,	(loose carpets)
stroke, incontinence, diabetes,	Slippery or uneven surfaces
Parkinson's disease, dementia	Psychoactive medications
Fear of falling	Improper use of assistive
	devices

Source: Adapted from Centers for Disease Control and Prevention. (2017). *Risk factors for falls.* https://www.cdc.gov/steadi/pdf/STEADI-FactSheet-RiskFactors-508.pdf.

Risk factors for falls can be categorized as intrinsic (person specific) or extrinsic (environmental specific). Some of these risk factors are presented in Table 12.1.

Older adults often have gait patterns that are stiffer and less coordinated (Pirker & Katzenschlager, 2017). Women with functional impairment and those who take medications are at a higher risk of falling than those who are not impaired or who do not take medications. Chronic diseases and periods of symptoms such as vertigo contribute to a high fall risk (Mota de Sousa et al., 2017; Bouccara et al., 2018). In inpatient settings, the most common causes of patient falls are inadequacies in patient assessment and communication, in footwear, and in environmental safety and security (Morris & O'Riodran, 2017). A relationship may exist between urinary tract infections and falls, particularly in LTC residents with dementia (Nicolle, 2016). In addition, insomnia is a fall risk factor for older adults in LTC homes who may get out of bed during the night while drowsy (Jiang et al., 2019).

Even if a fall does not result in injury, it contributes to a loss of confidence that leads to reduced physical activity, increased dependency, and social withdrawal. Fear of falling may restrict a person's life space (the area in which an individual carries on activities) and is an important predictor of general functional decline and a risk factor for future falls. Frequent falls contribute significantly to the downward spiral in frail older adults (Bartosch et al., 2020). Nursing staff may also contribute to their older patients' fear of falling by telling them not to get up by themselves or by using restrictive devices to keep them from independently moving about (King et al., 2018). A more appropriate nursing response would be to assess fall risk and design individual prevention interventions and safety plans that enhance mobility and independence and reduce the risk for falls (RNAO, 2017).

IMPLICATIONS FOR GERONTOLOGICAL NURSING AND HEALTHY AGING

Assessment

Comprehensive assessments (with attention to the conditions and situations noted earlier) and nursing observations of function are essential in assessing fall risk and premobilization safety. Nurses are the most likely to have greater opportunities to observe the older adults' functioning, whether in the community or in a health care facility. Older adults may be reluctant to share information about falls for fear of losing independence, so gerontological nurses must use judgement and empathy in eliciting information about falls, assuring the person that there are many ways to increase safety and maintain independence.

Assessment is an ongoing and comprehensive process that includes assessments of the older adult who is at risk for falls or who has had a fall, the environment and situational circumstances, and the person's knowledge about falls and their prevention (RNAO, 2017).

Assessment of Fall Risk

A variety of instruments for assessing fall risk are available. In Canada, hospitals often have their own fall risk scales that assist the health care team in determining who is at risk for falls. For example, some hospitals in Ontario have adopted the interRAI Acute Care Screener, which provides a comprehensive overview of older adults in acute care, including fall risk (Boscart et al., 2020). LTC homes use interRAI-specific fall risk assessment tools and protocols (Norman & Hirdes, 2020).

Assessments of fall risk provide general information about a person's risk factors, but must be combined with an individual assessment so that appropriate fall risk-reduction interventions can be developed, modifiable risk factors identified and managed, and all information

integrated in the care plan. In addition, any incident considered an "almost fall" or "near miss" needs to be assessed, as such an event could have led to an actual fall.

The Hendrich II Fall Risk Model (Fig. 12.1), an instrument that has been validated with skilled nursing and rehabilitation populations, provides a determination of the risk of falling (Miller, 2008). This determination is based on gender, mental and emotional status, symptoms of dizziness, and known categories of medications that increase risk (Hendrich, 2016). The tool screens for fall risk and has been integral to post-fall assessments for the prevention of falls (Hendrich, 2016).

The Morse Fall Scale (MFS) (Morse et al., 1989) is widely used in hospitals and other inpatient settings (https://networkofcare.org/library/Morse%20Fall%20 Scale.pdf). A rapid and simple method of assessing a patient's likelihood of falling, the MFS consists of six variables that are easy to score and has predictive validity and interrater reliability (Morse et al., 1989.).

The Berg Balance Scale measures balance ability in older adults whose balance function is impaired by assessing the performance of "functional tasks" (Alghwiri et al., 2018). It is an effective tool for assessing balance in older adults who have had a stroke (Alghadir et al., 2018) and is recommended by the RNAO (http://www.chiropractic.on.ca/wp-content/uploads/fp-berg-balance-scale.pdf). In the LTC setting, the minimum data set (MDS) calls for information about a history of falls and hip fractures in the previous 180 days, and the fall-related resident assessment protocol provides an excellent overview of fall risk and fall assessment (see Chapter 5).

It is recommended that all persons over 65 years of age be asked at least once a year about falls (Harris & Garcia, 2016) (Table 12.2). A history of falls is an important predictor of future falls, and any older adult who reports a fall should be observed with the brief, performance-based Fall Risk Assessment Tool (Nunan et al., 2018). The Tinetti balance scale has also been tested and validated to predict fall risk and was found to have 70% sensitivity and 52% specificity, indicating that it is a useful tool for preventative interventions (Tinetti, 2003).

An older adult who is seen after a fall, who shows abnormalities of gait or balance and impaired performance on any fall risk assessment test, or who has had recurrent falls should have a comprehensive fall evaluation (Box 12.2).

Hendrich II Fall Risk Model ™		
RISK FACTOR	**RISK POINTS**	**SCORE**
Confusion/Disorientation/Impulsivity	4	
Symptomatic Depression	2	
Altered Elimination	1	
Dizziness/Vertigo	1	
Gender (Male)	1	
Any Administered Antiepileptics (anticonvulsants): (Carbamazepine, Divalproex Sodium, Ethotoin, Ethosuximide, Felbamate, Fosphenytoin, Gabapentin, Lamotrigine, Mephenytoin, Methsuximide, Phenobarbital, Phenytoin, Primidone, Topiramate, Trimethadione, Valproic Acid)[1]	2	
Any Administered Benzodiazepines:[2] (Alprazolam, Chloridiazepoxide, Clonazepam, Clorazepate Dipotassium, Diazepam, Flurazepam, Halazepam[3], Lorazepam, Midazolam, Oxazepam, Temazepam, Triazolam)	1	
Get-Up-and-Go Test: "Rising from a Chair" If unable to assess, monitor for change in activity level, assess other risk factors, document both on patient chart with date and time.		
Ability to rise in single movement - No loss of balance with steps	0	
Pushes up, successful in one attempt	1	
Multiple attempts but successful	3	
Unable to rise without assistance during test If unable to assess, document this on the patient chart with the date and time.	4	
(A score of 5 or greater = High Risk)	**TOTAL SCORE**	
© 2013 AHI of Indiana, Inc. All rights reserved. United States Patent No. 7,282,031 and U.S. Patent No. 7,682,308. Reproduction of copyright and patented materials without authorization is a violation of federal law.		

On-going Medication Review Updates:

Levetiracetam (Keppra) was not assessed during the original research conducted to create the Hendrich Fall Risk Model. As an antieptileptic, levetiracetam does have a side effect of somnolence and dizziness which contributes to its fall risk and should be scored (effective June 2010).

The study did not include the effect of benzodiazepine-like drugs since they were not on the market at the time. However, due to their similarity in drug structure, mechanism of action and drug effects, they should also be scored (effective January 2010).

Halazepam was included in the study but is no longer available in the United States (effective June 2010).

Fig. 12.1 ■ The Hendrich II Fall Risk Model, a fall-risk assessment tool recommended by the Hartford Institute for Geriatric Nursing. © 2012 AHI of Indiana Inc. All rights reserved. US Patent Nos. 7,282,031 and 7,682,308. Federal laws prohibit the replication, distribution, or clinical use expressed or implied without written permission from AHI of Indiana, Inc.

TABLE 12.2

Clinical Assessment and Management of Fall Risk for Older Adults

Assessments	Management
Circumstances of previous falls*	Changes in environment and activity to reduce the likelihood of recurrent falls
Medication use ■ High-risk medications (e.g., benzodiazepines, other sleep medications, antipsychotics, antidepressants, anticonvulsants, or class IA antidysrhythmics)*[†‡] ■ Four or more medications[‡]	Review and reduction of medications
Vision ■ Acuity <20/60 ■ Decreased depth perception ■ Decreased contrast sensitivity ■ Cataracts	Ample lighting without glare; avoidance of multifocal glasses while walking; referral to ophthalmologist
Postural blood pressure (after ≥5 minutes supine, immediately after standing, and 2 minutes after standing)[‡] ≥20 mm Hg (or ≥20%) drop in systolic pressure, with or without symptoms, either immediately upon standing or after 2 minutes of standing	Diagnosis and treatment of underlying cause if possible; review and reduction of medications; modification of salt restriction; adequate hydration; compensatory strategies (e.g., elevation of head of bed, rising slowly, or dorsiflexion exercises); pressure stockings; pharmacological therapy if previously listed strategies fail
Balance and gait[†‡] ■ Person's report or observation of unsteadiness ■ Impairment on brief assessment	Diagnosis and treatment of underlying cause if possible; reduction of medications that impair balance; environmental interventions; referral to physiotherapist for assistive devices and for gait and progressive balance training
Targeted neurological examination ■ Impaired proprioception* ■ Impaired cognition* ■ Decreased muscle strength[†‡]	Diagnosis and treatment of underlying cause if possible; increase in proprioceptive input (with assistive device or appropriate footwear); reduction of medications that adversely affect cognition; caregivers' awareness of cognitive deficits; reduction of environmental risk factors; referral to physiotherapist for gait, balance, and strength training
Targeted musculo-skeletal examination ■ Legs (joints and range of motion) ■ Feet*	Diagnosis and treatment of underlying cause if possible; referral to physiotherapist for strength, range of motion, and gait and balance training (and assistive devices); appropriate footwear; referral to podiatrist
Targeted cardiovascular examination[†] ■ **Syncope** ■ Arrhythmia (if known cardiac disease, abnormal electrocardiogram, and/or syncope)	Referral to cardiologist; carotid-sinus massage ■ Syncope (in the case of syncope)
Evaluation of home hazards (after hospital discharge)[†‡]	Removal of loose rugs Use of night lights, nonskid bathmats, and stair rails Other interventions as necessary

*Recommendation is based on observational data indicating an association with an increased risk of falls.
[†]Recommendation is based on one or more randomized controlled trials of a single intervention.
[‡]Recommendation is based on one or more randomized controlled trials of a multifactorial intervention strategy that included this component.
Source: Tinetti, M. (2003). Clinical practice: Preventing falls in elderly persons. *New England Journal of Medicine, 348*(1), 42–49. doi:10.1056/NEJMcp020719.

BOX 12.2

RESEARCH FOR EVIDENCE-INFORMED PRACTICE: FALLS AND LONG-TERM CARE: A REPORT FROM THE CARE BY DESIGN OBSERVATIONAL COHORT STUDY

Objective: Researchers aimed to explore risk factors and potential prevention strategies for falls in elderly residents living in long-term care homes.

Methods: The researchers conducted a cross-sectional study. Researchers collected data before, during, and after the implementation of the Care by Design (CBD) intervention, which is designed to increase continuity of care and reduce unwanted and unnecessary transfers to the emergency department. Data collected included completing a chart review during a 6-month timeframe to determine the number of falls.

Findings: A total of 285 individuals participated in the study. The average age of participants was 85 years old.

Researchers found that falls were frequent, as more than half of residents in the study fell at least once (56.2%). Male gender, dementia diagnosis, and use of selective serotonin reuptake inhibitors or selective serotonin–norepinepherine reuptake inhibitors (SSRIs/SNRIs) were significantly associated with falls.

Conclusion: Falls are a significant concern among long-term care residents. It is important to understand the factors associated with an increased risk for falls. Nurses should work with the interprofessional team and screen for falls. Further research should identify risk factors and target interventions.

Source: Cameron, E. J., Bowles, S. K., Marshall, E. G., et al. (2018). Falls and long-term care: A report from the Care by Design observational cohort study. *BMC Family Practice, 19*(73). doi:10.1186/s12875-018-0741-6.

Environmental Assessment

Assessment of home safety and environmental factors should always be included in a comprehensive fall assessment of community-dwelling older adults.

A home safety assessment should include a fall, injury, fire, and crime risk assessment. Older adults with Alzheimer's disease may present with additional risk factors for injuries. The Alzheimer Society of Canada (2020) describes how to keep the environment safe for persons with Alzheimer's disease and their caregivers. Table 12.3 provides suggestions for assessment of safety in the home environment.

Environmental barriers often discourage ambulation in various settings. In the outside environment, steps and curbs may be too high. Buses, subway trains, elevators, revolving doors, and escalators may move too rapidly for a slower-moving older adult to enter and exit comfortably. Crossing the street may be difficult for older adults with mobility issues, as crossing time may be too short or crossing distance may be too long (Lachapelle & Cloutier, 2017). In their study, Lachapelle and Cloutier found that carrying loads, using walking aids, and posture (hunched back, looking towards the ground) were factors that may contribute to slowed walking and reduced situational awareness (Lachapelle & Cloutier, 2017).

Thus, the older adult may find the interactional world gradually shrinking as a result of factors that are beyond their control. Fortunately, the Canadian government has made a concerted effort to encourage the elimination of environmental barriers for persons with disabilities (e.g., by modifying public transit entrances and exits, sidewalk amenities), and this has had a beneficial effect on older adults and persons with disabilities as they navigate the environment. Accessibility standards can be found on the Canadian Standards Association Group website (http://www.csagroup.org/).

Assessment After a Fall Has Occurred

If an older adult does fall, the health care team must inform the family or significant other and conduct a post-fall assessment (PFA). A PFA is essential to the prevention of future falls and the implementation of risk-reduction programs, particularly in health care settings. If the older adult cannot tell you about the circumstances of the fall, information should be obtained from witnesses. The purpose of the PFA is to identify the underlying cause of the fall and to assist in implementing appropriate individualized risk-reduction interventions (Omer et al., 2018). Box 12.3 provides information for a PFA that can be used in health care settings.

Restraints

Restraints are "physical, chemical or environmental measures used to control the physical or behavioural

TABLE 12.3
Assessment and Interventions of the Home Environment for Older Adults

Assessment	Intervention
Bathroom	
Presence of unsafe bath rugs	Use a bath rug with nonskid bottom.
Lack of grab bars in the tub, shower area and near toilet	Add a bath grab bar on the wall or a clamp-on grab bar to the tub. Add grab bars to the wall near the shower and the wall where bath faucets are. Add a grab bar on the wall next to the toilet or toilet safety grab bars that attach at the toilet seat screws.
Toilet is too high/low	Too high: Consider a lower-profile toilet. Too low: Add a raised toilet seat.
Tub is slippery	Add a rubber mat or adhesive nonskid decals to the bottom of the tub.
Clutter	Remove clutter from all floor areas and place in drawers or closets. Inexpensive plastic cabinets or rolling units can be purchased to store bath items.
Staircase	
Poor lighting	Increase wattage to allowable limits in lights. Add additional overhead or wall lighting.
Lack of railings	Add at least one railing the entire length of the wall, ideally one on each side.
Clutter	Eliminate clutter on floors by removing or organizing items in areas near the stairs.
Steps too steep	Use railings for stability. Walk slowly up and down stairs with the lights on. Have others carry heavy or large items up or down the stairs. Reduce daily use of stairs to reduce risk of falls.
Slippery steps	Add adhesive stair treads or a carpet runner.
Bedroom	
Presence of clutter	Eliminate clutter on floor surfaces by placing items on shelves or storage. Consider donating or throwing out the items that are no longer used.
Presence of electric cords across the floor	Run cords behind furnishings. Use extension cords.
Unsafe carpet	Have carpet stretched or removed to eliminate wrinkles or bumps.
Presence of throw or scatter rug	Remove all scatter and throw rugs or use double-sided rug tape or a rug pad to secure rug to the floor.
Bed is too high/low	Too high (legs do not touch the floor when sitting at the edge of the bed): Remove bed frame or use a lower-profile mattress or box spring. Too low (knees are above the hips when sitting on edge of bed): Use bed risers below bed legs to raise height.
Lack of a telephone near the bed	Place a cordless type or cell phone next to the bed at night or during naps. Use a remote control for TV or VCR.
Lack of a nightlight	Place at least two nightlights in the bedroom to illuminate the room at night. Add additional nightlights along the hall or path to the bathroom. Also add one nightlight in the bathroom.
Kitchen	
Cabinet too high/low	Move items to the shelves closest to the counter. Add hooks to the wall for pots and pans used frequently.
Not enough counter space	Ensure available counter space is cleared of clutter. Move kitchen table closer to counter for additional workspace. Use a rolling cart for added workspace.

Continued

TABLE 12.3
Assessment and Interventions of the Home Environment for Older Adults—cont'd

Assessment	Intervention
Using a stool or a chair to reach things	Move items to lower shelves. Replace the stool with a sturdy step ladder.
Not enough room to manoeuvre	Eliminate clutter or excessive furniture to add space. Remove a leaf from the table and push it closer to the wall.
Presence of a throw or scatter rug	Remove a scatter rug or use double-sided rug tape or a rug pad to secure the rug to the floor.
Presence of slippery floor	Do not walk on a wet floor. Wear comfortable shoes that fit with a nonskid sole. Change flooring surface to one that is less slippery if possible.
Poor lighting	Increase wattage of bulbs to allowable level. Add under-counter lighting. Add additional overhead lighting.
Living room	
Presence of throw or scatter rug	Remove a scatter rug or use double-sided rug tape or rug pad to secure the rug to the floor.
Presence of clutter	Eliminate clutter on floor surfaces by placing items on shelves or storage. Consider donating or throwing out the items that are no longer used. Avoid carpets with confusing patterns.
Presence of electric cords across the floor	Run cords behind furnishings. Use extension cords. Rearrange items that must be plugged into areas near an outlet.
Poor lighting	Increase wattage to allowable limits in lamps/lights. Add additional lamps or wall/overhead lights.
Presence of unstable furniture	Place a block under the shorter leg. If the chair or table is broken, have it repaired or replaced.
Presence of unsafe chair	If the chair is too low, add a furniture leg riser to raise the height. A chair that is too high or without arms should not be used.
Light switches difficult to access	Add "clapper" light switch to control lamps or other use light-switching options.
Not enough space to move around	Remove clutter or excess furniture that prevents moving around easily. Some items may be arranged, donated, or thrown out.

Source: Adapted from Tomita, M. R. (2017). *Home safety self-assessment tool (HSSAT) v. 5.* Occupational Therapy Geriatric Group at the University at Buffalo. http://publichealth.buffalo.edu/rehabilitation-science/research-and-facilities/funded-research-archive/home-safety-training-to-prevent-falls-in-older-adults.html.

activity of a person or a portion of his/her body" (College of Nurses of Ontario [CNO], 2018). *Physical restraints* limit a person's movement (for example, bed rails that cannot be opened by the patient) (CNO, 2018). *Chemical restraints* use medication, particularly psychotropics, that are given without specific indications, given in excessive doses that affect functioning, used as sole treatment without behavioural interventions, or administered for the convenience of

staff. *Environmental restraints* control a person's mobility (e.g., seclusion, a secure unit or garden, or a time-out room.)

Restraints have been used historically for the "protection" of the patient and for the security of the patient and staff. Restraints were used to control the behaviour of individuals with mental illness who were considered to be a danger to themselves or others (Colaizzi, 2016). Some common reasons for restraining patients were to

BOX 12.3
POST-FALL ASSESSMENT

HISTORY

Ask the patient for or about the following:

- Description of the fall by the individual or witness
- Individual's opinion of the cause of the fall
- Circumstances of the fall (trip or slip, near miss)
- Individual's activity at the time of the fall
- Presence of comorbid conditions, such as a previous stroke, Parkinson's disease, osteoporosis, seizure disorder, sensory deficit, joint abnormalities, depression, or cardiac disease

MEDICATION REVIEW

Ask the patient for the following information:

- Associated symptoms (e.g., chest pain, palpitations, lightheadedness, vertigo, fainting, weakness, confusion, incontinence, or dyspnea)
- Time of day and location of the fall
- Presence of acute illness

PHYSICAL EXAMINATION

Observe or examine the following:

- Vital signs (postural blood pressure changes, fever, or hypothermia)
- Head and neck (visual impairment, hearing impairment, nystagmus, bruit)
- Heart (arrhythmia or valvular dysfunction)
- Neurological signs (altered mental status, focal deficits, peripheral neuropathy, muscle weakness, rigidity or tremor, and impaired balance)
- Musculo-skeletal signs (arthritic changes; reduced range of motion; podiatric deformities or problems; swelling, redness, or bruises; abrasions; pain on movement; shortening and external rotation of lower extremities)

FUNCTIONAL ASSESSMENT

Observe and inquire about the following:

- Functional gait and balance (rising from a chair, walking, turning, and sitting down)
- Balance test findings, mobility, use of assistive devices, mobility aids or personal assistance, extent of ambulation, use of restraints, and prosthetic equipment used
- Activities of daily living (bathing, dressing, transferring, and toileting)

ENVIRONMENTAL ASSESSMENT

Look for the following:

- Existing staffing patterns, unsafe practice in transferring, delay in response to call light
- Faulty equipment
- Incorrect use of bed and chair alarms
- Call light not within reach
- Wheelchair and bed unlocked
- Inadequate supervision
- Clutter (walking paths not clear)
- Dim lighting
- Glare
- Uneven flooring
- Wet, slippery floors
- Poorly fitting seating devices
- Inappropriate footwear or eyewear

---

prevent falls, altered mental status, the patient's harming of self or others, wandering, agitation, and interference with treatment. However, in recent years, the use of physical and chemical restraints has come under careful scrutiny, for both legal and ethical reasons, and they are now prohibited in some provinces and territories (Ontario Regulation 79/10, 2020). There is no evidence in the literature of the efficacy of physical restraints in maintaining safety, preventing the disruption of treatment, preventing falls, or controlling behaviour. In fact, research over the past 20 years, primarily in LTC settings, has shown that the practice of physical restraint is ineffective and hazardous (Bleijlevens et al., 2016). Physical restraints, intended to prevent injury, do not protect patients from falling, wandering, or removing tubes and other medical devices. Physical restraints may actually exacerbate many of the problems for which they are used and can cause serious injury as well as emotional and physical problems. Furthermore, research also indicates that physical restraints are associated with higher mortality rates, injurious falls, health care–associated infections, incontinence, contractures, pressure ulcers, agitation, and depression.

Although the prevention of falls is most frequently cited as the primary reason for using restraints, restraints do not prevent serious injury and may even increase the risk of injury and death. Injuries occur as a result of the patient's attempting to remove the restraint or attempting to get out of bed. The most common mechanism of restraint-related death is asphyxiation;

that is, the person is suspended by a restraint from a bed or chair, and the ability to inhale is inhibited by gravitational chest compression (Boltz et al., 2016). Restraints are a source of great physical and psychological distress to older adults, and they may intensify agitation and contribute to depression. A significant reduction in restraint use has largely resulted from a combination of research-based clinical evidence, increased knowledge about restraint alternatives, advocacy groups' efforts, and changed standards and regulations in regard to restraints. Restraint-free care is now the standard of practice and an indicator of quality care in all health care settings.

Because of the movement toward freedom from restraints and the promotion of the least restrictive environment, safety plans are essential. Many of the suggestions on safety and fall risk reduction in this chapter can be used to promote a safe and restraint-free environment. Implementing best-practice nursing care in a restraint-free environment calls for the recognition and assessment of physical and psychosocial concerns and for interventions to address those concerns. Consultation with advanced practice nurses when implementing alternatives to restraints has been most effective (Boltz et al., 2016). Alternatives to restraints are presented in Boxes 12.4 and 12.5.

BOX 12.4
ALTERNATIVES TO USING RESTRAINTS

- Work with the interprofessional team.
- Lower the bed to the lowest level, or use a bed that is specially designed to be low to the floor.
- Use a concave mattress.
- Use bed boundary markers to mark the edges of the bed (such as mattress bumpers, a rolled blanket, or "swimming noodles" under sheets).
- Place a soft floor mat or mattress by the bed to cushion any falls.
- Use a water mattress to reduce movement to edge of bed.
- Have the person at risk sleep on a mattress on the floor.
- Remove the wheels from the bed.
- Clear the floor of debris and excessive furniture, and make sure it is not wet or slippery.
- Place nonskid strips on the floor next to the bed, and ensure nonskid flooring.
- Place the call bell within the person's reach, and make sure the person can use it.
- Provide visual reminders to encourage the person to use the call bell.
- Use night lights in the room and bathroom.
- Use identification bracelets or door signs to identify persons at risk of falling.
- Inform all staff of fall risk, and put fall risk and fall risk–reduction interventions on the person's care plan.
- Involve family and all staff in fall risk–reduction education and activities.
- Assess ambulation ability; refer to physiotherapy for walking, strengthening, or both.
- Have ambulation devices within reach, and make sure the person knows how to use them properly.
- Use bed, chair, or wrist alarms, or use a patient-worn sensor alarm (a position-sensitive, lightweight alarm worn above the knee).
- Keep the person in a supervised area or room within view of the nursing station.
- Check for orthostasis (a systolic drop greater than 20 mm Hg, greater than 10 mm Hg after 2 minutes of standing, or both).
- If the person is able, they should walk at every opportunity possible.
- Establish a toileting plan, and take the person to the bathroom frequently.
- Make sure the person knows the location of the bathroom—leave the door open so they can see the toilet, or put a picture of a toilet on the door; clear a path to the bathroom.
- Know the person's sleeping patterns—if the person is usually up during the night, get the person up into a chair and keep them at the nursing station.
- Be especially alert at change-of-shift times.
- Understand that very few people spend all day in bed; activity is necessary.
- Provide diversional activities (catalogues, puzzles, busy box).
- Wedge cushions—or materials that promote sitting in an upright position without restraints—into the wheelchair; occupational therapy can be helpful.
- Arrange for a family member or a sitter to be with the person, especially at high-risk times.
- Ensure that the person wears their eyeglasses, hearing aids, or dentures.
- Have the person sleep wearing shoes, rubber-soled slippers, or socks with nonskid treads.
- Ensure that pain is well managed.
- Provide a trapeze to enhance mobility in bed.

BOX 12.5
RESTRAINT ALTERNATIVES: TUBES, LINES, AND OTHER MEDICAL DEVICES

- Determine whether the device is really necessary.
- Show and explain the tubes to the patient preoperatively, which may be effective in decreasing anxiety about devices.
- Remove tubes and lines as soon as possible; Foley catheters should be used only if the person needs intensive output monitoring or has an obstruction.
- Use guided exploration and a mirror to help the person understand what is in place and why.
- Provide comfort care to the site (oral and nasal care, anchoring of tubing, topical anaesthetic).
- Consider alternatives (replace intravenous [IV] tubing with heparin lock, deliver medications intramuscularly, subcutaneously); consider intermittent IV administration, hypodermoclysis, or analgesic pumps.

- Use camouflage: clothing or elastic sleeves, a temporary air splint (occupational therapy can be helpful), or skin sleeves to prevent IV tube dislodgement.
- Use diversional activity aprons (zipping and unzipping, threading exercises, dials, and knobs), a busy box, or a therapeutic activity kit.
- Hang IV bags behind the person's field of vision.
- Replace a nasogastric (NG) tube with a percutaneous endoscopic gastrostomy (PEG) tube if necessary, but obtain a comprehensive speech therapy swallowing evaluation. If an NG tube is used, use as small a lumen as possible to minimize irritation; consider taping with occlusive dressings.
- Cover the PEG tube or abdominal incisions and other tubes with abdominal binder and sweatpants.
- Use a modified soft collar for tracheotomy protection.

Side Rails

The use of side rails is also coming under scrutiny through nursing research. Historically, side rails have been used to prevent falling from the bed, but careful evaluation has led to their use being discontinued. Side rails are no longer viewed as simply attachments to a patient's bed but are considered restraints accompanied with the concerns discussed mentioned earlier. When side rails impede the person's desired movement or activity, they meet the definition of a restraint. The proper use of side rails should be evaluated before they are applied.

FALL PREVENTION AND REDUCTION

The prevention and reduction of falls consists of eliminating or reducing the risk for the physical and psychological harm associated with falls in older adults. The most effective programs are often a combination of several interventions.

Fall Reduction Interventions

Successful approaches to fall risk reduction include education of health care providers about fall risk reduction, multifactorial assessment, and interventions directed at the identified risk factors (Ayton et al., 2017).

Fall risk reduction is the shared responsibility of all health care providers caring for older adults. It also calls for the patient (as well as informal and formal caregivers) to be educated about all aspects of environmental hazards and to become aware that falling may be an indication of underlying problems.

The choice of the most appropriate interventions to reduce the risk of falls depends on appropriate assessment at various intervals according to the person's changing condition. Best practice guidelines in falls prevention and management can be found at http://ltctoolkit.rnao.ca/clinical-topics/falls-prevention and https://hign.org/consultgeri/resources/protocols/fall-prevention.

The RNAO provides excellent resources on preventing falls in older adults, including the nursing best practice guideline entitled *Preventing Falls and Reducing Injuries From Falls* (http://www.rnao.org). The RNAO (2017) recommends the following interventions:

- Gait training and correct use of assistive devices
- Medication review (particularly psychotropics)
- Exercise programs that include balance training
- Assessment and treatment of **postural hypotension** and cardiovascular disorders
- Environmental hazard modification, and
- Staff education.

Exercise

Exercise programs have shown effectiveness in reducing falls and fall-related injuries in older adults who live in the community (Sibley et al., 2019). For older adults, the relationship between exercise and fall risk reduction is strong, particularly when combined with balance training. Although the best type, duration, and intensity of exercise have not been determined, exercise programs must be at least 10 weeks in duration, must be individualized, and must include balance training for benefit. Group exercises may also be effective. Further research is needed to evaluate the effect of exercise in LTC settings, as well as the effect of other programs, such as tai chi (see Chapter 10).

Environmental Modifications

Environmental modifications alone have not been shown to reduce falls, but they may be of benefit in risk reduction when included as part of a multifactorial program. However, research indicates that a home safety assessment and modifications to prevent injurious falls could produce considerable health gain and are highly cost effective for older adults (N. Wilson et al., 2017).

Medication Review

The reduction of medication use is an important component of effective fall-reducing programs in both community and LTC homes. Medications, including over-the-counter medications and herbals, should be reviewed, and only those that are essential should be used (see Chapter 21). The risk of falls increases with the use of four or more medications, particularly antipsychotics and benzodiazepines (both long- and short-acting).

Behaviour and Education Programs

Used alone, behaviour and education programs do not reduce falls, but they are recommended as part of multifactorial intervention programs. Information on fall risk factors and risk-reduction strategies should be provided to older adults, health care providers, and caregivers. Many excellent sources of information on interventions to reduce fall risks are available for both consumers and professionals (see the Resources at the end of this chapter).

Assistive Devices

Research on multifactorial interventions, including the use of assistive devices, has indicated that they are of benefit in fall risk reduction. It is important to provide instruction in the correct use of assistive devices and to supervise their use. Many devices are designed for specific benefits. When the correct device is obtained, the older adult will need assistance in learning how to use it correctly; this assistance should be provided by specialists in occupational therapy or physiotherapy. Nurses can supervise older adults' use of assistive devices. Some of these devices can also be used to facilitate safe transfers from one location to another; for example, a correctly used walker or a sit-to-stand device can reduce the risk of falls when an older adult is being transferred from a bed to a chair or vice versa.

The following principles and recommendations should be followed when caring for persons who are using assistive devices:

- Advise the person who is using a cane to do the following: Place the cane firmly on the ground before taking a step, ensuring that the cane is not placed too far ahead. Put all the weight on the unaffected leg, and then move the cane and the affected leg a comfortable distance forward. With the weight supported by the cane and the affected leg, step through with the unaffected leg.
  Older adults should always wear low-heeled, non-skid shoes. It is best to have people wear the kind of shoes they are accustomed to wearing. Consideration should be given to properly fitted orthotic shoes, as appropriate.
- Advise the person to do the following when using a cane on stairs: Step up with the unaffected leg and down with the affected leg. Use the cane as support when lifting the affected leg. Bring the cane up to the step just reached before climbing another step. When descending, place the cane on the next step down, move the affected leg down, and then move the unaffected leg down.
- Advise the patient who is using a walker to do the following: Stand upright and lift or roll the walker with both hands a step's length ahead. Lean slightly forward and hold the arms of the walker for support. Step toward it with the weaker leg,

and then bring the stronger leg forward. Do not climb stairs with a walker.

- Every assistive device must be adjusted to the individual's height; the top of a cane should align with the crease of the wrist.
- Choose a size and shape of cane handle that fits comfortably in the person's palm; like a tight shoe, it will be a constant irritant if it is not properly fitted.
- Cane tips are most secure when they are flat across the bottom and have a series of concentric rings. Replace tips frequently because they wear out, and a worn tip is insecure.
- Wheelchairs are a necessary adjunct at some level of immobility. General safety tips for preventing fall-related injuries can be applied to both power and manual wheelchairs. Caregivers and wheelchair users need to remember to always lock the brakes of the chair when transferring to or from another location. Inform the user never to reach for an object if they have to move to the edge of the seat to reach it. Also, instruct the user not to reach for an object that is on the floor. These actions may cause a fall. It is important that a professional evaluate the wheelchair for proper fit and provide training in its proper and safe use. Often, physiotherapists and occupational therapists can assist in wheelchair mobility programs.
- Discuss safety in regard to the use of motorized scooters or wheelchairs and the use of helmets.

Other Interventions

Other interventions include assessment and treatment of osteoporosis to reduce fracture rates (see Chapter 18). Older adults with osteoporosis are more likely to sustain serious injury from a fall. The use of hip protectors for the prevention of hip fractures in high-risk persons may be considered, but further research is needed to determine their effectiveness (Korall et al., 2019). Formal vision assessment is also an important intervention to identify remediable visual problems. Poor visual acuity, reduced contrast sensitivity, decreased visual field, cataracts, and use of nonmiotic glaucoma medications have all been associated with falls. Although there is a significant relationship between visual problems and falls, little research has been done on intervention for visual problems as a part of fall risk-reduction programs.

ENVIRONMENTAL SAFETY

A safe environment is one in which a person is capable (with reasonable caution) of carrying out activities of daily living and instrumental activities of daily living, as well as life-enriching activities, without fear of attack, accident, or imposed interference. It is the responsibility of nurses, other health care team members, and all community members to ensure a safe environment for older individuals. Table 12.3 describes home environment assessments and interventions.

Vulnerability to environmental risks increases as people become less physically or cognitively able to recognize or cope with real or potential hazards. Older adults and their caregivers need to be knowledgeable about risks and interventions to avoid unsafe behaviours and situations.

It is important for the nurse to also work with the older adult and family members to ensure that older adults who are at higher risk for falling are "checked in" on, whether through a phone call or a visit. For older adults who live alone and do not have family, many supports are available, such as personal support worker services or voluntary organizations such as Meals on Wheels, where someone can check in daily to ensure the older adult is safe.

Vulnerability to Environmental Temperatures

Given the growing problems with the supply and costs of energy, many older adults are exposed to temperature extremes in their own dwellings. Environmental temperature extremes pose a serious risk to older adults who are in declining physical health. Preventive measures entail paying attention to impending changes of season, as well as strategies to protect the person from extremes of temperature. Early intervention in extreme temperature exposure is crucial, because excessively high or low body temperatures further impair thermoregulatory function and can be lethal.

Sensorineural changes in thermoregulation diminish the older adult's awareness of temperature changes and may impair behavioural and thermoregulatory responses to dangerously high or low environmental temperatures (see Chapter 6). Furthermore, many of the medications taken by older adults affect thermoregulation by altering the ability of blood vessels to vasoconstrict or vasodilate, both of which are thermoregulatory mechanisms. Other medications inhibit neuromuscular activity, suppress metabolic heat generation, or dull awareness (e.g., tranquilizers and pain medications). Alcohol is notorious for inhibiting thermoregulatory function through its effect on vasomotor responses in either hot or cold weather.

Together, economic, behavioural, and environmental factors may create a dangerous thermal environment in which older adults are subjected to temperature extremes from which they cannot escape or that they cannot change. Caregivers and family members should be aware that older adults are vulnerable to temperature extremes if they are unable to shiver, sweat, take in sufficient liquids, move about, put on or take off clothing, adjust bedcovers, or adjust the room temperature. There may also be a lack of control of blood supply to the skin. A temperature that may be comfortable for a young and active person may be too cold or too warm for a frail older adult.

Economic conditions often determine whether an older adult living in the community can afford air conditioning or adequate heating. Older adults are the most vulnerable to adverse health effects due to prolonged heat exposure (Gagnon et al., 2016). Global warming is increasing the incidence of extreme heat–related events; local governments and communities must coordinate their response strategies to protect older adults.

Hyperthermia

When body temperature rises above normal ranges because of environmental or metabolic heat loads, a clinical condition called heat illness, or *hyperthermia*, occurs. Hyperthermia is a temperature-related illness and is classified as a medical emergency. The numerous deaths of older adults from high temperature extremes could be almost entirely prevented with education and caution. Most of these problems occur in the homes of people who do not have air conditioning, but older adults who are residing in LTC homes and have multiple physical problems may be especially vulnerable to high temperatures. Older adults with cardiovascular disease, diabetes, or peripheral vascular disease

and those taking certain medications (anticholinergics, antihistamines, diuretics, beta-blockers, antidepressants, or antiparkinsonian medications) are at risk. Instructions on how one can prevent hyperthermia when the ambient temperature exceeds 32°C are presented in Box 12.6.

Hypothermia

Hypothermia is a medical emergency necessitating comprehensive assessment of neurological activity, oxygenation, renal function, and fluid and electrolyte balance. The term "hypothermia" literally means "low heat," but it is used clinically to describe core temperatures below 35°C. A healthy individual exposed to a severely cold environment for a prolonged period will tend to become hypothermic. A person with impaired thermoregulatory ability is left without protection at room temperatures that may be comfortable for a younger person. The more prolonged the exposure or severe the impairment, the less thermoregulatory responses can defend against heat loss.

Older adults are particularly predisposed to hypothermia, because the opportunity for heat loss frequently coexists with the decline in heat generation and conservation responses. Such coexistence occurs frequently among persons who are homeless or cognitively impaired, persons injured in falls, and persons with cardiovascular, adrenal, or thyroid dysfunction. Other risk factors include excessive alcohol use, exhaustion, poor nutrition, inaccessible and inadequate housing, and the use of sedatives, anxiolytics, phenothiazines, and tricyclic antidepressants.

Unfortunately, a dulling of awareness accompanies hypothermia, and the person experiencing it rarely recognizes the problem or seeks assistance. For very old and frail persons, environmental temperatures below 18°C may cause a serious drop in core body temperature to 35°C or less. The numerous factors that increase the risk of hypothermia in older adults are listed in Box 12.7.

At normal room temperatures, heat in a person is produced in sufficient quantities by the cellular metabolism of food, the friction produced by contracting muscles, and blood flow. Paralyzed or immobile persons are unable to generate significant heat by muscle activity and become cold even at normal room temperatures. It is important to closely monitor body temperature in older

BOX 12.6
PREVENTING HYPERTHERMIA

- Keep out of the sun. If your house is cooler than out-doors, stay inside.
- If you must go out into the sun, shade yourself with an umbrella or a wide-brimmed hat that is well ventilated (to allow the sweat on your head to evaporate).
- Drink lots of water. How much water you should drink depends on how much you are sweating.
- If it is sunny, keep the house cooler by pulling down awnings or closing outdoor shutters over your windows, or keep the curtains or blinds closed.
- If the house has two stories, keep the upper-storey windows slightly open, to draw excess heat up and out.
- If the house is hot, try to spend a few hours in an air-conditioned space such as a shopping mall or a cooling centre. Rest in cool shade periodically.
- Take a cool bath or shower.
- At night, if the outdoor temperature is cooler, open all the windows. If you have fans that fit into the windows, use them to bring down the temperature faster.

- Use fans to evaporate sweat and cool the body; however, so may not be effective or may have the opposite effect if the temperature and humidity are both very high.
- Limit physical activity (especially if you are in an at-risk group), particularly during the middle of the day, when the heat is greatest.
- Avoid liquids that are high in sugar or alcohol, as they can increase the amount of water lost by the body.
- Consider taking in extra salt if you experience heat cramps, if so advised by your doctor, or if you have to work in the heat and are sweating a lot (even though most people's diets contain enough salt to make up for losses in sweat).
- Ask your doctor or pharmacist about the possible side effects of any medications you take during periods of extreme heat.
- Offer to check up on your neighbours, especially those who may be on their own and who may not be in a position to take these precautions.

Source: Adapted from Health Canada. (2011). *Extreme heat events guidelines: Technical guide for health care workers.* Water, Air and Climate Change Bureau, Healthy Environments and Consumer Safety Branch, Health Canada. https://www.canada.ca/en/health-canada/services/environmental-workplace-health/reports-publications/climate-change-health/extreme-heat-events-guidelines-technical-guide-health-care-workers.html.

BOX 12.7
FACTORS THAT INCREASE THE RISK OF HYPOTHERMIA

THERMOREGULATORY IMPAIRMENT

- Failure to vasoconstrict promptly on exposure to cold
- Failure to sense cold
- Failure to respond behaviourally to protect oneself against cold
- Diminished or absent shivering to generate heat
- Reduced cold-induced metabolic heat production

CONDITIONS THAT DECREASE HEAT PRODUCTION

- Hypothyroidism
- Adrenal insufficiency
- Sepsis
- Hypoglycemia
- Carbon monoxide poisoning
- Alcohol abuse

- Malnutrition
- Unintentional/intentional overdose

CONDITIONS THAT INCREASE HEAT LOSS

- Generalized inflammatory skin conditions such as psoriasis
- Burns

MEDICATIONS THAT INTERFERE WITH THERMOREGULATION

- Tranquilizers (e.g., phenothiazines)
- Sedative–hypnotics (e.g., barbiturates, benzodiazepines)
- Antidepressants (e.g., tricyclics)
- Vasoactive medications (e.g., vasodilators)
- Alcohol (causes superficial vasodilation; may interfere with carbohydrate metabolism and judgement)

Source: Adapted from Duong, H., & Patel, G. (2020). Hypothermia. *StatPearls.* https://www.ncbi.nlm.nih.gov/books/NBK545239/.

adults. When exposed to cold temperatures, older adults with some degree of thermoregulatory impairment are at high risk for hypothermia if they undergo surgery, are injured in a fall or accident, or are lost or left unattended in a cool place. Persons who are emaciated and have poor nutritional status lack insulation and fuel for metabolic heat-generating processes, so they may be chronically hypothermic.

IMPLICATIONS FOR GERONTOLOGICAL NURSING AND HEALTHY AGING

Recognition of the clinical signs and severity of hyperthermia and hypothermia is an important responsibility for nurses, who must keep frail older adults comfortable in order to prevent these problems. It is important to closely monitor body temperature in older adults and to pay particular attention to both lower and higher readings as compared with a person's baseline. The potential risk of hypothermia makes prevention important and early recognition vital.

Detecting hyperthermia and hypothermia among home-dwelling older adults is sometimes difficult (unlike detection in the clinical setting) because no one measures body temperature. For persons exposed to low temperatures in the home or outdoors, confusion and disorientation may be the first overt signs of hypothermia. As the person's judgement becomes clouded, they may remove clothing or fail to seek shelter, and hypothermia can progress to profound levels. For this reason, regular contact with home-dwelling older adults during cold or hot weather with extreme temperatures is crucial. Persons with pre-existing alterations in thermoregulatory ability should be monitored even in mildly cool weather. Specific interventions to prevent hypothermia are shown in Box 12.8.

TRANSPORTATION

Even though an older adult might be physically able to move about, there may be many hindrances to that person's full use of public space. Available transportation is critical to the ability of older adults to remain independent and functional. The lack of accessible transportation may contribute to other problems, such as social withdrawal, poor nutrition, or the neglect of

---

> ### BOX 12.8
> ### NURSING INTERVENTIONS TO PREVENT HYPOTHERMIA
>
> **SIGNS OF HYPOTHERMIA**
> - Shivering
> - Exhaustion or feeling very tired
> - Confusion
> - Fumbling hands
> - Memory loss
> - Slurred speech
> - Drowsiness
>
> **INTERVENTIONS**
> - Maintain a comfortably warm ambient temperature. Many frail older adults will require much higher temperatures.
> - Remove any wet clothing that the person is wearing.
> - Warm the centre of the person's body—chest, neck—using an electric blanket if available.
> - Warm drinks can help increase body temperature (tea or warm water).
>
> *Source:* Centers for Disease Control and Prevention. (2019). *Prevent hypothermia and frostbite*. https://www.cdc.gov/disasters/winter/staysafe/hypothermia.html.

---

health care. A "crisis in mobility" exists for many older adults because of their lack of access to an automobile, an inability to drive, limited access to public transportation, health factors, geographic location, or economic considerations. Culturally and ethnically diverse older adults and rural residents may experience more difficulty getting around.

Older adults may desire increased contact with friends and relatives. Even more crucial is the need to reach medical services, shopping areas, and service agencies. If mobility is hampered, both security and the sense of belonging to the mainstream of society may be blocked. The emphasis on a "barrier-free" (structurally revised) transportation system and reduced fares has been helpful to many older adults, but some cannot avail themselves of public transportation because of physical disability or because they live in a high-crime area.

Many provinces and territories provide subsidized transportation to help older adults reach social services, nutrition sites, health services, emergency or medical care facilities, recreational centres, mental health services, adult day programs, physical and vocational rehabilitation centres, continuing education classes, and library services. Although transportation can often be found for special needs (e.g., to attend health care appointments), transportation for pleasure or recreation may be virtually impossible to find. Senior centres offer a wide range of activities for older adults, as well as transportation services. Nurses can refer older adults to local services and aging-related organizations for information on resources and financial assistance.

Driving

Driving is one of the instrumental activities of daily living for most older adults, because it is often essential for obtaining necessities. Yet, driving is a highly complex activity that requires a variety of visual, motor, and cognitive skills (Lee et al., 2019). Assessments of functional capacities often neglect this important activity. Giving up driving is a major loss for an older adult in regard to independence, pleasure, and feelings of competence and self-worth. Giving up driving has been associated with decreased social integration, fewer out-of-home activities, increased depressive and anxiety symptoms, decreased quality of life, and a greater risk of being placed in an LTC facility (Musselwhite, 2018). Many older adults depend on driving to obtain basic needs, and the inability to drive can cause depression and isolation. For many, alternative transportation is not readily available; consequently, they may continue driving even when it is no longer safe for them to do so.

Age-related changes in driving skills—vision changes, cognitive impairment, and various medical illnesses and functional impairments—are all factors related to driving safety for older adults.

The procedures and regulations for driver's licence renewal vary across the country and may include repeated renewal, renewal in person rather than electronically or by mail, and vision and road tests.

The issue of older adults driving is the subject of a great deal of public discussion (Albert et al., 2018). Many older drivers and their families struggle with issues and conversations related to continued safety in driving. Each province and territory in Canada has specific laws on driving. For example, in Ontario and British Columbia, a person over the age of 80 years must renew their license every 2 years, undergo a medical examination or vision test, and undergo a driver record review (Government of

Ontario, 2020; Ministry of Transportation, 2020; Government of British Columbia, 2020). The Canada Safety Council offers a nonmandatory course called the 55 Alive Driver Refresher Course for those aged 55 years and older. Information on this course can be found at https://canadasafetycouncil.org/product/55-alive-driver-refresher-course/.

Older drivers typically drive fewer miles than younger drivers do, and they tend to drive less at night, less in adverse weather conditions, and less in congested areas. Generally, they choose familiar routes, and fewer older drivers speed or drive after drinking alcohol than do drivers of other ages. However, when compared with younger age groups, older adults have more accidents per mile driven, and older drivers and passengers are three times more likely than younger people to die after a motor vehicle crash.

IMPLICATIONS FOR GERONTOLOGICAL NURSING AND HEALTHY AGING

Gerontological nurses should encourage open discussions about driving with the older adult and their family, identify impairments that affect driving, correct these when possible, and offer alternatives for transportation. Vehicle modifications, sensory aids, driving training for older adults, and driving assessment programs are helpful in promoting safe driving.

Driving evaluations can help determine whether an older adult's driving ability is affected (Canadian Association of Occupational Therapists, n.d.). Evaluations of older adults include a screening evaluation and an on-road evaluation. The clinical evaluation consists of the following assessments:

- Visual screening—to check if a person's eyes meet the standards for driving, the person's ability to move their eyes, the person's ability to judge distance, and the person's peripheral vision.
- Movement and strength assessment—to ascertain whether the person's arms and legs have enough movement and strength to control all features of the car. The need for adaptive equipment is also assessed.
- Perceptual and cognitive screening—to measure the person's reaction time. Screening includes

other tests to assess the person's memory, problem-solving ability, and interpretation of what is seen.

The on-road evaluation involves assessing the following tests:

- Physical skill and endurance to drive and navigate the vehicle
- Awareness of and ability to identify potential hazards
- Efficiency with which the eyes move to take in necessary information, and
- Responses to traffic environments.

KEY CONCEPTS

- Mobility provides opportunities for exercise, exploration, and pleasure and is crucial to maintaining independence.
- Ease of mobility is thought to be the most visible measure of overall health and capacity for survival.

- Changes with aging in bones, muscles, and ligaments affect balance and gait and increase instability.
- Gait disorders are often an obvious index of systemic problems and should be investigated thoroughly.
- A thorough nursing assessment must include assessment of fall risk, balance, and gait, as well as intrinsic, extrinsic, and iatrogenic factors.
- Fall risk–reduction interventions are among the most important proactive measures for preserving the health and functioning of the older adult.
- Physical restraints have numerous negative consequences for the health and well-being of the older adult. Restraint-free care, fall risk–reduction interventions, and a safe environment are essential to providing the best care.
- Transportation for the older adult is critical to physical, psychological, and social health.

ACTIVITIES AND DISCUSSION QUESTIONS

1. Put your shoes on the wrong feet, then ask another student to analyze your gait.

2. Wear eyeglasses (or borrow a pair from someone), then walk up and down a flight of stairs.

3. Evaluate the safety of your living quarters, using Table 12.3 as a guide.

4. Discuss the activities you engage in that increase your vulnerability to falls.

5. Discuss falls you have had and their consequences. Consider how it might have been different if you were 80 years old.

6. Obtain a wheelchair and sit in it for 20 minutes with a restraining belt around your waist. Discuss

your feelings with a partner. Switch roles with your partner and have them do the same.

7. Discuss the risks for hypothermia and strategies for its prevention.

8. Discuss why the nurse might need to ensure safety for an older adult in hospital. Identify several alternative measures that might be appropriate for ensuring the person's safety.

9. Explore the transportation options in the person's community, and discuss how these may help or interfere with the older adult's independence and opportunities for social engagement.

RESOURCES

BC Ministry of Health. *Prevention of Falls and Injuries Among the Elderly: A Special Report from the Office of the Provincial Health Officer.*
http://www.health.gov.bc.ca/library/publications/year/2004/falls.pdf
Canadian Association of Occupational Therapists: Safe driving tips for older drivers

https://www.caot.ca/document/5640/SafeDrivingTips.pdf
Canadian Automobile Association (CAA). *Seniors driving.*
https://www.caa.ca/seniors/
Canadian Standards Association Group. *Safety standards.*
http://www.csagroup.org/
Health Canada. *Extreme heat events guidelines: Technical guide for health care workers.*

https://www.canada.ca/en/health-canada/services/environmental-workplace-health/reports-publications/climate-change-health/extreme-heat-events-guidelines-technical-guide-health-care-workers.html

National Institute for Health and Care Excellence. *Falls in older people: Assessing risk and prevention.* https://www.nice.org.uk/guidance/cg161

Public Health Agency of Canada. *Seniors' Falls in Canada: Second Report.* https://www.canada.ca/en/public-health/services/health-promotion/aging-seniors/publications/publications-general-public/seniors-falls-canada-second-report.html

Public Health Agency of Canada. *The Safe Living Guide—A Guide to Home Safety for Seniors.* https://www.canada.ca/en/public-health/services/health-promotion/aging-seniors/publications/publications-general-public/safe-living-guide-a-guide-home-safety-seniors.html

Registered Nurses' Association of Ontario. *Preventing Falls and Reducing Injury From Falls* https://rnao.ca/sites/rnao-ca/files/bpg/FALL_PREVENTION_WEB_1207-17.pdf

Veterans Affairs Canada. *Falls prevention* http://www.veterans.gc.ca/eng/services/health/promotion/fallsp

World Health Organization. *Prevention of Falls in Older Age. Falls Prevention: Policy, Research and Practice.* https://www.who.int/ageing/projects/5.Intervention,%20policies%20and%20sustainability%20of%20falls%20prevention.pdf

For additional resources, please visit *http://evolve.elsevier.com/Canada/Ebersole/gerontological/*

REFERENCES

Agahi, N., Fors, S., Fritzell, J., et al. (2018). Smoking and physical inactivity as predictors of mobility impairment during late life: Exploring differential vulnerability across education level in Sweden. *Journals of Gerontology. Series B, Psychological Sciences and Social Sciences, 73*(4), 675–683. doi:10.1093/geronb/gbw090.

Albert, G., Lotan, T., Weiss, P., & Shiftan, Y. (2018). The challenge of safe driving among elderly drivers. *Healthcare Technology Letters, 5*(1), 45–48. doi: 10.1049/htl.2017.0002.

Alghadir, A. H., Al-Eisa, E. S., Anwer, S., et al. (2018). Reliability, validity, and responsiveness of three scales for measuring balance in patients with chronic stroke. *BMC Neurology, 18*, 141. doi:10.1186/s12883-018-1146-9.

Alghwiri, A. A., Khalil, H., Al-Sharman, A., et al. (2018). Depression is a predictor for balance in people with multiple sclerosis. *Multiple Sclerosis and Related Disorders, 24*, 28–31. doi:10.1016/j.msard.2018.05.013.

Alzheimer Society of Canada. (2020). *Making your environment safe.* https://alzheimer.ca/en/help-support/im-caring-person-living-dementia/ensuring-safety-security/making-your-environment-safe.

Ayton, D. R., Barker, A. L., Morello, R. T., et al. (2017). Barriers and enablers to the implementation of the 6-PACK falls prevention program: A pre-implementation study in hospitals participating in a cluster randomised controlled trial. *PLOS One, 12*(2), e0171932. doi:10.1371/journal.pone.0171932.

Bartosch, P. S., Kristensson, J., McGuigan, F. E., et al. (2020). Frailty and prediction of recurrent falls over 10 years in a community cohort of 75-year-old women. *Aging Clinical and Experimental Research, 32*, 2241–2250. doi:10.1007/s40520-019-01467-1.

Berková, M., & Berka, Z. (2018). Falls: A significant cause of morbidity and mortality in elderly people. *Vnitrni Lekarstvi, 64*(11), 1076–1083.

Bleijlevens, M. H., Wagner, L. M., Capezuti, E., et al. (2016). Physical restraints: Consensus of a research definition using a modified Delphi technique. *Journal of the American Geriatrics Society, 64*(11), 2307–2310. doi:10.1111/jgs.14435.

Boltz, M., Capezuti, E., Fulmer, T. T., et al. (Eds.), (2016). *Evidence-based geriatric nursing protocols for best practice.* Springer.

Boscart, V., Sheiban Taucar, L., Heyer, M., et al. (2020). InterRAI acute care instrument for seniors in Canadian hospitals: Findings of an inter-rater reliability pilot study. *Canadian Journal of Nursing Research, 53*, 155–161. doi:10.1177/0844562120920513.

Bouccara, D., Rubin, F., Bonfils, P., et al. (2018). Vertiges et troubles de l'équilibre: Démarche diagnostique [Management of vertigo and dizziness]. *La Revue de Medecine Interne, 39*(11), 869–874. doi:10.1016/j.revmed.2018.02.004.

Canadian Association of Occupational Therapists. (n.d.). *Safe driving tips for older drivers.* https://www.caot.ca/document/5640/SafeDrivingTips.pdf.

Canadian Institute for Health Information. (2019). *Injuries among seniors.* https://www.cihi.ca/en/injuries-among-seniors.

Colaizzi, J. (2016). Seclusion and restraint: A historical perspective. *Journal of Psychosocial Nursing and Mental Health Services, 43*(2), 31–37.

College of Nurses of Ontario (CNO). (2018). *Understanding restraints.* https://www.cno.org/en/learn-about-standards-guidelines/educational-tools/restraints/.

DiPietro, L., Jin, Y., Talegawkar, S., et al. (2019). The joint associations of weight status and physical activity with mobility disability: The NIH-AARP Diet and Health Study. *International Journal of Obesity, 43*(9), 1830–1838. doi:10.1038/s41366-018-0294-8.

Gagnon, D., Romero, S. A., Cramer, M. N., et al. (2016). Cardiac and thermal strain of elderly adults exposed to extreme heat and humidity with and without electric fan use. *Journal of the American Medical Association, 316*(9), 989–991. doi:10.1001/jama.2016.10550.

Government of British Columbia. (2020). *Senior drivers.* https://www2.gov.bc.ca/gov/content/transportation/driving-and-cycling/roadsafetybc/medical-fitness/seniors.

Government of Ontario. (2020). *Seniors: Get around.* https://www.ontario.ca/page/seniors-get-around.

Harris, P., & Garcia, M. B. (2016). To fall is human: Falls, gait, and balance in older adults. In L. A. Lindquist (Ed.), *New directions in geriatric medicine* (pp. 71–90). Springer.

Hendrich. (2016). *Fall risk assessment for older adults: The Hendrich II Risk Model.* https://hign.org/consultgeri/try-this-series/fall-risk-assessment-older-adults-hendrich-ii-fall-risk-model.

Jiang, Y., Xia, Q., Wang, J., et al. (2019). Insomnia, benzodiazepine use, and falls among residents in long-term care facilities. *International Journal of Environmental Research and Public Health, 16*(23), 4623. doi:10.3390/ijerph16234623.

Kim, Y., & Lee, E. (2019). The association between elderly people's sedentary behaviors and their health-related quality of life: Focusing on comparing the young-old and the old-old. *Health and Quality of Life Outcomes, 17*(1), 131. doi:10.1186/s12955-019-1191-0.

King, B., Pecanac, K., Krupp, A., et al. (2018). Impact of fall prevention on nurses and care of fall risk patients. *Gerontologist, 58*(2), 331–340. doi:10.1093/geront/gnw156.

Korall, A. M., Feldman, F., Yang, Y., et al. (2019). Effectiveness of hip protectors to reduce risk for hip fracture from falls in long-term care. *Journal of the American Medical Directors Association, 20*(11), 1397–1403. doi:10.1016/j.jamda.2019.07.010.

Lachapelle, U., & Cloutier, M. (2017). On the complexity of finishing a crossing on time: Elderly pedestrians, timing and cycling infrastructure. *Transportation Research. Part A, Policy and Practice, 96,* 54–63. doi:10.1016/j.tra.2016.12.005.

Lee, S. C., Kim, Y. W., & Ji, Y. G. (2019). Effects of visual complexity of in-vehicle information display: Age-related differences in visual search task in the driving context. *Applied Ergonomics, 81,* 102888. doi:10.1016/j.apergo.2019.102888.

Miller, C. (2008). *Nursing for wellness in older adults.* Lippincott Williams & Wilkins.

Morris, R., & O'Riordan, S. (2017). Prevention of falls in hospital. *Clinical Medicine, 17*(4), 260–362. doi:10.7861/clinmedicine.17-4-360.

Morse, J., Morse, R., & Tylko, S. (1989). Development of a scale to identify the fall-prone patient. *Canadian Journal of Aging, 8*(4), 336–377. doi:10.1111/j.1440-172X.2006.00573.x.

Mota de Sousa, L. M., Marques-Vieira, C. M., Caldevilla, M. N., et al. (2017). Risk for falls among community-dwelling older people: Systematic literature review. *Revista Gaúcha de Enfermagem, 37*(4), e55030.

Musselwhite, C. (2018). Mobility in later life and wellbeing. In M. Friman, D. Ettema, & L. E. Olsson (Eds.), *Quality of life and daily travel* (pp. 235–251). Springer.

Nicolle, L. E. (2016). Urinary tract infections in the older adult. *Clinics in Geriatric Medicine, 32*(3), 523–538. doi:10.1016/j.cerg.2016.03.002.

Norman, K. J., & Hirdes, J. P. (2020). Evaluation of the predictive accuracy of the interRAI falls clinical assessment protocol, Scott Fall Risk Screen, and a supplementary falls risk assessment tool used in residential long-term care: A retrospective cohort study. *Canadian Journal on Aging, 39*(4), 521–532. doi:10.1017/S0714980820000021.

Nunan, S., Brown Wilson, C., Henwood, T., et al. (2018). Fall risk assessment tools for use among older adults in long-term care settings: A systematic review of the literature. *Australasian Journal on Ageing, 37*(1), 23–33. doi:10.1111/ajag.12476.

Omer, H. M. R. B., Hodson, J., Pontefract, S. K., et al. (2018). Inpatient falls in older adults: A cohort study of antihypertensive prescribing pre-and post-fall. *BMC Geriatrics, 18*(1), 58. doi:10.1186/s12877-018-0749-8.

Ontario Ministry of Transportation. (2020). *Senior driver's licence renewal program.* http://www.mto.gov.on.ca/english/driver/senior-driver-licence-renewal-program.shtml.

Ontario Regulation 79/10. (2020). *Long-Term Care Homes Act, 2007,* S.O. 2007, c. 8. https://www.ontario.ca/laws/regulation/100079/v58.

Panel on Prevention of Falls in Older Persons, American Geriatrics Society and British Geriatrics Society. (2010). Summary of the updated American Geriatrics Society/British Geriatrics Society clinical practice guideline for prevention of falls in older persons. *Journal of the American Geriatrics Society, 59*(1),148–157. doi:10.1111/j.1532-5415.2010.03234.x.

Pirker, W., & Katzenschlager, R. (2017). Gait disorders in adults and the elderly. *Wiener Klinische Wochenschrift, 129*(3–4), 81–95.

Public Health Agency of Canada (PHAC). (2016). *You CAN prevent falls!* https://www.canada.ca/en/public-health/services/health-promotion/aging-seniors/publications/publications-general-public/you-prevent-falls.html.

Registered Nurses' Association of Ontario (RNAO). (2017). *Preventing falls and reducing injury from falls* (4th ed.). https://rnao.ca/sites/rnao-ca/files/bpg/FALL_PREVENTION_WEB_1207-17.pdf.

Sibley, K. M., Touchette, A. J., Singer, J. C., et al. (2019). To what extent do older adult community exercise programs in Winnipeg, Canada address balance and include effective fall prevention exercise? A descriptive self-report study. *BMC Geriatrics, 19,* 201. doi:10.1186/s12877-019-1224-x.

Tinetti, M. E. (2003). Clinical practice. Preventing falls in elderly persons. *New England Journal of Medicine, 348*(1), 42–49. doi:10.1056/NEJMcp020719.

Wilson, D., Jackson, T., Sapey, E., et al. (2017). Frailty and sarcopenia: The potential role of an aged immune system. *Ageing Research Reviews, 36,* 1–10. doi:10.1016/j.arr.2017.01.006.

Wilson, N., Kvizhinadze, G., Pega, F., et al. (2017). Home modification to reduce falls at a health district level: Modeling health gain, health inequalities and health costs. *PLOS One, 12*(9). doi:10.1371/journal.pone.0184538.

World Health Organization. (2021, April 26). *Falls.* https://www.who.int/news-room/fact-sheets/detail/falls.

13

ASSESSMENT TOOLS IN GERONTOLOGICAL NURSING

Upon completion of this chapter, the reader will be able to:

- Discuss the advantages of using standardized assessment tools in gerontological nursing.
- Contrast different formats used to collect assessment data.
- Describe the range of tools used in a comprehensive gerontological assessment.
- Begin to develop the skills needed to select an evidence-informed and appropriate tool for a specific assessment situation and use it correctly.
- Identify key components of assessing older adults.

GLOSSARY

Activities of daily living (ADLs) Those tasks necessary to maintain one's health and basic personal needs.

Instrumental activities of daily living (IADLs) Those tasks necessary to maintain one's home and independent living, such as shopping, cooking, managing medications, using the phone, doing housework, driving or using public transportation, and managing finances.

Report by proxy One person (the proxy) answering questions or providing information for another person, based on the first person's knowledge of the second person.

THE LIVED EXPERIENCE

"After 2 months in [large rehab facility] I could not stay any longer, so they ship you home. But before they ship you home, they want to have somebody out here that's going to take over and look after you. They couldn't find anyone. So, I came home with nothing. I called several agencies. But I could not get anyone; they did not service this area. They couldn't help me. After 6 weeks, I found someone from Red Cross who came and gave me a shower. And they did that for once a week for 10 weeks. But after 10 weeks, I was on my own again. Then I went to my doctor and he asked me what I did for therapy. I said 'Nothing.' He said, 'That is ridiculous,' so he got on the phone with someone and then they called me from a community hospital that I should go there on Wednesday. But I have no way of getting all the way there. It's difficult being on your own."
A 70-year-old woman who had a stroke

ASSESSING OLDER ADULTS

One of the most important functions of gerontological nurses is to conduct skilled and detailed assessments of the older adult. Assessment of older adults differs from assessment of younger adults in that it is more complex and detailed and takes longer to complete. Comprehensive assessments are usually performed by a nurse-led interprofessional health care team. A gerontological assessment has a number of components, including the collection of physical data as well as the integration of biological, psychosocial, cognitive, and functional information.

Gerontological Assessment

Assessing the older adult requires that the nurse listens patiently, allows for pauses, asks questions that are not often asked, obtains data from all available sources, and recognizes the normal changes of aging (see Chapter 6). Furthermore, the assessment of older adults takes more time because older adults have increased medical and social complexity, and the assessment must therefore be paced according to the stamina of the person. Both the quality of the assessment and the time required to complete the assessment depend on the nurse's experience. Novice nurses should neither expect nor be expected to perform assessments proficiently, but the skills and information they acquire will increase over time. According to Benner (1984), assessment is a task for the expert. However, by following some basic guidelines and learning how to use select assessment tools, nurses at all skill levels can obtain reasonably reliable data.

Over the years, nurses and others have developed tools to facilitate and standardize the collection of assessment data. (A number of the tools used in the gerontological setting are presented in this chapter.) The use of these tools increases the likelihood of obtaining more reliable data. Data collection is followed by data analysis and identifying priority nursing diagnoses. The nursing diagnoses provide the basis for selecting nursing interventions to address the person's needs.

Assessments are conducted in every nursing setting. In most settings, a standardized electronic format is routinely used. For example, the minimum data set (MDS) is a standardized comprehensive geriatric assessment and is mandatory in most Canadian long-term care homes, rehabilitation settings, and home care settings (see Chapter 5). Which assessments are completed depends on both the setting and the purpose of the assessment. Some tools are derived directly from the gerontological literature; other tools are modified to meet the particular needs of the older adult in a particular setting.

Data Collection

Three approaches are used for collecting assessment data: self-report, **report by proxy**, and observation.

In the self-report approach, the person verbally answers direct questions (or responds to written questions) about their health status. Often, the person's ability to self-report is overestimated.

In the report-by-proxy approach, information is obtained indirectly by the nurse's asking another person (such as a spouse, child, or caregiver) to report their

observations. This approach is used when a person who is cognitively impaired requires an assessment, but it tends to underestimate the older adult's abilities and health.

In the observational approach, the nurse collects and records the data as observed. Physical examination and performance-based functional assessment are examples of observational measures. Observation is probably the most accurate data collection method, but it is limited in that it presents only a snapshot in time.

Regardless of the type or format of the tool used, the following guidelines should be observed:

- Whenever possible, collect the data at a time when the older adult is at their best.
- Use standardized tools correctly; training may be required.
- Do not direct the way the question is answered to avoid biasing the response; novice nurses need to ask questions in a way that avoids bias.
- Obtain more information only if necessary to complete the assessment.
- Be sensitive when asking questions of a more personal nature—for example, questions about sexual functioning.
- Record responses accurately, using the person's own words where possible; do not analyze data while they are being collected. (For example, if the person says, "I have a runny nose," do not record "Patient has a cold" until the analysis of the data is completed.)

Ideally, assessment tools should be used to gather baseline data before the older adult has a health crisis. Periodically, the person can be reassessed with the same tools. For example, a person with an altered mental status as a result of illness or medication should be reassessed when the underlying problem has been resolved.

HEALTH ASSESSMENT

Health History

The initiation of the health history marks the beginning of the nurse–patient relationship and the assessment process. This assessment begins with a review of what the person reports as the problem, known as the "chief complaint"; this is considered to be objective information recorded in the person's own words. With an older adult, the complaint is likely to be vague or less straightforward (for example, "I don't feel well").

The health history is best collected verbally during a face-to-face interview or by using the interview to review a written history completed by the person or the person's proxy beforehand; the latter method is usually faster. If the older adult has limited proficiency in the language in which the interview is being conducted, a trained interpreter is needed, and the interview will generally take about twice as long.

Any health history form or interview plan should include a profile, past medical history, review of symptoms and systems, medication history (prescribed and over-the-counter products such as herbals and dietary supplements), family history, and social history. The social history includes information about the person's living arrangements, economic resources to meet current health-related or food expenses, amount of support, community resources, and other social determinants of health. The health history also includes information on the person's functional status as measured by observation, self-report, or report by proxy.

When a more comprehensive assessment is indicated, additional information is collected on the person's cognitive and functional abilities, psychological well-being, caregiver support or burden, and patterns of health and health care. Areas frequently not addressed by the nurse or mentioned by the older adult include sexual dysfunction, depression, incontinence, alcoholism, hearing loss, memory loss, and confusion. See Chapter 23 for a discussion of the assessment of alcohol use and misuse. Although not usually conducted by a nurse, a driving assessment may be recommended (see Chapter 12).

Physical Assessment

The next step in the health assessment is the physical assessment, which includes the evaluation of vital signs, mobility, and laboratory results. The techniques used in the physical examination apply to any age group. However, because of the complexity of older adults, head-to-toe examination is more difficult with older adults and can be burdensome for them. When performing a physical assessment, gerontological nurses must be able to quickly determine what information is most necessary (based on the chief complaint) and then work from

there. When the chief complaint is unknown because of communication challenges (e.g., dementia or aphasia), a more thorough assessment is necessary.

A number of excellent tools have been developed specifically for assessing older adults who are frail, who exhibit signs or symptoms of common conditions, or who manifest both. Several tools are discussed or referred to in this chapter; however, these are some of the tools that are available. A list of additional evidence-informed tools is available at https://hign.org/ (see the Try This: Series).

Comprehensive Assessment for the Frail and Medically Complex Older Adult

A model for a comprehensive prioritized assessment that is especially useful for assessing frail older adults is FANCAPES (Fluids, Aeration, Nutrition, Communication, Activity, Pain, Elimination, and Socialization) (Ellison et al., 2015). This model emphasizes the determination of basic needs and the individual's functional ability to meet these needs independently. It can be used in all settings and may be used in part or in whole, depending on the need. The nurse obtains comprehensive information in each section, guided by the questions provided in Table 13.1.

AAPA and AINÉES are other tools used primarily in Quebec to help assess for functional decline in older adults. The Specialized Approach to Senior Care, or AAPA, stands for *Approche adaptée à la personne agée*. The AAPA is used in hospitals to monitor older adults, primarily those aged 75 years or older (Centre intégré universitaire de santé et de services sociaux [CISSS] de l'Ouest-de-l'Île-de-Montréal, 2016). The goal of the AAPA is to ensure that all measures are in place to prevent the physical deterioration of older adults (CISSS de Laval, 2020). The monitoring checklist for the AAPA includes functional independence, skin integrity, nutrition and hydration, toileting, cognitive status, and sleep (CISSS de Laval, 2020); mobility and delirium prevention is also emphasized.

AINÉES is an acronym used by care teams to observe aspects that are crucial to ensuring functional maintenance in older adults, the idea being that when one of these is disrupted, there is a risk for a negative spiral of other aspects being affected (CISSS de l'Ouest-de-l'Île-de-Montréal, 2016). AINÉES stands for (1) Autonomy and Mobility, (2) Integument of the Skin, (3) Nutrition, (4) Elimination, (5) Cognitive State (État cognitif) and

TABLE 13.1
FANCAPES Assessment

Acronym	Assessment
F (Fluids)	■ What is the person's current state of hydration? ■ Does the person have the functional capacity to consume adequate fluids to maintain optimal health, including the ability to sense thirst, obtain the needed fluids mechanically, and swallow and excrete fluids?
A (Aeration)	■ Is the person's oxygen exchange adequate for full respiratory functioning, including the ability to maintain an oxygen saturation >96%? ■ Is supplemental oxygen required, and if so, is it possible for the person to obtain it? ■ What is the respiratory rate and depth at rest and during activity (talking, walking, exercising, and performing activities of daily living)? ■ What sounds are auscultated, palpated, and percussed, and what do they suggest?
N (Nutrition)	■ What mechanical and psychological factors are affecting the person's ability to obtain and benefit from adequate nutrition? ■ What type and amount of food is consumed? ■ Does the person have the ability to bite, chew, and swallow? ■ What effect does oral health status or periodontal disease have on the person? ■ Do the dentures of an edentulous person fit properly, and does the person wear them? ■ Does the person understand the need for special diets? ■ Is the special diet designed to be consistent with the person's eating and cultural patterns? ■ Can the person afford the special foods needed? ■ Have preventive strategies been taught to persons who are at risk for aspiration, including those who are tube fed?
C (Communication)	■ Is the person able to communicate their needs adequately? ■ Do the care providers understand the person's form of communication? ■ What is the person's ability to hear in various environments? ■ Are there any environmental situations in which the patient's understanding of the spoken word is inadequate? ■ Is the vision of the person who depends on lip-reading adequate? ■ Does the person have either expressive or receptive aphasia? If so, has a speech pathologist been made available? ■ What are the levels of the person's reading comprehension and auditory comprehension?
A (Activity)	■ Is the person able to participate in the activities necessary to meet basic needs such as toileting, grooming, and meal preparation? ■ How much assistance does the person need, if any, and is someone available to provide such assistance? ■ Is the person able to participate in activities that address higher needs, such as the need for belonging or finding meaning in life? ■ Is the person able to voluntarily move about, either with or without assistive devices? ■ Does the person have the coordination, balance, ambulatory skills, finger dexterity, grip strength, and other capacities necessary to function fully in day-to-day life?
P (Pain)	■ Is the person experiencing physical, psychological, or spiritual pain? ■ Is the person able to express pain and the desire for relief? ■ Do any cultural barriers make the assessment or the expression of pain difficult for the patient? ■ How does the person customarily attain pain relief?
E (Elimination)	■ Is the person having difficulty with bladder or bowel elimination? ■ Does the person lack control of elimination? ■ Does the environment interfere with the person's elimination and related personal hygiene? ■ Does the person need any assistive devices, and if so, are they available and functioning? ■ How are problems, if any, affecting the person's social functioning?
S (Socialization and social skills)	■ Is the person able to negotiate relationships in society, give and receive love and friendship, and feel self-worth?

FANCAPES, fluids, aeration, nutrition, communication, activity, pain, elimination, and socialization.
Sources: Adapted from Jett, K. F. (2013). Health assessment. In T. A. Touhy & K. F. Jett (Eds.), *Ebersole and Hess' toward healthy aging: Human needs and nursing response* (8th ed., pp. 104–117). Mosby; Montgomery, J., & Mitty, E. (2008). Resident condition change: Should I call 911? *Geriatric Nursing, 29*(1), 15–26. doi:10.1016/j.gerinurse.2007.11.009.

(6) **S**leep (CISSS de l'Ouest-de-l'Île-de-Montréal, 2016). When a disruption is observed, quick and timely action can take place to prevent any further decline.

Functional Assessment

Whereas the emphasis of FANCAPES is on physical needs, a full functional assessment is broader. A thorough functional assessment will help gerontological nurses promote healthy aging by doing the following:

- Identifying specific areas in which help is needed
- Identifying changes in abilities from one period to another
- Helping to determine the need for specific services, and
- Providing information that may help determine the safety of a particular living situation.

Most functional assessment tools assess the individual's ability to perform the tasks needed for self-care and independent living. Self-care activities are known as **activities of daily living (ADLs)** and are most often identified as eating, toileting, ambulation, bathing, dressing, and grooming. Three of these activities (grooming, dressing, and bathing) entail higher cognitive function than the others.

Instrumental activities of daily living (IADLs) are tasks needed for independent living (e.g., cleaning, doing yard work, shopping, and managing money); they call for a higher level of cognitive and physical functioning than the ADLs do. Nurses must keep in mind that the interest and skills needed to perform specific ADLs and IADLs are influenced by social and cultural factors.

Numerous tools describe, screen, assess, monitor, and predict functional ability. Most of the tools yield a score of some kind—a rating of the person's ability (or inability) to complete the task alone or with assistance. However, ratings are not always sensitive enough to show small changes in function. The Katz Index, of which there are several versions, serves as a basic framework for most ADL measures (Katz et al., 1963). One version of the Katz Index is based on a three-point scale that scores persons as independent, assistive, dependent, or unable to perform. Another version of the Katz Index assigns one point to each ADL that the person can complete independently, with a zero recorded if the person is unable to perform these activities. Scores range from 0 (totally dependent) to 6 (totally independent). A score of 4 indicates moderate impairment, whereas a score of 2 or less indicates severe impairment (Table 13.2). This tool is useful because it creates a common language about patient function for all caregivers involved in care planning.

IADLs are considered to be activities that are more complex and that necessitate higher functioning than the ADLs. The original scoring tool for IADLs was developed by Lawton and Brody (1969). Both the original tool and its subsequent variations use self-reporting, reporting by proxy, and observation, with three levels of functioning (independent, assisted, and unable to perform). Box 13.1 gives an example of an instrument for rating IADLs.

In rehabilitation settings, the Barthel Index is commonly used to measure the amount of physical assistance required when a person can no longer carry out ADLs (Mahoney & Barthel, 1965). This index is especially useful for documenting the improvement in a person's abilities. It classes functional status as either "independent" or "dependent," then further classifies the former as either "intact" or "limited" and the latter as either "needing a helper" or "unable" to do the activity at all. Training in the correct use and scoring of this tool is required.

The widely used Functional Independence Measure (FIM) is the most comprehensive functional assessment tool used in rehabilitation settings (Chehata et al., 2018). It includes measures of mobility, cognition, social functioning, and the ability to carry out ADLs. It was developed through the work of a number of experts and has been thoroughly tested. The FIM is completed through the joint efforts of the interprofessional team and is used both for planning and for evaluating progress. Although considerable training is required to accurately use the FIM, its use is encouraged.

Performance Tests

The ADLs and IADLS can also be measured with performance tools. These tools overcome the problems associated with self-report and proxy report and yield a more objective measurement of performance. Performance tools take longer to use; again, the cut-offs are subjective and arbitrary. The three performance tests related to mobility are simple and quick: the ability to stand with feet together in a side-by-side manner and in tandem and semi-tandem positions; a timed walk of 2.5 m (8 feet); and a timed rise from a chair and return to a seated position, repeated five times (Box 13.2).

TABLE 13.2
Katz Index of Independence in Activities of Daily Living

Activities	Independence (1 Point)	Dependence (0 Points)
	No supervision, direction, or personal assistance	**With supervision, direction, personal assistance, or total care**
Bathing Points: ___	(1 point) Bathes self completely or needs help in bathing only one part of the body (i.e., back, genital area, or disabled extremity).	(0 points) Needs help with bathing more than one part of the body or with getting in or out of the tub or shower. Requires total bathing.
Dressing Points: ___	(1 point) Gets clothes from closets and drawers and puts on clothes and outer garments, complete with fasteners. May need help tying shoes.	(0 points) Needs help with dressing, or needs to be completely dressed by caregiver.
Toileting Points: ___	(1 point) Goes to toilet, gets on and off toilet, arranges clothes, and cleans genital area without help.	(0 points) Needs help going to the toilet or cleaning self, or uses a bedpan or commode.
Transferring Points: ___	(1 point) Moves in and out of bed or on and off chair unassisted. Mechanical transferring aids are acceptable.	(0 points) Needs help in moving from bed to chair, or requires a complete transfer.
Continence Points: ___	(1 point) Exercises complete self-control over urination and defecation.	(0 points) Is partially or totally incontinent of bowel, bladder, or both.
Feeding Points: ___	(1 point) Transfers food from plate to mouth without help. Preparation of food may be done by another person.	(0 points) Needs partial or total help with feeding, or requires parenteral feeding.
Total Points:	6 = High (independent)	0 = Low (totally dependent)

Source: Katz, S., Down, T. D., Cash, H. R. et al. (1970). Progress in the development of the index of ADL. *Gerontologist, 10*(1), 20–30.

BOX 13.1
INSTRUMENTAL ACTIVITIES OF DAILY LIVING

1. Using the telephone
   I: Able to look up numbers, dial, and receive and make calls without help
   A: Able to answer phone or call operator in an emergency, but needs a special phone or help in a getting number or dialing
   D: Unable to use telephone
2. Travelling
   I: Able to drive own car or travel alone by bus or taxi
   A: Able to travel but not alone
   D: Unable to travel
3. Shopping
   I: Able to take care of all shopping with transportation provided
   A: Able to shop but not alone
   D: Unable to shop
4. Preparing meals
   I: Able to plan and cook full meals
   A: Able to prepare light foods, but unable to cook full meals alone
   D: Unable to prepare any meals

5. Housework
   I: Able to do heavy housework
   A: Able to do light housework, but needs help with heavy tasks
   D: Unable to do any housework
6. Taking medications
   I: Able to take medications in the right dose at the right time
   A: Able to take medications, but needs reminding or someone to prepare them
   D: Unable to take medications
7. Managing money
   I: Able to manage buying needs, write cheques, and pay bills
   A: Able to manage daily buying needs, but needs help managing chequing account and paying bills
   D: Unable to manage money

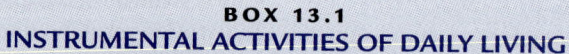

I, independent; A, assistance needed; D, dependent

Source: Duke University Center for the Study of Aging and Human Development. (1978). *Multidimensional Functional Assessment Questionnaire* (2nd ed.). Reprinted with permission of Duke University.

BOX 13.2
FUNCTIONAL PERFORMANCE TESTS

STANDING BALANCE

Instructions for Semi-Tandem Stand:

1. Demonstrate the task. (The heel of one foot is placed to the side of the first toe of the other foot.)
2. Support one arm of the older adult while they position the feet as demonstrated in step 1. The older adult can choose which foot to place forward.
3. Ask the person if they are ready, then release the support and begin timing.
4. Stop timing when the older adult moves the feet or grasps the nurse for support, or when 10 seconds have elapsed. Start with the semi-tandem stand. If it cannot be done for 10 seconds, then the side-by-side test should be done. If the semi-tandem stand can be done for the requisite 10 seconds, carry out the full-tandem stand, following the same instructions as above, except that the full-tandem stand calls for placing the heel of one foot directly in front of the toes of the other foot.

Score	Full-tandem stand	Semi-tandem stand	Side-by-side stand
0	_____	<10 seconds or unable	<10 seconds or unable
1	_____	<10 seconds or unable	10 seconds
2	<3 seconds or unable	10 seconds	_____
3	3–9 seconds	10 seconds	_____
4	10 seconds	10 seconds	_____

Standing Balance score: _____

WALKING SPEED

1. Set up a 2.5 m (8 ft.) walking course with an additional 60 cm (2 ft.) at both ends free of any obstacles.
2. Place a 2.5 m (8 ft.) rigid carpenter's ruler to the side of the course.
3. Instruct the older adult to "walk to the other end of the course at your normal speed, just like walking down the street to go to the store." Assistive devices should be used if needed.
4. Time two walks. The faster of the two is used as the score.

Score	Walking speed
0	Unable to complete course
1	>5.6 seconds
2	4.1–5.6 seconds
3	3.2–4.0 seconds
4	<3.2 seconds

Walking Speed score: _____

CHAIR SIT TO STANDS

1. Place a straight-backed chair next to a wall and ask the person to sit down.
2. Ask the person to fold their arms across their chest and stand up from the chair one time and sit down again. If successful, go to step 3.
3. Ask the person to stand and sit five times as quickly as possible.
4. Note and record the time taken for the person to go from the initial sitting position to the final standing position at the end of the fifth stand.
   Scores are for the five rise-and-sits only. If the person performs fewer than five chair stands, the score is 0.

Score	Time to complete five chair sit to stands
0	Unable to complete five chair sit to stands
1	>16.6 seconds
2	13.7–16.5 seconds
3	11.2–13.6 seconds
4	<11.2 seconds

Chair Stands score: _____

Total of all performance test scores (0–12): _____

Source: Adapted from Bennett, J. A. (1999). Activities of daily living: Old-fashioned or still useful? *Journal of Gerontological Nursing,* 25(5), 22–29.

Another performance test, the Timed Up and Go (TUG) test, is a basic evaluation of functional mobility. It measures the time needed to rise from a chair, walk 3 m (10 feet), turn around, and then return to a seated position. This test has been used extensively in the field of clinical geriatrics to assess gait and balance (Chen & Chou, 2017).

Mental Status Assessment

Increasing age is accompanied by an increased rate of illnesses that affect the person's cognition (for example, Alzheimer's disease). Cognitive ability is also easily threatened by any disturbance in health. Altered or impaired mental status may be the first sign of physical illness, from a heart attack to a urinary tract infection. Gerontological nurses must be aware of the tools that are used in the assessment of mental status, especially in regard to cognitive ability and mood (see Chapter 21). The interprofessional team plays an important role in collecting data for a cognitive assessment.

Cognitive Measures

Commonly used cognitive measures are the Mini-Mental State Examination, the clock drawing test, the Mini-Cog, the Montreal Cognitive Assessment, and the Cognitive Performance Scale and Cognitive Performance Scale 2.

Mini-Mental State Examination. The Mini-Mental State Examination (MMSE) was the first tool developed to screen for cognitive deficiencies such as those that occur with dementia or delirium (Folstein et al., 1975). It tests selected aspects of mental status, including orientation, short-term memory and attention, calculation ability, language, and construction. In general, a score of 30 suggests no cognitive impairment, and a score of 24 or less suggests potential dementia. It is important to note that adjustments are needed for educational level. A score of 22 or below for someone educated at a Grade 7 level or lower may indicate cognitive impairment. For those educated at a Grade 8 level or some high school, a score of 24 or below may suggest cognitive impairment. High school graduates who score 25 or below may suggest cognitive impairment. Finally, those with some college education or higher who score 26 or below may suggest cognitive impairment. A plethora of psychometric studies have indicated that the MMSE does not confirm dementia,

mild cognitive impairment, or delirium, but it can be used to rule out (screen) these conditions. The MMSE is neither the most accurate nor the more efficient tool with which to evaluate cognitive disorders, but it has provided a benchmark against which newer tools can be measured (Brossard, 2018).

Clock Drawing Test. The clock drawing test, which has been in use since 1992 (Tuokko et al., 1992), is a tool to identify the severity of cognitive impairment. This test requires the tested person to have some manual dexterity and thus would not be appropriate to use with persons who are limited in the use of their dominant hand or whose vision is impaired. The person is presented with a blank piece of paper or with a paper that has a circle drawn on it. The individual is then asked to draw the face of a clock and then indicate 1545 hours (3:45 p.m.) or some other selected time on the face of the clock. Scoring is based on both the position of the numbers and the position of the hands (Box 13.3). This tool does not establish criteria for dementia, but a poor performance indicates the need for further investigation.

Mini-Cog. The Mini-Cog is a tool used to determine a person's cognitive status. The Mini-Cog combines one

---

BOX 13.3
CLOCK DRAWING TEST

1. Ask the person to draw a circle on a blank piece of paper.
2. Ask the person to place the numbers 1 to 12 inside the circle, as they would appear on a clock.
3. Ask the person to place the clock hands to indicate 1545 hours (3:45 p.m.).

Performance	Score
Draws closed circle	1 point
Places numbers in correct positions	1 point
Includes all 12 correct numbers	1 point
Places hands in correct positions	1 point

Cognitively intact persons will rarely produce errors such as distorted contour or extraneous markings. Clinical judgement must be applied, but a low score indicates the need for further evaluation.

Source: Tuokko, H., Hadjistavropoulos, T., Miller, J. et al. (1992). The clock test: A sensitive measure to differentiate normal elderly from those with Alzheimer disease. *Journal of the American Geriatric Society, 40*(6), 579–584.

of the functions tested by the MMSE (short-term memory recall) with the executive function tested by the clock drawing test. Recent studies have found that the Mini-Cog has limited usefulness in primary care for detecting cognitive impairment (Seitz et al., 2018).

Montreal Cognitive Assessment. The Montreal Cognitive Assessment (MoCA) is designed to detect mild cognitive impairment. The MoCA consists of a brief 30-point test that takes about 10 minutes to complete (Julayanont & Nasreddine, 2017). The cognitive abilities it assesses include orientation, short-term memory, executive function, language ability, and visuospatial ability (Julayanont & Nasreddine, 2017). Scores on the MoCA range from 0 to 30; a score of 26 or higher is considered normal. The MoCA's advantages include its brevity, simplicity, and reliability as a screening test for Alzheimer's disease. In addition, it measures executive function, an important aspect of mental status that is affected in dementia. The MoCA also seems to work well in measuring executive functioning for those with Parkinson's disease or dementia and is free for nonprofit use (Kim et al., 2016; Julayanont & Nasreddine, 2017). The MoCA is available at http://www.mocatest.org.

Cognitive Performance Scale

The Cognitive Performance Scale (CPS) and the Cognitive Performance Scale 2 (CPS2) are assessment tools created by interRAI, an international collaborative group that focuses on creative comprehensive assessment systems (interRAI, 2017). The CPS, originally used in residential care, obtains scores that range from 0 (no memory impairment) to 6 (severe memory impairment). The CPS has been shown to be highly correlated with the MMSE (interRAI, 2017). The CPS2 is a more up-to-date version of the CPS and is typically used in conjunction with other assessment tools in acute care. The CPS2 is a reliable screening tool for assessing cognitive impairment in older patients in different sectors of care, including home care (de Almeida Mello et al., 2016).

Confusion Assessment Method

The Confusion Assessment Method (CAM) was developed by Inouye and colleagues (1990) to allow those not specialized in psychiatric care to diagnose delirium quickly and accurately. This tool is validated and detects the following key features of delirium: (1) acute onset and fluctuating course of symptoms, (2) inattention, (3) disorganized thinking, and (4) altered/impaired level of consciousness (Inouye et al., 1990). Delirium is diagnosed using the CAM if features 1 and 2 are present as well as either 3 or 4 (Inouye et al.,1990). In order to complete a proper assessment, the nurse must use subjective knowledge based on clinical observations and obtain information from family and objective testing of attention (Wong et al., (2018). The authors suggest that the nurse reflect on the following question while collecting subjective information: "Is the patient easily distractive or inattentive?" (Wong et al., 2018). The CAM is widely used in different settings, including hospitals and long-term care homes.

Delirium Index

The delirium index (DI), developed by McCusker and Cole, measures the severity of delirium based on observation of a patient. This index does not require any additional information from family members or other staff (McCusker et al., 2004). It was designed to be used in conjunction with the MMSE. The DI includes different categories measuring inattention, disorganized thinking, altered level of consciousness, disorientation in time and place, memory impairment, perceptual disturbances, psychomotor agitation, and psychomotor retardation (McCusker et al., 2004). The scoring is based on the sum of seven item scores.

Mood Measures

The aforementioned tools are measures of cognitive ability. Other tools are needed to assess mood and to screen for depression in particular—a common yet often unrecognized problem in older adults. Persons with untreated depression are more functionally impaired and will have prolonged periods in hospital, a lower quality of life, and earlier death (see Chapter 23). Persons with depression may appear as if they have dementia, and many persons with dementia are also depressed. The interconnection between the two syndromes calls for nurses' skill and sensitivity to ensure that older adults receive the most appropriate and effective care possible (Goodarzi et al., 2017). Commonly used mood measures include the Geriatric Depression Scale and the Cornell Scale for Depression in Dementia. (See Chapters 21 and 23 for further discussion of cognitive assessment.)

Geriatric Depression Scale. The Geriatric Depression Scale (GDS), developed by Yesavage et al. (1982–1983), measures mood. It is a 30-item tool designed for older adults and is based almost entirely on psychological factors. The GDS has been extremely successful in determining the presence of depression because it deemphasizes physical complaints, sex drive, and appetite—the factors that are most affected by medications. The GDS is thought to measure depression in older adults more accurately than any other tools do. It cannot be used for assessing persons who have dementia or cognitive impairment. An updated shorter (15-item) version is also available (Durmaz et al., 2018) (Fig. 13.1).

Cornell Scale for Depression in Dementia. The Cornell Scale for Depression in Dementia (CSDD) was developed specifically to assess the signs and symptoms of major depression in persons with dementia (Alexopoulos

et al., 1988). The CSDD evaluates a broad spectrum of depressive signs and symptoms and includes items from other depression scales. Information is obtained by interviewing a caregiver as well as by directly observing and interviewing the person with dementia. A total score of 8 or more suggests significant depressive symptoms.

Assessment of Social Supports

A comprehensive assessment includes an evaluation of the older adult's social networks and supports. Assessment of social supports considers an individual's network of significant others, friends, and family and their ability to provide companionship and assistance in times of need. Tools to adequately measure social networks have been in development for a number of years. However, the many nuances and configurations of social support networks make standardized measurements difficult. One tool that has shown some

---

Geriatric Depression Scale: Short Form

Choose the best answer for how you have felt over the past week:

1. Are you basically satisfied with your life?   YES / **NO**
2. Have you dropped many of your activities and interests?   **YES** / NO
3. Do you feel that your life is empty?   **YES** / NO
4. Do you often get bored?   **YES** / NO
5. Are you in good spirits most of the time?   YES / **NO**
6. Are you afraid that something bad is going to happen to you?   **YES** / NO
7. Do you feel happy most of the time?   YES / **NO**
8. Do you often feel helpless?   **YES** / NO
9. Do you prefer to stay at home, rather than going out and doing new things?   **YES** / NO
10. Do you feel you have more problems with memory than most?   **YES** / NO
11. Do you think it is wonderful to be alive now?   YES / **NO**
12. Do you feel pretty worthless the way you are now?   **YES** / NO
13. Do you feel full of energy?   YES / **NO**
14. Do you feel that your situation is hopeless?   **YES** / NO
15. Do you think that most people are better off than you are?   **YES** / NO

Answers in **bold** indicate depression. Score 1 point for each bolded answer.

A score > 5 points is suggestive of depression.
A score ≥ 10 points is almost always indicative of depression.

A score > 5 points should warrant a follow-up comprehensive assessment.

Fig. 13.1 ▪ Geriatric Depression Scale (short form). ***Source:*** Greenberg, S. A. (2012). The Geriatric Depression Scale (GDS). *The Hartford Institute for Geriatric Nursing, Try This: Series, 4*. https://hign.org/consultgeri/try-this-series/geriatric-depression-scale-gds.

usefulness is the Social Network and Support Scale in the International Mobility in Aging Study (Ahmed et al., 2018). This scale focuses on the emotional support and feelings of usefulness provided by the four cited types of social ties: friends, family members, children, and partners. Five Likert-scale questions about social support are asked for each type of social tie. The maximum total score for social support is 20 for each type of social tie (Ahmed et al., 2018).

Caregiver Burden

A number of tools are specifically designed to measure the burden of the caregiver role (see Chapter 21). Caregiver burden assessment is vital to prevent potential family burnout and elder abuse. One of the most frequently used measures is the Caregiver Strain Index (CSI) (Fig. 13.2) (Gerritsen & Van Der Ende, 1994). The CSI identifies families that have potential caregiving concerns. The tool comprises 13 questions that

I am going to read a list of things that other people have found to be difficult. Would you tell me if any of these apply to you? (Give examples.)

	Yes = 1	No = 0
Sleep is disturbed (e.g., because is in and out of bed; wanders around at night)		
It is inconvenient (e.g., because helping takes so much time; it's a long drive over to help)		
It is a physical strain (e.g., because of lifting in and out of a chair; effort or concentration is required)		
It is confining (e.g., helping restricts free time; cannot go visiting)		
There have been family adjustments (e.g., because helping has disrupted routine; there has been no privacy)		
There have been changes in personal plans (e.g., had to turn down a job; could not go on vacation)		
There have been other demands on my time (e.g., from other family members)		
There have been emotional adjustments (e.g., because of severe arguments)		
Some behavior is upsetting (e.g., because of incontinence; has trouble remembering things; accuses people of taking things)		
It is upsetting to find has changed so much from his/her former self (e.g., he/she is a different person than he/she used to be)		
There have been work adjustments (e.g., because of having to take time off)		
It is a financial strain		
Feeling completely overwhelmed (e.g., because of worry about _____; concerns about how to manage)		
TOTAL SCORE (Count yes responses. Any positive answer may indicate a need for intervention in that area. A score of 7 or higher indicates a high level of stress.)		

Fig. 13.2 ▓ Caregiver Strain Index. *Source:* Robinson, B. C. (1983). Validation of a caregiver strain index. *Journal of Gerontology, 38*(3), 344–348.

measure strain related to care provision within employment, financial, physical, social, and time domains. Positive responses to seven or more items on the index indicate a greater level of strain. The CSI can be used to assess individuals of any age who have assumed the role of caregiver for an older adult.

Environmental and Safety Assessment

Environmental safety is an issue at all ages. Safety is especially important for persons who have limitations in cognition, mobility, vision, or hearing or who are at risk for a fall-related injury (see Chapters 12 and 19). Nurses in every setting are responsible for promoting the safety of the persons in their care. The most commonly used tools related to safety are (1) the listing of potential dangers and the status (present or absent) of the dangers and (2) the provision of suggestions or opportunities for reducing the potential dangers. Often, nurses think of safety as related to the risk of falling, but safety hazards include fires, poisoning, and problems with temperature (hypothermia or hyperthermia) as well. Unfortunately, many older adults who have lived in their homes for many years also face potential dangers from increased crime and victimization. See Chapter 12 for a detailed discussion of mobility and environmental safety, including premobilization assessment. See Chapter 19 for a description of several strategies and assessments to promote safety related to vision or hearing impairments.

Integrated Assessments

In some cases, an integrated approach is used rather than a collection of separate tools and assessments. The most well known of these integrated tools is the Duke Older Americans Resources and Service (OARS) Program (Fillenbaum & Smyer, 1981), which was taken into consideration in the development of the MDS currently used in most facilities (see Chapter 5).

Older Americans Resources and Service

The classic Duke OARS instrument was designed to evaluate ability, disability, and the capacity level at which the person is able to function (Fillenbaum & Smyer, 1981). Each of its subscales—social resources, economic resources, physical health, mental health, and the ability to perform ADLs—can be used separately.

The person's functional capacity in each area is rated on a scale of 1 (excellent) to 6 (completely impaired). At the conclusion of the assessment, a cumulative impairment score ranging from 6 (most capable) to 30 (total disability) is established. The information considered in each domain is briefly described next.

Social Resources. The social resources domain addresses the person's social skills and ability to negotiate and make friends. Is the person able to seek help from friends, family, and strangers? Is a caregiver available if needed? Who is the caregiver, and how long are they available? Does the person belong to any social network or group? How is the person's need for belonging met?

Economic Resources. Data about monthly income and sources are needed to determine the adequacy of income compared to the cost of living, including costs of food, shelter, clothing, medications, and small luxury items. This information can provide insight into the person's relative standard of living and can point to needs that might be alleviated by the use of additional resources.

Mental Health. Consideration is given to intellectual function, the presence or absence of psychiatric symptoms, and the amount of enjoyment and social interaction the person gets from life.

Physical Health. Diagnoses of major diseases, the type of prescribed and over-the-counter medications the person is taking, and the person's perception of their health status are evaluated. Physical health includes participation in regular vigorous activity (such as walking, dancing, or biking) daily or at least twice a week. Seriously impaired physical health is the result of the presence of one or more illnesses or disabilities that are severely painful or life-threatening or that require extensive care.

Activities of Daily Living. The ADLs included in the OARS are walking, getting into and out of bed, bathing, combing hair, shaving, dressing, eating, and getting to the bathroom on time by oneself. The IADLs include using the telephone, driving a car, hanging up clothes, obtaining groceries, taking medications, and having correct knowledge of the required medication dosages.

Fulmer SPICES

The Fulmer SPICES is a tool for the overall assessment of older adults (Fulmer, 2019). This tool has proved reliable and valid for persons in later life, whether in health or illness, living in acute or residential care homes, or living at home. The acronym "SPICES" refers to six common syndromes of the older adult that require nursing interventions: **S**leep disorders, **P**roblems with eating or feeding, **I**ncontinence, **C**onfusion, **E**vidence of falls, and **S**kin breakdown. Several of these domains can be assessed in greater depth with specific tools that assess sleep (see Chapter 10), nutrition (see Chapter 8), continence (see Chapter 9), cognition (see Chapter 21), mobility (see Chapter 12), and skin (see Chapter 11). Nurses are encouraged to make an index card (3 inches × 5 inches) with the SPICES acronym to use as a reference when caring for older adults. The SPICES acronym can also be found online (https://hign.org/).

SUMMARY

This chapter is a brief overview of the standardized assessment tools that are commonly used in gerontological nursing. Whether using a standardized tool or a new measure to make an assessment, the goal is always to collect the most accurate data in the most efficient yet caring manner possible. Meeting this goal requires strong collaboration within the interprofessional team. The tools organize the collected data necessary for assessment and make it possible to compare the data over time. Some of the factors that complicate the assessment of the older adult are the difficulty of differentiating the effects of aging from those of disease, the coexistence of multiple diseases, the underreporting of symptoms by older adults, atypical or nonspecific presentation of illness, and the increase in iatrogenic illnesses.

Overdiagnoses and underdiagnoses occur when normal age changes, both physical and psychosocial, are not considered. Underdiagnosis is far more common in gerontological nursing. Many symptoms or complaints are ascribed to normal age-related changes rather than to a health problem that may be developing. Assessing the older adult who has multiple chronic conditions is also a challenge; the symptoms of one condition can exacerbate or mask the symptoms of another. The goal of gerontological nurses is to achieve the highest level of excellence in the care of older adults; the use of validated assessment tools facilitates the attainment of this goal.

KEY CONCEPTS

- Assessment of the person's physical, cognitive, psychosocial, and environmental status is essential to meet the specific needs of the older adult and to implement appropriate interventions.
- Collecting the data through self-report, report by proxy, or observation will affect the quality and quantity of the data.
- Knowledge of how to use a particular gerontological assessment tool is needed for its accurate use.
- Most comorbidities complicate the obtaining and interpreting of assessment data.

ACTIVITIES AND DISCUSSION QUESTIONS

1. Discuss the importance of the measurement of ADLs and IADLs for older adults.

2. Develop for each ADL a plan of interventions that could be used to compensate for ADL deficits and that would still foster an older adult's independence.

3. Describe what makes an assessment tool effective.

4. Consider the limitations and challenges of using assessment tools for older adults.

5. Determine which tools would be most appropriate for assessing cognition in older adults who live in the community, in hospital, or in a long-term care home, and state the rationale for the choices.

RESOURCES

Geriatric Depression Scale
http://www.stanford.edu/~yesavage/GDS.html
Hartford Institute for Geriatric Nursing. Evidence-informed geriatric assessment tools in the Try This: Series of assessments (cost-free, web-based resources, including demonstration videos and a corresponding print series).
https://hign.org/consultgeri-resources/try-this-series
Registered Nurses' Association of Ontario. *Best practice guidelines and fact sheets on the assessment of pain, pressure ulcers, fall risk, delirium, dementia, depression, incontinence, and constipation.*
http://rnao.ca/bpg

For additional resources, please visit *http://evolve.elsevier.com/ Canada/Ebersole/gerontological/*

REFERENCES

Ahmed, T., Belanger, E., Vafaei, A., et al. (2018). Validation of a social networks and support measurement tool for use in international aging research: The International Mobility in Aging Study. *Journal of Cross-Cultural Gerontology, 33*(1), 101–120. doi:10.1007/s10823-018-9344-x.

Alexopoulos, G. S., Abrams, R. C., Young, R. C., et al. (1988). The Cornell Scale for Depression in Dementia. *Biological Psychiatry, 23*(3), 271–284.

Benner, P. (1984). *From novice to expert.* Addison-Wesley.

Brossard, B. (2018). Objectifying dementia: The use of the Mini-Mental State Exam in medical research and practice. In P. Le Moigne (Ed.), *Measuring mental disorders* (pp. 127–154). Elsevier.

Centre intégré de santé et de services sociaux de Laval. (2020). *Specialized approach to senior care.* https://www.lavalensante.com/en/care-and-services/list-of-care-and-services/hospitalization-and-surgery/specialized-approach-to-senior-care/.

Centre intégré universitaire de santé et de services sociaux (CISSS) de l'Ouest-de-l'Île-de-Montréal. (2016). *L'Approache adaptée à la personne âgée.* https://santemontreal.qc.ca/fileadmin/fichiers/actualites/2016/sept/COMTL_AAPA.pdf.

Chehata, V. J., Shatzer, M., & Cristian, A. M. (2018). Inpatient rehabilitation outcome measures in persons with brain and spinal cord cancer. In A. Cristian, *Central nervous system cancer rehabilitation* (pp. 19–25). Elsevier.

Chen, T., & Chou, L. S. (2017). Effects of muscle strength and balance control on sit-to-walk and turn durations in the timed up and go test. *Archives of Physical Medicine and Rehabilitation, 98*(12), 2471–2476.

de Almeida Mello, J., Declercq, A., Cès, S., et al. (2016). Exploring home care interventions for frail older people in Belgium: A comparative effectiveness study. *Journal of the American Geriatrics Society, 64*(11), 2251–2256. doi:10.1111/jgs.14410.

Durmaz, B., Soysal, P., Ellidokuz, H., et al. (2018). Validity and reliability of geriatric depression scale-15 (short form) in Turkish older adults. *Northern Clinics of Istanbul, 5*(3), 216–2020. doi:10.14744/nci.2017.85047.

Ellison, D., White, D., & Farrar, F. C. (2015). Aging population. *Nursing Clinics in North America, 50*(1), 185–213. doi:10.1016/j.cnur.2014.10.014.

Fillenbaum, G. G., & Smyer, M. A. (1981). The development, validity, and reliability of the OARS multidimensional functional assessment questionnaire. *Journal of Gerontology, 36*(4), 428–434. doi:10.1093/geronj/36.4.428.

Folstein, M. F., Folstein, S. E., & McHugh, P. R. (1975). "Mini-mental state": A practical method for grading the cognitive state of patients for the clinician. *Journal of Psychiatric Research, 12*(3), 189–198. doi:10.1016/0022-3956(75)90026-6.

Fulmer, T. (2019). Fulmer SPICES: An overall assessment tool for older adults. In T. Fulmer, K. Glassman, S. Greenberg, et al., *NICHE: Nurses Improving Care for Healthsystem Elders* (p. 393). Springer.

Gerritsen, J., & Van Der Ende, P. (1994). The development of a caregiving burden scale. *Age and Ageing, 23*, 483–491. doi:10.1093/ageing/23.6.483.

Goodarzi, Z. S., Mele, B. S., Roberts, D. J., et al. (2017). Depression case finding in individuals with dementia: A systematic review and meta-analysis. *Journal of the American Geriatrics Society, 65*(5), 937–948. doi:10.1111/jgs.14713.

Inouye, S. K., van Dyck, C. H., Alessi, C. A., et al. (1990). Clarifying confusion: The confusion assessment method. *Annals of Internal Medicine, 113*, 941–948. doi:10.7326/0003-4819-113-12-941.

interRAI. (2017). *Scales: Status and outcome measures.* http://www.interrai.org/scales.html.

Julayanont, P., & Nasreddine, Z. S. (2017). Montreal Cognitive Assessment (MoCA): Concept and clinical review. In A. J. Larner (Ed.), *Cognitive screening instruments: A practical approach* (pp. 139–195). Springer.

Katz, S., Ford, A. B., Moskowitz, R. N., et al. (1963). Studies of illness in the aged: The index of ADL: A standardized measure of biological and psychosocial function. *Journal of the American Medical Association, 185*, 914–919. doi:10.1001/jama.1963.03060120024016.

Kim, J. I., Sunwoo, M. K., Sohn, Y. H., et al. (2016). The MMSE and MoCA for screening cognitive impairment in less educated patients with Parkinson's disease. *Journal of Movement Disorders, 9*(3), 152–159. doi:10.14802/jmd.16020.

Lawton, M. P., & Brody, E. M. (1969). Assessment of older people: Self-maintaining and instrumental activities of daily living. *The Gerontologist, 9*(3), 179–186. doi:10.1093/geront/9.3_Part_1.179.

Mahoney, F. I., & Barthel, D. W. (1965). Functional evaluation: The Barthel Index. *Maryland State Medical Journal, 14*, 61–65.

McCusker, J., Cole, M. G., Dendukuri, N., et al. (2004). The delirium index, a measure of the severity of delirium: new findings on reliability, validity, and responsiveness. *Journal of the American Geriatrics Society, 52*(10), 1744–1749. doi:10.111/j.1532-5415.2004.52471.x.

Seitz, D. P., Chan, C. C., Newton, H. T., et al. (2018). Mini-Cog for the diagnosis of Alzheimer's disease dementia and other dementias within a primary care setting. *Cochrane Database of Systematic Reviews, 2*(2), CD011415. doi:10.1002/14651858. CD011415.pub2.

Tuokko, H., Hadjistavropoulos, T., Miller, J., et al. (1992). The clock test: A sensitive measure to differentiate normal elderly from those with Alzheimer disease. *Journal of the American Geriatric Society, 40*(6), 579–584. doi:10.1111/j.1532-5415.1992.tb02106.x.

Wong, E. K., Lee, J. Y., Surendran, A. S., et al. (2018). Nursing perspectives on the confusion assessment method: A qualitative focus group study. *Age & Ageing, 47*(6), doi:10.1093/ageing/afy107.

Yesavage, J. A., Brink, T. L., Rose, T., et al. (1982–1983). Development and validation of a geriatric depression screening scale: A preliminary report. *Journal of Psychiatric Research, 17*(1), 37–49.

14 SAFE MEDICATION USE FOR OLDER ADULTS

■ ■

LEARNING OBJECTIVES

Upon completion of this chapter, the reader will be able to:

- Explain age-related pharmacokinetic changes.
- Discuss potential use of chronotherapy for the older adult.
- Describe medication use patterns and their implications for the older adult.
- Explain the roles of the older adult, caregiver, and social network in promoting medication compliance.
- List interventions that can help promote medication compliance.
- Identify diagnoses or symptoms for which psychotropic medications are prescribed.
- Discuss issues concerning psychotropic medication management in the older population.
- Develop a nursing care plan for older adults who have been prescribed psychotropic medications.

GLOSSARY

Adverse effect or adverse event   A harmful and undesired consequence of a medication or procedure, or a consequence of a drug or procedure other than that for which it is used (e.g., dry mouth); formerly called a "side effect."

Bioavailability   The amount of medication available for effecting changes in target tissues.

Biotransformation   A series of chemical alterations of a medication that occur in the body.

Complementary and alternative medicine (CAM)   Health practices that are not traditionally part of the biomedical health care model, such as acupuncture, chiropractic, hypnosis, massage therapy, and natural health products, such as herbal remedies, vitamins, homeopathic medicines, and nutrition therapies.

Delusion   A false fixed belief that is not shared by others and guides the person's interpretation of events.

Half-life   The time it takes after medication administration to inactivate half of the medication.

Hallucination   A false sensory perception in the absence of a real stimulus (e.g., hearing voices that no one else can hear).

Iatrogenic   Pertaining to the result of something that is done or given to a person in the context of health care.

Pharmacokinetics   The movement of a medication in the body from its administration to its absorption, distribution, metabolism, and excretion.

Potentiation   The strengthening of the effect of one or more substances (e.g., food or another medication) when they are used in combination.

Regimen   A scheduled plan for taking medications (e.g., twice a day, with food).

Target tissue or target organ   Tissue or organ intended to receive the greatest concentration of a medication or to be most affected by the medication.

Therapeutic window   The range of the plasma concentration of a medication within which it is safe and effective.

Thought disorder   Disturbance in a person's thought processes or way of thinking.

THE LIVED EXPERIENCE

"It is so hard to keep track of my medications. I try arranging them in little cups to take with each meal, but then there are the ones that I take at odd times. Those are the easiest to forget. I get really confused and think sometimes I have taken them twice. I really wish I didn't have to take so many pills, but I'm not sure what would happen if I stopped any of them. I don't even know why I'm taking most of them."

Geraldo, 62 years old, living with hypertension and diabetes

MEDICATION USE FOR OLDER ADULTS

In Canada, persons who are 65 years of age and older are the largest users of prescription and over-the-counter (OTC) medications (Bernier, 2017). More than 80% of community-dwelling Canadians aged 65 years or more in 2007–2011 were found to be taking prescription medications, with 33% of this group taking five or more medications (Pannu et al., 2017). In a study by Fisher and colleagues (2020), participants took an average of 7.7 and 8.8 medications in the intervention and control groups, respectively. Another study found that up to 88% of older adults use **complementary or alternative medicine (CAM)** therapy (Groden et al., 2017). In this chapter, the term "medication" refers to prescription and OTC medications and herbal remedies. As people age, they are more likely to develop more complex health challenges, which is one reason the use of prescription medications tends to increase (Canadian Institute for Health Information [CIHI], 2018).

Unfortunately, the number of adverse drug reactions (ADRs) increases with the number of medications used. Also called adverse drug events, ADRs are a notable cause of hospital admission as well as a cause of **iatrogenic** mortality and morbidity for older adults (Jennings et al., 2019). How people use their prescribed medicines and other CAM or bioactive products depends on the person's unique characteristics, situations, beliefs, understanding of illness, function and cognition, perception of the necessity of the medications, severity of symptoms, reactions to the medications, finances, access to medications, and the compatibility of such products with their

lifestyle. Gerontological nurses have a responsibility to help minimize the risks of medication use for people in their care. Several resources on medication safety can be found at the Institute for Safe Medication Practices (ISMP), a nonprofit organization committed to the prevention of medication errors and advancing safe medication use (http://www.ismp.org/).

This chapter presents a review of changes in pharmacokinetics, pharmacodynamics, and medication use issues. The final section of this chapter discusses the use of psychotropic agents.

PHARMACOKINETICS

Pharmacokinetics refers to the movement of a medication in the body from the point of administration as it is absorbed, distributed, metabolized, and finally excreted. It is important for gerontological nurses to understand how pharmacokinetics may differ in older adults (Fig. 14.1). There is no conclusive evidence of an appreciable change in overall pharmacokinetics with aging; however, several changes with aging may have an effect on the process of pharmacokinetics (see Chapter 6). The four processes of pharmacokinetics (absorption, distribution, metabolism, and excretion) will be described in more detail.

Absorption

In order for a medication to be effective, it must be absorbed into the bloodstream, the tissue, or both. The amount of time between the administration of the medication and its absorption depends on a number of factors, including the route of introduction (i.e., intravenous, oral, parenteral, transdermal, or rectal), **bioavailability**, and the amount of medication that passes into the body. An intravenous route will deliver the medication immediately to the bloodstream. Other quick routes for medication absorption include parenteral and transdermal routes and through mucous membranes such as the rectum and the oral mucosa. Orally administered medications are absorbed through the gastro-intestinal tract.

A number of normal age-related physiological changes have implications for differences in both the prescription and the administration of medications for older adults (Petrovic et al., 2019). The commonly diminished gastric pH will retard the action of acid-dependent medications. Delayed stomach emptying

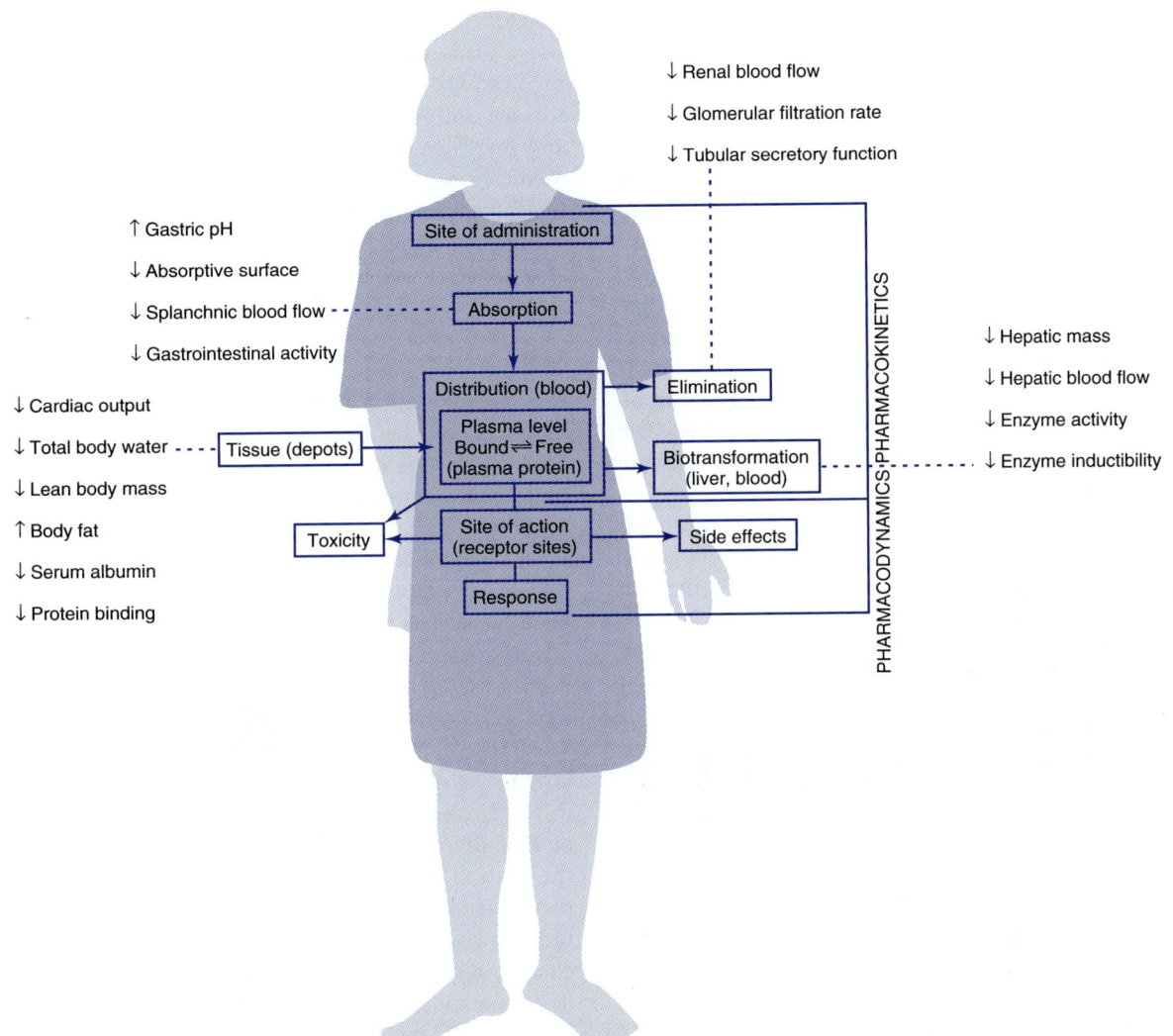

Fig. 14.1 ■ Physiological changes of aging and the pharmacokinetics and pharmacodynamics of medication use. **Sources:** Kane, R. L., Ouslander, J. G., & Abrass, I. B. (1984). *Essentials of clinical geriatrics.* McGraw-Hill; Lamy, P. P. (1984). Hazards of drug use in the elderly: Commonsense measures to reduce them. *Postgraduate Medicine, 76*(1), 50–53; Montamat, S. C., Cusack, B. J., & Vestal, R. E. (1980). Management of drug therapy in the elderly. *New England Journal of Medicine, 321*(5), 303–309; Roberts, J., & Tumer, N. (1988). Pharmacodynamic basis for altered drug action in the elderly. *Clinics in Geriatric Medicine, 4*(1), 127–149; Vestal, R. E., & Dawson, G. W. (1985). Pharmacology and aging. In C. E. Finch & E. L. Schneider (Eds.), *Handbook of the biology of aging* (pp. 744–819). Van Nostrand Reinhold.

may diminish or negate the effectiveness of short-lived medications that could become inactivated before reaching the small intestine. The absorption of enteric-coated medications—which are specifically meant to bypass stomach absorption—may be delayed so that their action begins in the stomach, which can lead to gastric irritation or nausea.

Absorption is also influenced by changes in gastro-intestinal motility. If there is increased motility in the small intestine, the medication effect is diminished because of shortened contact time and therefore decreased absorption and effectiveness. Conversely, slowed intestinal motility can increase the contact time and thus the amount absorbed, resulting in a change in the medication's effect. This increases the risk for adverse reactions or unpredictable effects.

Many prescription and OTC medications commonly taken by older adults can also affect the absorption of other medications. Antispasmodic medications slow gastric and intestinal motility. In some instances, the ingested medication's action may be useful, but when other medications are involved, it is necessary to consider the problem of changes in medication absorption due to medication–medication interaction. By binding the medication with elements and forming chemical compounds, antacids or iron preparations affect the availability of some medications for absorption. Medication–food interactions may either decrease or increase the amount absorbed. (Medication–herb interactions are presented in Table 14.1.) For example, when a bisphosphonate such as alendronate (Fosamax) is taken with food of any kind, absorption is reduced to only a few milligrams; therefore, the medication has no effect on the **target organ**, the bones.

Similarly, taking grapefruit juice with levothyroxine may delay the absorption of the medication (Ased et al., 2018).

Distribution

Once a medication is absorbed, it must be transported to the target organ to have any effect. Distribution depends on the availability of plasma protein in the form of lipoproteins, globulins, and especially albumin. As medications are absorbed, they bind with the protein and are distributed throughout the body. Normally, a predictable percentage of the absorbed medication is inactivated as it is bound to the protein. The remaining free medication is available in the bloodstream and has a therapeutic effect when an effective concentration is reached in the plasma.

Many older adults have an insignificant reduction in serum albumin. In others, especially those with prolonged illness or malnutrition (such as residents in long-term care [LTC] homes), the serum albumin may be diminished. When this occurs, toxic levels of available free drug may accumulate unpredictably, especially for highly protein-bound medications with narrow **therapeutic windows**, such as phenytoin and warfarin (Maher et al., 2020).

Potential alterations of medication distribution in late life are related to changes in body composition, particularly decreased lean body mass, increased body fat, and decreased total body water. Decreased body water leads to higher serum levels of water-soluble medications such as digoxin, ethanol, and aminoglycosides. Adipose tissue nearly doubles in older men and increases by one half in older women; therefore, medications that are highly lipid soluble are stored in the fatty tissue, extending and possibly elevating the medication effect. This includes medications such as lorazepam, diazepam, chlorpromazine, phenobarbital, and haloperidol (Haldol).

Metabolism

Biotransformation is the process by which the body modifies the chemical structure of medication. This process converts the compound to a metabolite that is more easily excreted later on. A medication will continue to exert a therapeutic effect as long as it remains in its original state or as an active metabolite. Active metabolites retain the ability to have a therapeutic effect, as well as the same or greater chance of causing **adverse effects or adverse events**. For example, the metabolites of acetaminophen (Tylenol) can cause liver damage with higher dosages (>4 g per 24 hours, or more than four extra-strength products) (Jiang et al., 2017). The duration of a medication's action is determined by the metabolic rate and is measured in terms of **half-life**, or how long the drug remains active in the body. The liver is the primary site of medication metabolism. With aging, the liver's activity, mass, volume, and blood flow are reduced (see Chapter 6). These changes result in a potential decrease in the liver's ability to metabolize medications such as benzodiazepines (e.g., lorazepam [Ativan] and diazepam [Valium]). These changes in the liver also result in a significant increase in the half-life of these medications. For example, the half-life of diazepam in a younger adult is about 37 hours but can be as long as 82 hours in an older adult. If the dose and timing of these medications are not adjusted, they can accumulate, and the administration of a single dose can have significantly more (and longer) effects in an older adult than in a younger person. Except in the rarest of circumstances, diazepam is typically not used in the older population (Greenblatt et al., 2020).

Excretion

Medications and their metabolites are excreted in sweat, saliva, and other secretions but are excreted primarily

TABLE 14.1
Significant Medication–Food Interactions

Medications	Food	Medication–Food Interaction Effects
Warfarin	High-protein diet	Raises serum albumin levels; decreases in INR
	Vegetables containing vitamin K	Interfere with effectiveness and safety of warfarin therapy
	Charbroiled vegetables and meat	Decrease warfarin activity
	Cooked onions	Increase warfarin activity
	Cranberry juice	Elevates INR without bleeding in older patient
	Leafy green vegetables	Potentiate development of thromboembolic complications
Monoamine oxidases	Tyramine-containing foods[1]	Cause hypertensive crisis
Propranolol	Protein-rich foods	Possibly increase serum level
Celiprolol	Orange juice	Inhibits intestinal absorption of drug
ACE inhibitors	(Empty stomach)	Increases absorption of drug
Ca^{2+} channel drugs	Grapefruit juice	Increases drug bioavailability
Antibiotics	Milk products[2]	Prevent the absorption of some antibiotics; reduce drug bioavailability
Acetaminophen	Pectin	Delays absorption and onset of acetaminophen
NSAIDs	Alcohol	Increases potential risk of liver damage or stomach bleeding
	Beverages	Increases C_{max} and $AUC_{0-alpha}$ significantly[3]
Theophylline	High-fat meal	Increases drug bioavailability
	Caffeine	Increases risk of drug toxicity
Esomeprazole	High-fat meal	Reduces drug bioavailability
Cimetidine, rupatadine	With food (any type)	Increases drug bioavailability
Isoniazide	Plants, medicinal herbs, oleanolic acid	Exert synergistic effect
Cycloserine	High-fat meals	Decrease serum concentration
Esomeprazole	High-fat meals	Reduce drug bioavailability
Glimepiride	With breakfast	Allows for absolute drug bioavailability
Acarbose	At start of each meal	Allows for maximum drug effectiveness
Mercaptopurine	Cow's milk[4]	Reduces drug bioavailability
Tamoxifen	Sesame seeds	Negatively interfere with tamoxifen in inducing regression of established mcf-7 tumour size, but beneficially interact with tamoxifen on bone in ovariectomized athymic mice
Levothyroxine	Grapefruit juice	Delays drug absorption[5]

ACE, angiotensin-converting enzyme; AUC, area under the curve; Ca^{2+}, ionized calcium; C_{max}, maximum concentration; INR, international normalized ratio; NSAIDs, nonsteroidal anti-inflammatory drugs.

[1]Frankel, E.H. (2003). Basic concepts. In B. J. McCabe, E. H., Frankel, & J. J. Wolfe (Eds.), *Handbook of food–drug interactions* (p. 2). CRC Press.

[2]Ayo, J. A., Agu, H., & Madaki, I. (2005). Food and drug interactions: Its side effects. *Nutrition & Food Science, 35*(4), 243–252. doi:10.1108/00346650510605630.

[3]Schmidt, L. E., & Dahloff, K. (2002). Food-drug interactions. *Drugs, 62*(10), 1481–1502. doi:10.2165/00003495-200262100-00005.

[4]Nekvindová, J., & Anzenbacher, P. (2007). Interactions of food and dietary supplements with drug metabolising cytochrome P450 enzymes. *Ceska a Slovenska Farmacie, 56*(4), 165–173.

[5]Hansten, P. D. (2004). Appendix II: Important interactions and their mechanisms. In B. G. Katzung, *Basic and clinical pharmacology* (9th ed., p. 1110). McGraw-Hill.

Source: Bushra, R., Aslam, N., & Khan, A. Y. (2011). Food-drug interactions. *Oman Medical Journal, 26*(2), 77–83. doi:10.5001/omj.2011.21. http://pubmedcentralcanada.ca/pmcc/articles/PMC3191675/.

through the kidneys. However, many older adults may have comorbidities that affect the rate of excretion, and just as kidney function declines significantly with aging, so does the ability to excrete or eliminate medications in a timely manner. The considerably decreased glomerular filtration rate leads to a prolonged half-life of medication (that is, the amount of time required to eliminate the medication), which again presents opportunities for accumulation and increases the potential for toxicity or other adverse events (see Chapter 6). Although renal function cannot be estimated according to serum creatinine, it can be approximated by the calculation of creatinine clearance. Reductions in dosages for renally excreted medications (e.g., allopurinol and vancomycin) are necessary when the creatinine clearance is reduced.

Pharmacodynamics

Pharmacodynamics refers to the interaction between a medication and the body. The older a person becomes, the more likely there will be an altered or unreliable response of the body to medication. Although it is not always possible to explain the change in response, several mechanisms are known.

The aging process causes a decreased response to beta-adrenergic receptor stimulators and blockers; decreased baroreceptor sensitivity; and increased sensitivity to a number of medications, especially anticholinergics, benzodiazepines, narcotic analgesics, warfarin (Coumadin), and the cardiac medications diltiazem and verapamil (Briggs, 2005). If food–medication interactions occur, the problems become worse. For example, drinking grapefruit juice while taking a statin such as Lipitor or taking any number of antibiotics may cause an unreliable response.

There is also a growing body of knowledge about the interaction of herbal preparations and currently prescribed medications. For example, the herbal extract of *Ginkgo biloba* is commonly thought to enhance cognitive function, but this herb will increase the potential for bleeding when an anticoagulant is used at the same time (Noori & Mehta, 2019) (see Table 14.1). In addition to causing expected dry mouth, medications with anticholinergic properties can cause confusion, constipation, blurred vision, or urinary retention, even at low doses (The University of British Columbia, 2018). The use of benzodiazepines is associated with an increased risk for accidental injury; thus, these medications are

on the "do not use" list for older adults (Canadian Coalition for Seniors' Mental Health, 2020).

CHRONOPHARMACOLOGY

The normal biorhythms of the body and their differences in men and women can also affect pharmacokinetics and pharmacodynamics. The relationship of biological rhythms to variations in the body's response to medications is known as *chronopharmacology*. Although chronopharmacology has not yet been explored in relation to aging, it is a developing science that may lead to more effective medication therapy (Çakmur, 2018). The best time to administer medications is thought to be influenced by the biorhythms of various physiological processes.

As discussed previously, absorption depends on gastric acid pH, the level of motility of the gastro-intestinal tract, and blood flow—all of which have been shown to have biorhythmic variations. The distribution of protein-bound medications depends on albumin and glycoproteins produced by the liver. During the day, albumin levels are high, but they are low in the early morning. Medication metabolism is also biorhythmic. Oxidation, hydrolysis, decarboxylation, and demethylation by liver enzymes demonstrate rhythmic variations. Renal elimination depends on kidney perfusion, glomerular filtration, and urine acidity and has shown rhythmic variation. The brain, heart, and blood cells also have varied rhythmicity, resulting in a cyclical response for beta-blockers, calcium channel blockers, angiotensin-converting enzyme (ACE) inhibitors, nitrates, and other similar medications. Medications such as Fosamax and risedronate (Actonel) must be taken upon waking in the morning for maximum effectiveness (Brown, 2017). Table 14.2 shows some of the rhythmic influences on diseases and physiological processes.

The potential for decreasing individual doses of medications, the frequency of administration, or both for older adults is the primary benefit of chronopharmacological therapy and may ultimately improve the therapeutic effect, decrease toxic effects, and improve compliance with a medication **regimen**. In addition, chronotherapeutics may be of financial benefit to the person (by reducing overall medication expense if lower or fewer doses are needed).

TABLE 14.2
Rhythmic Influences on Disease and Physiological Processes

Disease or Process	Rhythmic Influence
Allergic rhinitis	Symptoms worse in the morning
Arterial blood pressure	Circadian surge in the morning hours
Asthma	Greatest respiratory distress overnight (during sleep) Symptoms peak in early morning (0400–0500 hours)
Blood plasma	Plasma volume falls at night, and thus hematocrit increases
Cancer	Tumour cells proliferate when normal cell mitosis is low
Cardiac disease	Angina, myocardial infarction, and thrombolytic stroke occur in the first 4 hours after waking (peak at 0900 hours) (Prinzmetal's angina—during sleep).
Catecholamines	Increase in early morning
Fibrinolytic activity	Increases in early morning
Platelet activation	May result from abnormality in circadian rhythm, which affects cortisol levels, body temperature, and sleep–wake cycle
Gastric system	Gastric acid secretion peaks every morning (0200–0400 hours); circannual variability—incidence of gastric ulcers greater in winter
Osteoarthritis	Pain more severe in morning
Potassium excretion	Lowest in morning; highest in late afternoon
Rheumatoid arthritis	Pain more severe in late afternoon
Systemic insulin	Highest in afternoon

MEDICATION ISSUES FOR OLDER ADULTS

Polypharmacy

The number of administered medications that is considered "too many" is controversial. *Polypharmacy* is the use of a large number of medications (pills, patches, injections, etc.), contraindicated or potentially inappropriate medications, or medications that are duplicated or unnecessary (Guillot et al., 2019) (Fig. 14.2). The use of prescription medication increases with age (Morin et al., 2016). A Canadian study found that almost 27% of the older adults surveyed took more than five medications. Older adults who are subjected to polypharmacy are twice as likely as older adults who are taking one or two medications to report medication errors (Kim & Parish, 2017). Polypharmacy may be "accidental" when an existing medication regimen is not considered when new medications are prescribed or when any number of the thousands of OTC preparations and supplements are added to prescribed medications. The two major concerns with polypharmacy are the increased risks for medication interactions and adverse events. Assessment and management of polypharmacy are competencies expected by the Canadian gerontological nursing standards of practice (Canadian Gerontological Nursing Association, 2020).

Medication Interactions

The more medications a person takes or applies, the greater the possibility that one or more of the medications will interact with another medication, an herbal product or nutritional supplement, food, or alcohol. When two or more medications are taken close together in time, the medications may **potentiate** one another, making one more effective or making one or both less effective.

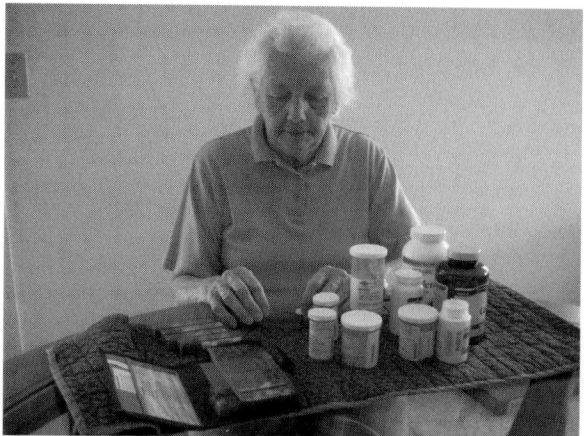

Fig. 14.2 ■ Polypharmacy. Courtesy Shannon Perry, Phoenix, Arizona.

An interaction may result in altered pharmacokinetic activity or alterations in the absorption, distribution, metabolism, or excretion of one or more of the medications. Absorption can be delayed by medications that exert an anticholinergic effect. Tricyclic antidepressants (TCAs) act in this manner, decreasing gastro-intestinal motility and interfering with the absorption of other medications. More than one medication may also compete to simultaneously occupy the necessary binding receptors, preventing one or the other from reliably reaching the target organs and creating a varied bioavailability of one or both.

Interactions can also occur when two medications or foods are mixed together before administration. For example, medications are often crushed and delivered simultaneously through an enteral tube, yet the appropriate administration requires the nurse to know which medications are crushable and which medications can be administered together. For example, Fosamax and other bisphosphonates must be taken with a full glass of water 1 hour before any other medication, beverage, or food is ingested.

In 2018, the *Cannabis Act* came into effect, legalizing cannabis use for recreational purposes (with restrictions) for those 18 years and older (Government of Canada, 2019). Cannabis is also used for medicinal purposes, with authorization from a health care provider. Cannabis can be inhaled or ingested. Medical cannabis is typically used to alleviate pain. However,

there is limited evidence available on the use of medical cannabis' effect on acute pain and modest effects for chronic, noncancer pain (Government of Canada, 2018). Note that cannabis can interact with other prescribed and OTC medications, such as pain medications, blood thinners, antidepressants, and sleeping pills (Canadian Centre on Substance Use and Addiction, 2020). For some, cannabis use may increase the risk of psychosis, worsen anxiety or depression, and affect memory, including concentration and the ability to make decisions (Canadian Centre on Substance Use and Addiction, 2020). More information on cannabis can be found in Chapter 16.

In pharmacodynamic interactions, one medication alters the body's response to another medication. This can be especially dangerous for older adults when two or more medications with the same effect are additive (that is, more potent taken together than when taken separately). Unless attention is paid to what the overall medication list includes, to when each medication is administered, and to what other products are taken, a harmful polypharmacy situation will occur. Nurses can lessen the likelihood of such an outcome by monitoring the medications administered and by encouraging the older adult to do the same.

Adverse Drug Reactions

ADRs are unwanted pharmacological effects that range from minor annoyances to death; they include allergic reactions. ADRs can sometimes be predicted from the pharmacological action of the medication (e.g., bone marrow depression from cancer chemotherapy; bleeding from Coumadin). Predictable ADRs can also occur when a person is started on a medication at a dosage that is inappropriately high or one that necessitates laboratory monitoring and adjustment (e.g., lithium or Coumadin).

All settings in which people take or are administered medications can have occurrences of ADRs. In 2016, older adults prescribed 10 to 14 different drug classes were five times more likely to be hospitalized than those prescribed 4 or fewer drug classes (CIHI, 2018). Those who took 10 or more different medications from different drug classes accounted for close to 60% of all ADR-related hospital admissions (CIHI, 2018). Among the most common medications that lead to adverse reactions are anticoagulants, antibiotics, antineoplastic

TABLE 14.3

Examples of Drugs Considered Inappropriate for Older Adults

Drug	Concern
Alprazolam (Xanax)	Rapid addiction, prolonged sedation effects, potential for confusion and falling
Amitriptyline (Elavil)	Strong anticholinergic and sedating properties, little effect on depression; at low dose, sometimes effective for neurogenic pain
Chlorpropamide (Diabinese)	Long lasting; danger of hypoglycemia is increased in older adults
Cimetidine (Tagamet)	Significant risk for ADRs with many substances and medications
Cyclobenzaprine (Flexeril)	Anticholinergic side effects, sedation, weakness
Diazepam (Valium)	Prolonged sedation, increasing fall risk and confusion risk
Diphenhydramine (Benadryl)	Excessive sedation, dry mouth, urinary retention, confusion
Dipyridamole (Persantine)	Orthostatic hypotension; no demonstrated effect on cognition
Disopyramide (Norpace)	May induce heart failure; strong anticholinergic effect
Doxepin (Sinequan)	Strong anticholinergic and sedating properties
Meperidine (Demerol)	Metabolite accumulation in older adults; can cause tremors and seizures
Oxybutynin (Ditropan)	Strong anticholinergic effect, confusion
Temazepam (Restoril)	Confusion, prolonged half-life

ADRs, adverse drug reactions.
Source: Radcliff, S., Yue, J., Rocco, G., et al. (2015). American Geriatrics Society 2015 updated Beers Criteria for Potentially Inappropriate Medication Use in Older Adults. *Journal of the American Geriatrics Society, 63*(11), 2227–2246. doi:10.1111/jgs.13702.

medications, and opioids (CIHI, 2018). These medications are frequently prescribed to older adults. Because of the large number of medications taken by older adults in LTC settings and the high potential for residents to experience altered nutritional and fluid status, the risk for ADRs is of special concern to nurses working in these settings.

The use of medications that are considered inappropriate for older adults (Table 14.3) have also been found to increase the risk for ADRs and related hospitalizations. In a Canadian study by Morgan and colleagues, 37.2% of older adults were prescribed at least one inappropriate medication (Morgan et al., 2016).

ADRs are not always predictable. An older adult who is well controlled on a stable dose of a medication may undergo a change in physiology or environment that may alter the body's response to the medication. Changes in diet can also have a profound impact on medication effects. For example, decreased fluid intake can cause lithium toxicity (Chan et al., 2020), and an increased intake of leafy green vegetables will counteract

the anticoagulant effects of Coumadin and acetylsalicylic acid (Aspirin) (Di Minno et al., 2017). Some medications (e.g., antipsychotics, stimulants, anticholinergics) interfere with the body's ability to regulate temperature, such that exposure to hot weather can more easily lead to heat stroke (Gauer & Meyers, 2019). Other medications (e.g., sulfa medications, antidepressants, and many antipsychotics) are photosensitizing, and an increase in sun exposure can lead to sunburn more quickly than expected (Hinton & Goldminz, 2020). Older adults whose fluid intake is decreased because of illness, because they cannot access fluids, or because their intake is inadequate in hot weather may quickly become volume depleted and develop increased sensitivity to the orthostatic hypotensive effects of alpha-blockers (e.g., phenothiazines and terazosin) or toxicity to antipsychotics (Lei et al., 2020).

One of the most troublesome ADRs for the older adult is medication-induced delirium and confusion. Polypharmacy with several psychotropic medications that have anticholinergic actions is perhaps the greatest precipitator of delirium as an adverse reaction (Baruth et al., 2020). Too often, delirium goes unrecognized as an ADR and is instead perceived as a worsening of pre-existing dementia or even as new-onset dementia (see Chapter 21). Any time there is a change in an older adult's functional or cognitive abilities, the possibility of medication effect must be thoroughly evaluated. Box 14.1 contains a partial list of medications that have the potential to adversely affect cognitive functioning.

Another common adverse effect seen in older adults is lethargy, especially with the use of a number of cardiovascular agents and antidepressants. Lethargy can be misinterpreted as a symptom of worsening cardiac, respiratory, or neurological conditions rather than an ADR. Among other troublesome effects are those related to sexual functioning. Although they are not detailed in this chapter, many medications interfere with or contribute to sexual dysfunction in adults of any age. The medications that are most responsible are cardiovascular medications (antihypertensives and ACE inhibitors) and psychotropic medications (antidepressants).

Misuse of Medications

Medication misuse includes overuse, underuse, erratic use, and contraindicated use. Misuse of medications can occur for any number of reasons, including the inadequate skills of the prescribers or the nurses who administer the medications, the misunderstanding of instructions, or inadequate funds to purchase prescribed medications. Although misuse of medications is often referred to as noncompliance, the term "misuse" is more descriptive of what is happening (see Chapter 23). It is important that gerontological nurses realize that the greater the number of medications taken, the greater the potential for misuse. Wilcox et al. (1994) identified 20 medications that are considered inappropriate for older adults, including controversial cardiovascular agents (propranolol, methyldopa, and reserpine). The Beers Criteria identify medications that carry a higher-than-usual risk when used by older adults (Beers, 1997). The Beers Criteria have been recommended as a best practice by several Canadian regulating and professional organizations and by the Hartford Institute of Geriatric Nursing. The list can be found in the Resources at the end of this chapter.

The misuse of a medication by the person taking it may be accidental (e.g., through misunderstanding or the inability to read labels or understand instructions) or it may be deliberate (e.g., through an attempt to make a prescription medication last longer, for financial reasons; because of cultural differences; or owing to beliefs that the dose is too low or too high). When a person is labeled noncompliant, nurses may become frustrated with the individual for their inability to follow the plan of care and medication regime. Yet, care providers tend to forget or ignore the reality that a person cannot and will not comply with a prescription or treatment plan under certain circumstances, such as when it is incompatible with the person's day-to-day life. For example, an individual cannot follow the instruction to "take medication three times per day with meals" if they eat only two meals each day (which is often the case with older adults).

Memory failures related to noncompliance with medication regimens are generally of two types: (1) the person forgets to take the medications correctly (e.g., dose, route) or (2) the person experiences "prospective" recall failure, whereby they forget to take the medication at the correct times, resulting in missed doses. The more frequently a medication must be taken, the less likely it will be taken as prescribed. With more and more medications available in once-a-day doses rather than doses to be taken three or four times each day, more people can take their medications as instructed.

BOX 14.1
COMMON CATEGORIES OF MEDICATION WITH THE POTENTIAL TO CAUSE COGNITIVE IMPAIRMENT

Alcohol
Analgesics
Antidepressants*
Antihistamines*
Antiparkinsonian agents
Antipsychotics*
Benzodiazepines*
Beta-blockers
Digitalis, Lanoxin
Diuretics
Muscle relaxants
Sedatives, hypnotics

*May be associated with falls, delirium, and cognitive and physical impairment. Anticholinergic reactions may also be confused with behaviours associated with worsening psychosis.

Health literacy also influences a person's ability to correctly take medications (see Chapter 7). Many older adults, especially those from minority groups, have low levels of literacy; thus, written instructions should be at the Grade 3 level or lower. Limitations in vision will interfere with the reading of instructions, especially those on bottle labels; pharmacists can use large type or symbols to avoid this problem. The practice of nurses, physicians, and pharmacists giving rapid-fire directions is not effective when addressing most older adults, especially those with hearing impairments or normal age-related changes. It is also common for care providers to explain the treatment and give directions concerning medications when the person is physically uncomfortable or is about to be discharged from a care facility; to explain instructions in English even when the person has limited English proficiency; and to explain medication regimens while in a noisy or busy environment. All of these practices can significantly reduce the clarity of the message and lead to consequent misuse of medications.

IMPLICATIONS FOR GERONTOLOGICAL NURSING AND HEALTHY AGING

Assessment

The initial step in ensuring that older adults use their medications safely and effectively is to conduct a comprehensive medication assessment. In some settings, a clinical pharmacist collects the medication history, but this assessment is more often completed through the combined efforts of the nurses and the prescribing health care provider (a nurse practitioner or physician).

Medication reconciliation is a formal process of comparing the prescribed medications, patches, or injections to the medications the person is actually taking or applying by completing a systematic and comprehensive review of all medications (Canadian Patient Safety Institute, 2020). This process typically involves the pharmacist and other members of the care team, including the nurse and physician. Medication reconciliation is designed to prevent ADRs that occur as a result of miscommunication at times of transition in care (e.g., from one health care setting to another or from a health care setting to home) or when more than one physician is prescribing medication. Medication reconciliation on admission to, discharge from, or transfer between services is required by Canadian hospital accreditation standards. A medication reconciliation kit is available from the Institute for Safe Medication Practices website (http://www.ismp.org).

As the nurse learns the type and number of prescribed medications, herbs, supplements, and OTC medications the person takes, the assessment can continue. There is a great deal of information needed, but this assessment is vital to promoting the health and well-being of the older adult (Box 14.2). Through this assessment, nurses can learn of discrepancies between the prescribed dosage and the actual dosage, potential medication–medication and food–medication interactions, and potential or actual ADRs. Key nursing actions include monitoring and education as well as facilitating communication and collaboration with the older adult's community pharmacist and community physician to enhance safety.

Monitoring and Evaluation

A significant part of a gerontological nurse's responsibilities consists of monitoring and evaluating the effectiveness of prescribed treatments and observing for signs of problems or iatrogenic complications. Monitoring and evaluating a situation involves observing and documenting observations, noting changes in physical and functional status (e.g., vital signs, performance of activities of daily living, sleeping, eating, hydrating, and eliminating)

BOX 14.2
COMPONENTS OF A COMPREHENSIVE MEDICATION ASSESSMENT

- Allergies
- Adverse interactions with any medication in the past
- Medical conditions
- Lifestyle factors (smoking, nicotine use, cannabis use, caffeine use, alcohol use, diet, exercise regime)
- Prescription medications
- Over-the-counter medications
- Natural health products, herbal remedies
- Changes to patient's health status
- Indication for medication

Source: Adapted from Pharmacy Connection. (2018). *The importance of patient assessment.* https://pharmacyconnection.ca/patient-assessment-spring-2018/.

and changes in mental status (attention and alertness, memory, orientation, behaviour, mood, emotional display and affect, and content and characteristics of interactions). Monitoring also means ensuring that blood levels (such as fluids and electrolytes, albumin, and creatinine) are measured as needed. The following must be monitored on a schedule: thyroid-stimulating hormone levels for individuals taking thyroid replacement medication; international normalized ratios for those taking warfarin; periodic hemoglobin A1c levels for people with diabetes; serum digoxin level for individuals taking digoxin; and serum lithium levels for those prescribed lithium. Nurses need to promptly communicate their findings of potential problems to the person's nurse practitioner or physician.

Patient Education

Nurses are responsible for educating patients (individually or in small groups) about medication use, by way of setting goals and creating a treatment plan (Box 14.3). Older adults should be encouraged to ask questions and know what medications they are taking, how it will affect them, and what alternatives are available to them. Pamphlets and booklets written in lay terms, in appropriate language, and at an appropriate reading level should be available; if none are available, the nurse can develop a booklet or information sheet for the particular person. Information is best presented in point-form lists rather than in paragraph form, and the type should be large and boldfaced. (See Chapter 7 for additional information about health education for older adults.)

Because of the complex needs of older adults, educating them about medications can be particularly challenging. The following tips may be helpful:

1. *Identify key persons:* Find out who, if anyone, manages the person's medications or assists with decision making. When applicable, and with the

---

BOX 14.3
QUESTIONS AND RECOMMENDATIONS FOR OLDER ADULTS TAKING MEDICATIONS

- What is the name of each medication?
- What is the purpose of each medication?
- What is the dose per administration?
- What is the number of doses every day?
- What is the best time to take the medication?
- How should the medication be taken?
- Do food or fluid choices influence the absorption or metabolism of the medication?
- Can the medication be taken with other medications?
- Which medications can and cannot be taken together?
- Are any special techniques, devices, or procedures necessary to administer the medication?
- For how long should the medication be taken?
- What are the common side effects?
- If side effects occur, what should be done? What changes in administration are necessary? When should the medication be stopped? When should the physician or pharmacist (or both) be called?
- What can be done at home to watch for a therapeutic medication response?
- What should be done if a dose is missed?
- How many refills are allowed?
- How should the medication be stored?
- Are other nonprescription medications or herbal remedies also being taken?
- What nonprescription preparations should not be used with the present medication?

- Are you taking cannabis/marijuana for medicinal or recreational purposes?
- Take all medications prescribed unless the physician states otherwise.
- If any new or unusual problems occur—such as shortness of breath, nausea, diarrhea, vomiting, sleepiness, dizziness, weakness, skin rash, or fever—stop taking the medication and report the problem.
- Never take medication prescribed for another person.
- Do not take medication that is more than 1 year old or past the expiration date on the container.
- Talk to your health care provider if you are taking prescription medications as well as cannabis for medicinal or recreational purposes, as this may cause adverse interactions.
- Store medications in a safe place, preferably in the kitchen rather than in the bathroom, where moisture from bathing and (especially) showers may affect them.
- Do not keep medicines, especially sedatives and hypnotics, on the bedside stand; when you are sleepy, you may forget that you have already taken the medication.
- Do not place different medicines in the same container.
- Take a sufficient supply of all medicines in their individual containers when travelling away from home.
- Use a chart to keep track of medications.

person's permission, make sure that the support person is present during the education or teaching session.

2. *Ensure good environment:* Minimize distractions, and avoid competing with television or other sources of sound for the person's attention. Make sure the person is comfortable and is not hungry, thirsty, tired, too warm or too cold, in pain, or in need of the bathroom.

3. *Determine best time:* Teach during the best time of the day for the person (i.e., when they are most alert, engaged, and energetic), and keep the sessions short and succinct.

4. *Communicate:* Ensure that you are understood. Make sure that the older adult has their eyeglasses or hearing aids on if these are used. Use simple and direct language, and avoid medical or nursing jargon (e.g., "intake"). Remain respectful at all times, and do not allow negative stereotypes to cloud communication. Encourage questions.

5. *Reinforce teaching:* Provide memory aids to reinforce teaching. Have actual medications or containers handy to visually illustrate directions. If appropriate, use written charts and lists with large letters and simple language, or charts with pictures of the medications and symbols for times of day. After discharge, a follow-up phone call can help with assessing accurate medication usage or other problems with medications. A nurse's home visit to people at high risk for problems, such as those with cognitive deficits or those who have many medications for new conditions, reinforces education and provides assessment information.

6. *Evaluate teaching:* Have the person repeat back the instructions and each medication's name, purposes, side effects, and times for administration. Have the patient describe their method for remembering to take the medicines and to mark off their ingestion.

7. *Avoid medication interactions:* Older adults should be taught to obtain all their medications from the same pharmacy if possible, so that the pharmacist is able to watch for medication duplications and interactions. Additional information about recognizing and responding to early signs of ADRs may save lives.

Medication Administration

Most older adults self-administer their medications; others receive them from family, friends, or health care providers. In LTC homes, the administration of medications is carried out by nurses. Regardless of the setting or the persons involved, several skills are needed for safe administration.

To ensure optimal safety, everyone who administers medication needs to take the "10 rights" into account. These 10 rights are right medication, right patient, right dose, right time and frequency, right route, right reason, right documentation, right to refuse, right patient education, and right evaluation.

Several other factors need to be taken into consideration when administering medication or providing education to the older adult.

Because of the high rate of arthritis and other debilitating conditions among older adults, it may be difficult or impossible for the older adult to open a medication bottle, remove a medication bottle's cap, or break a tablet. Either the person or the nurse can ask the pharmacist to break the pills, dispense a smaller dose, or provide blister packages that are easy to open.

Many tablets and capsules are difficult to swallow because of their size or because they stick to the tongue, especially if the mouth is dry. A medication in liquid form is sometimes preferable and allows for flexible dosing; concentrations can be varied so that quantities of solution can be prepared and taken with a teaspoon or tablespoon—simple and commonly used household measurements. Crushing tablets or emptying the powder from capsules into fluid or food should not be done, unless specified by the pharmaceutical company or approved by a pharmacist; doing so may interfere with the effectiveness of the medication (causing either underdose or toxicity), create problems in administration, or injure the mouth or gastro-intestinal tract.

Some people have difficulty swallowing capsules. They can be advised to place the capsule onto the front of the tongue and swallow a fluid; this should wash the capsule to the back of the throat and down. Other persons do better taking pills or capsules with a semisolid food—such as applesauce, chocolate syrup, or peanut butter—as long as the substances do not interact.

Enteric-coated, extended-release, and sustained-release products allow absorption at different parts of the gastro-intestinal tract. Capsules containing these medications should never be broken, opened, or otherwise altered before administration, nor should pills be crushed before being taken. A transdermal patch, also called a transdermal delivery system, provides for a more constant rate of medication absorption and eliminates concern for gastro-intestinal absorption variation, gastro-intestinal tolerance, and medication interaction. Transdermal delivery systems are not recommended for persons who are noticeably underweight because absorption is unpredictable owing to reduced body fat.

Several supports are available for the older adult who is self-administering medication. Pharmacists can prepare weekly doses of the required medication prepackaged in daily doses in easily opened containers, dossettes, or blister packs. Weekly calendars or tear-off daily calendars will remind the older adult to take daily medication. Clear envelopes or sandwich bags containing the medication can be affixed to the square on a calendar; each envelope or bag should state the medication's name, dose, and times it is to be taken that day. Commercial medication boxes are available for single or multiple doses by the day, week, or month, and some have medication administration alarms.

PSYCHOTROPIC MEDICATIONS

Psychotropic medications are those that alter brain chemistry, emotions, and behaviour. They include antipsychotics (formerly known as neuroleptics), antidepressants, mood stabilizers, anti-anxiety agents (anxiolytics), and sedative–hypnotic medications. This section provides an overview of psychotropic medications used to treat symptoms of disorders of behaviour, cognition, arousal, and mood in the gerontological population. This chapter also provides information on treating the movement disorders that may occur as a side effect of the use of antipsychotics.

Psychotropic Medication for Older Adults

Gerontological nurses, especially in LTC settings, are likely to care for older adults with mental health problems or cognitive impairment, especially depression, anxiety, and psychosis. The rate of depression for older adults aged 65 years or older living in the community is about 10% to 15%; the rate is up to 44% in LTC settings (Government of Canada, 2016). Treatment for depression and other mental health issues has both pharmacological and nonpharmacological components.

Psychotropic medications can alter some behaviours and emotions; these medications can be prescribed only after thorough medical, psychological, and social assessments. These assessments should be done quickly to enable the individual to receive the appropriate treatment as soon as possible. Pharmacological interventions need to be supplemented by nonpharmacological measures such as counselling. Nursing assessment before medication intervention contributes knowledge and baseline information that can optimize the patient's medical and psychological improvement. Issues to consider include the patient's medical status (and medications that might interact with psychotropics), mental status, ability to carry out activities of daily living and instrumental activities of daily living, and ability to participate in social activities and maintain satisfying relationships with others. Pharmacological treatment can include antidepressants, anti-anxiety medications or antipsychotics, or any combination of these medications.

Antidepressants

Antidepressants are medications used to treat depression. In the past, the major antidepressants were monoamine oxidase inhibitors (MAOIs) and TCAs, especially amitriptyline and doxepin (Sinequan). These medications had significant side effects, such as dry mouth, constipation, sedation, and urinary retention. The development of newer antidepression medications, such as selective serotonin reuptake inhibitors (SSRIs) and nonselective serotonin reuptake inhibitors (NSSRIs), has decreased the use of MAOIs and TCAs.

The SSRIs (e.g., Zoloft, Prozac) and NSSRIs are highly effective but have been implicated in serotonin syndrome, a potentially life-threatening ADR (Foong et al., 2018). Serotonin syndrome manifests as changes in autonomic function and mental status as well as other neurological findings within hours to one day of starting or increasing serotonergic medications (Foong et al., 2018). Taken in combination with St. John's wort (an herbal preparation taken for mild depression), SSRIs can also cause serotonin syndrome (Apaydin et al., 2016). Recognition and discontinuation of the causative medication is essential. Table 14.4 outlines the mild, moderate, and severe signs and symptoms of serotonin syndrome. Most SSRIs and NSSRIs cause

TABLE 14.4				
Signs and Symptoms of Serotonin Syndrome				
Severity	**Autonomic Symptoms**	**Neurological Symptoms**	**Mental Status**	**Other**
Mild	■ Afebrile or low-grade fever ■ Tachycardia ■ Mydriasis ■ Diaphoresis or shivering	■ Intermittent tremor ■ Akathisia ■ Myoclonus ■ Mild hyper-reflexia	■ Restlessness ■ Anxiety	
Moderate	■ Increased tachycardia ■ Fever (up to 41°C) ■ Diarrhea with hyperactive bowel sounds ■ Diaphoresis with normal skin colour	■ Hyper-reflexia ■ Inducible clonus ■ Ocular clonus (slow continuous lateral eye movements) ■ Myoclonus	■ Easily startled ■ Increased confusion ■ Agitation and hypervigilance	■ Rhabdomyolysis ■ Metabolic acidosis ■ Renal failure ■ Disseminated intravascular coagulopathy (secondary to hyperthermia)
Severe	■ Temperature often greater than 41°C (secondary to increased tone)	■ Increased muscle tone (lower limbs greater than upper limbs) ■ Spontaneous clonus ■ Substantial myoclonus or hyper-reflexia	■ Delirium ■ Coma	■ As above

Sources: Adapted from Botros, M., Wood, K., Negatu, Y., et al. (2016). Serotonin syndrome and critical care: A case report. *CHEST Journal,* *150*(4S), 384A–384A. doi:10.1016/j.chest.2016.08.397; Werneke, U., Jamshidi, F., Taylor, D. M., et al. (2016). Conundrums in neurology: Diagnosing serotonin syndrome—A meta-analysis of cases. *BMC Neurology, 16*(1), 97. doi:10.1186/s12883-016-0616-1.

initial problems with nausea or dry mouth. One side effect of the SSRIs that does not resolve with time is sexual dysfunction. The NSSRIs and other antidepressants, such as venlafaxine (Effexor), and trazodone (Desyrel), are less likely to cause this problem and may be preferred by older adults who are sexually active.

Many older adults experience a therapeutic effect and significant relief from depression at lower doses of SSRIs because of age-related changes that affect the metabolism of medication. More than one trial of a medication, as well as some time, is often needed to find the optimal dose. Nurses can help older adults and their support persons monitor target symptoms and advocate for continued dose adjustments or changes until relief is obtained (see Chapter 23).

Gradually tapering doses is recommended when discontinuing SSRIs, because withdrawal effects that are self-limiting yet uncomfortable and distressing can occur, especially when medications are abruptly discontinued (Ruhe et al., 2020). Discontinuation symptoms can include disequilibrium (e.g., dizziness, vertigo, ataxia), gastro-intestinal issues (e.g., nausea and vomiting), flulike symptoms (e.g., myalgia, fatigue), sensory disturbances (e.g., paresthesia), and sleep disturbances (e.g., insomnia, vivid dreams). Other psychological symptoms, such as anxiety and irritability, can occur (Ruhe et al., 2020). When discussing the possibility of starting SSRIs, nurses can educate and inform the person about the side effects and possible withdrawal symptoms. This information is important in helping the person understand that these symptoms could be normal and that the medication is not an addictive substance.

Anti-Anxiety Agents

Medications designed for the treatment of anxiety are referred to as anti-anxiety agents, or *anxiolytics*. The decision to treat anxiety pharmacologically is based on the degree to which the anxiety interferes with the person's ability to function and on the person's feelings of discomfort.

Anxiolytics include benzodiazepines, buspirone, and beta-blockers. Antihistamines, especially diphenhydramine (Benadryl), are often used but are not recommended owing to their anticholinergic effects. Antidepressants are usually the first-line pharmacological treatment for anxiety in older adults because of the risks associated with the use of benzodiazepines.

The most frequently used anxiolytic agents are the benzodiazepines. Older adults metabolize these medications slowly; thus, the medications remain in the bloodstream for long periods and can easily reach toxic levels. Adverse effects include drowsiness, dizziness, ataxia, mild cognitive deficits, and memory impairment. Signs of toxicity include excessive sedation, unsteady gait, confusion, disorientation, cognitive impairment, memory impairment, agitation, and wandering. Because these symptoms resemble those of dementia, people can easily be misdiagnosed once they start taking benzodiazepines. Benzodiazepines are highly addicting but are often prescribed because of their quick sedating effects for the highly anxious person. Because of the aforementioned problems, however, they should be avoided except in extreme cases.

Lorazepam (Ativan), when prescribed in very low doses and for short periods, appears to be the least problematic benzodiazepine. It has the shortest half-life of the benzodiazepines and no active metabolites. Buspirone, which is not a benzodiazepine, is a safer alternative. Although dizziness is a side effect, it is often dose related and resolves with time. Buspirone is best used for chronic anxiety and is not indicated for acute needs (see Chapter 23).

Antipsychotics

The term "psychosis" refers to a break with reality and may include **delusions, hallucinations,** and **thought disorders**. The person's behaviour is a response to this private reality—a reality that may be distressing and problematic for the person and those around them. Characteristically, psychosis occurs in schizophrenia as part of the typical presentation of the illness; however, some psychotic symptoms can also occur as part of mania, depression, some paranoid states, delirium, infection, and dementia.

Psychosis manifests as delusional beliefs, hallucinations, and thought disorders, which can cause extreme anxiety and bizarre behaviour. Antipsychotics, also known as neuroleptics, are medications used to treat psychotic symptoms. Older antipsychotics, referred to as *typical antipsychotics* or *first-generation antipsychotics*, include haloperidol, perphenazine, and chlorpromazine. The newer antipsychotics, referred to as *atypical antipsychotics* or *second-generation antipsychotics*, include risperidone, olanzapine, and quetiapine (Seroquel). When

antipsychotics are prescribed to older adults, the atypical antipsychotics should be the first-line treatment because they cause fewer side effects. However, haloperidol is the first-line treatment when antipsychotics are used in the treatment of delirium if there is no previous evidence of Parkinson's disease or Lewy body dementia (Grover & Avasthi, 2018).

Unfortunately, antipsychotics are often misused by caregivers and health care providers in an attempt to control disruptive behaviours; they are also used without a careful assessment of the underlying cause of the behaviours.

When used appropriately and cautiously for psychotic illnesses, antipsychotics can provide a person with relief. Medications with the lowest side effects profile and at the lowest dose possible should be prescribed. Prescribing and using antipsychotics for persons with dementia is never recommended as a first-line treatment; nonpharmacological approaches should be considered as first-line treatments, even in conjunction with antipsychotics if necessary (Kaminishi et al., 2019). In such a case, low doses, small increases in dose, and careful monitoring by an experienced nurse, nurse practitioner, or physician are necessary.

Although the atypical antipsychotics have a better side effect profile (e.g., fewer anticholinergic effects) than the typical antipsychotics, older adults who take them may experience side effects (Chacko et al., 2018). Some typical and atypical antipsychotics can cause orthostatic hypotension, thereby increasing the risk for falls. Anticholinergic effects are more likely with typical antipsychotics and are mild with atypical antipsychotics (except clozapine, which is strongly anticholinergic). Anticholinergic side effects include dry mouth, constipation, urinary retention, hypotension, and confusion. Careful nursing observation is essential for monitoring side effects and medication interactions whenever any of these medications is given.

Owing to the effects of antipsychotics on the thermoregulatory centre of the brain, persons who take antipsychotics cannot tolerate excess environmental heat. Even mild elevations of core temperature can result in liver damage known as *neuroleptic malignant syndrome* (NMS), a serious complication of taking antipsychotic medications. Owing to increased awareness and detection, mortality from NMS has been significantly reduced from 30% to less than 10% (Simon et al., 2020). When diagnosing NMS, the most common symptoms are exposure to a dopamine-blocking agent, severe muscle rigidity, and fever (Simon et al., 2020). Other symptoms include diaphoresis, dysphagia, tremors, incontinence, and tachycardia (Simon et al., 2020). Common laboratory test findings include elevated creatine kinase levels due to rhabdomyolysis and leukocytosis (Simon et al., 2020). The person taking antipsychotics must avoid or be protected from hyperthermia by staying in a cool environment, maintaining adequate hydration, being in a cool area when engaging in activity, and using a fan or taking a sponge bath should overheating occur. The person may or may not communicate their discomfort, so an assessment of body temperature is essential. Diuretics, coffee, alcohol, lithium, and uncontrolled diabetes decrease vascular volume, thereby decreasing the body's ability to sweat. Anticholinergics inhibit sweating and lead to further heat retention.

Movement Disorders

The most significant potential side effects of antipsychotics are movement disorders, also referred to as *extrapyramidal syndrome* (EPS) reactions—acute dystonia, akathisia, parkinsonian symptoms, and tardive dyskinesia. Although the risk of these side effects is lower with atypical antipsychotics, some people do experience these effects.

Acute Dystonia. An acute dystonic reaction is an abnormal involuntary movement consisting of a slow and continuous muscular contraction or spasm. Involuntary muscular contractions of the mouth, jaw, face, and neck are common. The jaw may lock (trismus), the tongue may roll back and block the throat, the neck may arch backward (opisthotonos), or the eyes may close or be fixed in one position. These effects often create a feeling of needing to look up constantly without the ability to lower the eyes. Dystonias can be painful and frightening. An acute dystonic reaction may occur hours or days after antipsychotic medication administration or dosage increases and may last for minutes to hours.

Caregivers or others who are unfamiliar with EPS reactions often become alarmed. Although frightening, acute dystonia is usually not dangerous and is quickly relieved by anticholinergic medication such as benztropine, trihexyphenidyl, or diphenhydramine (Benadryl). These medications should be readily available to treat dystonic reactions in persons who are taking antipsychotics.

Akathisia. *Akathisia* refers to the compulsion to be in motion. Akathisia may occur at any time during therapy. People who are diagnosed with akathisia report feeling restless, unable to be still, or an unrelenting desire to move. Often this symptom is mistaken for worsening psychosis instead of the ADR that it is. Pacing, aimless walking, fidgeting, shifting weight from one leg to the other, and marked restlessness are characteristic behaviours for a person experiencing akathisia.

Parkinsonian Symptoms. The use of antipsychotics may cause symptoms that mimic Parkinson's disease. A bilateral tremor (as opposed to the unilateral tremor characteristic of true Parkinson's disease), bradykinesia, and rigidity that may progress to the inability to move may be observed. The person may have an inflexible facial expression and appear bored and apathetic and be mistakenly diagnosed as depressed. More common when higher-potency typical antipsychotics are given, parkinsonian symptoms may occur within weeks to months of the initiation of antipsychotic therapy.

Tardive Dyskinesia. People who have used antipsychotics continuously for at least 3 to 6 months are at risk for developing an irreversible movement disorder called *tardive dyskinesia* (TD). The risk of TD is considerably lower with the use of atypical antipsychotics. It usually appears first as wormlike movements of the tongue; grimacing, blinking, and frowning are other facial movements that occur. Slow, maintained, involuntary twisting movements of the limbs, trunk, neck, face, and eyes (involuntary eye closure) have been observed. It is essential that nurses be attentive for early detection so that changes to the psychotropic regimen can be made promptly.

Response to treatment is the most important consideration when psychotropics are taken. The person's subjective comments about feelings and symptoms and caregivers' observations of the person's behaviour are important data for evaluating the effectiveness of a medication.

Mood Stabilizers

Mood stabilizers are agents used for the treatment of bipolar disorders (formerly known as manic depression), which are characterized by periods of mania or hypomania and periods of depression affecting the person's functioning. The symptoms of mania are euphoria (elation), disinhibition, impulsivity, distractibility, grandiosity, labile affect, pressured speech and flight of ideas, increased psychomotor activity, irritability that can result in anger, and decreased need for sleep. Hypomania, which is less extreme, is characterized by the same symptoms, but they last for a shorter time than they do in mania and do not markedly impair the person's functioning. For the older adult, the symptoms of bipolar disorders are easily confused with the symptoms of moderate dementia (e.g., wandering, emotional lability) (see Chapter 23).

Lithium carbonate (Lithium), divalproex sodium (Epival), and carbamazepine (Tegretol) are mood-stabilizing medications. When a person who has bipolar disorder or who is taking a mood stabilizer is being cared for, guidance from a psychiatrist is required. It is important to monitor patients who are taking lithium, as this medication interacts with other medications and certain foods. Lithium has a narrow therapeutic window, and toxicity can develop quickly. A low-salt diet will elevate serum lithium, and a high-salt diet will decrease it. Likewise, thiazide diuretics and non-steroidal anti-inflammatory medications will elevate serum lithium. The side effects of lithium include fine resting tremor, fatigue, polyuria, and polydipsia. Nausea, vomiting, diarrhea, vertigo, muscle weakness, and sleepiness may occur when the medication is initiated, but these symptoms resolve. Symptoms of toxicity include gastro-intestinal symptoms, drowsiness, ataxia, tinnitus, blurred vision, confusion, muscle twitching, hyper-reflexia, and seizures; eventually, coma and death occur.

SUMMARY

This chapter reviewed age-related pharmacokinetic changes, medication compliance, and the use of psychotropic medications in the older population. All medications have indications, side effects, and interactions, as well as individual reactions. The nurse's advocacy role includes educating the older adult and the family and determining whether the side effects are minimal and tolerable or whether they are serious. Asking the person about their experience and observing interactions, behaviour, mood, emotional responses, and daily habits provide data to delineate the problem, develop nursing diagnoses and interventions, and decide outcome criteria.

Medications occupy a central place in the lives of many older adults; cost, acceptability, interactions, unacceptable side effects, and the need to schedule medications appropriately all combine to create many difficulties. Nurses need to have a strong understanding of issues specific to the safe administration and consumption of medications in the older population in order to reduce the use of inappropriate medications and prevent or treat side effects and interactions. The nurse might also increase compliance through providing personally and culturally appropriate instructions.

Nurses in all health care settings are responsible for monitoring the overall health of older adults, being alert to the need for laboratory tests, and other measures to ensure the correct dosage of several medications. Nurses are often the first care providers to assess medication use, evaluate outcomes, and teach older adults about safe medication use and self-administration.

KEY CONCEPTS

- The aging body responds to medication changes.
- Any medication has side effects. The therapeutic goal is to reduce the targeted symptoms without undesirable side effects.
- The likelihood of medication–medication and medication–food incompatibilities increases with aging.
- Polypharmacy is of serious concern for older adults.
- Medication misuse may be triggered by prescriber practices, individual self-medication and physiology, altered biodegradability, nutritional and fluid states, and inadequate assessment before prescribing.
- Nurses must consider the occurrence of a possible medication side effect immediately if they observe changes in the person's condition, including functional changes and changes in cognitive status.

- Chronotherapy uses the biorhythms of the body to ensure the most effective medication therapy; it has the potential to decrease the dose, frequency, and cost of medication regimens and to improve compliance with medication therapy.
- The side effects of psychotropic medications vary significantly; thus, great care must be taken when selecting and prescribing these medications for the older adult.
- The responses of the older adult to treatment with psychotropic medications should be reduced distress, clearer thinking, and more appropriate behaviour.
- Older adults are particularly vulnerable to developing movement disorders with the use of antipsychotics.
- Any time a behavioural change in a person is noted, reversible causes must be sought and treated before medications are used.
- Dosages of medications must be carefully titrated for the individual, and the individual's responses must be accurately and consistently recorded.

ACTIVITIES AND DISCUSSION QUESTIONS

1. Describe the age-related changes that occur in the pharmacokinetics of the older adult.

2. Explain the meaning of "chronotherapeutics." How applicable is chronotherapeutics to older adults?

3. Describe the medication use patterns of the older population. What can be done to correct or improve them?

4. Explain the role of the older adult, the care provider, and the social network in medication compliance.

5. List a variety of measures that nurses can suggest to assist older adults with their medication use and compliance with their medication regimen.

6. List the most troublesome side effects of antipsychotic medications.

7. Describe what you would do to manage the following situation: Mrs. J. is calling out repeatedly for a nurse; although other patients are complaining, you simply cannot be available for long periods to quiet her.

8. Review the medications taken by an older adult in the clinical setting. Use the Beers Criteria for Potentially Inappropriate Medication Use in Older Adults to determine whether any of the medications are potentially contraindicated. Discuss your findings.

RESOURCES

2019 American Geriatrics Society Updated Beers Criteria for Potentially Inappropriate Medication Use in Older Adults
https://hign.org/consultgeri/try-this-series/2019-american-geriatrics-society-updated-beers-criteria-r-potentially

Alzheimer's Association. *Medications for memory, cognition, and dementia-related behaviours.*
https://www.alz.org/alzheimers-dementia/treatments/medications-for-memory

Canadian Coalition for Seniors' Mental Health. *Guidelines on the assessment and treatment of depression, delirium, dementia, and suicide risk in older adults.*
http://www.ccsmh.ca

Canadian Patient Safety Institute. *Medication safety.*
https://www.patientsafetyinstitute.ca/en/Topic/Pages/Improving-Medication-Safety.aspx

Government of Canada. *Medication matters: How you can help seniors use medication safely.*
http://publications.gc.ca/site/eng/9.646877/publication.html

Government of Canada. *Sleeping pills and tranquilizers: Important information for seniors.*
http://publications.gc.ca/site/eng/112429/publication.html

Institute for Safe Medication Practices
http://www.ismp.org/about/default.aspx

Institution for Safe Medication Practices Canada (ISMP Canada). *Medication reconciliation in acute care: Getting started kit.*
https://www.ismp-canada.org/download/MedRec/Medrec_AC_English_GSK_V3.pdf

For additional resources, please visit *http://evolve.elsevier.com/Canada/Ebersole/gerontological/*

REFERENCES

Apaydin, E. A., Maher, A. R., Shanman, R., et al. (2016). A systematic review of St. John's Wort for major depressive disorder. *Systematic Reviews, 5*(1), 148. doi:10.1186/s13643-016-0325-2.

Ased, S., Wells, J., Morrow, L. E., et al. (2018). Clinically significant food–drug interactions. *Consultant Pharmacist, 33*(11), 649–657. doi:10.4140/TCP.n.2018.649.

Baruth, J. M., Gentry, M. T., Rummans, T. A., et al. (2020). Polypharmacy in older adults: The role of the multidisciplinary team. *Hospital Practice, 48*(Suppl. 1), 56–62. doi:10.1080/21548331.2019.1706995.

Beers, M. H. (1997). Explicit criteria for determining potentially inappropriate medication use by the elderly: An update. *Archives of Internal Medicine, 157*(14), 1531–1536.

Bernier, N. F. (2017). *Improving prescription drug safety for Canadian seniors.* http://irpp.org/wp-content/uploads/2017/01/study-no61.pdf.

Briggs, G. C. (2005). Geriatric issues. In E. Youngkin, K. J. Sawin, J. Kissinger, et al. (Eds.), *Pharmacotherapeutics: A primary care clinical guide* (pp. 189–194). Prentice-Hall.

Brown, P. (2017). Osteoporosis and fracture prevention in primary care. In A. Connolly & A. Britton (Eds.), *Women's health in primary care* (pp. 230–241). Cambridge University Press.

Çakmur, H. (2018). Circadian rhythm and chronobiology. In M. A. El-Esawi (Ed.), *Circadian rhythm: Cellular and molecular mechanisms.* doi:10.5772/intechopen.75928.

Canadian Centre on Substance Use and Addiction. (2020). *A guide to cannabis for older adults.* https://www.ccsa.ca/guide-cannabis-older-adults.

Canadian Coalition for Seniors' Mental Health. (2020). *Benzodiazepine use among older adults.* https://ccsmh.ca/wp-content/uploads/2020/04/FINAL_CCSMH_BZRA_brochure_ENG.pdf.

Canadian Gerontological Nursing Association. (2020). *Gerontological nursing standards of practice and competencies* (4th ed.). https://cgna.net/standards.

Canadian Institute for Health Information (CIHI). (2018). *Drug use among seniors in Canada, 2016.* https://www.cihi.ca/sites/default/files/document/drug-use-among-seniors-2016-en-web.pdf.

Canadian Patient Safety Institute. (2020). *Getting started kit: Medication reconciliation.* https://www.patientsafetyinstitute.ca/en/toolsResources/pages/med-rec-resources-getting-started-kit.aspx.

Chacko, E., Boyd, S., & Murphy, R. (2018). Metabolic side effects of atypical antipsychotics in older adults. *International Psychogeriatrics, 30*(10), 1557–1566. doi:10.1017/S1041610218000273.

Chan, B. S., Cheng, S., Isoardi, K. Z., et al. (2020). Effect of age on the severity of chronic lithium poisoning. *Clinical Toxicology (Philadelphia, Pa.), 58*, 1023–1027. doi:10.1080/15563650.2020.1726376.

Di Minno, A., Frigerio, B., Spadarella, G., et al. (2017). Old and new oral anticoagulants: Food, herbal medicines and drug interactions. *Blood Reviews, 31*(4), 193–203. doi:10.1016/j.blre.2017.02.001.

Fisher, K., Markle-Reid, M., Ploeg, J., et al. (2020). Self-management program versus usual care for community-dwelling older adults with multimorbidity: A pragmatic randomized controlled trial in Ontario, Canada. *Journal of Comorbidity, 10*, 1–18. doi:10.1177/2235042X20963390.

Foong, A. L., Grindrod, K. A., Patel, T., et al. (2018). Demystifying serotonin syndrome (or serotonin toxicity). *Canadian Family Physician, 64*(10), 720–727.

Gauer, R., & Meyers, B. K. (2019). Heat-related illnesses. *American Family Physician, 99*(8), 482–489.

Government of Canada. (2016). *Report on the social isolation of seniors.* https://www.canada.ca/en/national-seniors-council/programs/publications-reports/2014/social-isolation-seniors/page05.html.

Government of Canada. (2018). *Information for health care professionals: Cannabis (marihuana, marijuana) and the cannabinoids.* https://www.canada.ca/en/health-canada/services/drugs-medication/cannabis/information-medical-practitioners/information-health-care-professionals-cannabis-cannabinoids.html#a4.7.1.

Government of Canada. (2019). *Cannabis legalization and regulation.* https://www.justice.gc.ca/eng/cj-jp/cannabis/.

Greenblatt, D. J., Harmatz, J. S., & Shader, R. I. (2020). Diazepam in the elderly: Looking back, ahead, and at the evidence. *Journal of Clinical Psychopharmacology, 40*(3), 215–219. doi:10.1097/JCP.0000000000001213.

Groden, S. R., Woodward, A. T., Chatters, L. M., et al. (2017). Use of complementary and alternative medicine among older adults: Differences between baby boomers and pre-boomers. *American Journal of Geriatric Psychiatry, 25*(12), 1393–1401. doi:10.1016/j.jagp.2017.08.001.

Grover, S., & Avasthi, A. (2018). Clinical practice guidelines for management of delirium in elderly. *Indian Journal of Psychiatry, 60*(Suppl. 3): S329–S340. doi:10.4103/0019-5545.224473.

Guillot, J., Maumus-Robert, S., & Bezin, J. (2019). Polypharmacy: A general review of definitions, descriptions and determinants. *Therapie, 75*, 407–416. doi:10.1016/j.therap.2019.10.001.

Hinton, A. N., & Goldminz, A. M. (2020). Feeling the burn: Phototoxicity and photoallergy. *Dermatologic Clinics, 38*(1), 165–175. doi:10.1016/j.det.2019.08.010.

Jennings, E., Gallagher, P., & O'Mahony, D. (2019). Detection and prevention of adverse drug reactions in multi-morbid older patients. *Age and Ageing, 48*(1), 10–13. https://doi.org/10.1093/ageing/afy157.

Jiang, L., Ke, M., Yue, S., et al. (2017). Blockade of Notch signaling promotes acetaminophen-induced liver injury. *Immunologic Research, 65*(3), 739–749. doi:10.1007/s12026-017-8913-3.

Kaminishi, K., Sutherland, E., Youngblood, E., et al. (2019). Challenging behaviors on inpatient medical units: Integrated, non-pharmacological approach for patients with dementia. *American Journal of Geriatric Psychiatry, 27*(3), S131–S133. doi:10.1016/j.jagp.2019.01.084.

Kim, J., & Parish, A. L. (2017). Polypharmacy and medication management in older adults. *Nursing Clinics, 52*(3), 457–468. doi:10.1016/j.cnur.2017.04.007.

Lei, L. Y., Chew, D. S., & Raj, S. R. (2020). Differential diagnosis of orthostatic hypotension. *Autonomic Neuroscience: Basic & Clinical, 228*, 102713. doi:10.1016/j.autneu.2020.102713.

Maher, D., Ailabouni, N., Mangoni, A. A., et al. (2020). Alterations in drug disposition in older adults: A focus on geriatric syndromes. *Expert Opinion on Drug Metabolism & Toxicology, 17*, 41–52. doi:10.1080/17425255.2021.1839413.

Morgan, S. G., Hunt, J., Rioux, J., et al. (2016). Frequency and cost of potentially inappropriate prescribing for older adults: A cross-sectional study. *Canadian Medical Association Journal, 4*(2), E346–E351. doi:10.9778/cmajo.20150131.

Morin, L., Laroche, M. L., Texier, G., et al. (2016). Prevalence of potentially inappropriate medication use in older adults living in nursing homes: A systematic review. *Journal of the American Medical Directors Association*, *17*(9), 862.e1. doi:10.1016/j.jamda.2016.06.011.

Noori, S. A., & Mehta, N. (2019). Anticoagulation. In A. Abd-Elsayed (Ed.), *Pain* (pp. 435–442). Springer.

Pannu, T., Sharkey, S., Burek, G., et al. (2017). Medication use by middle-aged and older participants of an exercise study: Results from the Brain in Motion study. *BMC Complementary and Alternative Medicine*, *17*(1), 105. doi:10.1186/s12906-017-1595-5.

Petrovic, M., Somers, A., Marien, S., et al. (2019). Optimization of drug use in older people: A key factor for a successful aging. In Fernandez-Ballesteros, R., Benetos, A., & Robine, M. (Eds.), *The Cambridge handbook of successful aging* (pp. 237–262). Cambridge: Cambridge University Press.

Ruhe, H. G., Horikx, A., van Avendonk, M. J. P., et al. (2020). Het afbouwen van SSRI's en SNRI's [Discontinuation of SSRIs and SNRIs]. *Nederlands Tijdschrift Voor Geneeskunde*, *164*, D4004.

Simon, L.V., Hashmi, M. F., & Callahan, A. L. (2020). *Neuroleptic malignant syndrome*. StatPearls. https://www.ncbi.nlm.nih.gov/books/NBK482282/.

The University of British Columbia. (2018). How well do you know your anticholinergic (antimuscarinic) drugs? *Therapeutics Letter*, *113*. https://www.ti.ubc.ca/wordpress/wp-content/uploads/2018/09/113.pdf.

Wilcox, S. M., Himmelstein, D. U., & Woolhandler, S. (1994). Inappropriate drug prescribing for the community-dwelling elderly. *Journal of the American Medical Association*, *272*(4), 292–296. http://www.citizen.org/documents/1343.pdf.

15

LIVING WITH CHRONIC ILLNESS

LEARNING OBJECTIVES

Upon completion of this chapter, the reader will be able to:

- Define chronic illness and explain the differences between chronic illness and acute illness.
- Explain the concept of wellness in chronic illness.
- Discuss explanatory models of chronic illness.
- Discuss the factors that influence the experience of chronic illness.
- Explain strategies that have been used successfully to maintain maximal function and increase an individual's ability for self-care.
- Discuss nursing interventions to maximize wellness in the presence of chronic illness.

GLOSSARY

Care coordination   An approach to health care in which all of a person's needs are coordinated with the assistance of a primary point of contact to make sure that the person gets the most appropriate treatment.

Case management   The coordination of services on behalf of the patient or resident to ensure that the appropriate care is provided.

Exacerbation   Worsening; in medicine, the term may refer to an increase in the severity of a disease or its signs and symptoms.

Exorbitant   Exceeding that which is usual or proper.

Frailty   A clinically recognizable state of increased vulnerability.

Iatrogenesis   A complication or side effect of the health care intervention, advice given, or the environment itself.

Trajectory   The path followed by a body or an event moved along by the action of certain forces.

THE LIVED EXPERIENCE

"Because you understand my disease, you don't understand me. To understand that I am ill does not mean that you understand how I experience my illness. I am unique. I think and feel and behave in a combination that is unique to me. You do not understand me because you have a label for my disease or a plan for my treatment. It is not my disease or treatment that you need to understand. It is me."
(Jevne, 1993, p. 121)

CHRONIC ILLNESS

Chronic illnesses are "conditions that last a year or more and require ongoing medical attention and/or limit activities of daily living" (Centers for Disease Control and Prevention [CDC], 2019). From a nursing perspective, chronic illness has no quick fix (Eastern Michigan University, 2018). Chronic illnesses often require ongoing treatments over time. Regular check-ups are required to keep the illness from becoming life threatening (Eastern Michigan University, 2018).

The rising prevalence and associated costs of chronic illness are a global health concern. Chronic illness accounts for over half of the global health burden (World Health Organization [WHO], 2021). Noncommunicable diseases (NCDs) are collectively responsible for 71% of all deaths and over 80% of all NCD-related deaths worldwide (WHO, 2021). In Canada, it is estimated that up to 60% of older adults living in the community have two or more chronic conditions (Canadian Institute for Health Information [CIHI], 2016; Mokraoui et al., 2016). A host of social determinants—especially education, income, gender, and ethnicity—influence levels of chronic illness (WHO, 2021). Chronic illnesses also exact significant personal costs and burdens owing to a diminished quality of life for both the individual and their family and significant others. This chapter discusses chronic illness and its implications for gerontological nursing and healthy aging. (For information on specific chronic illnesses, see Chapters 16 through 22.)

Chronic Illness and Aging

Although new cases of chronic illnesses have decreased, older adults are still disproportionately affected (Public Health Agency of Canada, 2019). The life expectancy of Canadians continues to rise and has now reached 79.8 years for men and 83.9 years for women (Statistics Canada, 2018). Unfortunately, a longer life often means living longer with a chronic illness, especially for women, whose life expectancy is longer. Illnesses such as cancer, Alzheimer's disease, and diabetes; mental health challenges; and human immunodeficiency virus (HIV) and acquired immunodeficiency syndrome (AIDS) are becoming chronic illnesses with which people will live for extended periods.

Chronic illnesses are common among older adults in Canada. Approximately one-quarter (24%) of Canadian older adults reported having received a diagnosis of three or more chronic conditions (multimorbidity) (CIHI, 2011). By the time a person has lived 50 years, they are likely to have at least one chronic condition. The most common chronic conditions for Canadians aged 65 years and older are high blood pressure (47%) and arthritis (27%) (CIHI, 2011). Those conditions also accounted for the three most common combinations of chronic conditions in older adults—14% had both high blood pressure and arthritis; 12% had both high blood pressure and heart disease; and 11% had both high blood pressure and diabetes (CIHI, 2011). Chronic illnesses in older adults can be categorized as follows:

1. Nonfatal chronic illness—conditions such as osteoarthritis or hearing or vision impairments. These conditions contribute to disability and increased health care costs, but most individuals can live with them for many years.
2. Serious, potentially fatal chronic conditions—cancers, organ system failures, dementia, and stroke.

3. Frailty—a condition in which the body has few reserves left and in which any disturbance can cause multiple health conditions and costs (Kojima et al., 2019).

For the older adult, having a chronic illness is not as important as its effect on functioning. The effect may be as little as an inconvenience or as great as an impairment of a person's ability to perform activities of daily living (ADLs) or instrumental activities of daily living (IADLs). Limitations in the ability to perform ADLs and IADLs occur more frequently among individuals over the age of 75 years, but recent trends show that the disability rate among older adults has declined and that the incidence of long-term disability has dropped dramatically (http://www.statcan.gc.ca). However, the health disparities that exist for many members of minority groups can reduce these gains (Ng et al., 2019) (see Chapter 4).

Acute Versus Chronic Illness

Chronic disorders and acute illnesses cannot really be separated because many conditions are intricately intertwined. Some acute disorders have chronic sequelae, and many commonly identified chronic disorders tend to intermittently flare up into acute problems and then move back into remission. Acute illnesses are those that occur suddenly, often without warning (e.g., stroke, myocardial infarction, hip fracture, or infection), and show signs and symptoms related to the disease process. These illnesses are usually treated aggressively and end in a relatively short time. Acute problems in later life can quickly cause death; at other times, the sequelae of the acute episode constitute a new or exacerbated chronic condition.

A chronic illness, on the other hand, continues indefinitely, is managed rather than cured, and requires the person to learn to live with the condition (Boscart et al., 2020). If not triggered by an acute event, the onset of a chronic illness may be insidious and identified only during a health screening. Symptoms of the effects of the illness or condition, including disabilities, may not appear for years. For example, a person with hypertension can develop enough heart damage to cause an acute episode of heart failure years later.

A person with a chronic illness may have episodic **exacerbation**, or the illness may remain in remission, with no symptoms for a long period of time (Touhy et al., 2018). People with chronic illness often continue to work and perform their usual activities early in their disease. Later, and with increasing age or frailty, the effects of the limitations increase. Many older adults have several chronic disorders simultaneously (i.e., comorbidities) and have great difficulty managing the complexity of overlapping and often contradictory demands. Symptoms of chronic illness can interfere with many regular activities and routines, require medical regimens, disrupt patterns of living, and frequently make it necessary for the person to make significant lifestyle changes. Physical suffering, loss, worry, grief, depression, functional impairment, and increased dependence on family or friends for support are among the negative consequences of chronic illness (Nierenberg et al., 2016; Warner et al., 2017). One of the greatest fears of older adults is the fear of being dependent on others as a result of chronic illness (Morse et al., 2021).

Frailty Syndrome

Frailty is an independent geriatric syndrome that may be seen in older adults with multiple comorbidities. It is "a clinically recognizable state in which the ability of older adults to cope with everyday or acute stressors is compromised by an increased vulnerability brought by age-associated declines in physiological reserve and function across multiple organ systems" (WHO, 2017). Frailty includes both physical and mental decline and leads to an increased risk for morbidity and mortality (Sieber, 2017). Frailty has also been linked to acute illness, falls, and hospitalization (Sieber, 2017).

Seven percent of older adults are classified as frail; however, the prevalence of frailty increases up to 40% in persons aged 80 years and older. With the dramatic increase in the "oldest old" population, frailty is becoming common (Chinda et al., 2019). Other factors associated with frailty include being female, living below poverty status, having less education, having a greater body mass index, and taking more than six prescription medications (Griffin et al., 2018).

Factors responsible for the pathogenesis of frailty include sarcopenia and related metabolic pathogenic factors, atherosclerosis, cognitive impairment, and malnutrition (Umegaki, 2016). Weight loss, fatigue, muscle weakness, slow or unsteady gait, and declines in activity are signs and symptoms of frailty (Sieber, 2017).

Frailty often goes unnoticed, as the symptoms are attributed to the aging process. Frailty can be assessed by using the Clinical Frailty Scale (accessed at the website listed in the Resources at the end of this chapter). The identification of frailty during an early stage is important because specific interventions may prevent functional decline and other negative consequences. Interventions are aimed at maintaining homeostatic balance. They focus on resistance and balance exercises; nutritional support; treatment of depression, delirium, diabetes, osteoporosis, and hypertension; appropriate social support; aggressive treatment of pain; and treatment of early cognitive impairment (Zengarini & Cherubini, 2019).

PREVENTION OF CHRONIC ILLNESS

Research has shown that chronic illness and poor health are not inevitable consequences of aging. Many chronic illnesses are preventable through lifestyle choices or early detection and management of risk factors. Yet much remains to be learned about the distribution, risk factors, and effective measures to prevent or delay the onset of certain chronic conditions. Some of these conditions can be managed with improved diet, exercise, medical treatment, or a combination of these. Health promotion activities and attention to healthy lifestyle habits can postpone and reduce morbidity for older adults. Key strategies for improving the health of older adults are presented in Box 15.1.

The common modifiable risk factors for most chronic illnesses are poor diet, inactivity, and smoking (Cancer Care Ontario & Public Health Ontario, 2019). Public health efforts have traditionally focused on physical health, but health also includes mental health. The promotion of cognitive health is an emerging public health priority and an essential feature of health-related quality of life (see Chapter 21). Public health efforts can help individuals avoid preventable illness and disability as they age. These efforts include the increased use of preventive health strategies and improved approaches to effectively treating health problems for all persons, regardless of age, ethnicity, or income. As a result of these efforts, older adults have the potential to live longer and in better health. A focus on healthy aging requires nurses to implement health promotion and disease prevention activities.

BOX 15.1

KEY STRATEGIES FOR IMPROVING THE HEALTH OF OLDER ADULTS

1. Promote the awareness of and access to information on existing services and supports available to older adults.
2. Promote the importance of collaborations to address the identified needs of older adults across rural, urban, and northern locations.
3. Support planning to create environments supportive of mobility by identifying potential barriers and risks prior to and during planning.
4. Support multi-sectoral collaboration to identify opportunities to enhance physical activity and mobility.
5. Identify and promote strategies that address diversity of experiences.
6. Develop a framework to measure, monitor, and report on interventions that support rural healthy aging in place.

Source: Adapted from Saskatchewan Population Health and Evaluation Research Unit. (2018). *An overview of healthy aging strategies in rural and urban Canada.* https://spheru.ca/publications/files/Healthy%20Aging%20Enviro%20Scan%20Report%20June%202018%20FINAL%2026-Sep-2018.pdf.

BOX 15.2

COMPETENCIES TO IMPROVE CARE FOR CHRONIC CONDITIONS

1. Patient-centred care
   - Interviewing and communicating effectively
   - Assisting changes in health-related behaviours
   - Supporting self-management
   - Using a proactive approach
2. Partnering
   - Partnering with patients
   - Partnering with other providers
   - Partnering with communities
3. Quality improvement
   - Measuring care delivery and outcomes
   - Adapting to change
   - Translating evidence into practice
4. Information and communication technology
   - Designing and using patient registries
   - Using electronic patient records
   - Using computer technologies
   - Communicating with partners
5. Public health perspective
   - Providing population-based care
   - Thinking in terms of systems
   - Working across the care continuum
   - Working in primary health care–led systems

Source: Data from World Health Organization. (2005). *Preparing a health care workforce for the 21st century: The challenge of chronic conditions.* http://www.who.int/chp/knowledge/publications/workforce_report.pdf.

Care Delivery System

The current health care system, with its focus on immediate medical needs to manage acute events (such as accidents, severe injury, and sudden bouts of illness), does not meet the needs of individuals with chronic illness, nor does it support health promotion and disease prevention. Each component of the health care system views the person from its own narrow window of care. No single entity, practice, organization, or agency is managing the entire disease, and certainly none is managing the illness experience of the person and family. Health insurance coverage for preventive health care services and rehabilitation, long-term care, and home care needed by persons with chronic illnesses is often limited. (See Chapters 24 and 28 for a discussion of health care costs and funding for older adults, as well as transitions in care across the continuum.)

In addition to the previously mentioned challenges, health care providers sometimes lack the knowledge, awareness, and skills to care for the growing numbers of people with chronic illnesses. Most education programs for health care workers focus on episodic care in acute care settings (Fazio et al., 2016). The WHO (2005) report *Preparing a Health Care Workforce for the 21st Century: The Challenge of Chronic Conditions* presents a training model and competencies for all health care workers for the care of people with chronic illness (Box 15.2).

THEORETICAL FRAMEWORKS FOR CHRONIC ILLNESS

Several theoretical frameworks—including the Chronic Illness Trajectory (Strauss & Glaser, 1975; Corbin & Strauss, 1988; Woog, 1992) and the Shifting Perspectives Model of Chronic Illness (Paterson, 2001)—have been used to understand the effect of chronic illness on wellness and to organize nurses' responses in order to help persons with chronic illness. First, however, it is crucial that nurses caring for older adults with chronic illness have a good understanding of wellness.

Wellness in Chronic Illness

A person's feeling of wellness is important when they are living with chronic illness. "Wellness in chronic illness" suggests that the person has an optimal level of functioning for achieving well-being and a good and satisfactory existence. Even for people who have a chronic illness or are dying, an optimum level of wellness and well-being should be strived for.

Nurses working within a wellness model or approach focus on moving in a positive direction instead of a downward negative trajectory and the deterioration of the person's health. The older adult may reach plateaus in their ascension to a higher level of wellness. The person may also regress because of an illness event, but the event can also be a stimulus for growth and a return to moving up the wellness continuum (see Chapter 1). Wellness is not a given; rather, it is a state of being and feeling that one strives to achieve through motivation and health practices.

The greatest factor in establishing wellness is adaptation. The maximization of life satisfaction requires an adaptation of lifestyle. The results of a qualitative study that explored the perceptions of nurses, older adults, and families about living with a chronic illness in the community offered insight into the complexity of their lives and adaptation (Ploeg et al., 2017). Participants spoke about the complexity of their experience of chronic illness and multi-comorbidity, which included physical conditions and psychological conditions such as depression and anxiety; about the impacts of these conditions on the physical, psychological, and social domains of health; about managing many different medications for multiple conditions; about seeing numerous health and social care providers; and about health-related crises that led to transitions to and from the acute care sector. Participants described how they had to accept the realities of gradual health decline and set realistic goals. One older adult explained, "I've adapted to it as it's happened . . . it's been a gradual thing. You know, you get this problem and then you get this problem and then you have another problem and . . . I've just dealt with it" (Ploeg et al., 2017). Building on the courage of older adults who are coping with

chronic illnesses, disabilities, and other challenges is a good starting point for gerontological nurses.

Some wellness strategies include helping those who are living with a chronic illness to remain active, independent, and involved in their community as long as possible; providing resources to help care partners stay healthy and deliver quality care to their care recipients; increasing early assessment and diagnosis, risk reduction, and prevention and management of chronic diseases; and promoting physical activity programs to reduce the risk of dementia, arthritis pain, and falls (CDC, 2020).

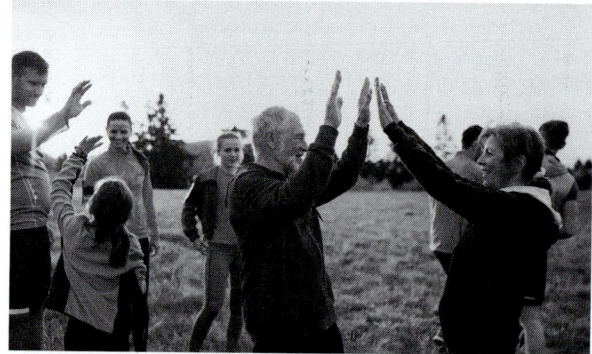

Staying active in later life can aid in the prevention and management of chronic illnesses. © Can Stock Photo / halfpoint.

Chronic Illness Trajectory

The **trajectory** model of chronic illness, conceptualized by Strauss and Glaser (1975), has long helped health care providers better understand the realities of chronic illness. Corbin and Strauss (1988) viewed the course of chronic illness as being on a trajectory that moved forward through eight phases: a preventive phase (pretrajectory), a definitive phase (trajectory onset), a crisis phase, an acute phase, a stable phase, an unstable phase, a downward phase, and a dying phase (Table 15.1). The shape and stability of the trajectory is influenced by the combined efforts, attitudes, and beliefs held by the person, family members, significant others, and the involved health care providers. The key points of the model are based on the theoretical assumptions listed in Box 15.3. The person's perceptions of needs that are met and basic biological functional limitations are paramount to predicting the person's movement along the illness trajectory (Corbin & Strauss, 1992).

TABLE 15.1
The Chronic Illness Trajectory: Definitions of Phases and Goals

Phase	Definition
1. Pretrajectory	Before the illness course begins; the preventive phase; no signs or symptoms present
2. Trajectory onset	Signs and symptoms are present; includes diagnostic period
3. Crisis	Life-threatening situation
4. Acute	Active illness or complications that require hospitalization
5. Stable	Illness course—symptoms controlled by regimen
6. Unstable	Illness course—symptoms not controlled by regimen but not requiring hospitalization
7. Downward	Progressive deterioration of physical status, mental status, or both, characterized by increasing disability, symptoms, or both
8. Dying	Immediate weeks, days, and hours preceding death

Examples of Goals That Nurses Might Establish

1. To assist the person in overcoming a plateau during a comeback phase, by increasing the person's compliance with a regimen so that they might reach the highest level of functional ability possible within limits of the disability.

2. To assist a person in making the attitudinal and lifestyle changes needed to promote health and prevent disease.

3. To assist a person who is in a downward trajectory to make the adjustments and readjustments in everyday activities that are necessary to adapt to increasing physical deterioration.

4. To assist the person in an unstable phase to gain greater control over symptoms that are interfering with their ability to carry out everyday activities.

5. To assist a person in maintaining illness stability by finding a way to blend illness management activities with everyday life activities. Goals can be broken down into specific person-oriented objectives. Built into the objectives are the criteria that will be used to evaluate the effectiveness of each intervention.

Source: Woog, P. (1992). *Chronic illness trajectory framework: The Corbin and Strauss nursing model.* Springer.

BOX 15.3
KEY POINTS IN THE CHRONIC ILLNESS TRAJECTORY FRAMEWORK

- The majority of health problems in late life are chronic.
- Chronic illnesses may be lifelong and entail lifestyle adaptations.
- Chronic illness and its management often profoundly affect the lives and identities of both the person and the person's family or significant others.
- The management of the acute phase of illness is designed to stabilize physiological processes and promote a recovery (comeback) from the acute phase.

- The management of other phases of illness is designed primarily to maximize and extend the period of stability in the home, helped by family members and augmented by visits to and from health care providers.
- Maintaining stable phases is central to the work of managing chronic illness.
- The primary care nurse is often the coordinator of the numerous resources that may be needed to promote quality of life along the trajectory.

The Shifting Perspectives Model of Chronic Illness

The Chronic Illness Trajectory model just described views living with a chronic illness as a progression of phases that follow a predictable trajectory. The Shifting Perspectives Model of Chronic Illness (Paterson, 2001), derived from a synthesis of qualitative research findings, views living with chronic illness as an ongoing, continually shifting process in which the person moves between the perspectives of wellness in the foreground and illness in the foreground.

The Shifting Perspectives Model is more reflective of an "insider" perspective on chronics illness, as opposed to the more traditional "outsider" view. The model also changes the traditional view of the patient—from seeing the patient as a client to seeing them as a partner in care—and focuses on health within illness rather than on loss and burden (Larsen et al., 2006). People's perspectives on their chronic illnesses are neither right nor wrong but rather reflect their needs and situations. How people perceive the chronic illness at any given time influences how they interpret and respond to the disease, to themselves, to caregivers, and to situations affected by the illness (Paterson, 2001).

Chronic illness contains elements of both illness and wellness, and people with chronic illness live in the "dual kingdoms of the well and the sick" (Donnelly, 1993, p. 6). The illness-in-the-foreground perspective is characterized by a focus on sickness, suffering, loss, and burden caused by the illness. This perspective occurs when a person is newly diagnosed, when new disease-related symptoms appear, when the illness is in an acute phase, or when there are perceived threats to the person's control (signs of disease progression, lack of skills to manage the symptoms, disease-related stigma, or interactions with others that emphasize dependence and hopelessness). The illness-in-the-foreground perspective has a protective function, may assist in conserving energy, and helps a person learn more about the illness and come to terms with it (Paterson, 2001).

Returning to the wellness perspective calls for courage and resilience as well as the development of strategies and resources to adjust to the changes. Nurses can assist by understanding the person's perspective and providing education and support. The shift from illness to wellness is an active process triggered by the need to return to the wellness perspective.

In the wellness-in-the-foreground perspective, the focus is centred more on the self than on the disease and its consequences. The illness becomes part of who a person is but does not define the person. The illness is seen as an opportunity for growth and meaningful changes in relationships with the environment and others. This perspective is fostered by the patient's learning as much as possible about the illness, creating supportive environments, paying attention to their own patterns of response to the illness, and sharing knowledge of the disease with others.

With this perspective, the person is able to focus on the emotional, spiritual, and social aspects of life while still attending to disease management and the effects of the illness on their life. That the participants in a study of men with advanced prostate cancer were reluctant to describe themselves as ill suggests that having the wellness-in-the-foreground perspective is a desirable state (Lindqvist et al., 2006). Paterson (2001) has suggested that the Shifting Perspectives Model calls for an understanding of the person's perspective and why the person varies in their attention to symptoms. Health care providers who see the person with chronic illness as sick focus only on the disease and its symptoms and may not provide opportunities or support for wellness. Gerontological nurses must support persons with either perspective to optimize and sustain the wellness-in-the-foreground perspective.

Like the Shifting Perspectives Model of chronic illness, the person-centred care model focuses on partnership and on setting goals that are tailored to the individual person and their lifestyle. Person-centred care was conceptualized by Tom Kitwood (1997) as a way to care for persons with dementia. Person-centred care considers each person's needs and preferences from a holistic perspective that includes associated relationships and the effect that other people or the physical environment (or a combination of these) may have on the person. Thus, this model of care emphasizes the person living with chronic illness rather than the chronic illness itself.

IMPLICATIONS FOR GERONTOLOGICAL NURSING AND HEALTHY AGING

Chronic illnesses are illnesses that a person must live with, and nursing's response is one of long-term caring. The focus of treatment for chronic illness is seldom on cure; rather, the focus is care for the person. Nursing for chronic illness requires a different focus from that of acute care nursing, in which the emphasis is on attention to immediate and life-threatening needs and attempts to cure.

Assessment

Assessment of the older adult with a chronic illness involves the selection of appropriate tools, ongoing evaluation of responses and outcomes, careful observation, periodic monitoring, alert watchfulness, and most importantly, discussion and collaboration with the older adult about their perceptions and the meaning of the illness. In the case of chronic illness and the great variability in its presentation and impact on individual lifestyle, adequate assessment is critical. Assessment focuses on function and how the chronic illness affects function and well-being.

Functional assessments strive to identify the quantity and quality of disability in chronic illness. These assessments, although sometimes not specific to the medical treatment regimen, are often a good measure of the person's response and adaptation to persistent health problems. Disability assessment helps identify the gap between existing self-care abilities and needed self-care resources. The difference between abilities and needed resources identifies areas on which nursing care should focus. In this approach to assessment, nurses embrace the idea of illness as persistent; patients can achieve various degrees of adaptation, and nurses can help maximize people's function and therefore their quality of life. (See Chapter 13 for a discussion of comprehensive assessment and assessment instruments.)

Since many people with chronic illness manage their conditions in a community setting and may need assistance from different caregivers, assessment must also focus on the ability of family or significant others to assist and cope with caregiving. (See Chapter 25 for a discussion of the caregiving role.)

Interventions

Interventions in the care of chronically ill persons must take into consideration the person's emotional responses, perspectives on the illness, individual needs, self-care ability, support from family and friends, and available resources, as well as the trajectory experience. Chronic illness affects all aspects of a person's life, and interventions must be holistic. Nursing recommendations for the care of persons with chronic illnesses are presented in Box 15.4.

Caring

Caring has historically been the foundation of nursing. The concept of caring has been studied by many nursing scholars. Roach's "five Cs" of caring offer a framework for understanding the meaning of caring. The five Cs are a way of understanding what the nurse is doing when they are caring, and they provide a

> **BOX 15.4**
> ## NURSING RECOMMENDATIONS FOR THE CARE OF PERSONS WITH CHRONIC ILLNESS
>
> - Come to know the person and what gives their life meaning.
> - Provide education about the illness and its management.
> - Provide ongoing assessment, focusing on the prevention of complications.
> - Relieve symptoms that interfere with functioning and quality of life.
> - Help the person set realistic goals and expectations.
> - Focus on potential rather than limitations.
> - Teach the skills required for effective self-care.
> - Ensure the delivery of needed care and support for both the person and the person's family or significant others.
> - Encourage the verbal expression of feelings.
> - Provide support for losses, and facilitate the grieving process.
> - Provide access to resources.
> - Provide timely and appropriate referrals to suitable providers (or resources).
> - Help the person balance the effects of treatment on quality of life.
> - Maintain hope for the person through a supportive environment and by developing a caring, reciprocal relationship with the person.
> - Help the person die with dignity and comfort.

comprehensive view of caring (Roach, 1992). The five Cs are as follows:

- Competence: Having the ability and skills to provide required nursing care
- Compassion: Sensitivity to the pain and brokenness of others
- Conscience: Moral awareness, practising within the moral framework, doing what "ought" to be done, and advocating for conditions of justice
- Commitment: Staying with the person on the journey; nursing as a lifelong commitment and way of life; doing the work of nursing because you want to, not because you have to
- Confidence: Inspiring trust through caring

All five Cs must be actualized in caring. In other words, being competent in skills without compassion or being compassionate without adequate skills and knowledge does not demonstrate caring. Older adults with chronic illnesses are not seeking a cure; rather, they need care of the highest quality. Practising within this framework, nurses bring expertise in caring to meet the needs of older adults with chronic illnesses. Nursing's response of caring applies this expertise to helping people to adapt, continue to grow, and attain a level of wellness and wholeness despite chronic illnesses and functional limitations. Gerontological nurses know that understanding and caring for an older adult who has a chronic illness and is facing long-term challenges requires them to develop a close caring relationship and to accompany the person on their journey, day after day, with a focus on quality of life.

Special Considerations in Chronic Illness

Regardless of the nature of chronic conditions, special considerations need attention and must be actively addressed by nurses. The following is not a comprehensive discussion of these considerations but a touchstone for further examination and discussion. This chapter will discuss fatigue and grieving in more depth. (For a discussion of pain, which is common in most conditions, see Chapter 16, Chapter 26 for a discussion of sexuality, Chapter 16 for information about complementary and alternative resources, and Chapter 27 for further descriptions of palliative care, loss, grief, dying, and death.)

Fatigue

Fatigue is a common complaint of persons living with chronic illness, yet it is different from the normal feeling of being tired from activity. Fatigue from chronic illness affects every aspect of the person's life and may interfere with self-care as well as performing family and societal roles. Fatigue is often variable and unpredictable and is either ignored or assumed to be an inevitable part of the aging process. Instead, fatigue may be a symptom of the illness, a side effect of a medication, a symptom of depression, or all of these.

The goal of nursing interventions is to find ways to decrease fatigue and help the person manage its effects on daily life. The most important intervention is to acknowledge the person's experience of fatigue and any effects that this may cause in their daily life. The following instruments are available to assess fatigue: the Multidimensional Assessment of Fatigue scale, the Functional Assessment of Chronic Illness Therapy – Fatigue scale, and the Profile of Mood States. It is also important to assess and treat depression that may be superimposed on the fatigue of chronic illness.

Discussing patterns of fatigue and identifying the precipitants is important. Gerontological nurses can encourage the person with a chronic illness to keep a health diary. The health diary may help the person develop self-awareness in regard to the perception and management of a chronic illness. It is also helpful to emphasize the signals of the body and to balance rest and activity (within limitations) in order to help the person conserve their energy for the most important or necessary activities. The diary may also assist the nurse in understanding the experience of the illness from the person's perspective so that interventions can be tailored to the person's unique journey. Interventions for the person with fatigue include strategies for energy conservation, an appropriate balance of exercise and rest, and adequate nutrition (Box 15.5). Nurses should listen carefully to what is most important to the older adult, as well as to what responses are most useful. People with chronic illnesses are the experts on managing their illnesses and lifestyles.

Grieving

Grieving the loss of independence, control, status, activities, social roles, appearance, comfort, and one's identity as a healthy person may initially occupy much of a person's time when they are adapting to a chronic illness. Grieving can be more pronounced if the onset of the illness is abrupt and if the losses interfere directly with a major source of pleasure. The older adult may begin to memorialize the "perfect" self that no longer exists.

Nursing interventions for loss and grief should focus on encouraging the person to talk about their losses, providing support through active listening, and recognizing the stages of grief that may be occurring. Clearly, the reaction to loss and grief will depend on the significance of the loss to the person and the number of additional losses with which they are attempting to cope. It is important to come to know the person, what is most meaningful in the person's life, and the impact of the losses on that person. The number of losses, and any other recent losses in the person's life, may have depleted their psychic reserves (see Chapter 27).

BOX 15.5
INTERVENTIONS FOR PERSONS EXPERIENCING FATIGUE

- Set priorities, and make a list of daily activities, identifying which activities are essential, optional, desirable, and transferable.
- Delegate activities and learn to accept help when needed.
- Anticipate needed resources, and determine the most efficient way to carry out important activities.
- Act during periods of peak energy.
- Pace activities by planning for rest and activity, breaking big tasks into smaller and more manageable ones, spreading activities out over the day and week, and resting for short periods before activity.
- Use relaxation strategies.
- Exercise appropriately to increase muscle strength and endurance. Consult a physiotherapist for specific therapeutic exercises that are appropriate for the type of illness.
- Consume a healthy, nutritious diet, and maintain normal body weight.

Source: Mueller-Schotte, S., Bleijenberg, N., van der Schouw, Y. T., et al. (2016). Fatigue as a long-term risk factor for limitations in instrumental activities of daily living and/or mobility performance in older persons after 10 years. *Clinical Interventions in Aging, 11,* 1579. doi:10.2147/CIA.S116741.

There often seems to be a subversive sense of failure or weakness in people who have developed a chronic disorder. The suffering that a chronic illness entails is compounded by a sense of responsibility for remaining healthy, especially in the current climate of wellness. There is often the persistent thought that hard work and compliance with a strict treatment regimen will bring about a cure, and when that does not occur, a sense of shame develops. This may affect an older adult's willingness to seek and accept help.

Fostering Self-Care

In the day-to-day life of a person with chronic illness, self-care skills are of the greatest importance. Nurse theorist Orem provided a useful language and taxonomy for both understanding and responding to persons with self-care needs (Orem, 1980, 1995).

According to Orem, each person has self-care needs, called "universal self-care requisites." Each person also develops self-care capacity—that is, the ability to meet these requisites. However, under some circumstances, the needs exceed the person's capacity to meet them, and a self-care deficit ensues. These deficits can be the result of pathophysiological disorders, but they can also have a psychological or spiritual origin. Those with chronic illness are strong, responsible, and able to take care of their health and self-care as needed (Khademian et al., 2020). If people need assistance with self-care, this is where the nurse can play an important role.

Nursing interventions include assessments of self-care abilities and deficits. The appropriate approach is highly individualized and may involve changing the environment, modifying the treatment, or teaching the person strategies to compensate for the changes caused by the chronic illness. It may also involve teaching others how to provide the needed care or teaching the older adult how to direct the provision of care by others.

Rehabilitation and Restorative Care

Many individuals who are experiencing chronic illness will require short- or long-term rehabilitation and restorative care. The goal of such care is to capitalize on the individual's needs and strengths in a manner that will help them achieve the highest practicable level of function. Rehabilitation seeks to restore or maintain physical functioning and strives to recover a person's ability to perform ADLs and improve their quality of life (McGlinchey et al., 2020).

Rehabilitation and restorative services take place in acute care settings, outpatient clinics, rehabilitation and skilled-care facilities, and the home. The rehabilitation plan often begins in the acute care setting and can continue into long-term care settings, the community, and people's homes. The following issues should be considered in rehabilitation planning:

1. The person is often in a crisis when admitted to acute care, and personal strengths are not always evident or easily assessed.
2. Interprofessional discharge planning must begin upon admission, and a nurse or case manager should be assigned to each person.
3. Rehabilitation focuses on abilities, not disabilities; it maximizes strengths and supports limitations.

Comprehensive interprofessional assessment is critical to the rehabilitation plan, which involves working alongside the older adult, family, and significant others.

The total assessment includes a comprehensive biopsychosocial history, functional and cognitive assessment, and a plan of care that includes long- and short-term goals. Weekly joint conferences of the interprofessional team, the older adult, and the older adult's family are held to evaluate the person's progress, revise goals as needed, and develop discharge plans. (See Chapter 28 for additional information on rehabilitative and restorative care and transitional care.)

Prevention of Iatrogenic Disturbances

While health care providers are aiming to reduce the complications of chronic illnesses, a secondary risk, that of **iatrogenesis**, increases. Iatrogenesis is defined as a complication or byproduct of a health care intervention or of the environment (Box 15.6). Sometimes, the treatment of an illness can be more devastating than the illness itself.

The older adult may become incontinent not because of a new physiological problem but because of a prescribed diuretic, and the person may consequently experience an increase in urinary frequency but have no increased access to toilet facilities. A new medication can cause depression, poor appetite, or fatigue while it is simultaneously improving control of the underlying illness. Nurses have to be vigilant for a negative change occurring after an intervention or medication administration. Working proactively, the older adult and the care team can identify the potential or actual effect of a treatment, and the treatment can be reassessed from a benefit-versus-burden perspective. The goal is to treat the illness-related problems without compromising function and quality of life. (See Chapter 2 for a discussion of some models used to prevent iatrogenesis in hospitalized older adults.)

Assistive Technology

Advances in all types of technology hold promise for improving quality of life, reducing the need for personal care services, and enhancing independence and the ability to live safely at home or in another environment. *Assistive technology* refers to any device or system that allows a person to perform a task independently or that makes the task easier and safer to perform. Health care technologies, telehealth, mobility and ADL aids, virtual video appointments and consultations, and environmental control systems (such as "smart" houses) are some examples of assistive technology. (See Chapter 12 for a discussion of mobility and ADL aids.) *Gerotechnology* (assistive technologies for older adults) is expected to significantly influence how older adults live in the future.

BOX 15.6

COMMON IATROGENIC PROBLEMS ASSOCIATED WITH HOSPITALIZATION

- Loss of mobility because of insufficient ambulation
- Incontinence caused by inattention, immobility, or both
- Confusion or delirium caused by medications, treatments, anaesthesia, or translocation
- Pressure injury caused by immobility and reduced sensation
- Dehydration caused by limited access to fluids
- Fluid overload caused by improper use of intravenous fluids
- Health care–associated infections caused by infectious agents in surroundings
- Urinary tract infections caused by catheter use
- Upper respiratory tract infections caused by immobility, shallow breathing, and aspiration of oral secretions
- Fluid and electrolyte imbalances caused by medications and treatments
- Falls because of unfamiliar environment, weakness, positional instability, or medications
- Impaired sleep due to treatments and environment
- Malnutrition caused by anorexia and insufficient assistance with eating

---

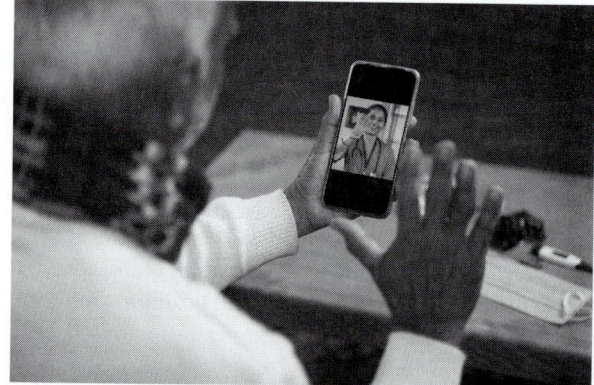

Virtual appointments allow older adults to easily access health care services from the comfort and safety of their own environment. © Can Stock Photo / lakshmiprasad.

Telemedicine is another form of technology used in health care, including the remote diagnosing and electronic monitoring of people (AlDossary et al., 2017). In rural areas, telemedicine offers several possibilities in the home or in other settings—reducing health care costs, eliminating the need for transportation for people who need specialized health care services, and promoting the self-management of illness. For example, a home health nurse may see a person discharged home after an acute exacerbation of heart failure. The nurse completes a thorough assessment, records it on a handheld computer, and transmits it to other health care providers. The older adult is instructed to sit on a specialized chair each morning; blood pressure, pulse, and weight are measured by automation at the preset times; and the information is sent over the patient's phone line directly to the visiting nurse's office and the physician's or primary care office. The home health nurse is quickly alerted to potential problems, and the physician or nurse practitioner can make changes to the medical plan as needed. Telemedicine offers exciting possibilities for nursing at both the generalist and advanced practice levels.

In addition, artificial intelligence (AI) is a fast-growing field in health care, focusing on the development of systems that can perform tasks that would normally require humans. Some examples include problem solving, reasoning, and recognition. Within the past 20 years, AI has expanded tremendously and is expected to impact many areas of health care (Canadian Agency for Drugs and Technology in Health, 2020).

Some of the devices being used in hospital and in long-term care homes are wireless pendants that track people's movements, load cells built into beds to alert caregivers when a person gets out of bed, devices to monitor sleep and weight patterns, and bed lifts that help the person to go from lying down to standing up with the push of a button. Electronic health records improve care and are particularly important for people who have chronic illnesses and require multiple care providers across settings.

As each new generation ages, its comfort with technology increases, and people seek opportunities for better, safer, and more independent living in ways not yet imagined.

Models of Chronic Illness Care

Many efforts are underway to improve care for persons with chronic illness by providing cost-effective and care-efficient services that improve outcomes and quality of life. The traditional medical care model and public health models have not been effective in dealing with the complexity of chronic illness. Although not all people with a chronic illness have high care needs, the cost of care for those who do is increasingly **exorbitant**. The costs accrued by chronic illness (more than 75% of total medical expenditures), access to care, quality outcomes, and patient satisfaction remain issues of concern.

People with chronic illnesses often have to navigate a system that requires them to coordinate several disparate financing and delivery systems by themselves, making it more difficult for them to obtain the full range of appropriate services. People who need access to different programs are likely to find that each program has different eligibility criteria and sets of care providers and that there is little communication or coordination among health care providers. As a result, the health care delivery system is complex and confusing, and care is often fragmented, less effective, and more costly. A summary of the challenges in care for the older adult with chronic illness is presented in Box 15.7.

Managed care, **case management**, disease management, evidence-informed protocols for illness management, **care coordination**, and collaborative models of self-management are all care models to support an

---

BOX 15.7

CHALLENGES IN CARING FOR THE OLDER ADULT WITH CHRONIC ILLNESS

- The long-term and uncertain nature of the illness
- Costs associated with care
- Little coordination of care across the continuum
- Inadequate funding for preventive and long-term care
- Lack of health care providers with expertise in gerontology and in the care of persons with chronic conditions
- Acute and episodic focus in medical care
- The need for active partnership between the person, their family and significant others, and the health care provider

integrated system that ensures that the services needed by people with chronic illness are provided in a cost-effective manner. Elements essential to new models of care include coordination of care; identification of risk; improved access; prevention and health promotion; use of evidence-informed protocols to manage illness; holistic approaches; interprofessional focus; management of transitions across the continuum; and a collaborative approach that encourages self-management of the illness in a partnership between health care providers and the person living with the chronic illness (Holroyd-Leduc et al., 2016) (see Box 15.2).

Care management has been found to be beneficial for optimizing individualized treatment and care for persons living with dementia (Thyrian et al., 2017). In their study, Thyrian and colleagues (2017) completed a randomized clinical trial to look at the effectiveness of adopting a dementia care management strategy in primary care. This care management strategy aimed to provide care by keeping care individualized. The nurse conducts an in-depth assessment to determine the person's and caregivers' unmet needs. From there, a weekly case conference call with the interprofessional team takes place (including a neurologist, psychologist and pharmacist). The nurse and general practitioner then collaborate to establish an individualized care plan. Thyrian and colleagues (2017) found that this dementia care management strategy improved a person's behavioural and psychological symptoms, decreased caregiver burden, improved pharmacological treatment, and improved the quality of dementia care.

Small-Group Approaches to Chronic Illness

Early affiliation with a group of persons who are confronting similar issues may help some older adults who have chronic illnesses adapt to the altered role requirements and may also provide shared strategies for coping. Small-group meetings are among the most effective and economical ways of helping individuals meet informational and psychosocial needs. These groups can also be designed to provide family support and counselling. Self-help groups can be seen as support systems, consumer participant systems, advocacy–social influence groups, or homogeneously identified therapeutic groups. Support groups provide the opportunity to obtain information and share similar experiences and perspectives. Facilitating persons' adjustments to new roles and activities and facilitating the redefinition of self constitute a large part of working in these groups.

Many support services and opportunities for group work are available from organizations that are devoted to particular chronic illnesses (e.g., the Alzheimer Society of Canada, the Heart and Stroke Foundation of Canada, and Parkinson Canada), as well as many websites.

SUMMARY

Managing chronic illness in older adults is aimed toward achieving a healthier old age and enhancing health and wellness for those already in late life. Nurses must work with older adults to maximize their assets and abilities and minimize their limitations and disabilities.

This kind of nursing requires a different focus from that of acute care nursing, where the emphasis is on attention to immediate and life-threatening needs and attempts to cure. Chronic illnesses, on the other hand, are illnesses that the older adult must live with, and nursing's response is one of long-term caring. Progress is not measured by attempts to achieve cure, but rather in the maintenance of a steady state or regression of the condition, all the while remembering that the condition does not define the person. Understanding the meaning of the experience of chronic illness from the older adult's perspective, adopting a holistic approach, and working collaboratively with the person are of utmost importance.

KEY CONCEPTS

- Declines in mortality, increasing medical expertise, and sophisticated technological developments have resulted in a significant increase in the survival of older adults with multiple chronic disorders.
- The effects of chronic illness range from mild to life limiting, with each person responding to circumstances in a highly individual manner.
- The Chronic Illness Trajectory and the Shifting Perspectives Model of chronic illness offer useful frameworks for understanding chronic illness and designing nursing interventions.
- People with chronic illnesses can achieve wellness, and the role of the nurse is critical in its promotion.
- The goals of healthy aging include minimizing the risk for disease; encouraging health promotion; and, in the presence of disease, alleviating

symptoms, delaying or avoiding the development of complications, and maximizing function and quality of life.

▪ Loss and grief are common in chronic illness. Nursing interventions include encouraging the person to talk about their losses, providing support through active listening, and recognizing the grief process that may be occurring.

▪ New models of cost-effective care that increase access and improve outcomes and quality of life for persons with chronic illness are needed. Nurses are particularly well prepared to assume major roles in chronic illness care.

▪ The overall goal of rehabilitation for the older adult is to achieve the highest practicable level of functioning.

ACTIVITIES AND DISCUSSION QUESTIONS

1. What type of education and counselling might the nurse provide to a 40-year-old person to promote health and prevent chronic illness in their later life?

2. Discuss possible ways of modifying the living situation of a person whose energy is limited owing to chronic disorders.

3. What would be the most devastating loss in ADLs?

4. What are some nursing interventions that would help a person with chronic illness deal with loss? Practise or role play various ways in which this issue can be addressed.

5. How would you encourage a person toward maximal participation in self-care?

6. What would be the measures of wellness during chronic illness?

RESOURCES

Age in Place. Imagine the future of aging.
http://ageinplace.com/technology/imagine-future-aging-technology-video/
Canadian Study of Health and Aging
http://www.csha.ca
Chronic Disease Prevention Alliance of Canada
http://www.cdpac.ca
Canadian Nurses Association. *Chronic disease prevention and management.*
https://cna-aiic.ca/en/policy-advocacy/chronic-disease-prevention-and-management
Clinical Frailty Scale
https://www.bgs.org.uk/sites/default/files/content/attachment/2018-07-05/rockwood_cfs.pdf
Improving Chronic Illness Care
http://www.improvingchroniccare.org
Patient Safety Institute: Patient Safety in Canada
https://www.patientsafetyinstitute.ca/en/toolsResources/Documents/Patient%20Harm%20Awareness%20-%20Ipsos/CPSI%20-%20Patient%20Safety%20in%20Canada%20Baseline%20Report.pdf
Public Health Agency of Canada. *Aging and seniors.*
https://www.canada.ca/en/public-health/services/health-promotion/aging-seniors.html
Public Health Agency of Canada. *Healthy aging in Canada: A new vision, a vital investment. From evidence to action.*
http://www.health.gov.bc.ca/library/publications/year/2006/Healthy_Aging_A_Vital_latest_copy_October_2006.pdf

Registered Nurses' Association of Ontario. *Strategies to support self-management in chronic conditions: Collaboration with clients.*
http://rnao.ca/bpg/guidelines/strategies-support-selfmanagement-chronic-conditions-collaboration-clients
The LeadingAge Center for Aging Services Technologies
http://www.leadingage.org/center-aging-services-technologies
The Ontario Seniors' Secretariat. *Independence, Activity, and Good Health: Ontario's Action Plan for Seniors.*
https://dr6j45jk9xcmk.cloudfront.net/documents/215/ontarioseniorsactionplan-en-20130204.pdf
World Health Organization. *Noncommunicable diseases.*
https://www.who.int/health-topics/noncommunicable-diseases

For additional resources, please visit *http://evolve.elsevier.com/Canada/Ebersole/gerontological/*

REFERENCES

AlDossary, S., Martin-Khan, M. G., Bradford, N. K., et al. (2017). The development of a telemedicine planning framework based on needs assessment. *Journal of Medical Systems*, 41(5), 74. doi:10.1007/s10916-017-0709-4.

Boscart, V., Crutchlow, L. E., Taucar, L. S., et al. (2020). Chronic disease management models in nursing homes: A scoping review. *BMJ Open*, 10(2), e032316. doi:10.1136/bmjopen-2019-032316.

Cancer Care Ontario & Public Health Ontario. (2019). *The burden of chronic diseases in Ontario: Key estimates to support efforts in prevention*. https://www.ccohealth.ca/sites/CCOHealth/files/assets/BurdenCDReport.pdf.

Canadian Agency for Drugs and Technologies in Health. (2020). *An overview of clinical applications of artificial intelligence*. https://www.cadth.ca/sites/default/files/pdf/eh0070_overview_clinical_applications_of_AI.pdf.

Canadian Institute for Health Information (CIHI). (2011). *Seniors and the health care system: What is the impact of multiple chronic conditions?* https://secure.cihi.ca/free_products/air-chronic_disease_aib_en.pdf.

Canadian Institute for Health Information (CIHI). (2016). *Health spending*. https://www.cihi.ca/en/spending-and-health-workforce/spending.

Centers for Disease Control and Prevention (CDC). (2019). *About chronic diseases*. https://www.cdc.gov/chronicdisease/about/index.htm.

Centers for Disease Control and Prevention (CDC). (2020). *Promoting health for older adults*. https://www.cdc.gov/chronicdisease/resources/publications/factsheets/promoting-health-for-older-adults.htm.

Chinda, B., Song, X., Sarveswaran, S., et al. (2019). Frailty in healthy oldest old: Characterizing the frailty index of super-seniors. *Innovation in Aging*, 3(Suppl. 1), S913. doi:10.1093/geroni/igz038.3330.

Corbin, J. M., & Strauss, A. (1988). *Unending work and care: Managing chronic illness at home*. Jossey-Bass.

Corbin, J. M., & Strauss, A. (1992). A nursing model for chronic illness management based upon the trajectory framework. In P. Woog (Ed.), *The chronic illness framework: The Corbin and Strauss nursing model* (pp. 9–28). Springer.

Donnelly, G. F. (1993). Chronicity: Concept and reality. *Holistic Nursing Practice*, 8(1), 1–7.

Eastern Michigan University. (2018). *The nurse's role in chronic disease management*. https://online.emich.edu/articles/rnbsn/nurses-role-chronic-disease-management.aspx.

Fazio, S. B., Demasi, M., Farren, E., et al. (2016). Blueprint for an undergraduate primary care curriculum. *Academic Medicine: Journal of the Association of American Medical Colleges*, 91(12), 1628–1637. doi:10.1097/ACM.0000000000001302.

Griffin, F. R., Mode, N. A., Ejiogu, N., et al. (2018). Frailty in a racially and socioeconomically diverse sample of middle-aged Americans in Baltimore. *PLOS One*, 13(4), e01956637. doi:10.1371/journal.pone.0195637.

Holroyd-Leduc, J., Resin, J., Ashley, L., et al. (2016). Giving voice to older adults living with frailty and their family caregivers: Engagement of older adults living with frailty in research, health care decision making, and in health policy. *Research Involvement and Engagement*, 2, 23. doi:10.1186/s40900-016-0038-7.

Jevne, R. (1993). Enhancing hope in the chronically ill. *Humane Medicine*, 9(2), 121–130.

Khademian, Z., Ara, F. K., & Gholamzadeh, S. (2020). The effect of self-care education based on Orem's nursing theory on quality of life and self-efficacy in patients with hypertension: A quasi-experimental study. *International Journal of Community-Based Nurse Midwifery*, 8(2), 140–149. doi:10.30476/IJCBNM.2020.81690.0.

Kitwood, T. (1997). *Dementia reconsidered: The person comes first*. Open University Press.

Kojima, G., Liljas, A. E. M., & Iliffe, S. (2019). Frailty syndrome: Implications and challenges for health care policy. *Risk Management and Healthcare Policy*, 12, 23–30. doi:10.2147/RMHP.S168750.

Larsen, P., Lewis, P., & Lubkin, I. (2006). Illness behavior and roles. In I. Lubkin & P. Larsen (Eds.), *Chronic illness: Impact and interventions* (6th ed., pp. 25–41). Jones and Bartlett.

Lindqvist, O., Widmark, A., & Rasmussen, B. (2006). Reclaiming wellness—Living with bodily problems, as narrated by men with advanced prostate cancer. *Cancer Nursing*, 29(4), 327–337. doi:10.1097/00002820-200607000-00012.

McGlinchey, M. P., James, J., McKevitt, C., et al. (2020). The effect of rehabilitation interventions on physical function and immobility-related complications in severe stroke: A systematic review. *BMJ Open*, 2020(10), e033642. doi:10.1136/bmjopen-2019-033642.

Mokraoui, N. M., Haggerty, J., Almirall, J., et al. (2016). Prevalence of self-reported multimorbidity in the general population and in primary care practices: A cross-sectional study. *British Medical Council Research Notes*, 9(1), 314. doi:10.1186/s13104-016-2121-4.

Morse, J. M., Bowers, B. J., Charmaz, K., et al. (2021). *Developing grounded theory: The second generation*. Routledge.

Ng, J. H., Ward, L. M., Shea, M., et al. (2019). Explaining the relationship between minority group status and health disparities: A review of selected concepts. *Health Equity*, 3(1), 47–60. doi:10.1089/heq.2018.0035.

Nierenberg, B., Mayersohn, G., Serpa, S., et al. (2016). Application of well-being therapy to people with disability and chronic illness. *Rehabilitation Psychology*, 61(1), 32. doi:10.1037/rep0000060.

Orem, D. (1980). *Nursing: Concepts of practice* (2nd ed.). McGraw-Hill.

Orem, D. (1995). *Nursing: Concepts of practice* (5th ed.). Mosby.

Paterson, B. L. (2001). The shifting perspectives model of chronic illness. *Journal of Nursing Scholarship*, 33(1), 21–26. doi:10.1111/j.1547-5069.2001.00021.x.

Ploeg, J., Matthew-Maich, N., Fraser, K., et al. (2017). Managing multiple chronic conditions in the community: A Canadian qualitative study of the experiences of older adults, family caregivers and healthcare providers. *BMC Geriatrics*, 17(1), 40. doi:10.1186/s12877-017-0431-6.

Public Health Agency of Canada. (2019). *At-a-glance—How healthy are Canadians? A brief update. Health Promotion and Chronic Disease Prevention in Canada*, 38, 385–387. doi:10.24095/hpcdp.38.10.05.

Roach, S. (1992). *The human act of caring*. Canadian Hospital Association.

Sieber, C. C. (2017). Frailty—From concept to clinical practice. *Experimental Gerontology*, 87, 160–167. doi:10.1016/j.exger.2016.05.004.

Statistics Canada. (2018). *Health-adjusted life expectancy in Canada*. https://www150.statcan.gc.ca/n1/pub/82-003-x/2018004/article/54950-eng.htm.

Strauss, A., & Glaser, B. (1975). *Chronic illness and the quality of life*. Mosby.

Thyrian, J. R., Hertel, J., Wucherer, D., et al. (2017). Effectiveness and safety of dementia care management in primary care: A randomized clinical trial. *Journal of the American Medical Association*, 74(10), 996–1004. doi:10.1001/jamapsychiatry.2017.2124.

Touhy, T. A., Jett, K. F., Boscart, V., et al. (2018). *Ebersole and Hess' gerontological nursing and healthy aging in Canada*. Elsevier Health Sciences.

Umegaki, H. (2016). Sarcopenia and frailty in older patients with diabetes mellitus. *Geriatrics & Gerontology International, 16*(3), 293–299. doi:10.1111/ggi.12688.

Warner, C. B., Roberts, A. R., Jeanblanc, A. B., et al. (2017). Coping resources, loneliness, and depressive symptoms of older women with chronic illness. *Journal of Applied Gerontology, 38*(3), 295–322. doi:10.1177/0733464816687218.

Woog, P. (1992). *The chronic illness trajectory framework: The Corbin and Strauss nursing model.* Springer.

World Health Organization (WHO). (2005). *Preparing a health care workforce for the 21st century: The challenge of chronic conditions.* http://www.who.int/chp/knowledge/publications/workforce_report.pdf.

World Health Organization (WHO). (2017). WHO Clinical Consortium on Healthy Ageing. Report of Consortium Meeting 1–2 December 2016 in Geneva, Switzerland. Geneva: WHO; 2017 (WHO/FWC/ALC/17.2). Licence: CC BY-NC-SA 3.0 IGO.

World Health Organization (WHO). (2021, 13 April). *Noncommunicable diseases.* https://www.who.int/news-room/fact-sheets/detail/noncommunicable-diseases.

Zengarini, E., & Cherubini, A. (2019). Frailty is not a fatality. In *Prevention of chronic diseases and age-related disability* (pp. 53–60). Springer.

16 PAIN AND COMFORT

LEARNING OBJECTIVES

Upon completion of this chapter, the reader will be able to:

- Define the concept of pain and recognize the older adult's interpretation of pain.
- Differentiate acute from persistent pain.
- Identify data to include in a pain assessment.
- Describe pharmacological and nonpharmacological measures to promote the comfort of the person in pain.
- Discuss the goals of pain management for the older adult.
- Develop a nursing care plan for an older adult in acute or persistent pain.

GLOSSARY

Adjuvant A medication that has a primary use other than pain relief (e.g., an antidepressant or anticonvulsant) but is also used to enhance the effects of traditional pain medication.

Titration The adjustment of the dosage of a given medication until the desired effect is produced.

THE LIVED EXPERIENCE

"Ms. S. had cancer of the stomach and was in pain most of the time. She was referred to the local hospice, and the nurse worked with her and her physician to make Ms. S. comfortable. First the nurse assessed potential causes for the pain, the level of pain, the type of pain, and what level of relief was desired. After a careful titration of her medications, it was found that only a long-acting morphine provided her with comfort and an improved quality of life. However, at the dose needed she also hallucinated, seeing several puppies in the room. When asked if she wanted to reduce the dosage to eliminate this side effect, she responded, "No—I'll keep the puppies, I know they are not real and they don't hurt anything. I'd rather have them with me than the pain."

Helen, a registered nurse

Comfort is a personal and intrinsic balance of the most basic physiological, emotional, social, and spiritual needs. Comfort is uniquely defined, experienced, and expressed by each person as a member of a family, community, and culture. A person comes to later life with many learned ways of promoting self-comfort and comforting loved ones. Without some level of comfort, wellness is beyond reach.

Pain, on the other hand, is a sensation of distress and can occur at a physical, psychological, and spiritual level. Pain is a multidimensional phenomenon, and usually one type of pain is intertwined with another. Physical pain and several chronic diseases (e.g., Parkinson's disease) can evoke the psychological pain of depression. Any type of pain can result in reduced socialization, impaired mobility, and a reconsideration of the meaning of life and self (Backe et al., 2018). This chapter describes acute and persistent pain, and explores assessments, interventions, and strategies to address pain and discomfort in older adults.

COMMUNICATION OF PAIN AND DISCOMFORT

How pain is expressed is highly influenced by the history of the individual and the meaning they ascribe to pain. It is not uncommon to express spiritual and psychological pain in somatic terms of "not feeling well." It is also important to realize that individuals respond in a way that reflects their own cultural expectations and understanding of acceptable behaviour. Simply put, pain is whatever a person says it is.

For those with cognitive and communication impairments (e.g., dementia or aphasia), pain is a particular challenge. Health care providers must interpret the person's expression of pain through subtle cues. Understanding what the person is trying to communicate through their behaviour is an essential skill in caring for older adults with and without communication difficulties (see Chapter 21). Other factors affecting the communication of pain include hearing loss, depression, sedating medications (which do not necessarily ease pain), the individual's personality, and the way discomfort is acceptably expressed. Nurses cannot assume that those who cannot or will not verbalize their pain do not have pain. Instead, nurses must be alert to the cues suggesting that pain and discomfort are present, and then initiate assessments and interventions that are appropriate and acceptable to the older adult.

Pain is now considered the fifth vital sign, which means that a pain assessment is part of any evidence-informed assessment (Kutlutürkan & Urvaylıoğlu, 2020). Providing comfort to persons in pain is a quality indicator—that is, a marker of quality care. Yet, even when best practice guidelines are followed, inadequate assessment and undertreatment of pain still occurs, especially when the patient is an older adult, a member of a minority group, or in a long-term care (LTC) home (Hunnicutt et al., 2017). Those who may not be able to communicate verbally may also not receive appropriate pain treatment (Achterberg et al., 2020). It is important to look for nonverbal cues as well (grimacing, pain expressions, wincing, etc.) (Browne et al., 2019).

Nurses have their own definitions and expectations of the expression of pain. These perceptions are drawn from nurses' personal and professional experiences, culture, and so on. Myths, stereotypes, and generalizations about aging influence the nurse's response (Box 16.1). Unfortunately, these beliefs make the undertreatment of pain more prevalent.

BOX 16.1
FACTS AND MYTHS ABOUT PAIN IN THE OLDER ADULT

Myth	Fact
Pain is a normal part of aging.	Pain is not part of the normal changes in aging; however, its occurrence increases with age.
Pain sensitivity and perception decrease with aging.	Not true. However, some older adults may have a greater tolerance for pain because of their adjustment to inadequate pain relief of long-standing pain.
If people don't complain of pain, they do not have pain.	People may not report pain for a variety of reasons; they may nonetheless have pain. Some persons feel that it is culturally inappropriate to complain of pain. Some feel that they are burdensome to those around them, including their nurses.
A person who has no functional impairment or who appears occupied is not in significant pain.	People have a variety of reactions and responses to pain. Some people are stoic and refuse to give in to their pain.
Narcotic medications are inappropriate unless used for short periods.	Opioid analgesics are often the best treatment for moderate to severe persistent pain in order to help restore the person's ability to function and quality of life.
Potential side effects of narcotic medication make these medications too dangerous to use with older adults.	Narcotics are safe to use with older adults.

Nurses have a responsibility to set aside their own expectations and promote the comfort of those who are suffering, regardless of the cause and manner of expression of their pain. Nurses should do so nonjudgementally and with the goals of understanding the person's pain and developing interventions to relieve, not just lessen, pain of all kinds. Gerontological nurses' skills in assessment and intervention are especially important.

ACUTE AND PERSISTENT PAIN

There are two main categories of pain: acute and persistent. Each category has subtypes (such as neuropathic and nociceptive pain).

Acute Pain

Acute physical pain is temporary pain that includes postoperative, procedural, and traumatic pain. Acute physical pain is usually easily controlled by analgesic medications. In the acute care hospital setting, patients can use a self-controlled analgesic pump for a restricted period. Acute pain is a universal experience for older adults because of lifespan, opportunities for traumatic injury, and pain-producing illnesses. At the same time, an older adult is more likely to have an adverse reaction to pain medication (see Chapter 14). For example, most analgesics cause sedation. Although use of the medication may be necessary, this adverse effect increases the risk for falls and delirium.

Acute pain may also be psychological or spiritual in nature (e.g., early bereavement or a major depressive episode). Because of the many losses in the lives of older adults (see Chapters 25 and 27), the risk for such acute pain is high.

Persistent Pain

One in five Canadians lives with *persistent pain* (Canadian Pain Task Force, 2019). The prevalence of persistent, or chronic, pain is higher in women and older adults (Canadian Pain Task Force, 2019). Lapane and colleagues (2012) have reported that between 33% and 83% of LTC residents experience persistent pain.

Persistent pain may be a sequela of an episode of acute pain, is not time limited, and may vary in intensity throughout the day or with changes in activity. For example, persons with persistent depressive disorder (formerly known as dysthymia) usually feel the most

sadness in the morning; however, their mood lifts as the day progresses (see Chapter 23). Higher age also creates a higher risk of developing health problems associated with persistent pain and iatrogenic side effects of treatment. Adverse iatrogenic events include falls and changes in cognitive function; these events are often the effect of different medications taken at the same time. Furthermore, loneliness and emotional pain from loss (see Chapter 27) decrease the ability to cope with physical pain. These psychosocial aspects of an older adult's pain experience are rarely (or superficially) assessed by nurses or included in the plan of care. Older adults may underreport their pain or "undertreat" themselves because of the cost of the medications, belief in an associated stigma, attribution of the pain to the normal burdens of "old age," or fear of addiction.

Conditions that are degenerative (e.g., osteoarthritis) or pathological (e.g., herpes zoster, stroke, or peripheral neuropathy) are common causes of pain.

Osteoarthritis

By 50 years of age, most adults have some level of degenerative abnormalities of the lower spine (see Chapter 18). One of the most typical abnormalities is the loss of support of the spinal column from osteoarthritis. Osteoarthritis—the destruction of the inner joint surfaces—is the most common form of joint disease. It is also the most common joint disorder in the world and one of the most common sources of pain and disability in advanced age (Vina & Kwoh, 2018). Joint pain and stiffness in osteoarthritis are initially intermittent and then become persistent. The pain is characterized by aching and stiffness in the joints with inactivity and by discomfort or acute pain with activity.

Relief from pain requires the skillful use of both nonpharmacological and pharmacological measures. Nonpharmacological pain management of osteoarthritis includes joint care and the application of moist heat to relieve pain, spasms, and stiffness. Joint care may include the use of orthotic devices such as braces and splints to support joints, weight reduction if necessary, physiotherapy, and the avoidance of overusing the affected joint. Complementary and alternative medicine (CAM) and cognitive behavioural measures may also be useful adjuncts.

Acetaminophen (Tylenol) remains the medication of choice for mild osteoarthritic pain. However, most people report better relief with nonsteroidal anti-inflammatory drugs (NSAIDs), such as naproxen or ibuprofen (Advil). These frequently used medications pose a considerable risk for interactions and adverse events (Vostinaru, 2017). Severe arthritis with unrelieved pain and extensive disability may necessitate the use of a local anaesthetic, such as a corticosteroid injected into the affected joints. Injections of hyaluronic acid have been found to improve joint lubrication in some persons. Both treatments are limited to three to five injections (Liu et al., 2018). In cases of extreme persistent pain, surgical intervention such as joint replacement may be performed. Long-acting narcotic pain relievers are also effective.

Herpes Zoster

Nearly 130,500 new cases of herpes zoster (HZ), or shingles, are diagnosed each year in Canada (Government of Canada, 2018a). This disorder occurs most often in persons between the ages of 50 and 70 years. About one in five people who have had chicken pox will develop shingles at some time in their lives (HealthLink BC, 2017). A viral infection of the nerves (see Chapter 11), HZ is characterized by an itching, stinging, burning rash along the pathway of the affected nerve (dermatome), followed by its eruption into serous vesicles. An acute episode lasts from days to weeks, whereas a chronic episode can last much longer (Devor, 2018). Involvement of the eye is considered a medical emergency owing to the high risk for blindness and brain involvement.

Although HZ causes acute pain, the pain may become persistent with what is diagnosed as postherpetic neuralgia (PHN), which is persistent pain from the damaged nerves after a case of HZ. The condition is difficult to treat once established; often, narcotics are necessary for pain relief. A combination of antiviral medications, steroids, Aspirin, and topical anaesthetics may be effective as well. Antiviral drugs such as acyclovir and famciclovir can shorten the duration of an acute outbreak and may prevent PHN when given promptly. Medications used to treat HZ and prevent PHN include Lyrica and gabapentin. Low doses of tricyclic antidepressants (e.g., desipramine and Elavil) have been used to treat PHN; however, some of these medications are contraindicated for use with older adults because of their anticholinergic effects (see Chapter 14).

IMPLICATIONS FOR GERONTOLOGICAL NURSING AND HEALTHY AGING

As always, care of the older adult who is in pain starts with an assessment and continues through to the evaluation of the interventions. Nurses are usually most attuned to the needs of older adults and are in a key position to work with the person until the pain is relieved. An advanced practice nurse or nurse practitioner with expertise in pain management can be consulted or requested to assist.

Assessment

A comprehensive assessment of pain includes a complete history and physical assessment, as well as an assessment specific to pain. Several organizations offer best practice guidelines for the assessment and management of pain. The Registered Nurses' Association of Ontario (http://www.rnao.ca) has developed best practice guidelines and a self-directed learning package for the assessment and management of pain in older adults. The Hartford Institute for Geriatric Nursing provides an evidence-informed guide in its Try This: Series, available on its website (https://hign.org/consultgeri-resources/try-this-series). The Canadian Pain Society also offers guidelines for the management of persistent neuropathic pain.

A number of factors should be considered when caring for older adults (Box 16.2). Assessment can be particularly challenging if the person has a cognitive or communication impairment.

When possible, assessment begins with a person's self-report of pain. Many times, older adults will not report pain unless directly asked specific questions, such as "Do you have pain now?," "Where is your pain?," "Do you have pain every day?," and "Does pain keep you from sleeping at night?" In some cases, using alternate words such as "ache," "hurt," or "discomfort" is necessary. Assessment includes a history of pain and detailed descriptions of pain intensity, frequency, quality, location, and aggravating and alleviating factors. Medication history includes prescribed medications, herbs and supplements, over-the-counter medications, and street medications. Figures 16.1 and 16.2 present a brief pain inventory and a standard pain assessment tool commonly used in hospitals and LTC homes.

BOX 16.2

FACTORS TO CONSIDER WHEN ASSESSING PAIN IN OLDER ADULTS

Function: How is the pain affecting the older adult's ability to perform activities of daily living and instrumental activities of daily living?

Expression of pain: Have there been recent changes in cognitive ability or behaviour, such as increased pacing, grimacing, or irritability? Have the number of complaints increased? Are the complaints vague and difficult to respond to? Has there been a change in sleep–wake patterns? Is the person resisting certain activities, movements, or positions?

Social support: What resources are available to help the person cope with and tolerate treatment? How is pain affecting the person's usual social role? How is pain affecting their relationships with others?

Pain history: How have previous experiences with pain been managed? What does the person perceive to be the meaning of the past and present pain? What cultural factors affect the person's belief in the meaning of the pain and the ability to express pain and receive relief?

For the person who is unable to express themself, assessment begins with the nurse's careful observation for any potential indicators of discomfort (Box 16.3). Written or visual analogue scales (Fig. 16.3) have also been found useful; most can be used cross-culturally or with individuals who have limited English proficiency. Visual analogue scales have been clinically tested and shown to be accurate and reliable tools in various health care settings (Delgado et al., 2018). However, their use for persons with dementia has varying results. Specific pain assessment tools such as the Pain Assessment in Advanced Dementia (PAINAD) scale can be used to assess people with cognitive impairments. (See the website in the Resources section at the end of the chapter). Another way to assess pain in those who have cognitive impairment or who cannot verbally express pain or discomfort includes having care staff complete an hourly observation for pain behaviours, tracked in a simple-to-use flowsheet. This observational assessment can be used with an analgesic trial to assess which, if any, pain behaviours are reduced with administration of pain medication or treatment.

Interventions

The goals of pain management for the older adult are to promote comfort and maintain the highest level of functioning and well-being possible. Careful use of nonpharmacological and pharmacological approaches helps to achieve both of these goals. To provide optimal care for the person in pain, attention needs to be given to the psychological and social consequences of physical pain. Reducing suffering calls for careful listening, unconditional positive regard, ongoing support, and mobilization of resources. Pillows for support or body positioning, appropriate and comfortable seating and mattresses, frequent rest periods, and pacing of activities to balance activity and rest are important for providing comfort.

Nurses should encourage older adults and their significant others to take an active role in their pain management. The person can keep a personal journal or pain diary that notes the times, types, and doses of medication taken; its effect; the duration of its benefit; and which activities increase or decrease the pain. This information helps to establish patterns that may improve pain management by adjusting activities, providing medications at the right times, and helping the person feel in control of some aspect of care. An example of a pain diary can be found at MyHealth.Alberta website (https://myhealth.alberta.ca/Health/Pages/conditions. aspx?hwid=abg7017). The diary should be reviewed with the health care provider and used to adjust dosages or timing for optimal relief.

Nurses should also encourage older adults to stay as active as possible within their comfort range. When a person experiences pain with a necessary activity (e.g., rehabilitation), anticipation anxiety may increase the pain. In this case, the plan of care should include both nonpharmacological and pharmacological interventions before the recommended activity. Administering an effective short-acting medication 20 to 30 minutes before the specific activity may lessen or eliminate the fear of discomfort and can greatly enhance the individual's capacity for that activity. Nurses should learn the older adult's ability to cope with pain and work within those parameters.

Nonpharmacological Measures for Pain Relief

Nurses have a long history of comforting patients using nonpharmacological measures in the form of a caring

Brief Pain Inventory

Date _____ / _____ / _____   Time: _____

Name: _____ _____ _____
          Last   First   Middle Initial

1) Throughout our lives, most of us have had pain from time to time (such as minor headaches, sprains, and toothaches). Have you had pain other than these everyday kinds of pain today?
   1. Yes   2. No

2) On the diagram, shade in the areas where you feel pain. Put an X on the area that hurts the most.

Right   Left   Left   Right

3) Please rate your pain by circling the one number that best describes your pain at its **worst** in the past 24 hours.

0	1	2	3	4	5	6	7	8	9	10
No pain								Pain as bad as you can imagine		

4) Please rate your pain by circling the one number that best describes your pain at its **least** in the past 24 hours.

0	1	2	3	4	5	6	7	8	9	10
No pain								Pain as bad as you can imagine		

5) Please rate your pain by circling the one number that best describes your pain on the **average.**

0	1	2	3	4	5	6	7	8	9	10
No pain								Pain as bad as you can imagine		

6) Please rate your pain by circling the one number that tells how much pain you have **right now.**

0	1	2	3	4	5	6	7	8	9	10
No pain								Pain as bad as you can imagine		

7) What treatments or medications are you receiving for your pain?

_____

_____

8) In the past 24 hours, how much **relief** have pain treatments or medications provided? Please circle the one percentage that most shows how much relief you have received.

0%	10	20	30	40	50	60	70	80	90	100%
No relief										Complete relief

9) Circle the one number that describes how, during the past 24 hours, pain has **interfered** with your:

   A. General activity

0	1	2	3	4	5	6	7	8	9	10
Does not interfere										Completely interferes

   B. Mood

0	1	2	3	4	5	6	7	8	9	10
Does not interfere										Completely interferes

   C. Walking ability

0	1	2	3	4	5	6	7	8	9	10
Does not interfere										Completely interferes

   D. Normal work (includes both work outside the home and housework)

0	1	2	3	4	5	6	7	8	9	10
Does not interfere										Completely interferes

   E. Relations with other people

0	1	2	3	4	5	6	7	8	9	10
Does not interfere										Completely interferes

   F. Sleep

0	1	2	3	4	5	6	7	8	9	10
Does not interfere										Completely interferes

   G. Enjoyment of life

0	1	2	3	4	5	6	7	8	9	10
Does not interfere										Completely interferes

May be duplicated for use in clinical practice.

Fig. 16.1 ■ Brief pain inventory. © Charles S. Cleeland, PhD, Houston, Texas.

Pain Assessment Tool

Reason for assessment:
☐ New admission   ☐ Readmission ☐ Further assessment
☐ Change in condition ☐ Quarterly

Addressograph

1. Location of pain:

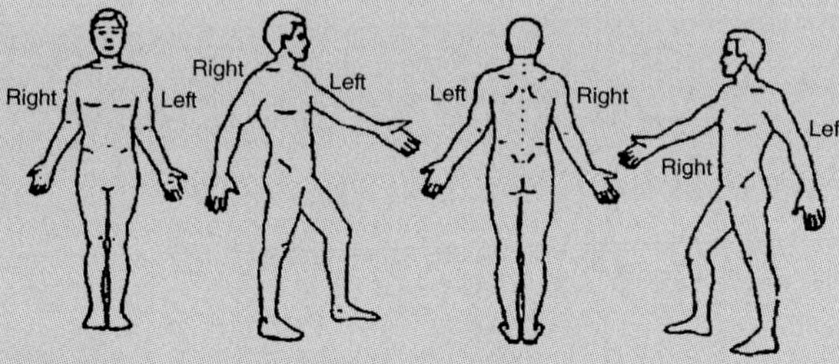

2. Severity of pain:

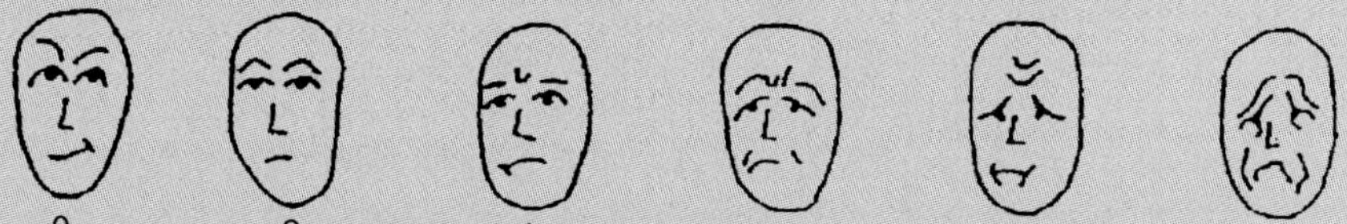

0	2	4	6	8	10
No pain	Mild	Discomforting	Distressing	Horrible	Excruciating

QUESTIONS	COMMENTS
What is the present level of pain? **(if no pain is present complete sections 6 and 7)**	
What is the rate when the pain is at its least?	
What makes the pain better?	
What is the rate when the pain is at its worst?	
What makes the pain worse?	
Is the pain continuous or intermittent?	
When did the pain start?	
What do you think is the cause of this pain?	
What level of pain are you satisfied with? (if 0 is unattainable)	

3. Quality: Indicate the words that describe the pain

☐ Aching	☐ Throbbing	☐ Shooting	☐ Stabbing	☐ Gnawing	☐ Sharp
☐ Burning	☐ Tender	☐ Exhausting	☐ Tiring	☐ Penetrating	☐ Numb
☐ Nagging	☐ Hammering	☐ Pins and needles	☐ Unbearable	☐ Tingling	☐ Stretching
☐ Pulling	☐ Other:				

Fig. 16.2 ▨ Pain assessment tool. ***Source:*** Brignell, A. (Ed). (2000). *Guideline for developing a pain management program: A resource guide for long-term care facilities* (3rd ed.). Grey Bruce Palliative Care Hospice Association. Reprinted with permission.

4. Effects of pain on <u>activities of daily living</u>

Activities of daily living	Yes	No	COMMENTS
Sleep and rest			
Social activities			
Appetite			
Physical activity and mobility			
Emotions			
Sexuality/intimacy			

5. Effects of pain on <u>quality of life</u>

What would you like to do now that you can't do because of the pain <u>or</u> What activity would improve your quality of life?

_____

_____

6. Symptoms: What other symptoms are being experienced?

☐ Constipation	☐ Nausea	☐ Vomiting	☐ Fatigue	☐ Insomnia	☐ Depression	☐ Drowsy
☐ Sore mouth	☐ Weakness	☐ Short of breath	☐ Other:			

7. Behaviours: What behaviours are present that may be a result of pain or treatment?

☐ Calling out	☐ Restlessness	☐ Disorientation	☐ Not eating	☐ Pacing
☐ Not sleeping	☐ Withdrawn	☐ Groaning/moaning	☐ Rocking	☐ New immobility
☐ Tense	☐ Distressed	☐ Distracted	☐ Crying	☐ Inexpressive
☐ Fists clenched	☐ Striking out	☐ Knees pulled up	☐ Frowning	☐ Facial grimacing
☐ Resistant to movement	☐ Pulling or pushing away	☐ Sad	☐ Frightened	☐ Other:

8. Past pain management

Has a significant degree of pain been experienced in the past? How was that managed?

_____

_____

Past use of pharmacological and nonpharmacological pain management?

_____

_____

9. Support system: _____

10. Other concerns related to pain _____

11. Nursing pain diagnosis:

☐ Visceral	☐ Somatic (muscle or bone)	☐ Raised intracranial pressure
☐ Naturopathic	☐ Mixed	☐ Unknown

Date Care Plan updated: _____

Signature: _____   **Assessment date:** _____

Fig. 16.2, cont'd

BOX 16.3

PAIN CUES IN THE PERSON WITH COMMUNICATION DIFFICULTIES

BEHAVIOURAL CHANGES

Restlessness, agitation (or both), or reduction in movement
Repetitive movements
Physical tension, such as clenching teeth or hands
Unusually cautious movements, guarding

ACTIVITY CHANGES

Sudden resistance to help from others
Decreased appetite
Decreased sleep

VOCALIZATION CHANGES

Groaning, moaning, or crying for unknown reasons
Increases or decreases in the usual vocalizations

PHYSICAL CHANGES

Pleading expression
Grimacing
Pallor or flushing
Diaphoresis (sweating)
Increased pulse, respirations, or blood pressure

---

and supportive relationship or specific techniques. A combination of pharmacological and nonpharmacological interventions appears to be most effective in the relief of both acute and persistent pain (Edmond et al., 2018). The basic approach to pain control is to encourage whatever strategies have been effective in the past without causing harm. This applies particularly to older adults with a lifetime of experience managing their own pain. In some cases, what is now referred to as CAM is actually the formalization of approaches that people have used for years.

Physical Approaches

The methods of pain reduction briefly reviewed here are only a small sample of what is available.

Touch. Touch is a natural way of providing noninvasive pain management and comfort (Mueller et al., 2019). When combined with purposeful relaxation, touch may lessen anxiety, reduce muscle tension, and help relieve pain. Touch is now placed in the category of "energy medicine," which includes approaches such as reiki. Reiki is a complementary therapy that can be implemented alongside other techniques. During a reiki session, the practitioner's hands are placed in contact with or slightly above the person receiving treatment to encourage the proper flow of spiritual energy (International Association of Reiki Professionals, 2021). Reiki has been shown to be effective in reducing heart rate and blood pressure and promoting relaxation (McManus, 2017). See the National Center for Complementary and Integrative Health website (https://nccih.nih.gov) for more information on touch.

Cutaneous Nerve Stimulation. Deep and superficial stimulation of nerves for the purpose of pain relief has been practised for centuries. The Chinese practices of acupuncture, acupressure, and moxibustion are examples of this approach. Scientific evidence of the effectiveness of acupuncture and acupressure in the treatment of persistent pain is growing (He et al., 2020; Yin et al., 2017). Nurses have long used massage, vibration, heat, cold, and ointments to treat pain. Heat and cold temporarily interrupt the transmission of pain impulses to the cerebral pain centre (Durham et al., 2015). However, caution must be used in consideration of the cause of the pain. Heat is effective for some pain, such as the deep pain of inflammatory musculo-skeletal conditions (e.g., rheumatic arthritis). On the other hand, heat increases circulation to the area and therefore is contraindicated in occlusive vascular disease and in nonexpansive tissue such as bursae (at some joints), where it may increase pain. At the same time, intermittent application of cold packs helps with low back pain and some instances of nerve irritation. Care must be taken when applying heat and cold to an older adult's skin to prevent skin damage due to normal age-related thinning (see Chapter 6).

Transcutaneous Electrical Nerve Stimulation. Other methods of cutaneous stimulation are transcutaneous electrical nerve stimulation (TENS), low-level laser therapy, and percutaneous electrical nerve stimulation (PENS). Electrodes taped to the skin over the pain site or on the spine emit a mild electrical current that is felt as a tingling, buzzing, or vibrating sensation. The electrical impulses are expected to prevent pain signals from reaching the brain. Both PENS and TENS have been helpful in treating phantom limb pain, PHN, and low back pain (Gibson et al., 2017).

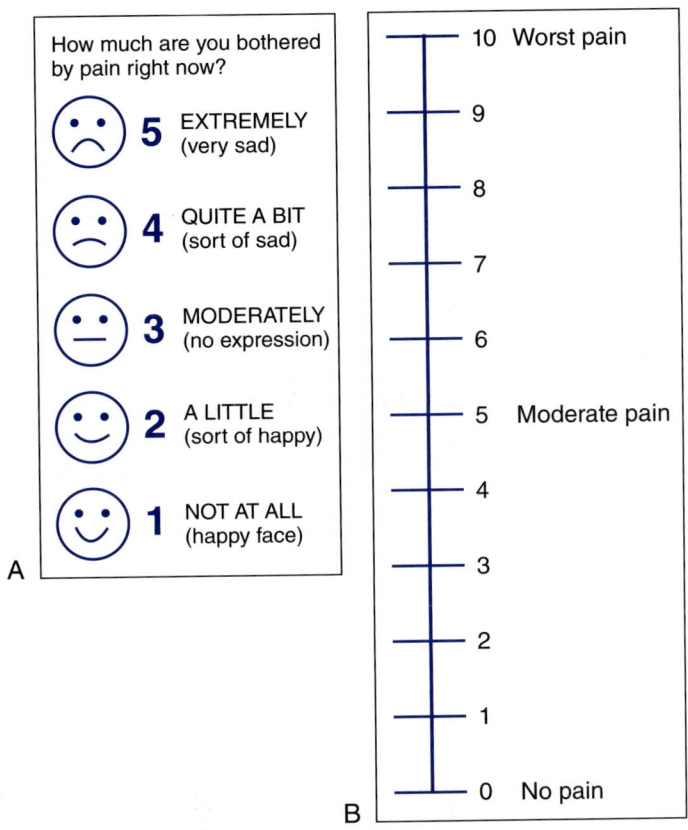

How much are you bothered by pain right now?

5 EXTREMELY (very sad)

4 QUITE A BIT (sort of sad)

3 MODERATELY (no expression)

2 A LITTLE (sort of happy)

1 NOT AT ALL (happy face)

A

10 Worst pain
9
8
7
6
5 Moderate pain
4
3
2
1
0 No pain

B

May be duplicated for use in clinical practice.

Fig. 16.3 ■ Visual analogue scales. (A) Example of a visual analogue scale. (B) Example of a numeric rating scale.

Cognitive Behavioural Approaches

Some of the cognitive behavioural approaches that can help relieve pain for older adults are biofeedback, distraction, relaxation, meditation, and imagery.

Biofeedback. In the biofeedback approach, a person can learn voluntary control over some bodily processes and alter them by changing the physiological correlates appropriate to them. Training and equipment of some type are needed to learn how to alter one's body response through biofeedback. Biofeedback requires full cognitive functioning and manual dexterity for self-treatment.

Distraction. Distraction is a behavioural strategy that lessens the perception of pain by drawing the person's attention away from the pain and relegating it to peripheral awareness. In some instances, the individual is completely unaware of the pain; in others, the intensity of pain is significantly diminished. Pain messages are more slowly transmitted to the pain centre in the brain, and thus less pain is felt.

Mild to moderate pain responds well to distraction. At times, if an individual concentrates intently on another subject, the acute pain may be relieved. The most common forms of distraction are breathing exercises, guided imagery, relaxation, and humour (Doody & Bailey, 2017).

Relaxation, Meditation, and Imagery. The behavioural strategy of relaxation enables the quieting of the mind and the muscles, providing the release of tension and anxiety. Relaxation should be adjunctive to all pharmacological interventions.

Meditation and imagery promote relaxation. Imagery uses the person's imagination to focus on settings that evoke happiness and relaxation rather than on stressful situations. Studies of guided imagery and other complementary therapies showed that these therapies decrease pain perception in cases of pain related to fibromyalgia and cancer (Zech et al., 2017; De Paolis et al., 2019).

Pharmacological Interventions for Pain Relief

Pharmacological pain relief is accomplished by using medication to alter sensory transmission to the cerebral cortex. This approach is most effective when the treatment regimen involves teamwork between the older person, health care providers, family members, and significant others. In some cultures, tribal elders, the oldest son, or others must be consulted first, with permission of the older adult (see Chapter 4).

A variety of pharmacological interventions are available for pain management. The World Health Organization (1996) recommends a "pain ladder" for managing analgesia for persistent pain and provides guidelines for selecting an analgesic and for stepping up the amount of it.

Non-narcotics, such as paracetamol (acetaminophen) and NSAIDs (e.g., ibuprofen) are used for mild pain. For mild to moderate pain, paracetamol and NSAIDs in combination with a weak opioid (e.g., hydrocodone) can be used.

The combination of long-acting medications and short-acting analgesics has been particularly effective. To relieve moderate to severe pain, narcotics (e.g., morphine, OxyContin) and **adjuvant** medications should be used. Adjuvant medications were originally developed to treat other medical conditions but have been found to have pain-relieving qualities. Some of the more frequently used adjuvant medications are antidepressants (to relieve nerve pain and insomnia), anticonvulsants (to relieve neuropathic pain), corticosteroids (to reduce inflammation), and bisphosphonates (to relieve bone pain).

The general principles of controlling pain in older adults are the same as those for controlling pain in younger adults. However, older adults may experience more medication side effects that are related to age-associated changes in the absorption, distribution, metabolism, and excretion of medication (see Chapter 14). Meperidine (Demerol),

frequently given for postoperative or post-traumatic injury pain, is absolutely contraindicated for use in older adults. A guideline for the management of pain in older adults has been developed by the Registered Nurses' Association of Ontario (https://rnao.ca/bpg/resources/assessment-and-management-pain-elderly-learning-package-long-term-care).

In gerontological nursing, it is essential that pain medications be started at the lowest dose possible. However, it is equally important for the dosages to be **titrated** to the point that pain is relieved and relief is continuous. Too often, a low dose is started but increases are delayed, unnecessarily prolonging the patient's suffering. The goal of pain management—particularly the management of persistent pain—is to prevent the pain, not simply relieve it.

Non-narcotic Analgesics. Acetaminophen is often adequate for mild to moderate pain. However 4 g (4 000 mg) is the maximum that can be taken every 24 hours. This maximum dose is reduced for persons with renal or hepatic dysfunction or who drink alcohol.

If acetaminophen is not effective or tolerated, one of the many available NSAIDs (e.g., Aspirin or ibuprofen) may be used. Commonly used over-the-counter NSAIDs must be used with caution because of the increased risk of negative side effects or death due to acute gastro-intestinal bleeding and cardiovascular events (McDonald, 2019).

The American Geriatrics Society (AGS) has long maintained an updated list of potentially inappropriate medication use in older adults called the AGS Beers Criteria. This comprehensive list allows health care providers to review which medications to avoid prescribing to older adults because they often present with a potentially life-threatening interaction (American Geriatrics Society Beers Criteria Update Expert Panel, 2019). One pain medication that is on the AGS Beers Criteria is Meperidine, as it may cause delirium and neurotoxicity. It is also recommended to avoid chronic use of noncyclooxygenase-selective NSAIDs such as Aspirin at a dose greater than 325 mg/day, diclofenac, and fenoprofen, as these may increase the risk of adverse reactions such as gastro-intestinal bleeding (American Geriatrics Society Beers Criteria Update Expert Panel, 2019).

Narcotic Analgesics. Narcotic medications, especially opioids, treat both acute and persistent pain effectively.

Opiates produce a greater analgesic effect, a higher peak, and a longer-duration effect in older adults than in younger adults. This is partly due to the prolonged half-lives of the medications (see Chapter 14). The recommendation to start with the lowest anticipated effective dose, monitor response frequently, and titrate slowly to the desired effect is especially applicable to the use of narcotic pain relievers. Pain relief should be planned for an "around the clock" approach, with a combination of long-acting or sustained-release analgesics and as-needed (PRN) medications. Regular use of breakthrough medication is an indication that the dosage of the long-acting medication should be adjusted.

Opioids used for persistent pain control over a long period should be convenient and easy to administer or take. The simplest medication regimen is the one most likely to be effective and easy to follow. The side effects of opioids include gait disturbance, dizziness, sedation, falls, nausea, pruritus, and constipation. Several of these effects will resolve on their own as the body becomes adjusted to the medication. The side effects may be lessened or prevented when the prescribing care provider works closely with the older adult and nurses to slowly titrate the dosage to the point at which the best relief is obtained with the fewest side effects. Sedation and impaired cognition do occur when opioid analgesics are started or when dosages are increased, which is often of great concern to older adults and their families. Both the older adult and their family should be cautioned about the potential for falls, and appropriate safety precautions should be taken.

Nurses should take careful note of the person's responses and needs in order to prevent and promptly treat side effects or negative drug reactions. Since constipation is almost universal when opioids are used, nurses need to ensure that an appropriate bowel regimen starts at the same time opioid administration starts. A daily dose of a combination stool softener and mild laxative may help, along with adequate fluid intake and exercise.

Medical Cannabis. Medical cannabis has been indicated to assist with pain relief. The two most common forms of cannabinoids are tetrahydrocannabinol (THC) and cannabidiol (CBD) (Canadian Centre on Substance Use and Addiction, 2020). THC is the primary psychoactive component of cannabis, which produces the "high" or euphoric feeling (Canadian Centre on Substance Use and Addiction, 2020). CBD does not produce a high but may cause drowsiness. More studies are being conducted on the effectiveness of CBD (Canadian Centre on Substance Use and Addiction, 2020).

There is limited evidence available on the use of medical cannabis to treat acute pain. Preclinical studies suggest that certain cannabinoids can block the response to experimentally induced acute pain in animal models (Government of Canada, 2018b). There is a modest effect for chronic, noncancer pain (studies have reported an analgesic effect of smoked cannabis) (Government of Canada, 2018b), and a modest or mixed effect for cancer pain (Government of Canada, 2018b).

People respond differently to medical cannabis. Acute effects of smoking or eating cannabis can include feelings of euphoria (a "high"). Others may experience anxiety (Government of Canada, 2018b). Side effects include heightened sensory perception, hallucinations, and misperceptions (Government of Canada, 2018b). Cannabis can interact with medications such as pain medications, blood thinners, antidepressants, and sleeping pills (Canadian Centre on Substance Use and Addiction, 2020). Health risks of daily cannabis use may include increased risk for psychosis, worsening anxiety or depression, and memory effects, including impaired concentration and ability to make decisions (Canadian Centre on Substance Use and Addiction, 2020).

Evaluation

Evaluation of pain relief outcomes requires a reassessment of the older adult's status. The ongoing reassessment includes the reevaluation of the frequency and intensity of pain; behavioural signs and symptoms that suggest pain; response to pharmacological and non-pharmacological interventions; and the impact of pain on mood, activities of daily living, sleep, functioning, and other measures of quality of life. Adjustments of treatment regimens and interventions are based on reassessment findings. Active involvement of the older adult, their family, and the interprofessional team is essential for the comprehensive assessment, management, and evaluation of pain.

SUMMARY

Pain should not be considered a normal part of aging. Gerontological nurses should promote appropriate pain management by first accurately assessing pain in their patients. Implementing and evaluating interventions to treat pain in older adults poses several challenges. Special considerations need to be taken for older adults with communication or cognitive difficulties, as they may express pain differently from those who are able to verbally describe their pain. Gerontological nurses also need to be able to accurately evaluate the effectiveness of their interventions and assess for complications.

KEY CONCEPTS

- The absence of expressed pain does not necessarily imply comfort. Comfort is a state of ease and the satisfaction of bodily needs, as well as freedom from pain and anxiety.
- Pain is not limited to pain of physical origin. Pain from psychological or spiritual factors can have the same effect and is often combined with pain from physical causes.

- The assessment of pain is influenced by many misconceptions, myths, and stereotypes about pain. Inadequate treatment of pain is a major concern for older adults.
- Culture, ethnicity, family, and personal characteristics all influence a person's tolerance and expression of pain.
- Older adults with various degrees of cognitive impairment may demonstrate pain by increased levels of confusion, restlessness, or withdrawal.
- The nursing goal is to assist in pain relief. Some pain medications are more appropriate than others for older adults.
- Acute pain and persistent pain necessitate different therapeutic approaches. Persistent pain predominates in the lives of many older adults.
- Various combinations of pharmacological and nonpharmacological pain control measures can be effective but must be individually designed with the older adult's involvement in the decision making.

ACTIVITIES AND DISCUSSION QUESTIONS

1. What is pain?

2. Compare the features of acute and persistent pain.

3. List the data necessary for an accurate pain assessment.

4. What are the barriers that interfere with the assessment and treatment of pain in all adults? What barriers are associated with pain management in older adults?

5. How might pain be expressed in cognitively impaired older adults? How does the assessment of pain in cognitively impaired older adults differ from the assessment of pain in other people?

6. What pharmacological and nonpharmacological therapies are available?

RESOURCES

Arthritis Society
http://www.arthritis.ca
Canadian Pain Coalition. *Charter Of Pain Patient's Rights And Responsibilities.*
https://www.rsdcanada.org/parc/english/resources/coalition.htm
Canadian Pain Society
http://www.canadianpainsociety.ca
Canadian Skin Patient Alliance
http://www.skinpatientalliance.ca
The Hartford Institute for Geriatric Nursing. *Evidence-informed practice guidelines in its Try This: Series.*
https://hign.org/

National Center for Complementary and Integrative Health
https://nccih.nih.gov/
Pain Assessment in Advanced Dementia scale (PAINAD)
http://dementiapathways.ie/_filecache/04a/ddd/98-painad.pdf
Registered Nurses' Association of Ontario. *Assessment and Management of Pain in the Elderly—Learning Package Long-Term Care.*
https://rnao.ca/bpg/resources/assessment-and-management-pain-elderly-learning-package-long-term-care

For additional resources, please visit *http://evolve.elsevier.com/Canada/Ebersole/gerontological/*

REFERENCES

Achterberg, W., Lautenbacher, S., Husebo, B., et al. (2020). Pain in dementia. *Pain Reports, 5*(1), e803. doi:10.1097/PR9.0000000000000803.

American Geriatrics Society Beers Criteria Update Expert Panel. (2019). American Geriatrics Society 2019 Updated AGS Criteria for Potentially Inappropriate Medication Use in Older Adults. *Journal of the American Geriatrics Society, 67*(4), 674–694. doi:10.1111/jgs.15767.

Backe, I. F., Patil, G. G., Nes, R. B., et al. (2018). The relationship between physical functional limitations, and psychological distress: Considering a possible mediating role of pain, social support and sense of mastery. *SSM Population Health, 4*, 153–163. doi:10.1016/j.ssmph.2017.12.005.

Browne, E. M., Hadjistavropoulos, T., Prkachin, K., et al. (2019). Pain expressions in dementia: Validity of observers' pain judgments as a function of angle of observation. *Journal of Nonverbal Behavior, 43*, 309–327. doi:10.1007/s10919-019-00303-4.

Canadian Centre on Substance Use and Addiction. (2020). *A guide to cannabis for older adults.* https://www.ccsa.ca/guide-cannabis-older-adults.

Canadian Pain Task Force. (2019). *Chronic pain in Canada: Laying a foundation for action.* Health Canada. https://www.canada.ca/en/health-canada/corporate/about-health-canada/public-engagement/external-advisory-bodies/canadian-pain-task-force/report-2019.html/.

De Paolis, G., Naccarato, A., Cibelli, F., et al. (2019). The effectiveness of progressive muscle relaxation and interactive guided imagery as a pain-reducing intervention in advanced cancer patients: A multicentre randomised controlled non-pharmacological trial. *Complementary Therapies in Clinical Practice, 34*, 280–287. doi:10.1016/j.ctcp.2018.12.014.

Delgado, D. A., Lambert, B. S., Boutris, N., et al. (2018). Validation of digital visual analog scale pain scoring with a traditional paper-based visual analog scale in adults. *Journal of the American Academy of Orthopaedic Surgeons. Global Research & Reviews, 2*(3), e088.

Devor, M. (2018). Rethinking the causes of pain in herpes zoster and postherpetic neuralgia: The ectopic pacemaker hypothesis. *Pain Reports, 3*(6), 3702. doi:10.1097/PR9.0000000000000702.

Doody, O., & Bailey, M. E. (2017). Inventions in pain management for persons with an intellectual disability. *Journal of Intellectual Disabilities, 23*(1), 132–144. doi:10.1177/1744629517708679.

Durham, C. O., Fowler, T., Donato, A., et al. (2015). Pain management in patients with rheumatoid arthritis. *Nurse Practitioner, 40*(5), 38–45. doi:10.1097/01.NPR.0000463784.36883.23.

Edmond, S. N., Becker, W. C., Driscoll, M. A., et al. (2018). Use of non-pharmacological pain treatment modalities among veterans with chronic pain: Results from a cross-sectional survey. *Journal of General Internal Medicine, 33*(1), 54–60. doi:10.1007/s11606-018-4322-0.

Gibson, W., Wand, B. M., & O'Connell, N. E. (2017). Transcutaneous electrical nerve stimulation (TENS) for neuropathic pain in adults. *Cochrane Database of Systematic Reviews, 9*, CD011976. doi:10.1002/14651858.CD011976.pub2.

Government of Canada. (2018a). *Herpes zoster (shingles) vaccine: Canadian immunization guide.* https://www.canada.ca/en/public-health/services/publications/healthy-living/canadian-immunization-guide-part-4-active-vaccines/page-8-herpes-zoster-(shingles)-vaccine.html.

Government of Canada. (2018b). *Information for health care professionals: Cannabis (marihuana, marijuana) and the cannabinoids.* https://www.canada.ca/en/health-canada/services/drugs-medication/cannabis/information-medical-practitioners/information-health-care-professionals-cannabis-cannabinoids.html.

He, Y., Guo, X., & May, B. H. (2020). Clinical evidence for association of acupuncture and acupressure with improved cancer pain: A systematic review and meta-analysis. *JAMA Oncology, 6*(2), 271–278. doi:10.1001/jamaoncol.2019.5233.

HealthLink BC. (2017). *Shingles.* https://www.healthlinkbc.ca/health-topics/hw75433.

Hunnicutt, J. N., Ulbricht, C. M., Tjia, J., et al. (2017). Pain and pharmacologic pain management in long-stay nursing home residents. *Pain, 158*(6), 1091–1099. doi:10.1097/j.pain.0000000000000887.

International Association of Reiki Professionals. (2021). *Reiki in Ontario hospitals.* https://iarp.org/reiki-in-ontario-hospitals-3/.

Kutlutürkan, S., & Urvaylıoğlu, A. E. (2020). Evaluation of pain as a fifth vital sign: Nurses' opinions and beliefs. *Asia-Pacific Journal of Oncology Nursing, 7*(1), 88. doi:10.4103/apjon.apjon_39_19.

Lapane, K. L., Quilliam, B. J., Chow, W., et al. (2012). The association between pain and measures of well-being among nursing home residents. *Journal of the American Medical Directors Association, 13*(4), 344–349. doi:10.1016/j.jamda.2011.01.007.

Liu, S. H., Dubé, C. E., Eaton, C. B., et al. (2018). Long-term effectiveness of intra-articular injections on patient-reported symptoms in knee osteoarthritis. *Journal of Rheumatology, 45*(9), 1316–1324. doi:10.3899/jrheum.171385.

McDonald, D. D. (2019). Predictors of gastrointestinal bleeding in older persons taking nonsteroidal anti-inflammatory drugs: Results from the FDA adverse events reporting system. *Journal of the American Association of Nurse Practitioners, 31*(3), 206–213. doi:10.1097/JXX.0000000000000222.

McManus, D. E. (2017). Reiki is better than placebo and has broad potential as a complementary health therapy. *Journal of Evidence-Based Complementary & Alternative Medicine, 22*(4), 1051–1057. doi:10.1177/2156587217728644.

Mueller, G., Palli, C., & Schumacher, P. (2019). The effect of therapeutic touch on back pain in adults on a neurological unit: An experimental pilot study. *Pain Management Nursing, 20*(1), 75–81. doi:10.1016/j.pmn.2018.09.002.

Vina, E. R., & Kwoh, C. K. (2018). Epidemiology of osteoarthritis: Literature update. *Current Opinion in Rheumatology, 30*(2), 160. doi:10.1097/BOR.0000000000000479.

Vostinaru, O. (2017). Adverse effects and drug interactions of nonsteroidal anti-inflammatory drugs. *Nonsteroidal Anti-Inflammatory Drugs.* doi:10.5772/intechopen.68198.

World Health Organization. (1996). *Cancer pain relief: With a guide to opioid availability* (2nd ed.). http://apps.who.int/iris/bitstream/10665/37896/1/9241544821.pdf.

Yin, C., Buchheit, T. E., & Park, J. J. (2017). Acupuncture for chronic pain: An update and critical overview. *Anaesthesiology, 30*(5), 583–592. doi:10.1097/ACO.0000000000000501.

Zech, N., Hansen, E., Bernardy, K., et al. (2017). Efficacy, acceptability and safety of guided imagery/hypnosis in fibromyalgia–A systematic review and meta-analysis of randomized controlled trials. *European Journal of Pain, 21*(2), 217–227.

17

DIABETES MELLITUS

∎ ∎ ∎ ∎ ∎ ∎ ∎ ∎ ∎ ∎ ∎ ∎ ∎ ∎

LEARNING OBJECTIVES

Upon completion of this chapter, the reader will be able to:

- Explain the risks for and complications of diabetes in the older adult.
- Identify the unique aspects of diabetes management in older adults.
- Describe the assessment necessary in the screening and monitoring of individuals with diabetes.
- Explain the important components of diabetes management.
- Discuss the nurse's role in diabetes management.
- Develop a nursing care plan for an older adult with diabetes.
- Provide culturally safe and competent diabetes management to older adults.
- Discuss the evidence and rationale for a high rate of diabetes among those over 75 years of age.

GLOSSARY

Autoimmune   A term describing a condition where the immune system sees a part of the body as a foreign object and produces antibodies to attack it.

Glycosylated hemoglobin (Hb A1c) test   A blood test that measures the amount of glucose in the hemoglobin of red blood cells, averaged over the 90-day lifespan of the cells.

Hyperosmolar nonketotic syndrome   A metabolic complication of diabetes that often arises during periods of physiological stress and is characterized by a rise in blood glucose (hyperglycemia), dehydration, hyperosmolar plasma, and an altered level of consciousness.

Insulin   A hormone in the pancreas that controls blood glucose levels.

Insulin resistance   Insensitivity of the body's cells to the insulin produced by the pancreas, thus impairing glucose metabolism.

Intertriginous area   An area where two skin areas may touch or rub together. Examples are the axilla of the arm, the anogenital region, the nares, and the skinfolds of the breasts.

Macrovascular   Term referring to the larger, more prominent blood vessels in the body, such as the coronary arteries and the aorta.

Microvascular   Term referring to the smaller blood vessels in the body.

Polydipsia   Feelings of excessive thirst, often associated with diabetes.

Polyphagia   Feelings of excessive hunger, often associated with diabetes.

Polyuria   Abnormally excessive urine production and excretion, often associated with diabetes.

THE LIVED EXPERIENCE

"Today, I provided Rita with some more information on how to manage her diabetes. I realize there is a lot to learn, so we will do a little bit every day. She is really starting to understand it. I think she will do quite well."
Anna, gerontological clinical nurse specialist

DIABETES

Diabetes mellitus (DM), type 1 or type 2, is a syndrome of disorders of glucose metabolism that result in hyperglycemia. Although no direct genetic influence has been found in connection with the development of type 2 DM, genes that are related to the risk for type 1 DM have been identified. Type 1 DM (formerly called *insulin-dependent diabetes mellitus*) develops in early life and is a result of **autoimmune** destruction of the **insulin**-producing beta cells of the pancreas. The resulting absence of insulin is incompatible with life; without replacement of the insulin, the person will die.

Type 2 DM (formerly called *non–insulin-dependent diabetes mellitus*) develops later in life, when the pancreas makes insulin but not enough to keep up with the needs of the body. This inadequate supply of naturally occurring insulin is combined with the **insulin resistance** that is characteristic of type 2 DM. The onset is usually insidious, and up to one-half of all persons with type 2 DM may be undiagnosed (Box 17.1). These persons may go a number of years without treatment while they are developing serious complications.

The number of individuals with diabetes and the risk for diabetes vary by ethnicity, place of residence, and age (Box 17.2). Eleven million Canadians are living with diabetes or prediabetes (Diabetes Canada, 2020). People from some populations (e.g., people of South Asian, Asian, African, Latin American, or Indigenous descent) are at a higher risk for type 2 DM (Diabetes Canada, 2020). Various studies conducted throughout Canada reported extremely high rates of diabetes in some Indigenous communities. Specifically, type 2 DM is a major concern among the Indigenous population in Canada. Indigenous peoples in Canada are 2.25 to 3.5 times more likely to have type 2 DM than non-Indigenous people (Institute of Health Economics, 2018). Contributing factors to these high numbers include genetic susceptibility and rapid lifestyle changes over the past two or three generations, highlighted by a shift from traditional lifestyles toward more sedentary living and Western diets (Walker et al., 2020).

The question remains whether diabetes is a primary or secondary event when there is a coexisting illness. Coexisting illnesses, such as hypertension and dyslipidemia, are associated with a decrease in insulin sensitivity. Alcohol and drugs such as diuretics, glucocorticoids, and nonsteroidal anti-inflammatory drugs may also contribute to insulin resistance or the body's failure to use the insulin that is present. Owing to peripheral neuropathy and uncontrolled glucoses, persons with

---

BOX 17.1

SIGNS AND SYMPTOMS SUGGESTIVE OF DIABETES IN THE OLDER ADULT

1. General symptoms are polyphagia, polyuria, polydipsia, and weight loss. (As these symptoms are rarely seen in older adults, the nurse should also focus on additional symptoms that are more vague, such as fatigue and varied or recurrent infections.)
2. Recurrent infections (particularly those of bacterial or fungal origin) that involve the skin, **intertriginous areas**, or genito-urinary tract, and sores or wounds that tend to heal slowly.
3. Neurological dysfunction, including paresthesia, dysesthesia, or hyperesthesia; muscle weakness and pain (amyotrophy); cranial nerve palsies; autonomic dysfunction of the gastro-intestinal tract (diarrhea), cardiovascular abnormalities (orthostatic hypotension, dysrhythmias), reproductive system problems (erectile dysfunction), or bladder abnormalities (atony, overflow incontinence).
4. Arterial disease (macroangiopathy) involving the cardiovascular, cerebrovascular, or peripheral vasculature structures.
5. Small-vessel disease (microangiopathy) involving the kidneys (proteinuria, glomerulopathy, uremia) and eyes (macular disease, exudates, hemorrhages).
6. Lesions of the skin (Dupuytren's contracture, facial rubeosis, diabetic dermopathy).
7. Endocrine–metabolic complications (dyslipidemia, obesity, history of thyroid or adrenal insufficiency [Schmidt's syndrome]).

---

diabetes often have other health problems as well, including problems metabolizing lipids and proteins. Diabetes is the leading cause of end-stage renal disease and blindness and is especially prevalent among older adults over 65 years of age.

Complications

Complications occur over the long course of the disease and are **microvascular, macrovascular,** or both. The microvascular problems are loss of vision (diabetic retinopathy) and end-stage renal failure from diabetic nephropathy. Delayed wound healing, when combined with peripheral neuropathy, may necessitate amputation.

Macrovascular complications include myocardial infarction, stroke, peripheral vascular disease, and neuropathy. Combined macrovascular and microvascular

BOX 17.2
RISK FACTORS FOR DIABETES MELLITUS

- Ethnicity (Indigenous, Hispanic, Asian, and African descent)
- Increasing age (>40 years)
- Blood pressure ≥140/90 mm Hg
- First-degree relative (parent, sibling, or child) with diabetes mellitus (DM)
- History of impaired glucose tolerance or impaired fasting plasma glucose
- Obesity (>120% of desirable weight, or body mass index >30 kg/m^2)
- Previous gestational DM or having had a child with a birth weight >4.1 kg (9 lb)
- Undesirable lipid levels (high-density lipoproteins <0.90 mmol/L [35 mg/dL] or triglycerides >2.82 mmol/L [250 mg/dL])

damage can lead to erectile dysfunction as a result of reduced vascular flow, peripheral neuropathy, and uncontrolled circulating blood glucose. Persons with diabetes commonly have problems with their feet, which can have a considerable impact on their functional status (see Chapter 11). Warning signs of foot problems derive from different body systems and include cold feet and intermittent pain from claudication (vascular); burning, tingling, hypersensitivity, or numbness (neurological); a gradual change in shape or a sudden, painless change without trauma (musculoskeletal); and infections, changes of skin colour and texture, and slow-healing painful or painless wounds (dermatological) (Diabetes Canada, 2018).

Diabetes is often associated with a number of other health problems. Diabetes increases the risk of hypertension, atherosclerosis, coronary artery disease, and stroke (Heart and Stroke Foundation of Canada, 2020). The most common cardiovascular complications for people with diabetes are myocardial infarction or heart failure (Heart and Stroke Foundation of Canada, 2020). Those with diabetes are three times more likely to die of heart disease (Heart and Stroke Foundation of Canada, 2020).

Some of the barriers to the delivery of effective care for diabetes are related to the older adult's access to primary health care practitioners, especially in rural and remote areas and in Indigenous communities. Also, the

cost of test supplies is often an issue for people who do not have private health care insurance coverage. The gerontological nurse needs to collaborate with colleagues in the community, the diabetes educator, and social workers to find the best solution in these situations.

Treatment and Goals

Even in the best of circumstances, diabetes is a chronic disease that causes damage to the body's organs. When diabetes is untreated or undertreated, complications develop more quickly and are more severe. Therefore, holding back the progression of the disease is the major goal.

For younger adults (aged 18–60), the main goal of treatment is maintaining glycemic control most of the time, aiming for a blood sugar level of 4.4–6.1 mmol/L (82–110 mg/dL) and **glycosylated hemoglobin (Hg A1c)** at or below 7.0% (Punthakee et al. 2018). However, a consensus report on diabetes management of older adults has asserted that tight glycemic control is not always preferred (Sasso et al., 2018). Based on the results of several large studies, the American Diabetes Association modified its recommendations in 2020 for glycemic control in older adults (American Diabetes Association [ADA], 2020). It is now recommended that the degree of glycemic control be based on the condition of the person rather than on a universal number. For healthy older adults with a reasonably long life expectancy, the same evidence-informed practice as that for younger adults should be followed. However, for those who are medically fragile and whose life expectancy is limited, some flexibility may be more appropriate, along with an emphasis on quality of life rather than length of life. Tight control of glucose levels in these circumstances may lead to life-threatening hypoglycemia. A goal of an Hb A1c greater than 8% for the very frail may be adequate (Yanase et al., 2017).

As might be expected, anxiety, depression, and poor perceptions of one's health are often associated with diabetes, and these emotional states may reduce the person's motivation for self-management. Social support has a positive effect on the depression and anxiety surrounding the diagnosis of diabetes and living with diabetes (Williams et al., 2020). A holistic approach and more depth and breadth in nursing practice in the care of the diabetic patient facilitates improved health maintenance and adherence to recommended therapies.

IMPLICATIONS FOR GERONTOLOGICAL NURSING AND HEALTHY AGING

Gerontological nurses have great potential for helping individuals with diabetes, ranging from conducting screenings to educating and coaching the patient and their family. Nurses can participate in early detection through public screenings or by paying attention to the need for the screening of older adults residing in communal settings such as long-term care (LTC) homes, assisted-living facilities, and communities. Furthermore, nurses should promote healthy aging by helping people reach or maintain an ideal body weight, eat a healthy diet that provides adequate protein without excessive carbohydrates, exercise regularly, and keep cholesterol levels and blood pressure under control, all of which reduce the risk for diabetes.

For persons at higher risk for diabetes, especially those with impaired fasting glucose or impaired glucose tolerance, attention should be directed at reducing their risks for both diabetes and heart disease. This means education and the carrying out of interventions to help the older adult reach the following goals:

- No smoking
- Blood pressure ≤130/80 mm Hg
- Cholesterol <5.18 mmol/L (200 mg/dL)
- Low-density lipoprotein <2.56 mmol/L (100 mg/dL)
- High-density lipoprotein >1.03 mmol/L (40 mg/dL)
- Triglycerides <1.69 mmol/L (150 mg/dL)
- Fasting blood glucose <7 mmol/L (<126 mg/dL)

Screening for diabetes by fasting plasma and random blood glucose testing is important for the early identification of potential or actual disease. Annual screening of fasting plasma glucose measurements is recommended for all persons in high-risk groups, including all persons over 65 years of age.

Assessment

The nurse begins with an assessment for risk factors and a subjective report of signs and symptoms, including an evaluation of the presence or absence of hyperglycemia, **polydipsia**, **polyuria**, or **polyphagia**. Because these symptoms are rarely seen in older adults, it is important to also focus on symptoms that are more vague, such as fatigue, change in weight, and varied or recurrent infections.

When there are symptoms, their duration and character should be described. Family history is important because of genetic influence. Nutrition, weight, and exercise history can identify eating patterns, an active or sedentary lifestyle, and weight control measures, all of which can provide clues for realistic education. Assessing social determinants of health and economic resources help to establish the person's ability to purchase equipment, materials, and foods that may be needed to maintain diabetes control. This is important for older adults who may have a limited income. A history of alcohol and tobacco use provides information about the person's risk for complications.

The nursing assessment also includes the careful measurement of blood pressure, visual acuity, and gross neurological function. Distance vision can be checked with a Snellen chart, and near vision can be checked with a newspaper. The skin and feet should be thoroughly inspected for any injury, such as corns, calluses, blisters, cracks, or fungal infections. The use of the Semmes–Weinstein monofilament instrument is recommended to test for peripheral neuropathy. The test consists of a sensory assessment tool, with a set of monofilaments that vary in thickness and diameter. These monofilaments are used to map out sensory loss. Box 17.3 demonstrates monofilament testing.

Management

Promoting healthy aging in persons with diabetes requires an array of interventions and usually involves an interprofessional team that works together with the person. It is also important to involve care partners in the assessment and management of diabetes. Management of diabetes requires support for the person and expertise in medication use, diet and exercise, monitoring, and counselling. The interprofessional team may include nurses as well as dietitians, pharmacists, podiatrists, ophthalmologists, physicians, nurse practitioners, certified diabetic educators, and counsellors. If the disease is hard to control, endocrinologists are involved; as complications develop, more specialists (such as nephrologists, cardiologists, and wound care specialists) are called in.

Diabetes self-management, diabetes self-management education, and patient empowerment are now the cornerstones of disease management (Sherifali et al., 2018). The skills needed for self-management include

BOX 17.3
MONOFILAMENT TESTING IN THE DIABETIC FOOT

1. When performing the Semmes–Weinstein monofil-ament test, apply the monofilament perpendicular to the skin with enough force to cause the filament to bend. Skin contact and removal of the filament should take 2 seconds.
2. The filament should be applied along the perim-eter of an ulcer, scar, or neurotic tissue, not on

these tissues. Ask the patient whether they feel pressure (yes or no) and where they feel pressure (left foot or right foot).
3. Repeat this application twice at the same site, but alternate this with at least one "mock" application where no filament is applied.

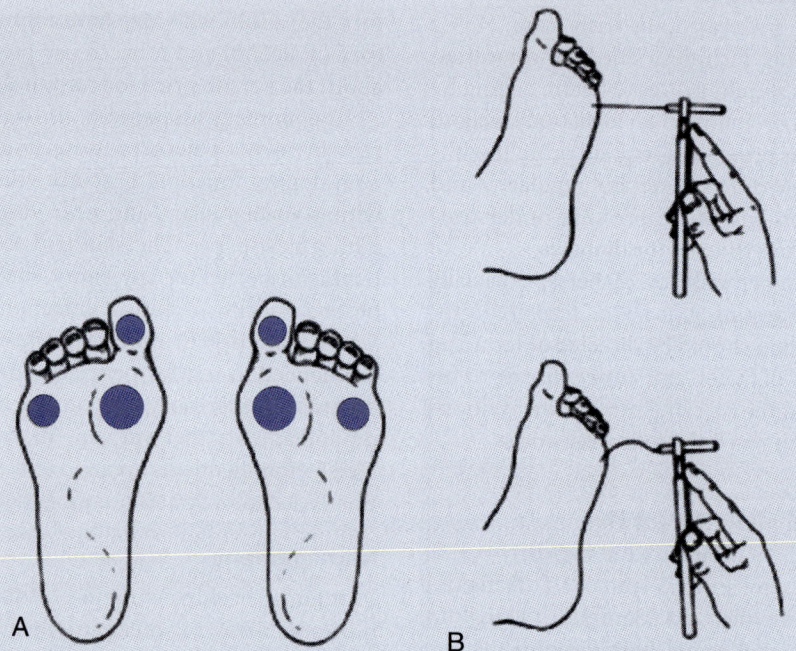

A   B

Semmes–Weinstein Monofilament. (A) Sites to be tested with the monofilament. (B) Application of the monofilament. *Protective sensation is present at each site if the patient correctly answers two out of three applications. Protective sensation is absent with two out of three incorrect answers. If protective sensation is absent, then the patient is considered to be at risk of ulceration.* **Source:** Adapted from Canadian Diabetes Association. (2018). Appendix 12: Monofilament testing in the diabetic foot. *Canadian Journal of Diabetes, 42,* S322.

knowledge of nutrition, the development of an exercise plan, the safe use of medication, what to do during peri-ods of other illness, attention to the psychological aspects of dealing with a chronic illness, the ability to use per-sonal glucose monitors, optimal care of the feet, and knowledge about the disease. These teachings should also include the care partners, especially if the person experi-ences difficulty with self-management resulting from conditions such as arthritis or dementia. The nurse is highly instrumental in the teaching of self-management

skills, encouraging patient and family empowerment, and supporting the person.

Standards of Care

Diabetes Canada has developed a set of clinical practice guidelines for the prevention and management of dia-betes in Canada (Diabetes Canada Clinical Practice Guidelines Expert Committee, 2018). The first and per-haps most important recommendation is that the care of the older adult with diabetes must be individually planned in order to consider the relative costs and benefits for the person. Among those recommendations are the following:

- When collecting the person's health history, the nurse should include smoking history, dietary habits, weight patterns, previous treatment programs, current treatment regimen, exercise and activity levels, infections, illnesses, and complications of diabetes. Information about the approaches that worked and those that failed will help the nurse design programs specific to the older adult.
- Annual physical examination includes blood pressure measurement; dilated eye examination; thyroid palpation; palpation of pulses; foot, periodontal, and skin examination; and neurological examination. Testing fine sensation with a monofilament is recommended.
- Laboratory tests should include both a fasting plasma glucose test and an Hb A1c test; fasting lipid profile; serum creatinine if proteinuria is present; urinalysis (including microalbuminuria) and urine culture if indicated; assessment of thyroid function (thyroxine [T_4] or thyroid-stimulating hormone); and an electrocardiogram (ECG).

Gerontological nurses have an important educational role in the treatment of diabetes and must encourage and help older adults obtain care that can delay or minimize complications. One of the most significant skills for the older adult to master is the technique for the self-monitoring of blood glucose (SMBG), including how to obtain a blood sample with glucose-monitoring equipment, troubleshoot when results indicate an error, and record the values from the machine. Older adults with arthritis, low vision, or peripheral neuropathy will have difficulties with the mechanics of SMBG and will require creative teaching and perhaps the help of others with the tasks that are necessary. New technologies and medication delivery systems (e.g., nasal sprays) are being designed to address some of these issues.

Daily foot care and foot examination should be discussed and demonstrated (Diabetes Canada Clinical Practice Guidelines Expert Committee, 2018). A person who is not particularly flexible will have difficulty reaching and inspecting the feet; a family member or a friend can be asked to do this. As long as the person's vision is adequate, they can place a mirror on the floor to reflect the sole of the foot for examination. Attention to foot care can reduce the risk of amputation. Also, it is essential that the person be aware of the need for shoes that fit well (see Chapter 11). Nurses should inspect the person's gait, foot and toe morphology, and skin for blisters, abrasions, calluses, ulcers, edema, or abnormal colour (Diabetes Canada Clinical Practice Guidelines Expert Committee, 2018).

Knowing about diabetes and its effects includes knowing what affects blood sugar. The older adult should have a list of warning signs for high and low blood sugar levels and know that extra SMBG is necessary any time they feel clammy or cold, sweaty, shaky, or confused—all signs of low blood sugar. Hypoglycemia is the most common challenge for older adults with diabetes, especially for those taking sulphonylureas. Sulphonylureas are antidiabetic medications that act by increasing the release of insulin from pancreatic beta cells. An identification bracelet is highly recommended, especially because of possible misdiagnosis if the person is found to be confused.

Experiential teaching, encouragement, and reinforcement of mastery are important factors that promote successful self-management. Some of the factors affecting diabetes control in older adults are identified in Box 17.4.

Nutrition

Adequate and appropriate nutrition is a key factor in the control of diabetes. An initial nutrition assessment with a 24-hour recall will provide some clues to the person's dietary habits, cultural preferences, intake, and style of eating. If the person is a member of a specific ethnic group or culture, the nurse will need to learn about that group's usual food ingredients and methods of food preparation in order to be able to give reasonable instructions. It is generally recommended that people with diabetes follow the healthy balanced diet presented in *Eating Well With Canada's Food Guide* (Diabetes Canada Clinical Practice Guidelines Expert Committee, 2018) (see Chapter 8). Ideally, all persons with diabetes should have annual medical nutrition therapy by a registered dietitian who is a certified diabetic educator. Diabetes Canada provides information, resources, and guidelines for a healthy diet, with attention to adequate variety, macronutrients, and foods with a low glycemic index (Diabetes Canada Clinical Practice Guidelines Expert Committee, 2018). The recommended daily caloric intake

BOX 17.4
INTERACTION BETWEEN DIABETES AND THE AGING PROCESS

1. A decline in visual acuity can affect the individual's ability to see printed educational material, medication labels, markings on a syringe, and the screen on blood glucose monitoring devices.
2. Auditory impairments can lead to difficulty hearing instructions.
3. Altered taste can affect food choices and nutritional status.
4. Poor dentition or changes in the gastro-intestinal system can lead to difficulties with food ingestion and digestion.
5. Altered ability to recognize hunger and thirst may lead to weight loss, dehydration, and increased risk for **hyperosmolar nonketotic syndrome**, a metabolic complication of diabetes that often arises during periods of physiological stress and is characterized by a rise in blood glucose (hyperglycemia), dehydration, hyperosmolar plasma, and an altered level of consciousness.
6. Changes in hepatic or renal function can affect the ability to absorb or excrete medications.
7. Arthritis or tremors can affect the ability to self-administer medications and use monitoring devices.
8. Polypharmacy complicates medication choices.
9. Depression affects motivation for self-management.
10. Cognitive impairment and dementia decrease self-care ability.
11. Inadequate education and poor literacy call for modifications in the method of teaching about diabetes care.
12. Level of income can affect the level of care sought or obtained.
13. Living alone without a resource person can have a negative effect on the person with diabetes.
14. A sedentary lifestyle and obesity can result in decreased tissue sensitivity to insulin.

ranges from 1 600 calories for women to a maximum of 2 200 calories for men. The goal is to keep the glucose level under control by balancing exercise with eating, weight loss (if overweight), and limiting saturated fats. Carbohydrates are included on the diabetes food pyramid but are restricted to whole grains. For details about all aspects of diet and diabetes, see the Diabetes Canada website at https://www.diabetes.ca/.

It is part of the nurse's responsibility to learn whether there is any difficulty with access to food (including fresh fruit and vegetables), shopping for food, and food preparation. Working with older adults, whose dietary habits have been formed over a lifetime, can be difficult but is not impossible.

Exercise

Exercise is an important aspect of therapy for type 2 DM because it increases insulin production and decreases insulin resistance. Walking is an inexpensive and beneficial way to exercise, and daily exercise is recommended. For older adults whose mobility is limited, chair exercises or exercise machines that permit sitting and holding on for support can be helpful.

In some cases, exercise in conjunction with an appropriate diet may be sufficient to maintain blood glucose within normal levels. A more intensive exercise program should not be started until the older adult has had a physical examination, including a stress test and an ECG. A physician or nurse practitioner and a diabetic educator will then have the information necessary to develop a safe exercise plan for and with the person. If the person is using insulin, exercise must be done on a regular rather than an erratic basis. To avoid hypoglycemia, blood glucose should be tested before and after exercise.

Medications

Antihyperglycemics include oral drugs (including the new inhalant insulin). Oral medications are prescribed according to the identified insulin deficit—insulin resistance, or inadequate or no secretion of insulin. The sulphonylureas (e.g., glyburide) and meglitinides (e.g., repaglinide and nateglinide) increase insulin secretion. Biguanides (e.g., metformin) or thiazolidinediones (e.g., glitazones) enhance insulin sensitivity by decreasing insulin resistance.

The mainstay of the treatment of type 2 DM in later life is oral medication. However, when blood sugar is greater than 11.11 mmol/L (200 mg/dL) and is difficult to control, additional insulin may be necessary. Note that the use of insulin by someone with type 2 DM does not "convert" the person to a type 1 diabetic, because the diagnosis is made on the basis of the type of disorder rather than on the treatment. Common types of insulin prescribed for older adults are rapid-acting insulin and long-acting insulin (Table 17.1). Most people need two or more types of insulin to reach their blood glucose targets. Insulin can be administered through subcutaneous injections (needle or insulin pen), an insulin pump, or an insulin jet injector, which sends a fine spray of insulin through the skin with high-pressure air).

TABLE 17.1
Types of Insulin

Insulin Type (Trade Name)	Onset	Peak	Duration
Bolus (preprandial or mealtime) insulins			
Rapid-acting insulin analogues (clear)			
■ Insulin aspart (NovoRapid)	9–20 min	1–1.5 hours	3–5 hours
■ Insulin glulisine (Apidra)	10–15 min	1–1.5 hours	3.5–5 hours
■ Insulin lispro (Humalog) U-100, U-200	10–15 min	1–2 hours	3–4.75 hours
■ Faster-acting insulin aspart (Fiasp)	4 min	0.5–1.5 hours	3–5 hours
Short-acting insulins (clear)			
■ Insulin regular (Humulin-R, Novolin)	30 min	2–3 hours	6.5 hours
■ Insulin regular (Entuzity (U-500)	15 min	4–8 hours	17–24 hours
Basal Insulins			
Intermediate-acting insulin (cloudy) ■ Insulin neutral protamine Hagedorn	1–3 hours	5–8 hours	Up to 18 hours
Long-acting insulin (clear) ■ Insulin detmir (Levemir) ■ Insulin glargine U-100 (Lantus) ■ Insulin glargine U-300 (Toujeo) ■ Insulin glargine biosimilar (Basaglar) ■ Degludec U-100, U-200 (Tresbia)	90 min	Not applicable	U-100 glargine: 24 hours Detemir: 16–24 hours U-300 glargine: >30 hours Degludec: 42 hours
Premixed insulins			
Premixed regular insulin NPH (cloudy) ■ Humulin 30/70 ■ Novolin ge 30/70, 40/60, 50/50	A single vial or cartridge contains a fixed ratio of insulin		
Premixed insulin analogues (cloudy) ■ Biphasic insulin aspart (NovoMix 30) ■ Insulin lispro/lispro protamine (Humalog, Mix 25, and Mix 50)	(% of rapid-acting or short-acting insulin to % of intermediate-acting insulin)		

Source: Adapted from Diabetes Canada. (2018). Appendix 6: Types of insulin. *Canadian Journal of Diabetes, 42*(1), S314.

If other medications are prescribed, they must be carefully reviewed. The effect of medications on blood glucose must be given serious consideration, because a number of medications commonly used for older patients adversely affect blood glucose levels (Box 17.5). Therefore, older adults who have diabetes should be advised to ask whether a particular prescribed medication affects their therapy, and they should check with their primary care provider before taking any over-the-counter medications.

Long-Term Care and the Older Adult With Diabetes

Many persons cared for by gerontological nurses in LTC homes have diabetes. According to data from the Continuing Care Reporting System maintained by the Canadian Institute for Health Information, the prevalence of diabetes in Ontario LTC homes is about 25% (in 2011); approximately 90% to 95% of diabetes cases are cases of type 2 DM (Osman et al., 2016).

In LTC homes, nurses are responsible for many of the activities that would otherwise fall to the older adult, a significant other, or a home caregiver to carry out. Meals, nutritional status, intake and output, and exercise and activity are monitored. The nurse assesses the resident for signs of hypoglycemia and hyperglycemia, as well as evidence of complications, and ensures that the standards of care are met. Having effective working relationships within the nursing team and ensuring that unregulated workers who provide care for residents with dementia know the signs

BOX 17.5

MEDICATIONS AFFECTING BLOOD SUGAR

MEDICATIONS THAT INCREASE BLOOD GLUCOSE LEVELS

- Corticosteroids
- Diazoxide
- Estrogens
- Furosemide and thiazide diuretics
- Glucagon
- Lithium
- Phenytoin
- Rifampin
- Sympathomimetics (antihistamines, decongestants, bronchodilators)
- Thyroid-replacement preparations
- Atypical antipsychotics (risperidone, olanzapine)

MEDICATIONS THAT DECREASE BLOOD GLUCOSE LEVELS

- Alcohol
- Anabolic steroids
- Beta blockers (antihypertensives)
- Salicylates (high doses)

MEDICATIONS THAT INTERACT WITH SULPHONYLUREAS (ORAL HYPOGLYCEMICS)

Increased Effects (Blood Glucose Levels Further Lowered)

- Allopurinol
- Beta blockers
- Clofibrate
- Histamine antagonists
- Imidazole antifungals
- Low-dose salicylates
- Monoamine oxidase inhibitors
- Probenecid
- Tricyclic antidepressants

MEDICATIONS NOT TO BE TAKEN IN COMBINATION WITH SULPHONYLUREAS

- Chloramphenicol
- Salicylates (high dose)
- Sulphonamides

MEDICATIONS THAT HAVE DECREASED EFFECTS (I.E., HINDER HYPOGLYCEMIC ACTION)

- Barbiturates
- Corticosteroids
- Diuretics
- Estrogens
- Rifampin

Source: Adapted from Freed, S. (2020). *443 drugs that can affect blood glucose levels.* http://www.diabetesincontrol.com/drugs-that-can-affect-blood-glucose-levels/.

of hypoglycemia and hyperglycemia are essential in providing the best care to residents with diabetes. The nurse monitors the effect and side effects of diet, exercise, and medication use; encourages self-care whenever possible; and administers medications or supervises their administration.

Box 17.6 presents an intervention to improve outcomes in patients with diabetes.

BOX 17.6

RESEARCH FOR EVIDENCE-INFORMED PRACTICE: EFFECTIVENESS OF A COMMUNITY PROGRAM FOR OLDER ADULTS WITH TYPE 2 DIABETES

Problem: Type 2 diabetes affects many older adults. Diabetes is associated with multi-morbidity and reduced quality of life. Lifestyle factors and self-management can improve health outcomes. This study evaluated the effect of a community-based intervention and compared it with usual care for older adults with type 2 diabetes.

Methods: Older adults living in the community who were diagnosed with type 2 diabetes and had two or more chronic conditions were invited to participate. Participants were allocated to the intervention or the control group. The intervention group received three in-home visits, a monthly group wellness program, monthly case conferencing, and care coordination over a period of 6 months. The control group received usual care. Outcome data was collected on all participants' physical and mental functioning, anxiety, depressive symptoms, self-efficacy, self-management, and the cost of health care service use.

Findings: The intervention did not show significant differences in improving physical or mental functioning between the two groups. However, the program does have the potential for significant improvements in mental functioning for participants who have lower baseline scores. The program was also shown to be cost neutral when compared with usual care.

Implications for Nursing Practice: Nurses can assist in implementing programs in diabetes clinics and community settings to support older adults with their diabetes management. It is also important to continue evaluating the impact of interventions such as exercise and diet on older adults' quality of life and ability to manage multi-morbidity.

Source: Miklavcic et al., (2020). Effectiveness of a community program for older adults with type 2 diabetes and multi-morbidity: A pragmatic randomized controlled trial. *BMC Geriatrics, 20*(1), 1–14. doi:10.1186/s12877-020-01557-0.

SUMMARY

Given the numerous complications and comorbidities associated with diabetes, gerontological nurses play an essential role in the prevention, early detection, and management of this disease. Nurses must be able to assess and identify older adults who are most at risk of developing diabetes or the complications associated with it. In addition, gerontological nurses help to educate patients about relevant health matters and provide accurate information about healthy lifestyle choices that can help slow the progression of diabetes and its associated conditions.

KEY CONCEPTS

- The signs and symptoms of diabetes in the older adult may be vague or suggestive of other medical conditions. They might be viewed as part of aging rather than symptoms of polyuria, polydipsia, and polyphagia.
- Close monitoring of blood glucose levels is the most effective way to prevent, delay, or slow the progression of macrovascular, microvascular, and neurological complications of diabetes.
- The management of diabetes is a comprehensive team effort and should include the older adult as much as possible. If this is not possible, the health care provider will need to ensure that the medical regimen is effective.
- Preventive foot care is essential for the prevention of future problems.

ACTIVITIES AND DISCUSSION QUESTIONS

1. What are the risks and complications of diabetes for the older adult?

2. State the components of diabetes management, and explain what each component entails.

3. Describe the nurse's role in the management of diabetes.

4. Develop a nursing care plan for an older Indigenous person with type 2 DM in the community.

RESOURCES

Diabetes Canada
http://www.diabetes.ca
Diabetes Canada. *Clinical guidelines for the prevention and management of diabetes in Canada.*
https://guidelines.diabetes.ca/cpg
Diabetes in Control. *443 drugs that can affect blood glucose levels.*
http://www.diabetesincontrol.com/drugs-that-can-affect-blood-glucose-levels/
Heart and Stroke Foundation of Canada
http://www.heartandstroke.ca
Public Health Agency of Canada. *Type 2 diabetes info sheet for seniors.*
http://carechat.ca/wp-content/uploads/2012/04/Type-2-Diabetes-Info-Sheet-for-Seniors.pdf
Registered Nurses' Association of Ontario. *Assessment and Management of Foot Ulcers for People with Diabetes* (2nd ed.).
http://rnao.ca/bpg/guidelines/assessment-and-management-foot-ulcers-people-diabetes-second-edition
Registered Nurses' Association of Ontario. *Best Practice Guideline for the Subcutaneous Administration of Insulin in Adults with Type 2 Diabetes.*
http://rnao.ca/sites/rnao-ca/files/BPG_for_the_Subcutaneous_Administration_of_Insulin_in_Adults_with_Type_2_Diabetes.pdf

For additional resources, please visit *http://evolve.elsevier.com/Canada/Ebersole/gerontological/*

REFERENCES

American Diabetes Association. (2020). Standards of medical care in diabetes—2020. *American Diabetes Care Diabetes Care, 43*(Suppl. 1), S1–S2. doi:10.2337/dc20-Sint.

Diabetes Canada. (2018). *Foot care: A step toward good health.* http://www.diabetes.ca/diabetes-and-you/healthy-living-resources/foot-care/signs-of-foot-problems.

Diabetes Canada. (2020). *Assess your risk of developing diabetes.* https://www.diabetes.ca/type-2-risks/risk-factors—-assessments.

Diabetes Canada Clinical Practice Guidelines Expert Committee. (2018). Diabetes Canada 2018 Clinical Practice Guidelines for the Prevention and Management of Diabetes in Canada. *Canadian Journal of Diabetes, 42*(Suppl. 1), S1–S325. http://guidelines.diabetes.ca/cpg.

Heart and Stroke Foundation of Canada. (2020). *Diabetes.* https://www.heartandstroke.ca/heart-disease/risk-and-prevention/condition-risk-factors/diabetes.

Institute of Health Economics. (2018). *Diabetes care and management in Indigenous populations in Canada: A pan-Canadian policy roundtable.* https://www.ihe.ca/advanced-search/diabetes-care-and-management-in-indigenous-populations-in-canada-summary-report-of-a-pan-canadian-policy-roundtable.

Osman, O., Sherifali, D., Stolee, P., et al. (2016). Diabetes management in long-term care: An exploratory study of the current practices and processes to managing frail elderly persons with type 2 diabetes. *Canadian Journal of Diabetes, 40*(1), 17–30. doi:10.1016/j.jcjd.2015.10.005.

Punthakee, Z., Goldenberg, R., & Katz, P. (2018). Diabetes Canada 2018 Clinical Practice Guidelines for the Prevention and Management of Diabetes in Canada: Definition, classification and diagnosis of diabetes, prediabetes, and metabolic syndrome. *Canadian Journal of Diabetes, 42*(1), S10–S15. https://guidelines.diabetes.ca/cpg/chapter3.

Sasso, F. C., Rinaldi, L., Lascar, N., et al. (2018). Role of tight glycemic control during acute coronary syndrome on CV outcome in type 2 diabetes. *Journal of Diabetes Research, 2018*, 3106056. doi:10.1155/2018/3106056.

Sherifali, D., Berard, L. D., Gucciardi, E., et al. (2018). Self-management education and support. Diabetes Canada 2018 Clinical Practice Guidelines for the Prevention and Management of Diabetes in Canada: Definition, classification, and diagnosis of diabetes, prediabetes, and metabolic syndrome. *Canadian Journal of Diabetes, 42*(1), S36–S41. https://guidelines.diabetes.ca/cpg/chapter7.

Walker, J. D., Slater, M., Jones, C. R., et al. (2020). Diabetes prevalence, incidence and mortality in First Nations and other people in Ontario, 1995–2014: A population-based study using linked administrative data. *Canadian Medicine Association Journal, 192*(6), E128–E135. doi:10.1503/cmaj.190836.

Williams, J. S., Walker, R. J., & Egede, L. E. (2020). The role of family and peer support in diabetes. In A. M. Delamater & D. Marrero (Eds.), *Behavioral diabetes: Social ecological perspectives for pediatric and adult populations* (pp. 391–401). Springer.

Yanase, T., Yanagita, I., Muta, K., et al. (2017). Frailty in elderly diabetes patients. *Endocrine Journal, 65*, 1–11. doi:10.1507/endocrj.EJ17-0390.

18

BONE AND JOINT HEALTH

LEARNING OBJECTIVES

Upon completion of this chapter, the reader will be able to:

- Describe the most common bone and joint problems affecting the older adult.
- Discuss the potential risks of osteoporosis.
- Recognize postural changes that suggest the presence of osteoporosis.
- Explain effective ways of preventing or slowing the progression of osteoporosis.
- Relate the differences between osteoarthritis, rheumatoid arthritis, and gout.
- Describe the nurse's responsibility in care for the person with osteoarthritis, rheumatoid arthritis, and gout.
- Name several methods of managing older adults' pain and disability resulting from joint and bone disorders.

GLOSSARY

Bone mineral density (BMD)   The mineral content of the bones.

Crepitus   The sound or feel of bone rubbing on bone.

Osteopenia   Loss of bone mineral density and structure at a mild to moderate level.

Osteophyte   Excessive bone growth.

Osteoporosis   Loss of bone mineral density and structure to a great degree.

Resorption   The loss of a substance or bone by physiological or pathological processes.

THE LIVED EXPERIENCE

"Halfway through the mall I had to sit because I couldn't go any further. I was just in agony with the pain; I was in agony. And so I just sat there and I had sunglasses on and I think tears were rolling out of my eyes because I couldn't—I just couldn't—go for a walk, and ugh, now I have to go back to the van. Can I drive back home? I had to call my daughter and I said, look, I'm not feeling good. So that's being dependent. You know, always not knowing, not trusting, that you can do something."

Maly, M. R., & Krupa, T. (2007). Personal experience of living with knee osteoarthritis among older persons. *Disability and Rehabilitation, 29*(18), 1423–1433.

MUSCULO-SKELETAL SYSTEM

A healthy musculo-skeletal system allows the human body to be upright and is necessary for comfortably carrying out the basic activities of daily living. For some older adults, later life is an opportunity to explore the limits of their ability and become more athletic. For others, later life is a time of significant restriction in movement. However, in both cases, older adults may have to deal with the challenges of one or more of the musculo-skeletal problems commonly encountered in later life. Gerontological nurses attend to the needs of older adults to promote healthy bones and joints. This chapter discusses osteoporosis and the different forms of arthritis and their implications for nursing interventions. For a discussion of health promotion, activity, and exercise to maintain musculo-skeletal health, see Chapter 10.

OSTEOPOROSIS

During the normal process of bone growth, bones build up mass (formation) and strength; at the same time, bones are losing mass and strength through **resorption**. In a healthy adult, formation and resorption are balanced, and peak bone mass is reached at 30 years of age. After that, the loss of **bone mineral density (BMD)** is minimal at first but then speeds up with age. For women, the period of the fastest overall loss of BMD is 5 to 7 years immediately following menopause. Severe loss of BMD is called **osteoporosis**.

Osteoporosis means "porous bone" and is characterized by reduced BMD, disrupted bone microarchitecture, and an altered amount and variety of proteins in the bone. Primary osteoporosis is sometimes thought to be a normal part of the aging process, especially in women. *Secondary osteoporosis* is the term used for porous bones caused by another disease, such as Paget's disease, or by medication, such as long-term steroids. Both types of osteoporosis are characterized by low BMD and subsequent deterioration of bone structure, as well as changes in posture. Approximately 2 million Canadians have osteoporosis (Osteoporosis Canada, 2021a). A negative consequence of osteoporosis is a high risk of fractures when a fall occurs. One in three women and one in five men will have an osteoporotic fracture in their lifetime (Osteoporosis Canada, 2021a). Approximately 28% of women and 37% of men with a hip fracture die within the following year (Osteoporosis Canada, 2021a).

Osteoporosis is a silent disorder. A person may have no symptoms of any kind for many years; another person may never show any symptoms. With the treatments and interventions now available, some osteoporosis can be prevented or treated and stabilized to some extent. Osteoporosis is diagnosed through a dual-energy X-ray absorptiometry (DXA) scan, but is presumed to be present in older adults who have non-traumatic fractures, a loss of 7.5 cm (3 inches) or more in height, or kyphosis (pathological curvature of the upper spine) (Fig. 18.1). Osteoporosis Canada recommends that all persons aged 65 years and older should have a BMD test (Osteoporosis Canada, 2021b). If the screening is positive, nurses can advocate that the older adult receive appropriate treatment.

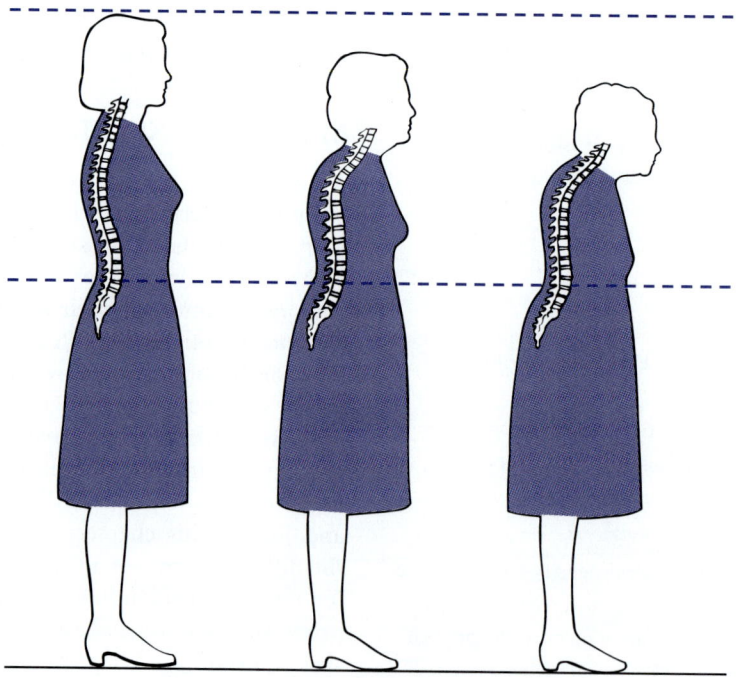

Fig. 18.1 ■ Osteoporosis spine alignment.

A number of other factors increase or decrease a person's risk for both **osteopenia**, a condition in persons whose BMD is lower than normal, and osteoporosis. Some of these factors cannot be changed (e.g., gender, race, or ethnicity), but others (e.g., calcium intake and exercise) are amenable to change (Box 18.1).

Reducing Osteoporosis-Related Risks and Injury

Measures to prevent osteoporosis-related injury or the progression of the disease include exercise, proper nutrition, and lifestyle changes. One major risk factor that can be changed is smoking. To prevent falls and fall-related injuries, home safety inspection and education regarding injury prevention strategies are essential (see Chapter 12). (An assortment of print and interactive educational materials for both a lay and professional audience can be found at https://www.osteoporosis.ca).

Weight-bearing physical activity and exercises help maintain bone mass. Brisk walking and working out with light weights apply mechanical force to the spine and long bones (see Chapter 10). Muscle-building exercises help maintain skeletal architecture by improving muscle strength and flexibility. Tai chi has been successfully used to strengthen the muscles and bones of older adults (Song et al., 2018). Tai chi and exercise have the added advantage of improving balance and stamina, which may prevent falls or limit the damage if a fall should occur. Examples of exercise can be found in Box 18.2.

Teaching for older adults includes teaching the key aspects of the prevention and treatment of osteoporosis. Information about the sites that are most vulnerable to injury through accidents, falls, back strain, and poor posture is important. Changes in the upper spine that occur when vertebrae are weakened should be explained, as should the pain that results from strain on the lower spine caused by the effort to compensate for changes of balance and height. Education also includes teaching the appropriate way to take medications and how to manage their side effects.

Fall prevention is especially important for decreasing the morbidity and mortality associated with osteoporosis. The nurse should emphasize the importance of living safely in the home (e.g., wearing shoes with good support and using handrails) and the risks of walking in poorly lit areas. Several fracture prevention strategies, such as wearing hip protectors and performing exercises for balance and agility, are listed on the Osteoporosis Canada website (https://www.osteoporosis.ca). Basic body mechanics, such as the mechanics of lifting heavy objects, can be discussed. The use of stepstools or chairs to reach things in high places should be discouraged. Walkways should be kept free of obstacles, and loose rugs and electrical cords should be arranged so that they do not cause falls (see Chapter 12).

Pharmacological Interventions

In the last decade, considerable progress has been made in the development of pharmacological interventions for both the prevention and treatment of osteoporosis.

BOX 18.1
RISK FACTORS FOR OSTEOPOROSIS

- Modifiable risk factors:
  - Inadequate nutritional absorption
  - Lack of physical activity or being a fall risk
  - Weight loss
  - Cigarette smoking
  - Alcohol consumption
  - Air pollution
  - Stress
- Nonmodifiable risk factors:
  - History of falls
  - Older age
  - Gender
  - White European ancestry
  - Prior fracture
  - Reproductive factors (family history of osteoporosis)
- Secondary causes of osteoporosis
  - Chronic use of certain medications (prolonged corticosteroid use, etc.)
  - Hypogonadism
  - Hyperparathyroidism
  - Chronic liver disease
  - Inflammatory diseases (rheumatoid arthritis, etc.)
  - Vitamin D deficiency
  - Renal disease or history of kidney stones
  - Cardiovascular disease
  - Diabetes mellitus
  - Dementia

Source: Pouresmaeili, F., Kamalidehghan, B., Kamarehei, M., et al. (2018). A comprehensive overview on osteoporosis and its risk factors. *Therapeutics and Clinical Risk Management, 14*, 2029–2049. doi:10.2147/TCRM.S138000.

BOX 18.2

FOUR EXAMPLES OF EXERCISES FOR HEALTHY BONES

1. Strength training*
   - ▪ Recommended frequency: At least 2 days/week
     - □ Exercises for your legs, arms, chest, shoulders, back.
     - □ Use body weight against gravity, bands, or weights.
     - □ 8–12 repetitions per exercise.
2. Balance exercises
   - ▪ Recommended frequency: Every day
     - □ Tai chi, dancing, walking on your toes or heels.
     - □ Have a sturdy chair, counter, or wall nearby, and try the following (from easier to harder): shift weight from heels to toes while standing; stand heel to toe; stand on one foot; walk on a pretend line.
3. Posture awareness
   - ▪ Recommended frequency: Every day
     - □ Gently tuck chin in and draw chest up slightly.
     - □ Imagining that your collarbones are wings, spread your wings slightly without pulling your shoulders back.
4. Aerobic physical activity
   - ▪ Recommended frequency: At least 150 minutes/week
     - □ Incorporate activity bouts of 10 minutes or more at moderate to vigorous intensity.
     - □ It should feel like your heart is beating faster and you are breathing harder.
     - □ You might be able to talk while doing it, but not sing.

*It is always a good idea to consult a physiotherapist/kinesiologist and other members of the health care team before the person uses weights and performs vigorous activity.
Source: Adapted from Osteoporosis Canada. (2020). *Exercises for healthy bones*. https://osteoporosis.ca/exercise/.

Adequate intake of calcium and vitamin D supplements is recommended for persons of all ages, and these supplements should be taken with all of the prescribed treatments currently available (Osteoporosis Canada, 2021c).

Ideally, optimal nutrition in late life follows a lifetime of good eating habits (see Chapter 8). Several common foods have high calcium content, such as cheese (between 400 and 500 mg of calcium per 50 g),

plain yogourt (between 260 and 270 mg of calcium per 0.75 cup), milk (between 290 and 320 mg of calcium per 1 cup), and other foods, including canned sardines and beans, tofu, almonds, and spinach. Canada's Food Guide recommends many foods that are rich in calcium (https://www.canada.ca/en/health-canada/services/nutrients/calcium.html). Calcium can be obtained from combined dietary and supplementary sources. If supplements are used, combined calcium and vitamin D (e.g., Caltrate-D) is recommended. The doses are best spread over the course of the day; for example, 400 mg of calcium is taken in the morning, 400 mg during the day, and another 400 mg before bed. However, this regimen might be difficult for older adults to keep track of (see Chapter 14). The current recommendation calls for 400 to 1000 international units (IU) of supplemental vitamin D for adults under the age of 50 years without osteoporosis or conditions affecting vitamin D absorption, and 800 to 2000 IU for those 50 years of age and older (Osteoporosis Canada, 2021c).

Nurses are also responsible for educating older adults about factors that inhibit calcium absorption (e.g., excess alcohol, protein, or salt) and enhance calcium excretion (e.g., caffeine; excess fibre; and phosphorus in meats, sodas, and preserved foods) and about the influence of the body's response to stress (decreased calcium absorption and increased excretion of calcium in the urine). Constipation is worsened by calcium supplements and may reduce the person's willingness to take them. Good nursing care includes developing, with the person, a preventive plan that includes extra fluid intake (if not contraindicated) and the use of stool softeners. Neither calcium nor calcium-enriched products can be taken at the same time as thyroid preparations are taken. Instead, calcium or calcium-enriched products should be taken at least 4 hours before or after thyroid preparations are taken (AbbVie Inc., 2020).

Estrogen has long been the medication of choice for increasing the BMD of women. However, estrogen also increases the rate of breast cancer, colon cancer, and heart disease, and thus it is no longer recommended (Levin et al., 2018).

Currently available medications include bisphosphonates, selective estrogen receptor modulators (SERMs), and parathyroid hormone. All increase bone mass, reduce bone turnover, or both. Bisphosphonates (e.g., Fosamax and Actonel) are often prescribed in daily, weekly, or monthly formulations. However, owing to the seriousness of the risk for esophageal erosion, the person must take them on an empty stomach, with a full glass of water, and must stay completely upright for half an hour after ingestion. Bisphosphonates are not appropriate for a person with memory loss or for anyone who cannot comply with directions. Some intravenously delivered bisphosphonates (e.g., Aclasta, Zometa) are being considered for use with older adults (Osteoporosis Canada, 2021d).

Evista, a type of SERM, is used as a substitute for estrogen and decreases the risk for breast cancer. It is approved for both prevention and treatment of bone loss, but it can cause hot flashes and coagulation disorders and is contraindicated for anyone who has a history of deep venous thrombosis or who is taking blood thinners.

A new treatment for osteoporosis consists of daily injections of parathyroid hormone in the commercial form of teriparatide (Forteo). It is recommended for men and women at risk for fractures; however, its use is also associated with an increased risk of developing osteosarcoma. Because of this, teriparatide is typically considered a second-line therapy; even then, it is not used for longer than 2 years (Lindsay et al., 2016). Denosumab (Prolia) is another new treatment from the class called human monoclonal antibody, which prevents osteoclast formation (Osteoporosis Canada, 2021e). Denosumab is administered as an injection. Since 2018, denosumab has been added as an osteoporosis treatment for postmenopausal women and men (Osteoporosis Canada, 2021e).

Another useful medication is calcitonin (Miacalcin), which is used to slow bone loss and increase spinal BMD in women who are at least 5 years past menopause; it is not indicated for men. Incidentally, calcitonin has been found to reduce back pain in some women. It is given either subcutaneously or as a nasal spray.

ARTHRITIS

The term *arthritis* refers to more than 100 diseases that involve damage to the joints of the body (Arthritis Society, 2019a). One in five Canadians live with arthritis, affecting 6 million Canadians and nearly half of older adults nationwide (Arthritis Society, 2019b).

By the year 2040, it is expected that arthritis will affect 9 million Canadians (Arthritis Society, 2019b). Arthritis is the number-one reason for activity limitations in older adults. The most common forms of the disease are osteoarthritis (OA), polymyalgia rheumatica (PMR), rheumatoid arthritis (RA), and gout.

Osteoarthritis

OA, also known as degenerative arthritis or degenerative joint disease, is a degenerative joint disorder that affects at least 4 million (one in seven) Canadians (Arthritis Society, 2021). Risk factors include age, obesity, a family history of OA, repetitive use of the joint, and trauma to the joint. It is likely that persons over 65 years of age will have radiographic evidence of OA even if they are asymptomatic. It should be noted that although OA is more common with increased age, it affects younger persons as well. The prevalence of OA is significantly higher among the First Nations population (Barnabe et al., 2017).

In an osteoarthritic joint, the normal soft and resilient cartilaginous lining becomes thin and damaged. This causes the joint space to narrow and the bones of the joint to rub together, causing joint and bone destruction, pain, swelling, and loss of motion. **Osteophytes** (bone spurs) may develop in the spaces, causing deformation and deterioration (Fig. 18.2). OA results from a complex interplay of many factors, including genetic predisposition, local inflammation, joint integrity, mechanical forces, and cellular and biochemical processes. Treatment is available to lessen pain and increase function (see Chapter 16).

Osteoarthritis presents with stiffness with inactivity, which is relieved by activity, and pain with activity, which is relieved by rest. The stiffness can be greater in the morning after disuse during sleep but normally resolves within 30 minutes of arising, but the pain is associated with the use of the joints. As the disease advances, there is pain at rest as well, and more joints become involved. There may be joint instability, and **crepitus** may be felt or heard, indicating the deterioration of the joint. The joint enlarges, and range of motion is reduced. The most common locations for OA are the knees, hips, neck (cervical spine), lower back (lumbar spine), fingers, and thumbs (Fig. 18.3).

At this time, OA cannot be "cured" without a joint replacement. Many older adults elect to undergo this

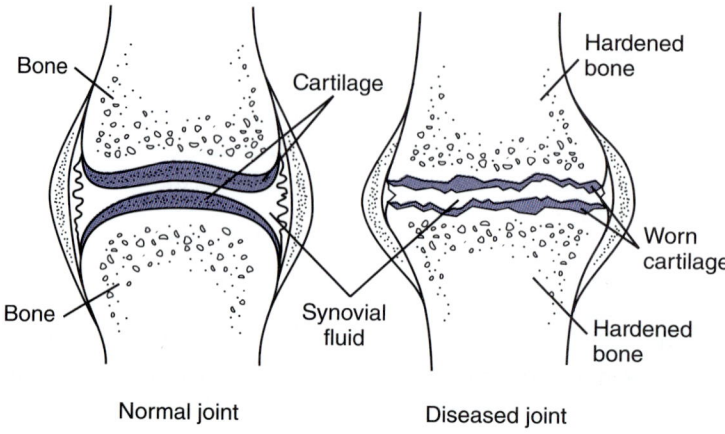

Fig. 18.2 ▪ A normal joint and a diseased joint.

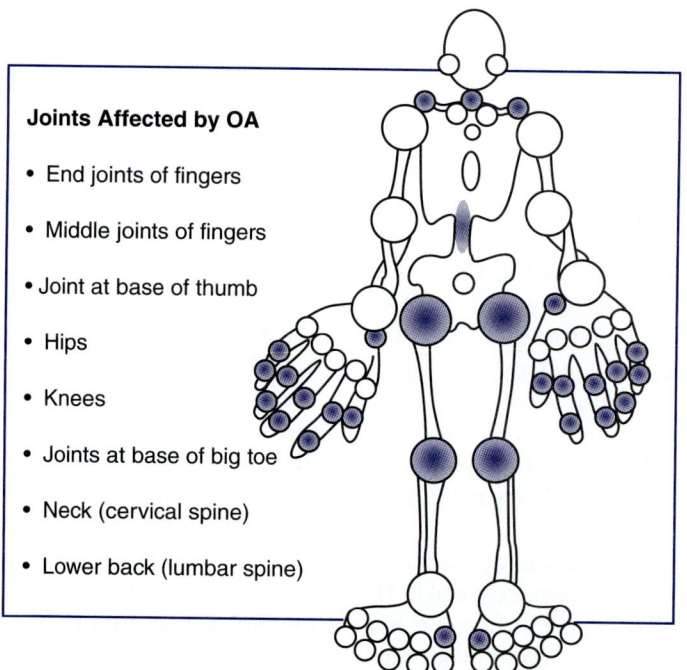

Fig. 18.3 ▪ Common locations for osteoarthritis. **Source:** Arthritis Society. (2007). *Osteoarthritis: Know your options.*

procedure for hips and knees when the pain becomes unbearable and the effect on function and quality of life becomes severe. The nurse is involved in the preoperative and perioperative periods and during rehabilitation (while the person is learning to use the new joint) and focuses on the treatment of pain.

Polymyalgia Rheumatica

PMR is one of the more common inflammatory diseases seen in older adults. It may occur at the same time as OA, and the two diseases may be difficult to distinguish from each other. The classic presentation of PMR is acute-onset pain beginning in the neck and upper arms and possibly spreading to the pelvic and pectoral girdles. The person may have a low-grade fever and feel fatigued. Pain is usually greatest at night and in the early morning.

This disorder causes stiffness, which occurs especially in the morning and lasts more than 1 hour, as well as severe stiffness and pain in the muscles (rather than the joints) of the neck, shoulders, lower back, buttocks, and thighs. The onset may be sudden or slow. Unlike OA, PMR resolves in 1 to 2 years and necessitates a different treatment. Symptoms may be quickly relieved by small doses of corticosteroids (Imai et al., 2019).

PMR rarely occurs in people under the age of 50 years, and women are at higher risk than men (Coelho et al., 2017). It is thought that PMR is the result of the inflammation of blood vessels (Arthritis Society, 2020). Its cause is unknown, but genetic factors are believed to play a role (González-Gay et al., 2017).

Rheumatoid Arthritis

RA is a chronic, systemic, inflammatory joint disorder. It is considered an autoimmune disease in which products from the inflamed lining of the joint invade and destroy the cartilage and bone within the joint. The cause is unknown. RA affects about 1 out of every 100 adult Canadians (300,000 adults) (Arthritis Society, 2017a). Women are twice to three times as likely to be affected by RA than men (Arthritis Society, 2017a).

RA is characterized by pain and swelling in multiple joints in a symmetrical pattern; for example, both hands will be affected at the same time. It generally affects the small joints of the wrist, knee, ankle, and hand, although it can affect large joints as well. Whereas morning stiffness from OA lasts less than 30 minutes, that resulting from RA lasts much longer. Since RA is a systemic disease, the person may feel generalized fatigue and malaise and have occasional fevers. The joints are warm and tender. Weight loss is common. The natural course of RA is highly variable, with good days and bad days. The disease may last a few months or years, or it may become a chronic condition with progressive damage to the joints, increasing the risk for fractures. Risk elements include environmental and genetic factors.

In the past, nonsteroidal anti-inflammatory drugs were used for treatment early in the disease, and the use of RA-specific medications was "saved" for later.

However, prompt efforts may halt or slow the damage (Niemantsverdriet et al., 2020). Persons diagnosed with RA usually come under a rheumatologist's care, with treatment involving aggressive therapy using disease-modifying antirheumatic drugs (DMARDs) such as methotrexate, sulfasalazine, and cyclosporine (Benjamin et al., 2020). Biological DMARDs (e.g., Enbrel and Remicade) are the newest class of medications that stimulate or restore the ability of the immune system to fight RA. Ongoing care of the person with RA includes monitoring the progression of the disease and effectiveness of treatment, as well as providing pain relief, comfort, and support. Support groups specifically for persons with RA may help to empower older adults, which in turn may improve their quality of life.

Gout

Gout is a common form of inflammatory arthritis that appears to result from the accumulation of uric acid crystals in a joint (Arthritis Society, 2017b). Uric acid is produced when the purines in food break down.

Gout typically starts with an acute attack. The person complains of exquisite pain in the affected joint, often starting in the middle of the night during sleep. The joint is bright purple—red, hot, and too painful to touch. The proximal joint of the great toe is the most typical site, although the ankle, knee, wrist, or elbow is sometimes involved. The development of gout and the body's response to uric acid accumulation differ from person to person. However, some people have elevated levels of uric acid and do not get gout, a condition called asymptomatic hyperuricemia.

After an acute attack, gout may become chronic, with periodic acute attacks. Risk factors include high blood pressure, a diet high in purines (Box 18.3), and certain medications, namely thiazide diuretics, salicylates (e.g., Aspirin), and cyclosporins (Lee et al., 2020).

The medical goal after the first acute attack of gout is to prevent another attack, prevent the systemic spread of the disease, and prevent the development of chronic gout. This may be accomplished through the patient's avoidance of alcohol and high-purine foods. Medications can be used to either decrease uric acid production (e.g., allopurinol, colchicine) or increase uric acid excretion (e.g., probenecid). Nurses need to ensure that the person takes in enough fluids to help flush the uric acid through the kidneys (2 L per day if not contraindicated).

BOX 18.3
**EXAMPLES OF FOODS
HIGH IN PURINES**

Asparagus
Beef kidneys
Cow, pig, or sheep brains
Sweetbread
Dried beans and peas
Gravy
Herring, mackerel, and sardines
Mushrooms
Scallops

The nurse's roles include educating the person about the side effects of medications, strategies to decrease the likelihood of another attack, and care of the joint. In administering medications for treating gout, the nurse will pay close attention to renal function and notify the physician or nurse practitioner of any change so that the dosage can be adjusted promptly.

IMPLICATIONS FOR GERONTOLOGICAL NURSING AND HEALTHY AGING

Assessment

When assessing the musculo-skeletal system, the nurse examines the joints and muscles for tenderness, swelling, warmth, and redness. For a person who has OA, crepitus is felt or heard in the affected joints. The hands are examined for osteophytes. If osteophytes appear in the distal joints as deformities of the fingers, they are called Heberden's nodes; if in the proximal joints, they are called Bouchard's nodes. The nurse has an important role in evaluating both passive and active range of motion. How far can the person reach, and bend all joints without assistance, and what are the person's reach, flexion, and extension when assisted? The testing of range of motion must go only to the point of discomfort and never to that of inducing pain. The functional ability of the arms is tested by asking the person to touch the back of the head and the mid-back with both hands. A referral to a physiotherapist might be needed. A pain assessment should always be included.

Interventions

The goals of intervention and management of the different forms of arthritis are to obtain treatment as soon as possible for inflammatory conditions, control pain, and minimize disability. Nurses are patients' primary advocates for adequate and prompt treatment, pain control, medication administration, evaluation, and education. (See Chapter 16 for a discussion of the pharmacological treatment of arthritis pain.)

Another pharmacological drug that may be used for pain control is capsaicin cream, made from pepper plants and available over the counter. Capsaicin cream is an effective and safe medication for reducing pain in persons with arthritis (Arthritis Society, 2021b). Creams with menthol or salicylates are also useful and are preferred by many older adults. Pain management and the minimization of disability are interconnected. To minimize disability for persons with OA and RA, the affected joint must be used, strengthened, and protected; the nurse has an important teaching role in this regard.

It cannot be overstated that ongoing physiotherapy is necessary to help persons with OA and RA retain joint use. Nurses and physiotherapists should collaborate in tailoring exercises for the person. Nurses should assist with range-of-motion activities. Weight loss (if necessary) and muscle building are highly recommended. For severe and disabling pain in the knees and hips from OA, surgical replacement of the joint (arthroplasty) may be highly successful in restoring the person's previous level of functioning. Nearly twice as many women as men have joint replacements. Surgical replacements are recommended for even very old persons in select cases. Outcomes of joint replacement depend on the timing of the surgery, the experience of the surgeon performing this surgery, the nursing care received, the patient's medical status before the surgery, and the person's ability to participate in rehabilitation.

For persons with OA or RA, exercise is the cornerstone of maintaining function and promoting physical functioning postfracture. Regular exercise can improve flexibility and muscle strength, which in turn help to support the affected joints, reduce pain, and reduce falls. Walking, swimming, and water aerobics are preferred by many; the last is often available at seniors' centres, public swimming pools, and YMCAs in many communities. More exercise recommendations are listed in Fig. 18.4.

TOP 10 EXERCISES

All exercises should be performed 20 times or as tolerated

1 Ankle Circles

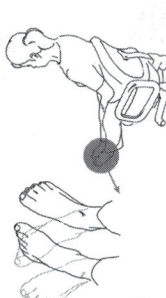

- Sit upright, keep abdominal muscles tight, chest high with legs stretched out in front
- Slowly circle your feet in one direction 20 times, then in the other direction 20 times (If you have difficulty try using one leg at a time)

2 Heel/Toe Lift

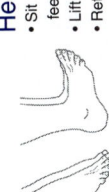

- Sit upright on the edge of a chair or stool with your feet flat on the floor
- Lift heels for 3 seconds, keeping toes on the floor
- Return feet to flat position then lift toes for 3 seconds

3 Knee Raises

- Sit upright on the edge of a chair or stool
- Keeping abdominal muscles tight, lift one knee as high as you can without bending your back (you can assist lifting your knee higher with your hands)
- Slowly lower your foot down to the floor

(Note: Avoid this exercise if you've had a total hip replacement)

4 Leg Lift with Ankle Movements

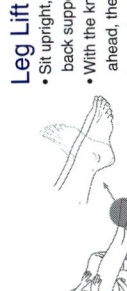

- Sit upright, keeping abdominal muscles tight and back supported, then slowly straighten your knee
- With the knee slightly bent, point your toes straight ahead, then reverse to point toes toward the ceiling
- Lower leg
- Repeat with other leg

5 Shoulder Stretches

- Sit or stand with good posture, forearms close together in front of the body **(Note: This start position is not suitable for those with osteoporosis)**
- Open arms at shoulder height, elbows bent and palms facing forward, squeezing shoulder blades together
- Stretch arms overhead, keeping elbows out in line with body

6 Forward Arm Reaches

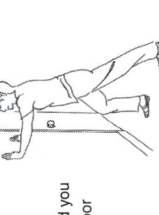 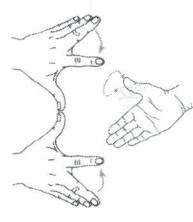

- Sit or stand upright with arms at your side, elbows bent and thumbs pointing back toward your shoulders
- Stretch arms overhead
- If one of your arms is weak, you can help it by placing your hand under the elbow and assisting the weak arm to the overhead position
- Lower arms slowly to the start position

7 Shoulder Squeeze & Wrist Stretch

- Put palms and fingers together
- Hold arms stretched out together in front of your body
- Pull hands in towards your chest, making your elbows point outwards to each side
- Press palms together as you move them closer to your body and squeeze shoulder blades together

8 Hip & Calf Stretch

- Stand upright, keep abdominal muscles tight with arms outstretched and hands against a wall, elbows straight and feet hip-width apart
- Keep shoulders and hips in a straight line as you place one leg behind you
- Bend the knee of the front foot keeping heel of the back foot on the floor to feel the stretch in the calf on the back of the leg
- Hold for 10 to 20 seconds, breathing deeply
- Alternate legs **(Note: If you cannot keep your heel on the floor bring your back foot forward more)**

9 Finger Walk & Thumb Circles

- Sit with hands on table, fingers pointing forward
- Slide thumbs toward each other
- Slide each finger one at a time towards the thumb
- After the little finger has completed the "walk", lift your hands and put them down straight
- Move the thumb in a large circle in each direction

10 Walking

- Take a walk every day; walking allows you to stretch your back and leg muscles and helps joints from becoming stiff due to inactivity
- Pay attention to good posture; stand tall, chest high and keep abdominal muscles tight

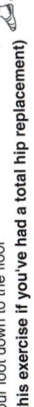 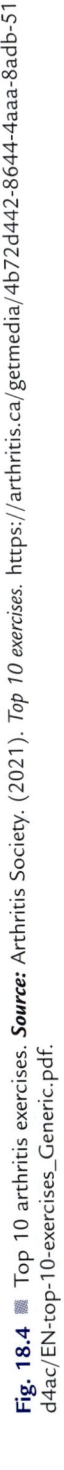

Fig. 18.4 ■ Top 10 arthritis exercises. **Source:** Arthritis Society. (2021). *Top 10 exercises.* https://arthritis.ca/getmedia/4b72d442-8644-4aaa-8adb-51b3041a-d4ac/EN-top-10-exercises_Generic.pdf.

Attention should also be given to diet, and a referral to a dietitian may be necessary (see Chapter 8). With the reduced activity associated with pain in all forms of arthritis, it is easy for the person to gain weight. Excess weight significantly increases the pressure and wear and tear on the body, leading to less activity and more weight gain. Weight reduction should be considered for all persons who are overweight. The nurse and registered dietitian can work with the person to identify realistic weight and caloric goals and develop meal plans that are personally and culturally acceptable but still balanced and healthy.

The therapeutic use of local heat and cold application in the management of pain in OA and RA patients is well known. The older adult's preference is important, but cold usually works best for an acute process—for example, to decrease muscle spasm, decrease swelling, and relieve inflammatory pain. Heat may be applied superficially or deeply. Ultrasound provides deep heat; hot packs, hydrotherapy, and radiant heat provide superficial heat. Liquid paraffin baths for submerging the hands to provide deep heat and temporary relief can be purchased in most pharmacies. A physiotherapist can determine the best course of therapy for each individual.

Devices are available to relieve some of the pressure to the joints and possibly decrease pain and improve balance and function. Canes, crutches, walkers, collars, shoe orthotics, and corsets are examples of devices that can help persons with OA or RA. A cane can reduce hip pressure by 60%; a shoe lift can improve lumbar pain. A knee brace is useful, especially in the case of lateral instability. If the hands are affected, the person can avoid carrying packages with the fingers and can use household equipment and utensils that have large rather than small grips. Not exposing the affected joints to cold temperatures may also help. The person is encouraged to wear leggings, gloves, or scarves as necessary when outdoors. An occupational therapist may be of help in identifying each individual's needs.

Complementary and Alternative Interventions for Osteoarthritis

A number of complementary and alternative interventions may provide pain relief for persons with arthritis. Among the most popular are the dietary supplements glucosamine and chondroitin sulphate, along with acupuncture and massage. While glucosamine and chon-droitin have been used for some time for self-treatment, research has found that their effect on pain is no better than that of placebos (Vasiliadis & Tsikopoulos, 2017).

Increasingly accepted in Canada is the centuries-old Chinese technique of acupuncture—the insertion of very fine needles into the body along what are called "meridians" in locations specific to a problem. Acupuncture can stimulate the natural pain-relieving endorphins produced by the nervous system, thereby temporarily relieving the pain caused by arthritis. For information about these and other techniques, see Chapter 16 and the Arthritis Society website (https://www.arthritis.ca).

SUMMARY

Older adults often have to deal with chronic bone and joint problems that affect their mobility, physical and emotional health, and overall quality of life. Gerontological nurses' assessment and interventions are necessary components of the management of these diseases. In caring for the person with osteoarthritis, rheumatoid arthritis, or gout, the nurse focuses on prevention (if possible), early detection, the optimization of mobility and function, and effective pain management. The nurse will use a number of approaches to teach and support the older adult and empower the person to participate in achieving the highest level of wellness possible.

KEY CONCEPTS

- Osteoporosis is a crippling problem for many older adults, especially women. Osteoporosis can be minimized through early interventions such as exercise, particularly weight-bearing exercise, and increased calcium and vitamin D intake.
- The most serious outcomes of osteoporosis are fractures, which are associated with high mortality.
- Most older adults will have some osteoarthritis, even though it may be asymptomatic.
- Rheumatoid arthritis produces swelling, inflammation, intense pain, and distortion of the joints.
- Gout is both an acute and a chronic condition. One of the goals of treatment is to minimize a future attack.
- Some complementary and alternative interventions are very helpful for individuals with joint disorders and persistent discomfort.

ACTIVITIES AND DISCUSSION QUESTIONS

1. What are the most effective ways of preventing osteoporosis?

2. What lifestyle issues would you discuss with a person who has advanced osteoporosis?

3. What are the differences in the appearance of osteoarthritis and rheumatoid arthritis?

4. What advice would you give someone who is experiencing joint pain and limited mobility?

5. Discuss your thoughts and experiences in regard to alternative methods of dealing with chronic pain.

RESOURCES

Arthritis Society
http://www.arthritis.ca
Osteoporosis Canada
https://www.osteoporosis.ca/
Public Health Agency of Canada
https://www.canada.ca/en/public-health/services/chronic-diseases/osteoporosis.html

Scientific Advisory Council of Osteoporosis in Canada. *Clinical practice guidelines.*
https://www.ncbi.nlm.nih.gov/pmc/articles/PMC2988535/

For additional resources, please visit *http://evolve.elsevier.com/Canada/Ebersole/gerontological/*

REFERENCES

AbbVie Inc. (2020). *Taking Synthroid the right way.* https://www.synthroid.com/starting/taking-synthroid-the-right-way.

Arthritis Society. (2017a). *Rheumatoid arthritis.* https://arthritis.ca/about-arthritis/arthritis-types-(a-z)/types/rheumatoid-arthritis.

Arthritis Society. (2017b). *Gout.* https://arthritis.ca/understand-arthritis/types-of-arthritis/gout.

Arthritis Society. (2019a). *What is arthritis.* https://arthritis.ca/about-arthritis/what-is-arthritis.

Arthritis Society. (2019b). *Arthritis facts and figures.* https://arthritis.ca/about-arthritis/what-is-arthritis/arthritis-facts-and-figures.

Arthritis Society. (2020). *Polymyalgia rheumatica with giant cell arteritis.* ht3tps://arthritis.ca/about-arthritis/arthritis-types-(a-z)/types/polymyalgia-rheumatica-with-giant-cell-arteritis.

Arthritis Society. (2021a). *Summary of special report: The burden of osteoarthritis in Canada.* https://arthritis.ca/getmedia/36cbffb1-f1d3-4689-8cad-39ef47954840/OAReportSummary_EN.pdf.

Arthritis Society. (2021b). *What are non-prescription medications?* https://arthritis.ca/treatment/pain-management/medications-to-manage-arthritis-pain.

Barnabe, C., Jones, C. A., Bernatsky, S., et al. (2017). Inflammatory arthritis prevalence and health services use in the First Nations and non–First Nations populations of Alberta, Canada. *Arthritis Care & Research, 69*(4), 467–474. doi:10.1002/acr.22959.

Benjamin, O., Bansal, P., Goyal, A., et al. (2020). *Disease modifying anti-rheumatic drugs* (DMARD). StatPearls. https://www.ncbi.nlm.nih.gov/books/NBK507863/.

Coelho, S., Magalhães, H., Correia, J., et al. (2017). Polymyalgia rheumatica and pulmonary adenocarcinoma: A case report and literature review. *Porto Biomedical Journal, 2*(3), 93–95.

González-Gay, M. A., Matteson, E. L., & Castañeda, S. (2017). Polymyalgia rheumatica. *Lancet, 390*(10103), 1700–1712.

Imai, Y., Tanaka, M., Fujii, R., et al. (2019). [Effectiveness of a low-dose corticosteroid in a patient with polymyalgia rheumatica associated with nivolumab treatment.] *Yakugaku zasshi: Journal of the Pharmaceutical Society of Japan, 139*(3), 491–495. Japanese.

Lee, J. S., Kwon, O. C., Oh, J. S., et al. (2020). Clinical features and recurrent attack in gout patients according to serum urate levels during an acute attack. *Korean Journal of Internal Medicine, 35*(1), 240–248. doi:10.3904/kjim.2018.205.

Levin, V. A., Jiang, X., & Kagan, R. (2018). Estrogen therapy for osteoporosis in the modern era. *Osteoporosis International, 29*(5), 1049–1055. doi:10.1007/s00198-018-4414-z.

Lindsay, R., Krege, J. H., Marin, F., et al. (2016). Teriparatide for osteoporosis: importance of the full course. *Osteoporosis International, 27*(8), 2395–2410. doi:10.1007/s00198-016-3534-6.

Niemantsverdriet, E., Dakkak, Y. J., Burgers, L. E., et al. (2020). TREAT early arthralgia to reverse or limit impending exacerbation to rheumatoid arthritis (TREAT EARLIER): A randomized, double-blind, placebo-controlled clinical trial protocol. *Trials, 21*, 862. doi:10.1186/s13063-020-04731-2.

Osteoporosis Canada. (2021a). *Fast facts.* https://osteoporosis.ca/about-the-disease/fast-facts/.

Osteoporosis Canada. (2021b). *Testing.* https://osteoporosis.ca/bone-mineral-density-testing/.

Osteoporosis Canada. (2021c). *Vitamin D.* https://osteoporosis.ca/vitamin-d/.

Osteoporosis Canada. (2021d). *Biophosphonates.* https://osteoporosis.ca/table-of-contents/bisphosphonates/.

Osteoporosis Canada. (2021e). *Denosumab.* https://osteoporosis.ca/denosumab/.

Song, Q., Wang, S., Wong, D. P., et al. (2018). Long-term Tai Chi exercise increases body stability of the elderly during stair ascent under high and low illumination. *Sports Biomechanics, 17*(3), 402–413. doi:10.1080/14763141.2017.1358761.

Vasiliadis, H. S., & Tsikopoulos, K. (2017). Glucosamine and chondroitin for the treatment of osteoarthritis. *World Journal of Orthopedics, 8*(1), 1–11. doi:10.5312.wjo.v8.i1.1.

19

VISUAL AND AUDITORY CHANGES

LEARNING OBJECTIVES

Upon completion of this chapter, the reader will be able to:

- Identify and discuss visual and auditory changes that may occur in older adults.
- Describe the importance of assessment, health education, and treatment of eye ailments or disorders to prevent unnecessary vision loss in older adults.
- Increase awareness of the resources available to assist older adults who experience visual and auditory impairments and changes.

GLOSSARY

Drusen Yellow deposits under the retina, often found in people over the age of 60 years.

Funduscopy Ophthalmoscopic examination of the fundus of the eye.

Keratoconjunctivitis sicca Diminished tear production with age.

Lipofuscin An age-related fatty brown pigment found in the liver, retina, kidneys, adrenals, nerve cells, and heart tissue.

Prelingual deafness Deafness that occurs before the acquisition of spoken language.

Tonometry Procedure used by eye care professionals to determine the intraocular pressure of the eye.

THE LIVED EXPERIENCE

My Eyes Are Failing

"For quite a while now, I've been pretending. That I was tired. That the light was bad. But my eyes are really getting worse. I'm afraid to go to the doctor because I'm afraid of what he'll say. Which is silly. Either there is something to be done. Or there is not. If it's glasses, hallelujah, and help me find the money. If it's an operation, see me through. If I am going blind, hold me. Help me put down the terror that rises in my gut at the word. Blind. There. I've said it. The ghost word that has been haunting me. Help me remember, if I have to walk in the dark, that I have had a lot of years of seeing clean and clear. I know the slender shape of a birch tree. I have seen thousands and thousands of things in my life. I can conjure them in my mind's eye. No matter what happens, I shall not be without beautiful sights. It is just that I may have to settle for the ones I have already seen."

Maclay, E. (1977). *Green winter: Celebrations of old age.* McGraw-Hill. (© 1977, Elise Maclay)

This chapter discusses illnesses that affect vision and hearing in older adults. Because visual and hearing impairments affect daily activities such as driving, reading, dressing, cooking, and engaging in social activities, it is important to assess the effect of these changes on the older adult's functional abilities, safety, and quality of life. Nurses need to know about age-related changes in vision and hearing as opposed to losses caused by disease or illness; conduct appropriate assessments; provide health teaching to help older adults prevent or cope with diseases and illnesses that affect vision and hearing; provide appropriate referrals for treatment; and help the older adult compensate for sensory losses by supplementing the remaining senses and abilities. The main goal is to augment and maximize sensory experiences when the senses are diminished and to help design a colourful, rewarding environment that fits the needs and abilities of the individual.

See Chapter 6 for a more detailed discussion of age-related changes in vision and hearing; Chapter 13 for information about the assessment of vision and hearing; Chapter 3 for a discussion of communication adaptations for older adults with vision and hearing loss; and Chapter 12 for information on safety precautions in the environment.

AGE-RELATED CHANGES IN VISION

It is important to distinguish between normal age-related changes and vision-related illness when assessing older adults. **Keratoconjunctivitis sicca**, or dry eyes, is a frequent complaint among older adults and is due to diminished tear production associated with age. The etiology is unclear, but researchers suspect that there may be age-related changes in the mucin-secreting cells that are necessary for surface wetting, changes in the lacrimal glands, or changes in the meibomian glands that secrete surface oil; all these changes may occur at the same time. Vitamin A deficiency or certain medications (such as antihistamines, diuretics, beta-blockers, and some sleeping pills) can also cause dry eyes. The condition occurs most commonly in women after menopause. Symptoms include a dry, scratchy feeling in mild cases (xerophthalmia) and discomfort and decreased mucus production in severe cases. The problem is diagnosed by an ophthalmologist using Schirmer's test, whereby filter paper strips are placed under the lower eyelid to measure the rate of tear production. Dry eyes are commonly treated with artificial tears; however, the eyes may be too sensitive to tolerate the preservatives in artificial tears. Other management methods include keeping the air in the living environment moist with humidifiers, avoiding wind and the use of hair dryers, and using artificial tear ointments at bedtime.

DISEASES THAT AFFECT VISION

Several diseases can affect the vision of the older population and result in blindness. An estimated one in nine Canadians over the age of 65 years will develop irreversible vision loss, as will one in four of those aged 75 years or older (Canadian Association of Optometrists, 2017).

A diagnosis of blindness does not equate to complete vision loss. The person may have some retained vision, and the nurse should be mindful and respectful of this difference. For older adults with visual impairment, the consequences for functional ability, safety, and quality of life can be profound. Therefore, it is important to identify older adults who have visual impairment and to provide appropriate assessment and treatment. Certain signs and behaviours that may indicate visual problems should prompt the nurse to act (Box 19.1).

The major diseases affecting the vision of older adults are glaucoma, cataracts, diabetic retinopathy, and macular degeneration.

BOX 19.1
SIGNS AND BEHAVIOURS THAT MAY INDICATE VISION PROBLEMS

REPORTED BY INDIVIDUALS

Squinting, greater sensitivity to light, or both
Choosing brightly coloured over dull-coloured objects or clothing
Misjudging where items are, resulting in spills
Having difficulty copying written texts
Having difficulty threading a needle or buttoning a shirt
Seeing flashes of light or rapid movement from the corners of the eyes
Having difficulties with driving at night
Experiencing uncontrolled eye movement
Making driving mistakes, such as missing street or traffic signs
Falling because of a missed step or an unseen object on the floor

NOTICED BY HEALTH CARE PROVIDERS

Mis-stepping
Mis-sitting
Walking into objects
Changes in ability to perform activities of daily living (e.g., brushing teeth)

Sources: Adapted from Health Canada. (2017). *Seniors and aging—vision care.* http://www.hc-sc.gc.ca/hl-vs/iyh-vsv/life-vie/seniors-aines_vc-sv-eng.php#sy; Kumar Dev, M., Paudel, N., Dev Joshi, N., et al. (2013). Impact of visual impairment on vision-specific quality of life among older persons living in nursing home. *Current Eye Research,* 39(3), 232–238. doi:10.3109/022713683.2013.838.973.

Glaucoma

Glaucoma is a major public health issue. It is estimated that more than 250,000 Canadians are living with glaucoma (Canadian National Institute for the Blind [CNIB], 2020a). The etiology of glaucoma is variable and often unknown. However, the progression of glaucoma indicates a process by which the natural fluids of the eye are blocked by ciliary muscle rigidity, causing a gradual build-up of intraocular pressure (IOP) and damage to the optic nerve.

Normal IOP is between 12 and 22 mm Hg (Glaucoma Research Society of Canada, 2021). Age, diabetes, steroid use, past eye injuries, and a family history of glaucoma are risk factors for the development of glaucoma. Age is the single most important predictor, and older women are affected twice as frequently as older men are. People of African, Asian, or Latin American ancestry have an increased risk of developing glaucoma (Glaucoma Research Society of Canada, 2021).

Among the several types of glaucoma are primary open-angle glaucoma, acute angle-closure glaucoma, and low-tension or normal-tension glaucoma. Glaucoma can be bilateral but occurs more commonly in only one eye.

Primary open-angle glaucoma accounts for about 80% of glaucoma cases. It is asymptomatic until very late in the disease, when there is noticeable loss in vision fields. This vision loss is irreversible; however, if detected early, glaucoma can be treated and blindness or severe vision loss can be prevented (CNIB, 2020a). The only symptom people tend to notice with open-angle glaucoma is loss of vision (HealthLink BC, 2019). Figure 19.1B illustrates the effects of glaucoma on vision.

Acute angle-closure glaucoma is characterized by a rapid rise in IOP accompanied by redness and acute

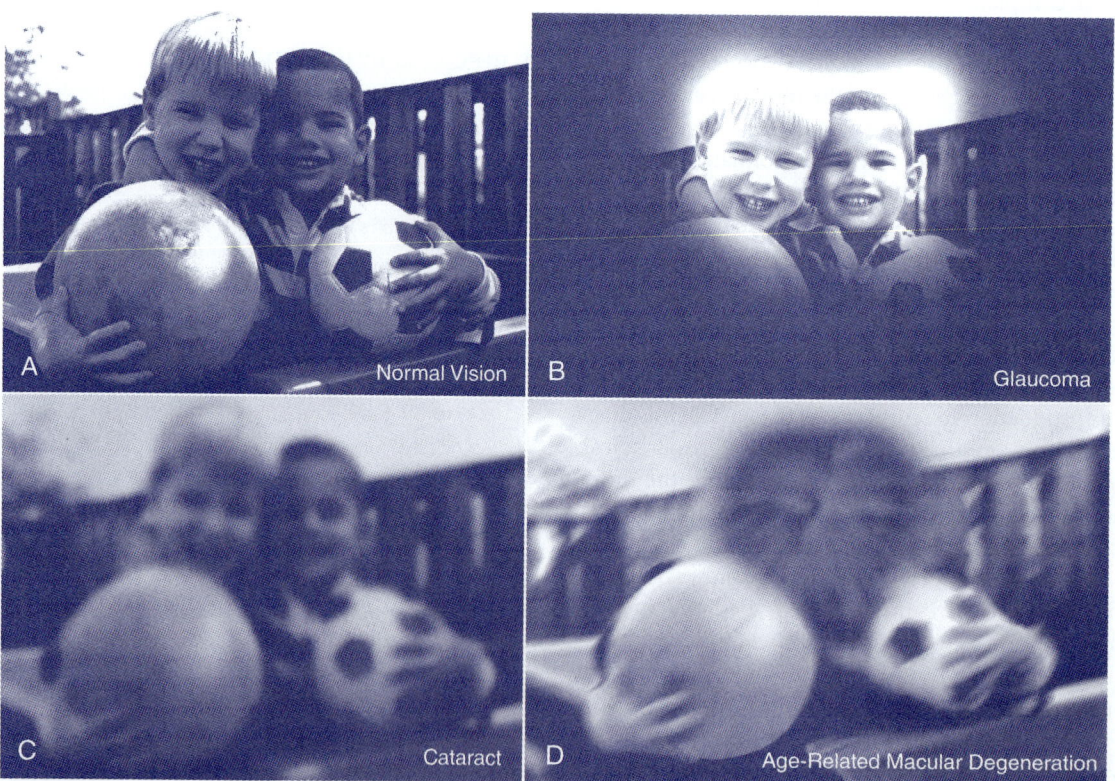

Fig. 19.1 ■ (A) Normal vision. (B) Simulated vision with glaucoma. (C) Simulated vision with cataracts. (D) Simulated vision with age-related macular degeneration (AMD). *Source:* National Eye Institute. (2012). *Age-related macular degeneration.* https://nei.nih.gov/photo/amd; https://courses.lumenlearning.com/suny-lifespandevelopment/chapter/sensory-changes-in-late-adulthood/.

pain in and around the eye, severe headache, nausea and vomiting, and blurred vision. These symptoms occur when the path of the aqueous humour (the thick, watery substance filling the space between the lens and the cornea) is blocked and the IOP builds up to more than 50 mm Hg. If the disease is untreated, blindness can occur within 2 days. Iridectomy, the surgical removal of part of the iris, can ease pressure. Risk factors for acute angle-closure glaucoma include female sex, increased age, Inuit or Asian ancestry, a shallow anterior chamber, and shorter axial length (Marchini et al., 2015; Harasymowycz et al., 2016; Glaucoma Research Foundation, 2017a). Many medications with anticholinergic properties, such as antihistamines, stimulants, vasodilators, clonidine, and sympathomimetics, are particularly dangerous for patients who are predisposed to angle-closure glaucoma. Older adults with glaucoma should be counselled to review all medications (both over the counter and prescribed) with their primary care provider.

Low-tension or normal-tension glaucoma is a third type of glaucoma occurring in older adults. In this type of glaucoma, the IOP is within the normal range (12–22 mm Hg), but there is damage to the optic nerve and a narrowing of the visual fields. The cause of this type of glaucoma is unknown, but its risk factors include a family history of any kind of glaucoma, Japanese ancestry, and cardiovascular disease. Management consists of the same medications and surgical interventions used to manage chronic glaucoma (Glaucoma Research Foundation, 2019).

Assessment

When caring for an older adult in hospital or in a long-term care home, the nurse must obtain a medical history to determine whether the person has glaucoma and to ensure that eye drops are given according to the person's treatment regimen. Eye drop medications help to lower eye pressure and prevent damage to the optic nerve (Glaucoma Research Foundation, 2019). Failing to administer eye drops at the prescribed times can cause eye pressure to rise, leading to an acute exacerbation of glaucoma (Boltz et al., 2016). Persons over the age of 65 years need annual eye examinations, and those with medication-controlled glaucoma should schedule follow-up appointments every 6 months. Annual screening is also recommended for persons of

African, Asian, or Latin American ancestry, as well as persons who are older than 40 years and have a family history of glaucoma (Glaucoma Research Society of Canada, 2021). The examination consists of a dilated-eye examination and **tonometry**, a procedure that measures IOP. These procedures can be performed by an optometrist, who will then refer the person to an ophthalmologist if glaucoma is suspected. In many cases, most provinces and territories cover the cost of annual eye examinations for older adults (FYidoctors, 2020).

Interventions

Glaucoma is managed with medications (i.e., oral medications or topical eye drops), laser surgery, or both. Eye drops and oral medications lower the IOP either by decreasing the amount of aqueous fluid produced within the eye or by improving the flow through the drainage angle.

Beta-blockers are the first-line therapy for glaucoma, and some people need combinations of several types of eye drops. Usually, medications can control glaucoma, but laser surgery (trabeculoplasty) may be recommended for some types of glaucoma. Surgery is usually recommended to prevent further damage to the optic nerve.

Some nonpharmacological or nonsurgical interventions that might be helpful for all types of vision loss include illumination, glare control, appropriate levels of magnification, and the use of colour contrast to identify or find objects.

Cataracts

A second major disease affecting the vision of older adults is cataracts, which are caused by oxidative damage to the lens protein and by fatty deposits, known as **lipofuscin**, in the ocular lens. Cataracts are a prevalent disorder among older adults; more than 2.5 million Canadians are living with cataracts (https://www.cnib.ca).

The most common causes of cataracts are heredity and advanced age. Cataracts may occur more frequently and at an earlier age in individuals who have been exposed to excessive sunlight or who have poor dietary habits, diabetes, hypertension, kidney disease, previous eye trauma, or a history of alcohol and tobacco use. Cataracts are also more likely to occur after surgery for glaucoma and after other types of eye surgery. There is evidence that a high dietary intake of lutein and zeaxanthin (compounds found in yellow or dark leafy vegetables), as well as vitamin C, vitamin E, copper, and zinc from food and supplements, lowers the risk for cataracts (McCusker et al., 2016).

Assessment

Cataracts are recognized by the clouding of the ordinarily clear ocular lens. The principal symptom of cataracts is the appearance of halos around objects. Other common symptoms include blurring, decreased perception of light and colour (giving a yellow tint to most things), and sensitivity to glare. Figure 19.1C illustrates the effects of a cataract on vision.

When lens opacity reduces visual acuity to 20/30 or less in the central axis of vision, the vision impairment is considered a cataract. Cataracts are categorized according to their location within the lens and are usually bilateral.

Interventions

When visual acuity decreases to 20/50 and the cataract affects the person's safety or quality of life, surgery is recommended (Casparis et al., 2017). Cataract surgery is the most commonly performed surgical procedure in developed countries. Most often, cataract surgery involves only local anaesthesia on an outpatient basis, and 95% of patients report excellent vision after surgery. The surgery involves the removal of the cloudy lens and its replacement with an artificial lens (called an intraocular lens, or IOL). If the person has bilateral cataracts, surgery is performed on one eye first; surgery on the other eye is performed 1 to 2 weeks later to ensure healing (Dickman et al., 2019). However, sometimes immediate sequential bilateral surgery is indicated for certain people. Persons who have cataracts or have had recent cataract surgery or trauma can have a detached retina; in some cases, the detachment occurs spontaneously. A detached retina manifests as a curtain coming down over the person's line of vision. It necessitates immediate emergency treatment.

Nursing interventions when caring for the person who will be undergoing cataract surgery include teaching and preparing the person for significant changes in vision and adaptation to light, discussing realistic postsurgical expectations, and assessing potential postsurgery infection. Postsurgical teaching includes teaching the patient to avoid heavy lifting, straining, and bending at the waist. Eye drops may be prescribed to aid healing and prevent infection.

Macular Degeneration

Age-related macular degeneration (AMD) is a degenerative eye disease that affects the macula, the central part of the eye responsible for clear central vision. The disease causes a progressive loss of central vision, leaving only peripheral vision intact. It usually starts in one eye but may affect the other eye later on (National Eye Institute, 2019). There are few symptoms in the early stages of AMD, and intermediate AMD may cause some vision loss (National Eye Institute, 2019). Therefore, it is important for adults to have their eyes examined regularly. Figure 19.1D illustrates the effects of AMD on vision.

Two million Canadians are affected by AMD; the majority are over the age of 50 years (Devenyi et al., 2016). The prevalence of AMD increases drastically with age, and its incidence is higher among women. Other nonmodifiable risk factors include genetic factors; the risk of developing AMD is greater if an immediate family member has the disease, and White persons are at higher risk than others (National Eye Institute, 2019). As the number of older adults affected is projected to increase over the next 20 years, AMD is considered a growing epidemic (Devenyi et al., 2016).

Although its etiology is unknown, AMD results from systemic changes in circulation, an accumulation of cellular waste products, tissue atrophy, and the growth of abnormal blood vessels in the choroid layer beneath the retina. Fibrous scarring disrupts the nourishment of photoreceptor cells, causing the death of the cells and the loss of central vision. Risk factors include genetic predisposition, smoking, obesity, family history, and excessive exposure to sunlight.

There are two forms of macular degeneration: dry AMD and wet AMD. Dry AMD accounts for 85% to 90% of all cases of AMD. This type of AMD has three stages, which may occur in one or both eyes (Box 19.2). Dry AMD occurs when the light-sensitive cells in the macula slowly break down and cause blurring in the central vision of the affected eye. As dry AMD gets worse, the person may see a blurred spot in the centre of their vision. One of the most common early signs of dry AMD is the presence of **drusen**, yellow deposits under the retina that are often found in people over the age of 60 years. The relationship between drusen and AMD is not clear, but an increase in the size or number of drusen increases the risk of developing advanced or wet AMD (CNIB, 2019).

Wet AMD occurs when abnormal blood vessels begin to grow under the macula and leak fluid or blood, which raises the macula from its normal place at the back of the eye. When the fluid or blood begins to accumulate in the macula, light-sensing cone cells degenerate and die. Damage to the macula occurs rapidly, sometimes within months, resulting in blurred or even lost central vision.

BOX 19.2
STAGES OF AGE-RELATED MACULAR DEGENERATION

1. Early age-related macular degeneration (AMD): Several small drusen; no symptoms; no vision loss
2. Intermediate AMD: Several medium-sized drusen, or one or more large drusen; blurred spot in the centre of vision; more light required for reading and other tasks
3. Advanced AMD: In addition to drusen, a breakdown of light-sensitive cells and supporting tissues in the central retinal area; expanding blurred spot in the centre of vision; difficulty reading or recognizing faces until they are very close

Source: Ruia, S., & Kaufman, E. J. (2020). *Macular degeneration. StatPearls.* https://www.ncbi.nlm.nih.gov/books/NBK560778/.

Peripheral vision usually remains normal, but the person will have difficulty seeing at a distance or doing detailed work such as sewing or reading. Faces may begin to blur, and it becomes harder to distinguish colours. An early sign may be distortion that causes edges or lines to appear wavy.

Assessment. There is no cure for AMD, and treatment options are limited to slowing the progression of the disease. Therefore, the focus is on screening, early detection, and prevention. People in the early stage of dry AMD may attribute their vision problems to normal aging or cataracts. Early diagnosis is the key, and individuals over the age of 40 years should have an eye examination at least every 2 years.

People diagnosed with AMD should check their eyes daily using an Amsler grid (CNIB, 2020b). The Amsler grid is used to determine the clarity of central vision (Fig. 19.2). The perception of wavy lines is diagnostic of the beginning of macular degeneration.

The National Eye Institute Age-Related Eye Disease Study (https://www.nei.nih.gov/research/clinical-trials/age-related-eye-disease-studies-aredsareds2) found that a high-dose formulation of antioxidants and zinc significantly reduced the risk of advanced AMD and associated vision loss. Individuals with intermediate AMD in one or both eyes or with advanced wet AMD in one eye but not

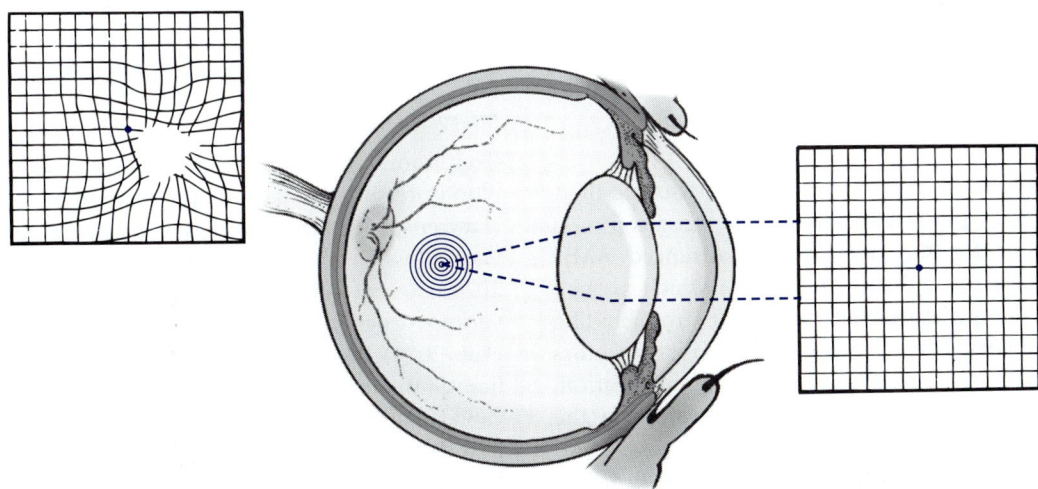

Fig. 19.2 ■ Macular degeneration: distortion of centre vision; normal peripheral vision. Illustration by Harriet R. Greenfield, Newton, Massachusetts.

BOX 19.3
AGE-RELATED EYE DISEASE STUDY 1 AND 2 (AREDS AND AREDS2) RECOMMENDED FORMULA

In the original AREDS trial (National Eye Institute, 2020), participants who took AREDS formula reduced the risk of AMD by 25% over a 5-year period. The second trial (AREDS2) found that adding omega-3s / lutein + zeaxanthin to the original AREDS formulation had no overall effect on reducing the risk of advanced AMD. However, participants who took AREDS containing lutein + zeaxanthin and no beta-carotene had a reduction in the risk of advanced AMD compared to those who took AREDS with beta-carotene.

Nutrient	AREDS formula	AREDS2 formula
Vitamin C	400 mg	400 mg
Vitamin E	400 IU	400 IU
Beta-carotene	15 mg	—
Copper	2 mg	2 mg
Lutein	—	10 mg
Zeaxanthin	—	2 mg
Zinc	80 mg	80 mg

Source: Adapted from National Eye Institute. (2020). *Taking the AREDS formula.* https://www.nei.nih.gov/research/clinical-trials/age-related-eye-disease-studies-aredsareds2/aredsareds2-frequently-asked-questions.

the other should consider taking the National Eye Institute's formulation (Box 19.3) (National Eye Institute, 2019). Because of some toxicity risks, these supplements are initiated by a physician or a nurse practitioner—people cannot start these on their own as a preventive measure.

Interventions

Treatment of wet AMD includes photodynamic therapy and laser photocoagulation. The most common medications for the treatment of advanced AMD include Lucentis and Avastin, both of which prevent vascular endothelial growth factor (VEGF) from binding to its receptors. The binding of VEGF to its receptors results in cell proliferation and increased vascularization, including vascular leakage, which contribute to the progression of AMD.

Abnormally high levels of a specific growth factor occur in eyes with wet AMD, promoting the growth of abnormal blood vessels. Anti-VEGF therapy blocks the effect of the growth factor. These medications are injected into the eye as often as once a month and can help slow vision loss from AMD and improve sight in some cases. Other treatments being researched are gene therapy, stem cell therapy, and retinal transplantation (Ludwig et al., 2019).

Diabetic Retinopathy

The deleterious effects of elevated blood sugar due to diabetes can cause diabetic retinopathy. Diabetic retinopathy is a disease of the retinal microvasculature that is characterized by increased vessel permeability. Blood and lipid leakage leads to macular edema and hard exudates (composed of lipids). Because of the vascular and cellular changes accompanying diabetes, other pathological vision conditions often worsen rapidly.

Diabetic retinopathy is the third leading cause of blindness in Canada, following macular degeneration and glaucoma. Approximately 500,000 Canadians live with diabetic retinopathy (CNIB, 2020c). Most people living with diabetes develop diabetic retinopathy within 20 years of diagnosis.

Assessment

There is little to no evidence of retinopathy until 3 to 5 years after the onset of diabetes. Early signs, which include microaneurysms, flame-shaped hemorrhages, cotton wool spots, hard exudates, and dilated capillaries, can be detected using a **funduscopy** examination. Annual dilated funduscopic examination of the eye, beginning 5 years after diagnosis of type 1 diabetes and at the time of the diagnosis of type 2 diabetes, is recommended.

Interventions

Continuous control of blood glucose, cholesterol, and blood pressure can halt the progression of the disease (Lawrenson et al., 2018). Laser treatment can reduce vision loss in about 50% of patients (Lupidi et al., 2020). Recent evidence indicates that treatment with various drugs may deliver a better outcome (Sharma et al., 2020). In many cases, pharmacotherapy is the first line of treatment (Mansour et al., 2020). Recent advancements in pharmacotherapy show that this method may be better than more invasive treatments at controlling diabetic retinopathy in a safe and effective manner (Mansour et al., 2020). The nurse should understand the different treatment options, ensure that the person understands the risks and benefits of treatment, and continue promoting person-centred care.

AUDITORY IMPAIRMENT AND LOSS

Hearing impairments can have severe consequences for an older adult's quality of life, well-being, and socialization, and may even be perceived as a social stigma. Two common auditory impairments that nurses caring for older adults will need to take into consideration are tinnitus and prelingual deafness. (See Chapter 3 for a discussion of presbycusis, a form of sensorineural hearing loss related to aging.)

Tinnitus

Tinnitus is the perception of sound in the absence of acoustic stimuli. It is characterized by ringing in the ear and may also manifest as buzzing; hissing; whistling; cricket-like chirping; bell sounds; and roaring, clicking, pulsating, humming, or swishing sounds. The sounds may be constant or intermittent and are more acute at night or in quiet surroundings. The most common type of tinnitus is high pitched with sensorineural loss; the root cause lies in the vestibulo-cochlear nerve, the inner ear, or the central processing centres of the brain. A less common type of tinnitus is low pitched and is associated with conduction loss—that is, loss of sound conductivity through the small, bony structures in the ear.

Tinnitus generally increases over time. It affects many older adults and can interfere with hearing, as well as become extremely irritating. Tinnitus affects 37% of the population (Canadian Hearing Society, 2020). Some people affected by tinnitus report that the presence of sound in their ear affects the carrying out of daily activities (Statistics Canada, 2019). The incidence of tinnitus peaks between the ages of 65 and 74 years and is higher in men than in women. (In men, the incidence seems to decrease after this period.) Tinnitus can be caused by loud noises, excessive cerumen (earwax) or other obstructions of the auditory canal, disorders of the cervical vertebrae or the temporomandibular joint, allergies, an underactive thyroid, cardiovascular disease, tumours, conductive hearing loss, anxiety, depression, degeneration of the bones in the middle ear, infections, and trauma to the head or ear. In addition, more than 200 prescription and nonprescription medications list tinnitus as a potential side effect. (Aspirin is the most common of these medications.)

Assessment

Tinnitus may be subjective (i.e., audible only to the affected person) or objective (i.e., audible to the examiner as well). The Tinnitus Handicap Questionnaire, developed by Newman et al. (1995), measures the physical, emotional, and social consequences of tinnitus. It also can be used to assess the changes the individual experiences with treatment. The Tinnitus Functional Index is another measure of the effects of tinnitus (Henry et al., 2016). The cause of tinnitus in some persons is never found. The problem may also arbitrarily disappear.

Interventions

Hearing aids can be prescribed to amplify environmental sounds to obscure tinnitus. There is a device that combines the features of a masker and a hearing aid and emits a competitive but pleasant sound that distracts from head noise. However, hearing aids can be costly (Ostevik et al., 2019), and therefore not all older adults find the investment worthwhile.

Some of the therapeutic modes of treating tinnitus are transtympanal electrostimulation, iontophoresis (use of a small electric charge to deliver local anaesthesia through the skin), biofeedback, tinnitus masking with alternative sound production (i.e., "white noise"), dental treatment, cochlear implants, and hearing aids. Hypnosis, acupuncture, and chiropractic, naturopathic, allergy, or medication treatment are effective for some people.

Nursing actions include having discussions with the older person about times when the noises are most irritating and asking them to keep a diary in order to identify patterns. There is some evidence that caffeine, alcohol, cigarettes, stress, and fatigue may exacerbate the problem. The nurse assesses medications for their possible contribution to the problem and discusses lifestyle changes and alternative methods that are effective.

Prelingual Deafness

Prelingual deafness in older adults is rarely addressed, because it is assumed that individuals who have been deaf since childhood learned to communicate early in life through the use of hearing aids and sometimes sign language. Until 50 years ago, deaf children were commonly placed in a school for the deaf to develop within a culture of their own; hence, many older adults with prelingual deafness will have had an entirely different childhood from those with normal hearing. Persons with prelingual deafness often learn audible speech, sign language, or both, as well as lip reading. However, their reading and writing skills may be impaired even though their intelligence is normal. For those who depend on visual cues, communication can also be compromised when vision changes occur. Often, older adults with prelingual deafness use signing as their first language and English as their second. Subtleties of verbal communication may be lost to them, although they often compensate and become extremely alert to nonverbal cues and feelings. At times, a certified and experienced interpreter will be needed.

IMPLICATIONS FOR GERONTOLOGICAL NURSING AND HEALTHY AGING

The older adult whose vision or hearing is impaired is deprived of major sensory input, which has a direct effect on everyday life. Sensory losses can lead to potential isolation, depression, withdrawal, and loss of self-esteem; raise personal safety issues; affect health; and (in some cases) influence the risk for or the experience of delirium. Nurses should take a leadership role in education related to visual and auditory diseases. To promote healthy aging and quality of life, gerontological nurses must be knowledgeable about regular screening for vision and auditory function, the impact of hearing and vision changes on the functional abilities and quality of life of older adults, vision and hearing assessment, prevention and treatment of diseases affecting vision and hearing, effective communication techniques, and ways to help the older adult adapt to these losses and compensate for them.

In the assessment of vision and hearing losses, the nurse should include the impact of these losses on the older adult's functional ability, mood, and quality of life. A recent study found that depression frequently develops after AMD is diagnosed (Casten & Rovner, 2018). A study reviewing problem-solving skills found that problem-solving interventions for emotional distress prevented depressive symptoms in the short term; yet no long-term improvements were noted (Holloway et al., 2015). The problem-solving sessions, led by a

nurse or counsellor in the patient's home, focused on identifying problems caused by loss of eyesight and on finding ways to compensate.

It is important that the nurse be considerate of potential vision or hearing loss when working with older adults. Care must be adapted to the person's needs, and environmental changes need to ensure the highest possible safety for the older adult (see Chapter 6). Especially in a health care setting where the environment is unfamiliar and constantly changing, close attention to environmental safety and the person's mobility is warranted. Ensuring that individuals with vision impairment have access to visual aids (i.e., appropriate eyeglasses, books on tape, or a variety of devices available through the Canadian National Institute for the Blind) and that persons with hearing impairment have access to their hearing aids will promote independence and social engagement.

SUMMARY

Hearing and vision impairments can contribute to challenges at all levels of the hierarchy of needs, from biological integrity needs (such as activity, safety, and security) to higher-level needs (such as self-esteem, self-actualization, and a sense of belonging). These impairments severely affect the person's quality of life. They also predispose the person to having negative health and quality-of-life outcomes. Whatever the person's age or impairments, both the task of aging and the continued growth and development toward self-actualization require interactions and environments in which the older adult is assured that basic needs are being met, compensations for losses are being made, and meaningful and satisfying experiences will continue to be part of life.

KEY CONCEPTS

- Vision and hearing impairment can significantly affect the functional ability, safety, and quality of life of older adults.
- Vision loss from an eye disease is a global concern; the screening, prevention, and treatment of eye diseases are important priorities for nurses and other health care providers.
- The major diseases and disorders that affect vision are glaucoma, macular degeneration, diabetic retinopathy, and cataracts, all of which can be identified

through proper screening and appropriately treated. All persons over the age of 65 years should have annual eye examinations.

- Hearing impairment often has severe consequences for a person's quality of life and socialization.
- Tinnitus is a common condition among older adults that can interfere with hearing and become extremely irritating. It is characterized by ringing in the ear and may also manifest as buzzing, hissing, whistling, clicking, pulsating, or swishing sounds.

- To promote healthy aging and a good quality of life, nurses must be knowledgeable about the following: the impact of hearing and vision changes on the functional abilities and quality of life of older adults, vision and hearing assessment, the prevention and treatment of diseases that affect vision and hearing, effective communication techniques, and ways to help persons adapt to and compensate for these changes and losses.

ACTIVITIES AND DISCUSSION QUESTIONS

1. How can nurses enhance awareness and education in regard to vision and hearing disorders?

2. What is the role of a nurse in community, acute care, or residential care settings in screening for and assessing eye and ear diseases?

3. Develop a teaching plan for an older adult with glaucoma.

4. What type of resources could a nurse in any setting offer to an older adult with vision or hearing loss?

5. Develop a plan of care for an older adult with diabetic retinopathy.

6. What are your local community resources for supporting older adults with low vision or hearing impairment?

7. What hearing and vision adaptive supports can be found on the Internet and used for free?

RESOURCES

Canadian Ophthalmological Society
https://www.cos-sco.ca
Eye care coverage in Newfoundland and Labrador
https://www.gov.nl.ca/hcs/mcp/healthplancoverage/
Eye care coverage in Ontario
https://www.ontario.ca/page/what-ohip-covers#section-5
Eye care coverage in Quebec
https://www.ramq.gouv.qc.ca/en/citizens/health-insurance/optometric-services
Health care coverage in Manitoba
http://www.gov.mb.ca/health/mhsip/
Health-related services in Saskatchewan
https://www.saskatchewan.ca/residents/health/accessing-health-care-services
Health services in Alberta
http://www.albertahealthservices.ca/default.aspx
Healthy Aging and Wellness Working Group. *Healthy aging in Canada: A new vision, a vital investment from evidence to action.*
http://www.health.gov.bc.ca/library/publications/year/2006/Healthy_Aging_A_Vital_latest_copy_October_2006.pdf
Medical and health benefits in British Columbia
http://www2.gov.bc.ca/gov/content/health/health-drug-coverage/msp

New Brunswick Provincial Health Plan
http://ucm.greatwestlife.com/web5/groups/group/@public/documents/web_content/s6_000282.pdf
Northwest Territories. *Extended health benefits for seniors program.*
https://www.hss.gov.nt.ca/en/services/supplementary-health-benefits/extended-health-benefits-seniors-program
Nova Scotia Health Authority
https://www.cdha.nshealth.ca/geriatric-medicine/centre-health-care-elderly
Nunavut Department of Health
https://gov.nu.ca/health/information/health-insurance-nihb-coverage
Prince Edward Island Seniors' Guide.
https://www.princeedwardisland.ca/sites/default/files/publications/web-seniors_guide.pdf
Simulation of glaucoma, cataracts, macular degeneration, and diabetic retinopathy
https://www.eyesiteonwellness.com/eye-diseases/
World Health Organization. *Vision 2020: The Right to sight: Global initiative for the elimination of avoidable blindness.*
http://www.who.int/blindness/Vision2020_report.pdf

For additional resources, please visit *http://evolve.elsevier.com/Canada/Ebersole/gerontological/*

REFERENCES

Boltz, M., Capezuti, E., Fulmer, T. T., et al. (2016). *Evidence-based geriatric nursing protocols for best practice* (5th ed.). Springer.

Canadian Association of Optometrists. (2017). *Canadian Association of Optometrists submission to the House of Commons Standing Committee on Human Resources, Skills and Social Development and the Status of Persons with Disabilities: Better vision for seniors: A public health imperative.*

Canadian Hearing Society. (2020). *Tinnitus and hyperacusis.* https://www.chs.ca/knowledge-centre/tinnitus-and-hyperacusis.

Canadian National Institute for the Blind (CNIB). (2019). *Age-related macular degeneration.* https://cnib.ca/en/sight-loss-info/your-eyes/eye-diseases/age-related-macular-degeneration?region=on.

Canadian National Institute for the Blind (CNIB). (2020a). *Glaucoma.* https://cnib.ca/en/sight-loss-infoyour-eyeseye-diseases/glaucoma?region=on.

Canadian National Institute for the Blind (CNIB). (2020b). *Check your vision: The Amsler grid.* https://cnib.ca/en/sight-loss-info/your-eyes/eye-diseases/check-your-vision-amsler-grid?region=on.

Canadian National Institute for the Blind (CNIB). (2020c). *Diabetic retinopathy.* https://www.cnib.ca/en/sight-loss-info/your-eyes/eye-diseases/diabetic-retinopathy?region=on.

Casparis, H., Lindsley, K., Kuo, I. C., et al. (2017). Surgery for cataracts in people with age-related macular degeneration. *Cochrane Database of Systematic Reviews, 13*(6), CD006757. doi:10.1002/14651858.CD006757.pub3.

Castin, R. J., & Rovner, B. W. (2018). Update on depression and age-related macular degeneration. *Current Opinion Ophthalmology, 24*(3), 239–243. doi:10.1097/ICU.0b013e32835f8e55.

Devenyi, R., Maberley, D., Sheidow, T. G., et al. (2016). Real-world utilization of ranibizumab in wet age-related macular degeneration patients from Canada. *Canadian Journal of Opthalmology, 51*(2), 55–57. doi:10.1016/j.jcjo.2015.11.008.

Dickman, M. M., Spekreijse, L. S., Winkens, B., et al. (2019). Immediate sequential bilateral surgery versus delayed sequential bilateral surgery for cataracts. *Cochrane Database of Systematic Reviews, 2019*(2), CD013270. doi:10.1002/14651858.CD013270.

FYidoctors. (2020). *Are eye exams in Canada covered by the government?* https://fyidoctors.com/en/blog/categories/health-and-wellness/eye-exams-and-eye-care-coverage-in-canada-a-guide-to-eye-care-in-every-province.

Glaucoma Research Foundation. (2017a). *Are you an angle-closure glaucoma suspect?* https://www.glaucoma.org/glaucoma/are-you-an-angle-closure-suspect.php.

Glaucoma Research Foundation. (2017b). *Understanding glaucoma eye drops.* https://www.glaucoma.org/news/blog/understanding-glaucoma-eye-drops.php.

Glaucoma Research Foundation. (2019). *Are you at risk for glaucoma?* http://www.glaucoma.org/glaucoma/are-you-at-risk-for-glaucoma.php.

Glaucoma Research Society of Canada. (2021). *Learning about glaucoma.* https://www.glaucomaresearch.ca/about/about-glaucoma/.

Harasymowycz, P., Birt, C., Gooi, P., et al. (2016). Medical management of glaucoma in the 21st century from a Canadian perspective. *Journal of Ophthalmology, 2016,* 6509809. doi:10.1155/2016/6509809.

HealthLink BC. (2019). *Glaucoma.* https://www.healthlinkbc.ca/health-topics/hw158191.

Henry, J. A., Griest, S., Thielman, E., et al. (2016). Tinnitus Functional Index: Development, validation, outcome research, and clinical application. *Hearing Research, 334,* 58–64. doi:10.1016/j.heares.2015.06.004.

Holloway, E. E., Xie, J., Sturrock, B. A., et al. (2015). Do problem-solving interventions improve psychosocial outcomes in vision impaired adults? A systematic review and meta-analysis. *Patient Education and Counseling, 98*(5), 553–564. doi:10.1016/j.pec.2015.01.013.

Lawrenson, J. G., Graham-Rowe, E., Lorencatto, F., et al. (2018). Interventions to increase attendance for diabetic retinopathy screening. *Cochrane Database of Systematic Reviews, 1*(1), CD012054. doi:10.1002/14651858.CD012054.pub2.

Ludwig, P. E., Freeman, S. C., & Janot, A. C. (2019). Novel stem cell and gene therapy in diabetic retinopathy, age related macular degeneration, and retinitis pigmentosa. *International Journal of Retina and Vitreous, 5*(1), 7. doi:10.1186/s40942-019-0158-y.

Lupidi, M., Gujar, R., Cerquaglia, A., et al. (2020). OCT-angiography as a reliable prognostic tool in laser-treated proliferative diabetic retinopathy: The RENOCTA study. *European Journal of Ophthalmology.* doi:10.1177/1120672120963451.

Mansour, S. E., Browning, D. J., Wong, K., et al. (2020). The evolving treatment of diabetic retinopathy. *Clinical Ophthalmology, 14,* 653–678. doi:10.2147/OPTH.S236637.

Marchini, G., Chemello, F., Berzaghi, D., et al. (2015). Chapter 10: New findings in the diagnosis and treatment of primary angle-closure glaucoma. *Progress in Brain Research, 221,* 191–212. doi:10.1016/bs.pbr.2015.05.001.

McCusker, M. M., Durrani, K., Payette, M. J., et al. (2016). An eye on nutrition: The role of vitamins, essential fatty acids, and antioxidants in age-related macular degeneration, dry eye syndrome, and cataract. *Clinics in Dermatology, 34*(2), 276–285. doi:10.1016/j.clindermatol.2015.11.009.

National Eye Institute. (2019). *Age-related macular degeneration (AMD) data and statistics.* https://www.nei.nih.gov/learn-about-eye-health/outreach-campaigns-and-resources/eye-health-data-and-statistics/age-related-macular-degeneration-amd-data-and-statistics.

Newman, C. W., Wharton, J. A., & Jacobsen, G. P. (1995). Retest stability of the tinnitus handicap questionnaire. *Annals of Otology, Rhinology, & Laryngology, 104*(9 Pt. 1), 718–723. doi:10.1177/000348949510400910.

Ostevik, A. V., Westover, L., Gynane, H., et al. (2019). Comparison of health insurance coverage for hearing aids and other services in Alberta. *Healthcare Policy, 15*(2), 72–84. doi:10.12927/hcpol.2019.26070.

Sharma, S., Wadhwa, S., Gulati, M., et al. (2020). Recent advances in intraocular and novel drug delivery systems for the treatment of diabetic retinopathy. *Expert Opinion on Drug Delivery, 18,* 553–576. doi:10.1080/17425247.2021.1846518.

Statistics Canada. (2019). *Tinnitus in Canada.* https://www150.statcan.gc.ca/n1/pub/82-003-x/2019003/article/00001-eng.htm.

20

CARDIOVASCULAR AND RESPIRATORY DISORDERS

LEARNING OBJECTIVES

Upon completion of this chapter, the reader will be able to:

- Identify common types of cardiovascular and respiratory diseases occurring in later life.
- Discuss assessment of and intervention for cardiovascular and respiratory diseases in the older population.
- Suggest ways to prevent cardiovascular and respiratory diseases to the extent possible.
- Differentiate infectious, obstructive, and restrictive lung disease.
- Discuss the signs and symptoms of pneumonia and influenza.
- Develop a tuberculosis surveillance plan for a long-term care home.

GLOSSARY

Arteriosclerosis Thickening and loss of elasticity of the arterial wall.

Comorbid Pertaining to a disease or other pathological process that occurs simultaneously with another.

Dyspnea The subjective report of shortness of breath.

Health care–associated infection An infection whose source is related to a particular setting or treatment.

Morbidity Disability as the result of a health condition.

Mortality Death as a result of a health condition or event.

THE LIVED EXPERIENCE

"When I first had that heart attack, I was so frightened it seemed I would die just from the fear. It was the first time I realized how comforting, calm, and efficient nurses could be."
Jerry, age 71 years

"When Dad had that heart attack, it really scared us all, and I know we were afraid we would say or do something that would bring on another. I think he was also afraid of everything. I'm so grateful for the nurses at the hospital. They seem to give him lots of attention and information about the things he needs to know. He seems quite relaxed with himself now."
Ruth, Jerry's youngest daughter

Caring for older adults means caring for persons with cardiovascular disease (CVD), respiratory problems, or both. These two systems are interconnected. When the nurse is helping a patient with a cardiac problem, such as heart failure (HF), the patient's respiratory system must be assessed as well; for example, pneumonia may trigger HF. Conversely, a patient who has a problem with their respiratory system can experience some consequences at the cardiac level. Therefore, nursing interventions frequently overlap. One carefully planned action can address several systems at the same time and achieve goals of homeostasis, energy conservation, and meeting basic physiological needs, and thereby reducing **mortality** and **morbidity**.

CARDIOVASCULAR DISORDERS

Although the number of deaths from heart disease has decreased, it remains the leading cause of death in Canada after cancer (Statistics Canada, 2020) (see Fig. 15.1). The rate of deaths per 100,000 persons increases dramatically with age owing to a combination of normal age-related changes (see Chapter 6) and the presence of risk factors (Box 20.1). CVD is the leading cause of death among Indigenous peoples in Canada (Prince et al., 2017). Older adults also undergo the majority of cardiovascular-related procedures, but treatment approaches are highly variable by ethnicity and sex.

CVD refers to diseases that affect the circulatory system, including the heart and blood vessels (Public Health Ontario, 2019). These diseases could affect organs such as the lungs, brain, kidneys, and liver. In 2017, two of the major cardiovascular-related causes of death included heart disease and stroke (Statistics Canada, 2019a). Table 20.1 presents information about CVD in Canada.

Risk factors for CVD are often part of a metabolic syndrome—namely, a combination of medical disorders that increase the risk of developing CVD and diabetes. Heart disease affects one in five people, and its prevalence increases with age.

Hypertension

Hypertension (HTN) is the most common chronic risk factor for CVD. Hypertension Canada provides guidelines for the assessment, diagnosis, and treatment of hypertension (https://www.hypertension.ca) (Box 20.2). HTN is diagnosed whenever the diastolic blood pressure (BP) is consistently ≥90 mm Hg or the systolic BP is consistently ≥140 mm Hg (Hermida et al., 2018) (Table 20.2). Older adults often have isolated systolic HTN, unlike younger people, who are more likely to have an elevation of just the diastolic BP or elevation indicated by both systolic and diastolic BP readings. The goals of therapy for HTN are to treat modifiable risk factors for persons with diabetes and other chronic diseases and to maintain a systolic BP <140 mm Hg and a diastolic BP <90 mm Hg (Leung et al., 2016). (Note that the Canadian guidelines for HTN vary depending on whether or not the person has diabetes.) The guidelines also provide annual recommendations, based on up-to-date research, for improving the care of people with HTN.

HTN is often treatable and preventable in some cases. Between 2012 and 2015, one in four Canadian adults were living with HTN (Statistics Canada, 2019b).

BOX 20.1
RISK FACTORS FOR HEART DISEASE

- Older age (>55 years for men; >65 years for women)
- Family history of premature CHD (<55 years for men; <65 years for women)
- Microalbuminuria or estimated GFR <60 mL/min
- Hypertension*
- Cigarette smoking
- Central obesity
- Physical inactivity
- Dyslipidemia*
- Diabetes, IGT, or IFG*

CHD, coronary heart disease; GFR, glomerular filtration rate; IGT, impaired glucose tolerance; IFG, impaired fasting glucose.
*Components of metabolic syndrome.

TABLE 20.1

Heart Disease in Canada

Death Rate	Men vs. Women	Risk-Reducing Factors
■ Three times higher among adults aged 20 years and over with diagnosed heart disease, compared with those without. ■ Four times higher among adults aged 20 years and over who have had a heart attack, compared with those who have not. ■ Six times higher among adults aged 40 years and over with diagnosed heart failure, compared with those without.	■ Men are two times more likely than women to have a heart attack. ■ Men are newly diagnosed with heart disease 10 years younger than women.	■ Smoking cessation ■ Physical activity ■ Healthy, balanced diet ■ Healthy weight ■ Limited alcohol intake

Source: Government of Canada. (2017). *Heart disease in Canada.* https://www.canada.ca/en/public-health/services/publications/diseases-conditions/heart-disease-canada.html.

BOX 20.2
KEY POINTS OF THE 2016 HYPERTENSION CANADA GUIDELINES

- The BP of all adults should be assessed at all appropriate visits to determine cardiovascular risk and to monitor antihypertensive treatment.
- If systolic BP is ≥140 mm Hg, diastolic BP is ≥90 mm Hg, or both, a follow-up is needed to assess for hypertension. If systolic BP is between 130 and 139 mm Hg, diastolic BP is between 85 and 89 mm Hg, or both, annual follow-up is recommended.
- Global cardiovascular risk, including both modifiable and nonmodifiable risk factors, should be assessed.
- Home BP monitoring should be encouraged for hypertensive adults, especially if they have diabetes mellitus, chronic kidney disease, suspected nonadherence to antihypertensive therapy, masked hypertension, or demonstrate white-coat effect.
- Thiazide diuretics should be the initial medication therapy, either alone or combined with other types of medication, unless compelling reasons to do otherwise are present. Hypokalemia should be carefully monitored when treating with thiazide diuretic monotherapy.
- Most patients require two or more antihypertensive medications to achieve the goal BP. The combination of an angiotensin-converting enzyme inhibitor and angiotensin II receptor blockers is not recommended.
- If BP is >20/10 mm Hg above goal, initiate therapy with two agents, one of which should usually be a diuretic of the thiazide type.

BP, blood pressure.
Source: Adapted from Leung, A. A., Nerenberg, K., Daskalopoulou, S. S., et al. (2016). Hypertension Canada's 2016 Canadian Hypertension Education Program Guidelines for blood pressure measurement, diagnosis, assessment of risk, prevention, and treatment of hypertension. *Canadian Journal of Cardiology, 32*(5), 569–588. doi:10.1016/j.cjca.2016.02.066.

TABLE 20.2
Blood Pressure Classification

Classification	Blood Pressure
Normal	<120 mm Hg systolic and <80 mm Hg diastolic
Prehypertension	120–139 mm Hg systolic or 80–89 mm Hg diastolic
Stage 1 hypertension	140–159 mm Hg systolic or 90–99 mm Hg diastolic
Stage 2 hypertension	>160 mm Hg systolic or >100 mm Hg diastolic

BOX 20.3
MODIFIABLE FACTORS THAT INCREASE THE RISK FOR ESSENTIAL HYPERTENSION

- Cigarette smoking or tobacco use
- Excessive alcohol intake
- Sedentary lifestyle
- Inadequate stress management, anger management, or both
- Unhealthy diet (high in sodium, trans fats, or both; low in fibre)

As indicated by the Canadian Community Health Survey, there are significant disparities in HTN among different ethnic groups (Elkind et al., 2020; Tan et al., 2019). Although a person's race, ethnicity, and family history of HTN cannot be changed, other factors are within the person's control to reduce the risk for HTN (Box 20.3).

Most HTN is discovered during screening or examination for another problem, when related complications may have already developed. The most important complication of HTN is long-term effects resulting in end-organ damage, especially to the heart. Older adults with HTN have an absolute higher risk for cardiac disease, such as coronary heart disease (CHD), atrial fibrillation, and HF, as well as acute cardiovascular and cerebrovascular events such as myocardial infarction, stroke, and sudden death. Poorly controlled HTN is also implicated in chronic renal insufficiency, end-stage renal disease, and peripheral vascular disease (Grams et al., 2017).

Coronary Heart Disease

Like all other muscles, the heart receives its oxygen from arteries within it; CHD is caused by a blockage of these vessels and may be referred to as **arteriosclerosis**, or "hardening of the arteries." CHD develops when cholesterol and other fats are deposited in the layers of the arteries, narrowing the channel through which blood flows and, combined with arteriosclerosis, limiting the amount of oxygen reaching the tissue (a process known as *isch-emia*). CHD is in part a direct consequence of chronic, untreated, or inadequately treated HTN (Hypertension Canada, 2018). Seventy-five percent of all cardiac-related deaths each year are attributed to CHD.

The symptoms of gripping chest pain, radiation to the shoulder, and so on that are usually thought to indicate acute ischemia caused by myocardial infarction are not usually seen in older adults. Instead, the older adult is more likely to have what is called a "silent myocardial infarction." Discomfort may be mild and be localized to the back, abdomen, shoulders, or one or both arms. Nausea and vomiting or merely a sensation like heartburn may be the only symptoms. Older women often present with weakness or lethargy as a sign of a myocardial infarction. According to the Heart and Stroke Foundation of Canada (2018), early signs of a heart attack are missed in 78% of women. Women may experience signs such as shortness of breath, weakness, fatigue, and dizziness. When they do have pain, women describe the feeling as tightness or pressure. They may also experience signs such as nausea, fatigue, and jaw pain. More often, there are no noticeable signs or symptoms at all, and the event is only noticed at the time of death or when an electrocardiogram (ECG) is performed for some other purpose. These vague symptoms are often not brought to the attention of a medical provider.

Heart Valve Disease

For seniors living with heart valve disease in the early stages and when not severe, their condition will most likely be monitored. For later stages of valve disease, some people may require a valve repair or replacement through surgery. Sometimes the aortic valve will not require a full replacement, but a tissue repair. Other times, mechanical values or tissues from an animal will be used to replace the valve (Heart Valve Voice Canada, 2020).

There are also less invasive treatments available such as the transcatheter aortic valve implantation (TAVI) procedure (Heart Valve Voice Canada, 2020). This procedure treats people with aortic stenosis. A catheter is inserted in the femoral artery in the groin and positions the valve in the heart under fluoroscopic guidance (Heart Valve Voice Canada, 2020). The new valve is made from cow tissue. This procedure uses local anesthetic and some sedation, and many people have a faster recovery time than from traditional open-heart surgery

(Heart Valve Voice Canada, 2020). TAVI is typically recommended for older adults with aortic stenosis, as it is less invasive with a shorter recovery time (Asgar et al., 2019). However, this is a newer procedure, and therefore little is known about the sustainability of TAVI procedures beyond 10 years (Asgar et al., 2019).

Heart Failure

The damage to the heart from CHD may lead to HF, which is the most frequent cause of hospitalization of older adults. Approximately 600,000 Canadians are living with HF (Heart and Stroke Foundation of Canada, 2020a). As the population ages, it is expected that hospitalization rates will also increase (Heart and Stroke Foundation of Canada, 2016).

HF is a progressive disorder of the heart muscle in which the muscle is damaged, malfunctions, and can no longer pump enough blood to meet the needs of the body. The severity of malfunctioning depends on whether the abnormality is mechanical or functional. Some causes of HF are previous myocardial infarction, HTN, excessive use of alcohol and drugs, diabetes, obesity, infection, high cholesterol, and other medical conditions (Heart and Stroke Foundation of Canada, 2020a). Over time, the heart is further damaged because of poor control of the underlying problem (e.g., arteriosclerosis, HTN, or CHD), leading to increasingly severe HF. An unhealthy diet, smoking, and a lack of exercise aggravate the development of heart disease and the extent of damage, especially for those who have a family (genetic) history of heart disease. There is no cure for HF, only the management of symptoms and the attempt to prevent worsening (Heart and Stroke Foundation of Canada, 2020a). About 50% of persons with HF will die within 5 years; most die within 10 years, depending on the severity of symptoms and other factors (Heart and Stroke Foundation of Canada, 2016).

Clinical HF is categorized as a left-sided, right-sided, or biventricular (i.e., both sides) failure. It can also be described as either systolic or diastolic dysfunction (American Heart Association, 2017). Left-sided and diastolic failures are the most common types of HF found in the older population. The American Heart Association (2020a) has presented recommendations for the assessment, diagnosis, and management of HF (Box 20.4).

Common signs and symptoms of HF in older adults include fatigue and **dyspnea** (shortness of breath)

nocturnal dyspnea). The dyspnea may be relieved by sitting up or by sleeping on multiple pillows or with the head of the bed elevated. If a cough is present, it is worse at night.

In addition, the nurse should be alert for the atypical clinical presentation of exacerbations of HF in the older adult. The person may appear confused or delirious; begin falling; or complain of insomnia or urinary frequency at night (nocturia). They may also complain of dizziness or may have syncope (i.e., may faint). More often, the nurse will notice that the person has "droops," or malaise, and a subtle decline in activity tolerance or in functional or cognitive abilities.

One major way in which cardiac conditions differ from other chronic problems is that they can become acute problems very rapidly and often necessitate acute hospitalization and intensive treatment followed by rehabilitation. Many other chronic disorders are managed at home.

IMPLICATIONS FOR GERONTOLOGICAL NURSING AND HEALTHY AGING

Assessment

A comprehensive review of the events leading up to and including the presentation of cardiovascular problems is essential. Monitoring of vital signs, laboratory results, and kidney function, as well as assessing the cardiac and respiratory function and cognitive status, are essential (see Chapters 13 and 21). The University of Iowa Gerontological Nursing Intervention Center offers an evidence-informed assessment tool that can be used as a basic assessment measure as well as one that indicates change in residents with HF in long-term care (LTC) homes (Harrington, 2019). The tool can be used to document status in the three following categories: activities of daily living, quality of sleep, and dyspnea.

Interventions

The goals of interprofessional treatment of persons with CVD are to provide relief of symptoms, improve quality of life, reduce mortality and morbidity, and slow or stop the progression of dysfunction through the use of aggressive medication therapy. Additional goals include maximizing the person's function and quality of life by

with exertion, an inability to lie flat without getting short of breath (orthopnea), waking up at night gasping for air, weight gain, and swelling in the lower extremities. Dyspnea may occur at rest or with exertion, or it may appear intermittently at night (paroxysmal

planning appropriate rest and energy management techniques (thus minimizing energy expenditure), and, when appropriate, providing expert palliative care. Concurrent and supportive therapies include diet optimization; exercise; education and symptom recognition; consideration for the psychological impact, including fear, isolation, anxiety, and depression; and family and social supports (Barbera et al., 2018). Collaboration with families and care partners as well as other professionals (such as physiotherapists, dietitians, respiratory therapists, and social workers) is crucial.

Several nursing interventions that help the person accomplish their goals are highly effective (Boscart et al., 2017; Heckman et al., 2018). Which specific interventions are used will depend on the person, the severity of disease, and the person's desire for either palliative or aggressive care. Nursing actions may include teaching the older adult and their support system about lifestyle changes, activity, and rest (see Chapter 10); looking for signs and symptoms of HF; or taking more acute measures, such as administering oxygen and medications. In general, the nurse needs to be knowledgeable about interventions related to the following:

- Noting responses to prescribed exercise
- Administering medication and evaluating medication effects
- Watching for signs and symptoms of HF
- Monitoring diet and fluid intake and output
- Monitoring weight (daily, biweekly, or weekly)
- Auscultating heart and lung sounds
- Monitoring laboratory values
- Educating the older adult and family about all these interventions, and
- Providing comfort (see Chapter 27).

The goal of management of HTN is to minimize the risk of complications and reduce or eliminate modifiable risk factors. This means keeping the BP at <140/90 mm Hg in otherwise healthy adults and <130/80 mm Hg in persons with diabetes. By doing so, many long-term complications (e.g., HF) can be avoided, minimized, or delayed (Boxes 20.5 and 20.6). To accomplish this goal, nurses have a responsibility to work with older adults and their families comprehensively.

It is also important to understand the risks and benefits of antihypertensive medication. When the

> **BOX 20.5**
> ## MINIMIZING RISK FOR HEART DISEASE
>
> Blood pressure ≤130/80 mm Hg
> Total cholesterol <5.18 mmol/L (200 mg/dL)
> LDL <2.56 mmol/L (100 mg/dL)
> HDL >1.03 mmol/L (40 mg/dL)
> Triglycerides <1.69 mmol/L (150 mg/dL)
>
> LDL, low-density lipoprotein; HDL, high-density lipoprotein.

> **BOX 20.6**
> ## BENEFITS OF CONTROLLING BLOOD PRESSURE: AVERAGE REDUCED RISK FOR NEW EVENTS
>
> - 35%–40% decreased risk for stroke
> - 20%–25% decreased risk for myocardial infarction
> - 50% decreased risk for heart failure

medication is misused or incorrectly dosed, frail older adults are at risk of experiencing lowered BP, which may have consequences such as falls (Odden et al., 2017; American Heart Association, 2020b). Orthostatic hypotension is associated with frailty, cognitive impairment, and CVDs including stroke (Canadian Geriatrics Society, 2017). Orthostatic hypotension occurs when BP falls quickly after a person sits or stands upright. This can cause adverse events such as falls (Shaw et al., 2019).

Frail older adults with CVD and those who reside in LTC homes or at home require appropriate treatment and a careful risk–benefit analysis regarding treatment and outcomes (Heckman et al., 2016). Limited food choices and the significant side effects of some medications may result in an unnecessary reduction in quality of life for a person with a limited life expectancy. When aggressive treatment is no longer effective, a referral to hospice or palliative care services in the community may be a possibility.

The potential for wellness after older adults have experienced a major cardiac event or procedure is increased when they participate fully in any available cardiac rehabilitation program. Otherwise, disability can progress rapidly, especially if the person believes that any exertion overtaxes the heart and will cause acute HF, another myocardial infarction, or death. To prevent this, cardiac-exercise rehabilitation programs are designed to address the physical, mental, and spiritual needs and overall health of the person and their family. Cardiac-exercise rehabilitation programs consist of exercise, education and counselling to help one recover. Such programs typically include a medical assessment, physical activity such as cardiovascular and muscular fitness activities, lifestyle education, and psychosocial support (Heart and Stroke Foundation of Canada, 2020b). Typically, these programs are prescribed by the physician or nurse practitioner and begin with self-managed education and light activity, progressing to moderate activity under the supervision of a rehabilitation nurse and physiotherapist. If the person is more physically compromised, it is necessary to identify energy-conserving measures applicable to their daily tasks.

The nurse and the person with CVD must be cautious with exercise. In a person who has had a myocardial infarction, exercise-related orthostatic hypotension is more likely to occur. This hypotension is a result of age-related decreases in baroreceptor responsiveness, which controls the body's ability to respond to the need for changes in BP (see Chapter 6). Because the person's thermoregulation is also impaired, the intensity of exercise must be reduced in hot, humid climates (see Chapter 12). A healthy alternative is "mall walking" in local, covered, and climate-controlled shopping centres. In some locations, this becomes a social event as well as a safe way to exercise.

Risk-reduction programs should be instituted with a clear understanding of the difficulties involved in attempts to alter harmful lifestyle practices such as smoking, overeating, habitual anger or irritation, and a sedentary lifestyle. These practices may have been going on for all of the person's life and are not easily changed by education. The nurse's role in these instances is to discuss these practices in a nonjudgemental manner, providing acceptance, encouragement, resources, knowledge, and affirmation of both the difficulty of making lifestyle changes and the person's right to choose.

RESPIRATORY DISORDERS

The normal physical changes of aging (see Chapter 6) result in a higher risk for respiratory problems; when such problems occur, older adults have a higher risk of death than younger persons. Diseases of the respiratory system involve the upper or lower respiratory tract and are identified as infectious, acute, or chronic. Infections are further defined as either obstructive (preventing airflow out as a result of obstruction or narrowing of the respiratory structures) or restrictive (causing a decrease in total lung capacity as a result of limited expansion). Almost all chronic obstructive pulmonary disease (COPD) that occurs in late life arises from tobacco use or exposure to tobacco and other environmental pollutants earlier in life. Although asthma may be triggered by environmental factors, strong genetic and allergic factors contribute to its occurrence. In addition to being vigilant for signs of infection, the nurse should focus on helping the person maintain function and quality of life.

Chronic Obstructive Pulmonary Disease

COPD consists of a group of conditions that affect airflow, including asthma, bronchitis, and emphysema. COPD affects 2 million Canadians (Government of Canada, 2019a). In 2012–2013, 15% of older adults between the ages of 65 and 69 were living with COPD, with incidence increasing to 26% in those aged 85 years and older (Government of Canada, 2018). It is estimated that the prevalence of COPD is approximately three times higher in the Indigenous population (Turner et al., 2020). Cigarette smoking is the underlying cause of approximately 80% to 90% of COPD cases (Public Health Agency of Canada [PHAC], 2019).

COPD contributes to severe activity limitations. The 2009–2010 Canadian Community Health Survey found that 45% of Canadians with self-reported COPD reported their health as "fair or poor" (PHAC, 2019).

The signs and symptoms vary with the type of COPD. For example, persons with emphysema have little sputum production, and they appear pink because they are receiving adequate oxygen. On the other hand, persons with bronchitis have chronic sputum production, frequent cough, and are pale and somewhat cyanotic. Thorough discussions of these symptoms can be found in medical-surgical nursing and pathophysiology texts. What is crucial to gerontological nursing is the need to watch the person with COPD very closely for signs of worsening infection and aggravation of any underlying heart disease.

When respirations exceed 30 breaths per minute, the person's COPD is worsening, and prompt response is necessary. An acute episode of emphysema or bronchitis is characterized by significantly worsened dyspnea, coughing, shortness of breath at rest, sleepiness, and increased volume and change in the colour of sputum (Healthline, 2020). An acute episode of asthma is characterized by shortness of breath and wheezing. A number of factors—for example, viral or bacterial infections, exposure to polluted air or other environmental pollution, or changes in the weather—may trigger a change in the person's respiratory health. Persons with advanced COPD, as seen in most older adults with the disease, can expect to have periods of worsening symptoms and functioning between periods of control. During periods of illness, medication changes are usually needed. Persons with well-developed skills in self-management often will begin to deal with the changes before consulting a health care provider. Hospitalization is always a possibility with COPD exacerbations, especially when the person has or is suspected of having an acute infection.

Pneumonia

Pneumonia is a bacterial or viral infection of the lower respiratory tract that causes inflammation of the lung tissue. Pneumonia and influenza are the seventh and eighth leading causes of death for men and women, respectively, over the age of 65 years (Statistics Canada, 2019a). Particularly susceptible are older adults with **comorbid** conditions (such as alcoholism, asthma, COPD, or heart disease) and older adults who live in institutional settings. Older adults residing in LTC homes (for any reason) have a 10-fold greater incidence of pneumonia. Other factors that increase the risk of acquiring pneumonia are related to normal age-related respiratory system changes, such as a diminished cough reflex, increased residual volume, and decreased chest compliance (see Chapter 6). Many cases of pneumonia can be either prevented by immunization or treated effectively. The pneumococcal vaccine is a one-time vaccine that can prevent pneumonia and other infections and is recommended for people who are at high risk, who are older than 65 years, or both. More information can be found on the Health Canada website (https://www.hc-sc.gc.ca).

Pneumonia is classified as either a community-acquired infection or a **health care–associated infection**; that is, it is acquired either as a consequence of living in the community or as a result of medical treatment or hospitalization. In LTC homes, the most frequent causes of aspiration pneumonia are reflux of colonized oral secretions either from an enteral tube or from simply eating.

The usual signs and symptoms of pneumonia, such as cough, fatigue, and dyspnea, may easily be attributed to something else initially, such as medications or underlying COPD. In older adults, other signs of pneumonia may be seen, such as falling, mental status changes or signs of confusion, general deterioration, weakness, anorexia, rapid pulse, and rapid respirations. When a person appears to have pneumonia, an abnormal chest X-ray, fever, and an elevated white blood count are expected. However, these signs may be delayed in an older adult, and treatment that is not started until these signs are present may be too late, resulting in death. For the best possibility of survival, a frail older adult with pneumonia requires very prompt interventions. For the frail and medically compromised, interventions may be necessary as soon as an infection is determined to be a reasonable explanation for a sudden change.

One of the most important questions a nurse needs to consider is whether recommendation and advocacy for hospitalization are appropriate. Fortunately, several evidence-informed indicators help the nurse make this decision (Box 20.7).

For the older adult, especially a person who is frail or decompensated, the decision to hospitalize or not will be determined by the person's wishes regarding aggressive treatment. It is always imperative to make sure that the person and the person's significant others realize

---

BOX 20.7
INDICATORS OF PNEUMONIA-RELATED DEATH

The indicators of an increased likelihood of pneumonia-related death for persons in the community are as follows: (1) aggravation of another health condition at the same time, (2) respiratory rate >25, and (3) elevated C-reactive protein (if known).

The indicators of an increased risk for death within 30 days for persons residing in LTC homes are as follows: respiratory rate >30, pulse >125, altered mental status, and history of dementia.

the severity of the situation and that there are always options, such as treatment in the facility (e.g., intravenous antibiotics or oxygen per cannula) and comfort measures. The decision will always be a personal one.

Influenza

In Canada, influenza causes 500 to 1,500 deaths and thousands of hospitalizations each year. The greatest morbidity and mortality occur in those aged 65 years and older, owing to comorbid conditions and complications (Government of Canada, 2017a). In addition to medical complications, an older adult can experience a significant decline in functional ability as a result of a bout with the flu (Demicheli et al., 2018). Multiple studies report higher prevalence of seasonal and pandemic influenza in Indigenous populations, including COVID-19 (Alves et al., 2021).

The influenza vaccine remains the cornerstone of prevention. The Government of Canada (2020) suggests that everyone older than 6 months of age get a flu vaccine once a year. An annual flu vaccine is especially important for those who are more likely to have complications from the flu, such as people who are 65 years and older, people who are living in a home or a residential facility, people with CVD or respiratory disease, and people with a health condition that requires regular medical care or hospitalization (Demicheli et al., 2018). If used accordingly, the vaccine could prevent 70% of hospitalizations and 80% of deaths due to influenza among older individuals living in the community. The National Advisory Committee on Immunization (NACI) provides important guidelines on immunization strategies, surveillance, and the early identification and isolation of persons with influenza.

IMPLICATIONS FOR GERONTOLOGICAL NURSING AND HEALTHY AGING

Assessment

The nursing assessment of the person with respiratory problems focuses on (1) objective observations of oxygen saturation, sputum production, and coughing and (2) subjective reports of dyspnea and its effect on functional status and quality of life. Only persons experiencing a problem can really tell us what it is like for them. Visual analogue scales and numerical rating scales similar to those used to assess pain may be helpful (see

Chapter 16). Persons can be asked how they would rate their breathing from 1 (no dyspnea) to 10 (worst dyspnea possible), and so on.

When an infection is suspected, a "wait and see" approach is never appropriate; elevations in temperature or white blood cell count may not occur until the person is in a septic state, and chest X-ray examinations in chronically ill persons are often falsely negative at the beginning of the infection or when dehydration is present. Patients and their families should be told about the seriousness of this or any infection in older adults. More timely diagnosis calls for sensitive clinical assessments by both the nurse and the other health care providers.

Assessment includes detailed information about a cough. When did it start? How long are the episodes of coughing? Is there any associated pain? What seems to make it better, and what makes it worse? Is the person using anything to treat the cough? Is the person smoking (and how much) or exposed to smoke or other respiratory irritants? If the cough is productive, what is the colour, texture, and odour of the mucus? Does the colour change according to the time of day?

The remaining physical examination is the same as that for persons with cardiac disease since it is not always clear whether symptoms such as fatigue and shortness of breath are cardiac or respiratory in nature. Observation of airway clearance, breathing patterns, and mobility; measurement of pulse oximetry; mental status examination; and functional assessment can provide a clear picture of the person's health status. Pulmonary function testing is most definitive in terms of lung capacity; along with a chest X-ray examination, such testing can show the extent of respiratory damage from acute or chronic conditions. Box 20.8 presents the key components of a respiratory assessment.

Interventions

For pneumonia and influenza, the focus of intervention is on prevention and vaccination. As with HF, many respiratory diseases in later life cannot be cured. Nursing interventions are instead focused on optimizing self-care and support systems, health promotion strategies to minimize complications, and palliative goals, namely stabilizing the disease, reducing the risk of exacerbations and hospitalizations, promoting maximal functional capacity, and preventing premature disability.

BOX 20.8
PERFORMING A RESPIRATORY ASSESSMENT

Obtain the following histories:
  Family and support system
  Past medical
  Symptoms
Assess the following:
  Overall body configuration (e.g., posture, chest symmetry, shape)
  Respirations, including ease of ventilation, use of accessory muscles, and so forth
  Level of dyspnea per activity, in detail
  Oxygenation (pulse oximetry, skin colour, capillary refill, and pallor)
  Sputum (colour, amount, and consistency)
  Palpation, percussion, and auscultation
  Functional status
  Cognitive status (if indicated)
  Mood (if indicated)
  Advance planning and patient's wishes for treatment
  Presence or absence of a living will and a designated health care surrogate

Education always includes teaching smoking cessation, secretion clearance techniques, the identification and management of exacerbations, breathing retraining, management of depression and anxiety, nutritional support, the proper use and administration of medications, and dealing with supplemental oxygen therapy if and when necessary (Healthline, 2020). Except in severe cases, treatment can be done at home or in an LTC home, as long as oxygen therapy, parenteral fluids, and antibiotics can be administered by nursing staff.

Oxygen therapy can have a significant impact on a person's quality of life. It takes the person receiving oxygen, the care partners, and the entire care team to ensure that oxygen is being used safely. If a person does not need oxygen therapy, the air will typically provide 21% of oxygen, which is adequate if one's airway is not compromised. In those with compromised airways such as with pneumonia, the person must have higher concentrations of oxygen to ensure that all body tissues receive enough oxygen to sustain life (Alberta Health Services, 2019).

If someone is available to assume a caregiver role, the older adult's care and treatment can be carried out in their home with temporary home health service support. If the older adult fails to improve or deteriorates,

then hospitalization is often necessary, unless this is against the wishes of the older adult. A change to active palliative care may be appropriate at any time. If the person is hospitalized, a prolonged rehabilitation may be necessary, whether at home, in a rehabilitation facility, or both (see Chapter 28). Pharmacological and mechanical interventions for the treatment of infection are based on the health status of the person before the infection, the expected outcomes of treatment, where treatment will be provided, and the wishes of the patient (as noted previously).

Interdisciplinary Care

Education is a part of every aspect of pulmonary care (Box 20.9). The person and their support system are taught to recognize the signs and symptoms of respiratory infection; how to maintain adequate nutrition; how to use and clean an inhaler, nebulizer, and peak flow meter; how to use oxygen safely; how to tell which type of exercise is beneficial; how to pace activities; and how to use coping strategies. Each of these areas (and any other issues, such as sexual function) calls for teaching and indicates specific interventions that will help older adults and their support system participate in the management.

Diet education should address the reasons for monitoring weight and the signs of malnutrition. Weight loss can occur rapidly because of the energy expenditure needed to breathe while eating. A sense of being full early in the meal is caused by congestion in the abdomen because of a flattened diaphragm. Anorexia or decreased appetite occurs as a result of sputum production and gastric irritation from the use of bronchodilators and steroids.

Activity and exercise tolerance should be assessed by the occupational and respiratory therapists, and activities should be prescribed to increase endurance and improve respiratory status. Exercise may be done with or without supplementary oxygen to control symptoms so that the older adult can spend enough time in exercise to benefit from it. The person should be informed that sexual activity is still possible, and education and counselling should be provided, either by the rehabilitation nurse or a professional counsellor.

Medications are used to treat infection and control dyspnea, cough, and sputum production. When teaching about any medication, the nurse needs to make

consist of medication therapy, reconditioning exercises, and counselling. An interprofessional team of health care providers works to help the older adult do the following:

- Increase the level of independence
- Maintain individuality and autonomy
- Improve function in their environment
- Decrease the number of hospitalizations and the need for hospitalization
- Increase exercise tolerance
- Increase self-esteem and self-care skills, and
- Improve quality of life and comfort.

The number of goals achieved depends on many factors, including the extent of illness and coexisting conditions. Rehabilitation may be prolonged for persons recovering from pneumonia.

Economic issues are always a concern for persons with chronic disease (see Chapter 15). Not all prescription medication costs are covered by the health system, and the amount of coverage varies across provinces and territories. Medications can be very expensive, especially when needed for an indefinite period of time.

Mouth care is essential, especially for people who are receiving supplemental oxygen and those who are medically or physically debilitated. Inadequate mouth care leads to the propagation of bacteria, which compounds an already serious situation and may lead to aspiration pneumonia. Sputum is considered potentially infectious and must be handled appropriately.

Monitoring nutrition and obtaining nutritional consultation as necessary are the responsibility of the nurse in all settings. The nurse will also ensure that the person recovering from pneumonia or influenza is adequately nourished and—while monitoring fluid volume—is adequately hydrated. Overload is a risk for persons with coexisting heart disease. As soon as the condition allows, the older adult should be mobilized and referred for physiotherapy and occupational therapy to prevent or stop functional decline.

Tuberculosis

Tuberculosis (TB) is a communicable infectious disease caused by *Mycobacterium tuberculosis*, a bacterium that affects one-third of the world's population (Centers for Disease Control and Prevention, 2019). *Tuberculosis infection* is identified by a positive TB skin test result with no evidence of active disease. The term

sure that the person knows the purpose and correct dosage and regimen of any medication they are taking, its side effects, and what to do if these side effects occur (see Chapter 14). Inhalers are difficult to use for persons with limited manual dexterity, strength, or both (such as people with arthritis in their hands). Special adaptive devices are available if needed.

Rehabilitation is an important aspect of maximizing quality of life for the person with respiratory problems, as it is for those with cardiovascular problems. An older adult with COPD would be considered a candidate for pulmonary rehabilitation as long as they have pulmonary reserve and as long as any heart disease is stable. Rehabilitation programs for the older adult with COPD

"tuberculosis disease" refers to cases in which a person has a positive acid-fast smear or culture for *M. tuberculosis* or has radiographic and clinical evidence of TB.

Mycobacterium tuberculosis was considered to be conquered in the 1950s with the development of the isoniazid. Many older adults were treated following infections contracted during the Second World War; many others were infected as children. However, if older adults become immunocompromised as a result of chemotherapy, extreme old age, or human immunodeficiency virus (HIV) infection, the bacterium could be reactivated.

In 2017, there were 1,796 cases of TB reported, a 2.6% increase since 2016 (Government of Canada, 2017b). The majority of TB cases in Canada are reported in those who are born in other countries (71.8% of cases), followed by the Canadian-born Indigenous population (17.4%) (Government of Canada, 2017b). In 2017, 313 cases of TB were reported (or 21.5 cases per 100,000 population) among Indigenous peoples. In those aged 75 years or older, males are twice as likely to be diagnosed with TB (13.2 versus 7.2 cases per 100,000) (Government of Canada, 2017b).

Gerontological nurses working in areas where TB rates are high must be particularly knowledgeable about this potentially life-threatening disease and must protect themselves and others. Persons who are immunosuppressed, persons who are from areas with high infection rates, and persons who live in group settings are at particular risk. Older residents in congregate living settings are more likely to acquire the disease than those who live in the community (Dhaolakia & Mistry, 2017). Improvements in socioeconomic conditions is a priority to achieve a decrease in TB prevalence in Indigenous communities (Canadian Public Health Association, 2021).

The symptoms of TB, regardless of age group, include unexplained weight loss or fever and a cough lasting more than 3 weeks. The person may experience night sweats and generalized anxiety. In more advanced stages, the person will also experience dyspnea, chest pain, and hemoptysis. Laboratory results for older adults may show an increased sedimentation rate and lymphocytopenia. Because these signs and symptoms are associated with many disorders common in older adults, diagnosis is often made during a health screening (Dheda et al., 2017).

Testing for active TB is indicated in everyone who has signs and symptoms of TB or is considered to be at high risk for TB disease. Every effort should be made to obtain a microbiological diagnosis, which requires demonstration of acid-fast bacilli on smear microscopy or culture of *Mycobacterium tuberculosis*, or it requires amplification and detection of *M. tuberculosis* complex (MTBC) nucleic acids using nucleic acid amplification tests (NAATs). For persons with positive skin test results, it is necessary to confirm the diagnosis with a chest X-ray and a sputum culture (Rastoder et al., 2019). At least three sputum specimens should be collected and tested with microscopy as well as culture. Where feasible, three sputum specimens (either spontaneous or induced) can be collected on the same day, a minimum of 1 hour apart.

IMPLICATIONS FOR GERONTOLOGICAL NURSING AND HEALTHY AGING

In promoting healthy aging in the context of TB, the nurse has a responsibility to both the public and the patient. The nurse must be proactive in the prevention of contagious disease and in the prompt treatment of persons who are ill or become ill; this responsibility is especially important in a communal care setting, where older adults are at higher risk for TB because of the shared living situation and a high rate of frailty. To ensure the prompt identification of persons with TB and to limit its spread, especially in LTC homes, Indigenous communities, and other high-risk populations (shelters), nurses must develop and implement an appropriate surveillance plan in collaboration with these communities (Box 20.10). The Public Health Agency of Canada and the Canadian Lung Association provide guidance, and Health Canada's strategy outlines the mandate to provide TB services to First Nations and Inuit communities (Health Canada, 2012).

TB is a reportable condition, which means that all suspected and confirmed cases are reported to the appropriate health authorities (Government of Canada, 2019b). The local public health nurses must conduct investigations to ensure that all potentially infected people have been tested and that all persons with the disease receive treatment. The nurse actively participates in health screenings that may include TB testing.

BOX 20.10

SURVEILLANCE GUIDELINES FOR TUBERCULOSIS IN THE LONG-TERM CARE SETTING

- Each long-term care (LTC) home should have an individual responsible for tuberculosis (TB) infection control and an infection prevention and control plan.
- Each LTC home should conduct regularly scheduled TB risk assessments that consider the residents and staff.
- Determine the need for TB screening as indicated by the results of the risk assessments. Most LTC homes are low-risk settings.
- Screen all new residents on admission and employees on hire for symptoms, and consider using the two-step tuberculin skin test for *Mycobacterium tuberculosis*. Repeat the tests annually.
- For persons who test positive or have had a positive test result in the past, perform one chest X-ray examination, then review the symptoms annually.
- No person with a diagnosis of TB should remain in an LTC home unless adequate administrative and environmental controls and a respiratory protection program are in place.

Source: Public Health Agency of Canada (PHAC), Canadian Lung Association/Canadian Thoracic Society. (2014). *Canadian tuberculosis standards* (7th ed.). https://www.canada.ca/en/public-health/services/infectious-diseases/canadian-tuberculosis-standards-7th-edition/edition-13.html#a6_.

As a health care provider, the nurse is also at risk for acquiring the infection and needs to be screened regularly to keep from becoming a carrier.

In regard to persons with TB, nurses have a role in monitoring laboratory values, assessing any medication side reactions, and monitoring medication adherence in persons with TB, all of which are crucial to the treatment's effectiveness and the person's well-being. The gerontological nurse participates in screening, educating the person about the seriousness of the infection, and helping the person obtain the appropriate treatment.

KEY CONCEPTS

- Heart disease is the most common cause of death for persons in Canada.
- The underlying cause for the majority of cardiovascular and pulmonary diseases is smoking; therefore, smoking cessation can have a significant impact on improving people's health.
- Pneumonia and influenza are particularly important health problems for persons over 65 years of age and are significantly more so for persons who are frail or immunocompromised, have HIV infection, or are otherwise decompensated.
- The mortality associated with pneumonia and influenza can be minimized through vaccination.
- The goal of therapy for cardiac and respiratory disorders is to relieve symptoms, improve quality of life, reduce mortality, stabilize and slow the progression of the disease, reduce the risk of exacerbation, and maximize functional capacity.
- Continued careful attention to the early detection and prompt treatment of TB within Indigenous communities, as well as addressing social determinants of health, is necessary to eradicate this communicable disease.

ACTIVITIES AND DISCUSSION QUESTIONS

1. What is heart failure?

2. Compare and contrast the types of heart failure and chronic obstructive pulmonary disease.

3. Discuss the assessment of and interventions for older adults with a diagnosis of heart failure, chronic obstructive pulmonary disease, or pneumonia.

4. Discuss why pneumonia and influenza are so dangerous to the older adult.

5. What preventive measures can be instituted to prevent or lessen the severity of pneumonia, influenza, and tuberculosis among the older population?

6. Develop a nursing care plan for an older adult with heart failure or a respiratory condition.

7. Discuss the implications of cardiovascular disease and respiratory illness for an older adult's ability to live independently.

RESOURCES

Canadian Cardiovascular Society. *Recommendations for the assessment, diagnosis, and management of cardiovascular disease.*
https://www.ccs.ca

Canadian Heart Failure Society
https://heartfailure.ca

Canadian Hypertension Education Program. *Educational tools for patients and families.*
https://guidelines.hypertension.ca

Canadian Lung Association
https://www.lung.ca

Government of Canada. *Tuberculosis in Indigenous communities.*
https://www.sac-isc.gc.ca/eng/1570132922208/1570132959826

Health Canada. *Information on vaccinations and immunization policy for pneumonia and influenza.*
http://www.hc-sc.gc.ca

Heart and Stroke Foundation of Canada
https://www.heartandstroke.ca

Heart and Stroke Foundation of Canada. *Helping to close the gap in Indigenous health.*
https://www.heartandstroke.ca/what-we-do/our-impact/helping-to-close-the-gap-in-indigenous-health

Hypertension Canada
https://www.hypertension.ca

For additional resources, please visit *http://evolve.elsevier.com/Canada/Ebersole/gerontological/*

REFERENCES

Alberta Health Services. (2019). *Oxygen therapy for acute adult inpatients.* https://www.albertahealthservices.ca/assets/info/hp/edu/if-hp-edu-ahc-oxygen-therapy-learning-module-cat-1and2.pdf.

Alves, D. E., Rogeberg, O., & Mamelund, S. (2021). Indigenous groups and influenza: Protocol for a systematic review and meta-analysis. *Research Square.* doi:10.21203/rs.3.rs-616894/v1.

American Heart Association. (2017). *Types of heart failure.* http://www.heart.org/HEARTORG/Conditions/HeartFailure/About-HeartFailure/Types-of-Heart-Failure_UCM_306323_Article.jsp#.WMvgwxIrJmA.

American Heart Association. (2020a). *Classes of heart failure.* https://www.heart.org/en/health-topics/heart-failure/what-is-heart-failure/classes-of-heart-failure.

American Heart Association. (2020b). *Dropping blood pressure may predict frailty, falls in older people.* https://www.heart.org/en/news/2020/03/30/dropping-blood-pressure-may-predict-frailty-falls-in-older-people.

Asgar, A. W., Ouzounian, M., Adams, C., et al. (2019). 2019 Canadian Cardiovascular Society position statement for transcatheter aortic valve implantation. *Canadian Journal of Cardiology, 35*, 1437–1448. doi:10.1016/j.cjca.2019.08.011.

Barbera, M., Mangialasche, F., Jongstra, S., et al. (2018). Designing an internet-based multidomain intervention for the prevention of cardiovascular disease and cognitive impairment in older adults: The HATICE trial. *Journal of Alzheimer's Disease, 62*(2), 649–663. doi:10.3233/JAD-170858.

Boscart, V. M., Heckman, G. A., Huson, K., et al. (2017). Implementation of an interprofessional communication and collaboration intervention to improve care capacity for heart failure management in long-term care. *Journal of Interprofessional Care, 31*(5), 583–592. doi:10.1080/13561820.2017.1340875.

Canadian Geriatrics Society. (2017). *Treatment of orthostatic hypotension in older patients: The geriatric perspective.* http://canadiangeriatrics.ca/wp-content/uploads/2017/07/TREATMENT-OF-ORTHOSTATIC-HYPOTENSION-IN-OLDER-PATIENTS.pdf.

Canadian Public Health Association. (2021). *TB and Aboriginal people.* https://www.cpha.ca/tb-and-aboriginal-people.

Centers for Disease Control and Prevention. (2019). *Tuberculosis: Data and statistics.* https://www.cdc.gov/tb/statistics/default.htm.

Demicheli, V., Jefferson, T., Di Pietrantonj, C., et al. (2018). Vaccines for preventing influenza in the elderly. *Cochrane Database of Systematic Reviews, 2*(2), CD004876. doi:10.1002/14651858.CD004876.pub4.

Dhaolakia, Y., & Mistry, N. (2017). Tuberculosis in congregate settings: Policies and practices in various facilities in Mumbai, India. *Indian Journal of Tuberculosis, 64*(1), 10–13. doi:10.1016/j.ijtb.2016.11.006.

Dheda, K., Gumbo, T., Maartens, G., et al. (2017). The epidemiology, pathogenesis, transmission, diagnosis, and management of multidrug-resistant, extensively drug-resistant, and incurable tuberculosis. *The Lancet Respiratory Medicine, 5*(4), 291–360. doi:10.1016/S2213-2600(17)30079-6.

Elkind, M. S. V., Lisabeth, L., Howard, V. J., et al. (2020). Approaches to studying determinants of racial-ethnic disparities in stroke and its sequelae. *Stroke, 51*(11). doi:10.1161/STROKEAHA.120.030424.

Government of Canada. (2017a). *FluWatch report: January 8 to January 14, 2017 (Week 2).* http://www.healthycanadians.gc.ca/publications/diseases-conditions-maladies-affections/fluwatch-2016-2017-02-surveillance-influenza/index-eng.php.

Government of Canada. (2017b). *Tuberculosis in Canada, 2017.* https://www.canada.ca/en/public-health/services/reports-publications/canada-communicable-disease-report-ccdr/monthly-issue/2019-45/issue-2-february-7-2019/article-4-tuberculosis-in-canada.html.

Government of Canada. (2018). *Asthma and chronic obstructive pulmonary disease (COPD) in Canada, 2018.* https://www.canada.ca/en/public-health/services/publications/diseases-conditions/asthma-chronic-obstructive-pulmonary-disease-canada-2018.html.

Government of Canada. (2019a). *Data blog: Chronic obstructive pulmonary disease (COPD) in Canada.* https://health-infobase.canada.ca/datalab/copd-blog.html.

Government of Canada. (2019b). *Tuberculosis: For health professional.* https://www.canada.ca/en/public-health/services/diseases/tuberculosis/health-professionals.html.

Government of Canada. (2020). *Flu (influenza): Get your flu shot.* https://www.canada.ca/en/public-health/services/diseases/flu-influenza/get-your-flu-shot.html.

Grams, M. E., Yang, W., Rebholz, C. M., et al. (2017). Risks of adverse events in advanced CKD: The chronic renal insufficiency cohort (CRIC) study. *American Journal of Kidney Diseases, 70*(3), 337–346. doi:10.1053/j.ajkd.2017.01.050.

Harrington, C. C. (2019). Assessing heart failure in long-term care facilities. *Journal of Gerontological Nursing, 45*(7), 18–24. doi:10.3928/00989134-20190409-01.

Health Canada. (2012). *Health Canada's strategy against tuberculosis for First Nations on-reserve*. https://www.canada.ca/en/public-health/services/publications/diseases-conditions/summary-health-canada-strategy-against-tuberculosis-first-nations-reserve.html.

Healthline. (2020). *COPD exacerbation*. https://www.healthline.com/health/copd/exacerbation-symptoms-and-warning-signs.

Heart and Stroke Foundation of Canada. (2016). *The burden of heart failure*. https://www.heartandstroke.ca/-/media/pdf-files/canada/2017-heart-month/heartandstroke-reportonhealth-2016.ashx?la=en.

Heart and Stroke Foundation of Canada. (2018). *Ms.Understood: Women's hearts are victims of a system that is ill-equipped to diagnose, treat and support them*. https://www.heartandstroke.ca/-/media/pdf-files/canada/2018-heart-month/hs_2018-heart-report_en.ashx.

Heart and Stroke Foundation of Canada. (2020a). *Heart failure*. https://www.heartandstroke.ca/heart/conditions/heart-failure.

Heart and Stroke Foundation of Canada. (2020b). *Cardiac rehabilitation (cardiac rehab)*. https://www.heartandstroke.ca/heart-disease/recovery-and-support/cardiac-rehabilitation.

Heart Valve Voice Canada. (2020). *Heart valve disease*. https://www.heartvalvevoice.ca/heart-valve-disease-1.

Heckman, G. A., Boscart, V. M., D'Elia, T., et al. (2016). Managing heart failure in long-term care: Recommendations from an interprofessional stakeholder consultation. *Canadian Journal on Aging*, 35(4), 447–464. doi:10.1017/S071498081600043X.

Heckman, G. A., Shamji, A. K., Ladha, R., et al. (2018). Heart failure management in nursing homes: A scoping literature review. *Canadian Journal of Cardiology*, 34(7), 871–880. doi:10.1016/j.cjca.2018.04.006.

Hermida, R. C., Ayala, D. E., Fernandez, J. R., et al. (2018). Hypertension: New perspective on its definition and clinical management by bedtime therapy substantially reduces cardiovascular disease risk. *European Journal of Clinical Investigation*, 48(5), e12909. doi:10.1111/eci.12909.

Hypertension Canada. (2018). *VI. Assessment of overall cardiovascular risk in hypertensive patients: diagnosis and assessment*. https://guidelines.hypertension.ca/diagnosis-assessment/ambulatory-measurement/.

Leung, A. A., Nerenberg, K., Daskalopoulou, S. S., et al. (2016). Hypertension Canada's 2016 Canadian Hypertension Education Program Guidelines for blood pressure measurement, diagnosis, assessment of risk, prevention, and treatment of hypertension. *Canadian Journal of Cardiology*, 32(5), 569–588. doi:10.1016/j.cjca.2016.02.066.

Odden, M. C., Beilby, P. R., & Peralta, C. A. (2017). Blood pressure in older adults: The importance of frailty. *Current Hypertension Reports*, 17(7), 55. doi:10.1007/s11906-015-0564-y.

Prince, S. A., McDonnell, L. A., Turek, M. A., et al. (2017). The state of affairs of cardiovascular health research in Indigenous women in Canada: A scoping review. *Canadian Journal of Cardiology*, 34(4), 437–449. doi:10.1016/j.cjca.2017.11019.

Public Health Agency of Canada (PHAC). (2019). *Chronic obstructive pulmonary disease (COPD)*. https://www.canada.ca/en/public-health/services/chronic-diseases/chronic-respiratory-diseases/chronic-obstructive-pulmonary-disease-copd.html.

Public Health Ontario. (2019). *Cardiovascular disease*. https://www.publichealthontario.ca/en/diseases-and-conditions/chronic-diseases-and-conditions/cardiovascular-disease.

Rastoder, E., Shaker, S. B., Naqibullah, M., et al. (2019). Chest X-ray findings in tuberculosis patients identified by passive and active case finding: A retrospective study. *Journal of Clinical Tuberculosis and Other Mycobacterial Diseases*, 14, 26–30. doi:10.1016/j.jctube.2019.01.003.

Shaw, B. H., Borrel, D., Sabbaghan, K., et al. (2019). Relationships between orthostatic hypotension, frailty, falling and mortality in elderly care home residents. *BMC Geriatrics*, 19(80). doi:10.1186/s12877-019-1082-6

Statistics Canada. (2019a). *Causes of death, 2017*. https://www150.statcan.gc.ca/n1/daily-quotidien/190530/dq190530c-eng.htm.

Statistics Canada. (2019b). *Blood pressure and hypertension*. https://www150.statcan.gc.ca/n1/pub/82-003-x/2019002/article/00002-eng.htm.

Statistics Canada. (2020). *Leading cause of death, total population, by age group*. https://www150.statcan.gc.ca/t1/tbl1/en/tv.action?pid=1310039401.

Tan, S. M., Han, E., Chin Quek, R. Y., et al. (2019). A systematic review of community nursing interventions focusing on improving outcomes for individuals exhibiting risk factors of cardiovascular disease. *Journal of Advanced Nursing*, 76(1), 47–61. doi:10.1111/jan.14218.

Turner, J., Holyk, T., Bartlett, K., et al. (2020). "Bayis Ilh Tus—A strong breath" a community-based research project to estimate the prevalence of chronic obstructive pulmonary disease in remote and rural First Nations communities in Canada: Research protocol. *International Journal of Equity Health*, 19, 123. doi:10.1186/s12939-020-01240-1.

COGNITIVE IMPAIRMENT

LEARNING OBJECTIVES

Upon completion of this chapter, the reader will be able to:

- Differentiate between dementia, delirium, and depression.
- Discuss the different types of dementia and appropriate diagnosis.
- Describe nursing models of care for persons with dementia and cognitive impairment.
- Discuss common concerns in caring for persons with dementia.
- Develop a nursing care plan for a person with delirium.
- Develop a nursing care plan for a person with dementia.

GLOSSARY

Agnosia Inability to recognize common objects, familiar faces, or sounds, despite intact sensory abilities.

Aphasia Loss of the ability to use and understand spoken and written language.

Apraxia Impaired ability to manipulate objects or perform purposeful acts.

Cognitive functioning "Comprises perception, memory, and thinking. The processes by which an individual perceives, stores, retrieves, and uses information" (Fick et al., 2020).

Computed tomography (CT) An X-ray technique that produces an image representing a detailed cross-section of tissue; used primarily to diagnose space-occupying lesions.

Electroencephalogram (EEG) A recording of the electrical activity of the brain by means of electrodes attached to the scalp.

Hallucinations Perceptions of sensory experiences with no external stimuli.

Magnetic resonance imaging (MRI) A noninvasive technology that uses magnets (not radiation) and radiofrequency current to produce an image of the soft tissues of the body, including the brain.

Milieu Environment or setting.

THE LIVED EXPERIENCE

"I have dementia and I'm going to reach a stage whereby I can no longer think as a logical person or do things in a logical way."

"Dementia also includes, as I say, organizational skills, erm, coordination skills, and memory skills, and I never used to use, consider these."

"I'll stand my ground and fight it at the moment, in my own way on my own."

"You can't do anything about it."

"I'm giving up various activities because I have the onset of Alzheimer's disease."

"I'm misconstrued and misunderstood until I . . . blow."

"If I'm a patient, nobody seems to care."

"People tend to talk about them behind your back rather than to your face." (Comments made by participants in a research study about living with early stages of dementia.)

Harman, G., & Clare, L. (2006). Illness representations and lived experience in early-stage dementia. *Qualitative Health Research, 16*, 484–502. doi:10.1177/1049732306286851.

HEALTHY AGING CARE PLAN

About M.R.

M.R. (pronouns he/him) is a 76-year-old who lives alone in an apartment. He was admitted to the hospital with pyelonephritis; his symptoms are improving after 36 hours of intravenous therapy, and discharge planning is in progress. M.R. repeatedly asks the nurses where he is. He left the unit, was unable to find his way back, and was escorted back by a security officer. He has no family nearby, but a close friend visits daily. The friend tells you that they've been worried about M.R. because his ability to take care of himself and his home has deteriorated over the past year. He's gotten lost when driving, and recently he left the stove on and burned a pot. The friend has been helping out for several months but is very concerned about M.R.'s safety.

QUESTIONS TO CONSIDER

1. What could explain M.R.'s symptoms?
2. What nursing interventions are a priority, given M.R.'s symptoms and the friend's concerns?
3. Which members of the interprofessional team should be involved in discharge planning for M.R.?

This chapter focuses on cognitive impairment, particularly delirium, Alzheimer's disease, and other dementias. The chapter also presents nursing interventions for people experiencing delirium and dementia, as well as caregiving for persons with dementia. (See Chapter 7 for a discussion of cognitive function in aging, Chapter 13 for a discussion of instruments for cognitive assessment, and Chapter 3 for a discussion of communication with persons experiencing cognitive impairment.)

COGNITIVE IMPAIRMENT

The term *cognitive impairment* describes a range of disturbances of **cognitive functioning**, including disturbances in memory, orientation, attention, and concentration. Other disturbances of cognition may affect intelligence, judgement, learning ability, perception, problem solving, psychomotor ability, reaction time, and social intactness.

The Three Ds

Delirium, dementia, and depression, which occur frequently in older adults, have been called the "three Ds" of cognitive impairment. These important geriatric syndromes are not normal consequences of aging, although their incidences increase with age. Because cognitive and behavioural changes characterize all three "Ds," it can be difficult to diagnose delirium, delirium superimposed on dementia, or depression. The inability to concentrate, along with the resulting memory impairment and other cognitive dysfunction, can occur in late-life depression (see Chapter 23).

Delirium is characterized by a relatively rapid onset, usually over hours or days, with symptoms that fluctuate throughout the day. The other key features of delirium are disturbances in consciousness and attention, and changes in cognition (memory deficits and perceptual disturbances). Perceptual disturbances are often accompanied by delusional (paranoid) thoughts and behaviour and by disturbances of the sleep–wake cycle, psychomotor behaviour, and emotions. In contrast, dementia typically has a gradual onset and a slow, steady pattern of decline without alterations in consciousness (Blevins, 2020).

Dementia, delirium, and depression are manifestations of serious pathology and require urgent assessment and intervention (Fick et al., 2020). However, changes in the cognitive function of older adults are often seen as "normal" and are thus not investigated. Any change in mental status in an older adult requires appropriate assessment. Knowledge about cognitive function in aging and appropriate assessment and evaluation are the keys to differentiating the three syndromes. Table 21.1 presents the clinical features of and differences in cognitive and behavioural characteristics between delirium, dementia, and depression.

Cognitive Assessment

An older adult with a change in cognitive function needs a thorough assessment to identify the presence

TABLE 21.1			
Differentiating Delirium, Depression, and Dementia			
Characteristic	**Delirium**	**Depression**	**Dementia**
Onset	Sudden, abrupt	Recent, may relate to life change	Insidious, slow (over years), often unrecognized until deficits are obvious
Course over 24 hours	Fluctuating, often worse at night	Fairly stable, may be worse in the morning	Fairly stable, may change with stress
Consciousness	Disturbed	Clear	Clear
Alertness	Increased, decreased, or variable	Normal	Generally normal
Psychomotor activity	Increased, decreased, or mixed	Variable, agitated, or slowed down	Normal, may have apraxia or agnosia
Duration	Hours to weeks	Variable, at least 2 weeks and may be chronic	Years
Attention	Disordered, fluctuates	Little impairment	Generally normal but may have trouble focusing
Orientation	Usually impaired, fluctuates	Usually normal; may answer "I don't know" to questions, or may not answer	Often impaired
Thinking	Disorganized, rambling, illogical, or incoherent	May be slow; hopelessness, helplessness	Difficulty finding words, **perseveration**, impoverished thoughts, difficulty with abstraction, delusions in severe cases
Perception	Disturbed; illusions, hallucinations, misperceptions	Misperception usually absent	Intact, hallucinations in severe cases
Affect	Variable but may look disturbed, frightened	Flat	Slowed response, may be labile

Sources: Adapted from Fick, D. M., Heeren, P., & Milisen, K. (2020). Assessing cognitive function. In M. Boltz, E. Capezuti, T. Fulmer, et al. (Eds.). *Evidence-based geriatric nursing protocols for best practice* (6th ed., pp. 119–132). Springer; American Psychiatric Association. (2013). *Diagnostic and statistical manual of mental disorders: DSM-5* (5th ed.). Author.

of specific pathological conditions, as well as to rule out potentially reversible causes of cognitive impairment. Pathological conditions causing impairment of cognition include delirium, dementia, depression, Parkinson's disease, and stroke. During the assessment, the physical environment should be comfortable and free from distractions that could affect the older adult's performance.

Cognitive assessment is a component of the mental status examination conducted by nurses and other health care providers (see Chapter 23). Mental status is assessed through observation and careful interviewing, and the examination may also include standardized assessments.

Screening instruments provide some information about cognitive status and may indicate a need for a more comprehensive cognitive assessment.

The components of a cognitive assessment are level of consciousness; orientation; immediate, short-term, recent, and long-term memory; attention and concentration; abstract reasoning; and problem solving. In addition, **aphasia**, **apraxia**, and **agnosia** are assessed when there is an indication of cognitive disturbance.

The literature reveals that both nurses and physicians in all settings routinely fail to appropriately assess cognitive functioning. Pathological conditions are often undiagnosed, reversible causes are not identified, and opportunities for early intervention are missed. As a result, the affected person experiences greater impairment and functional decline (Fick et al., 2020). There are several excellent resources to assist nurses in assessing cognition (Box 21.1). Many of these resources are available as streaming videos or as e-learning instructions.

Screening for Cognitive Impairment

Screening can determine whether cognitive impairment exists, but basic screening methods are insufficient to diagnose specific pathological conditions. If impairment is identified through screening, the person should be referred for a more comprehensive evaluation to confirm a diagnosis of dementia, delirium, depression, or some other health problem (Fick et al., 2020). Screening for depression should be conducted with instruments such as the Geriatric Depression Scale (see Chapter 13). A comprehensive evaluation includes a complete assessment, including a laboratory workup, to rule out any medical causes of cognitive impairment. Formal cognitive testing, neuro-psychological examination, interview (of family and patient), observation, and functional assessment are additional components of a comprehensive assessment. **Computed tomography (CT)**, **magnetic resonance imaging (MRI)**, and an **electroencephalogram (EEG)** may be indicated in the diagnostic process. Several evidence-informed guidelines are available for the assessment of changes in cognition, including the Registered Nurses' Association of Ontario best practice guideline entitled *Delirium, Dementia, and Depression in Older Adults: Assessment and Care* (https://rnao.ca/bpg/guidelines).

The Short Portable Mental Status Questionnaire, the Mini-Cog, the Confusion Assessment Method, the Neecham–Champagne Confusion Scale (NEECHAM), and the Montreal Cognitive Assessment are examples of screening instruments (see Chapter 13). These instruments may also be used to monitor and evaluate cognitive status. However, the use of cognitive screening instruments across cultures may require adjustment (O'Driscoll & Shaikh, 2017; MacDonald et al., 2018). Box 21.1 presents suggestions for the assessment and screening of cognitive impairment.

Considerations in Cognitive Assessment

Cognitive functioning assessments are often stressful experiences for older adults. Many older adults worry about developing memory problems or dementia. Cognitive tests and poor performance on memory tests often cause great anxiety. Assessment of cognitive functioning can be perceived by the person as "intrusive, intimidating, fatiguing, and offensive; characteristics that can seriously and negatively affect performance" (Fick et al., 2020, p. 124). Too often, assessments are done when a person is not wearing their hearing aids or eyeglasses, or the person is rushed through a series of questions in a noisy, distracting environment, without any preparation or explanation.

It is important to attend to these concerns by establishing rapport and developing a therapeutic relationship, ensuring comfort (pain relief), accommodating physical impairments such as hearing and vision loss, creating an environment free of distractions, and putting

---

BOX 21.1
RESOURCES FOR ASSESSMENT OF COGNITION

TRY THIS: SERIES

- Issue 3: Mental status assessment of older persons: The Mini-Cog (article and video)
- Issue 13: Confusion Assessment Method (article and video)
- Issue 25: The Confusion Assessment Method for the intensive care unit
- Issue D3: Brief evaluation of executive dysfunction—An essential refinement in the assessment of cognitive impairment
- Issue D8: Assessing and managing delirium in persons with dementia https://hign.org/consultgeri-resources/try-this-series

OTHER RESOURCES

Canadian Coalition for Seniors' Mental Health:
National Guidelines: The Assessment and Treatment of Delirium;
Clinician's Pocket Card: Delirium: Assessment & Treatment for Older Adults (interactive, case-based tutorial) https://www.ccsmh.ca

BC Guidelines:
Cognitive Impairment—Recognition, Diagnosis and Management in Primary Care http://www2.gov.bc.ca/gov/content/health/practitioner-professional-resources/bc-guidelines/cognitive-impairment

Registered Nurses' Association of Ontario:
Best Practice Guideline: Delirium, Dementia, and Depression in Older Adults: Assessment and Care (guide and e-learning course) (http://www.rnao.ca)

the person in the best environment to ensure that performance is truly reflective of ability. The challenge is to stress the importance of the assessment without creating undue anxiety for the person. Fick et al. (2020, p. 124) warn that "it is essential to avoid counterproductive statements that describe the assessment as consisting of 'simple,' 'silly,' or 'stupid' questions. These tend to diminish motivation to perform and heighten anxiety when errors are committed."

Timing is also important; cognitive assessments should not be conducted immediately upon the person's awakening from sleep or immediately before or after meals or medical diagnostic and therapeutic procedures (Fick et al., 2020). What seems to be a routine procedure to health care providers can be very intimidating for an older adult, especially one who is ill or frail.

DELIRIUM

Etiology

Delirium is most often the result of complex interactions among predisposing factors (e.g., vulnerability due to predisposing conditions, such as cognitive impairment, severe illness, and sensory impairment) and precipitating factors or insults (e.g., medications, procedures, restraints, iatrogenic events) (Inouye, 2018). Although a single factor, such as an infection, can trigger an episode of delirium, several coexisting factors are also likely to be present. A highly vulnerable older adult requires fewer precipitating factors to develop delirium (Inouye, 2018).

The exact pathophysiological mechanisms involved in the development and progression of delirium remain uncertain, and further research is needed to understand its neuro-pathogenesis. Several neurophysiological processes have been identified, including inflammatory processes, oxidative stress, and disturbances in neurotransmitters such as glutamate, acetylcholine, and GABA (Oldham et al., 2018). The precipitants of delirium are in most cases reversible; therefore, accurate assessment and diagnosis are critical.

Incidence and Prevalence

Delirium is a prevalent, serious, and often preventable disorder that occurs in older adults across the continuum of care. Delirium may affect 20% of older adults in the emergency department (Émond et al., 2018), more than half of hospitalized older adults, and as many as 90% of older adults in intensive care units (Lau et al., 2019). Delirium can significantly affect functional outcomes and mortality in long-term care (LTC) homes, where over 40% of residents experience delirium at some point during their stay (Cheung et al., 2018).

Patients with dementia are at higher risk for delirium, and it is less likely to be recognized when delirium is superimposed on dementia (Schnitker et al., 2020). Delirium superimposed on dementia is associated with high mortality and worse functional outcomes among hospitalized older adults (Morandi et al., 2017). Changes in the mental status of older adults with dementia are often attributed to underlying dementia, or "sundowning," and are thus not investigated. This is particularly significant because between 20% and 40% of all patients in acute care settings have dementia (McGilton & Lemay, 2020).

Recognition of Delirium

Delirium is a medical emergency and one of the most significant geriatric syndromes. However, it is often not recognized by nurses and other health care providers. Studies indicate that delirium is unrecognized in 34% to 90% of patients and residents in acute and LTC settings (Boucher et al., 2019). Failure to recognize delirium, identify the underlying causes, and implement timely interventions contributes to higher mortality and worse outcomes.

Factors that contribute to the lack of recognition of delirium by nurses include inadequate knowledge about delirium and assessment approaches, lack of understanding of the relationship between dementia and delirium, and ageist attitudes (Brooke, 2018; Dahlke et al., 2019; Mukaetova-Ladinska et al., 2019; Kagan, 2020). Workplace factors such as time constraints and support for assessing and documenting mental status also contribute to lack of recognition of dementia (Voyer et al., 2017).

Risk Factors for Delirium

Identification of risk factors, prompt and appropriate assessment, and continued surveillance are the cornerstones of delirium prevention. The model developed by Inouye (2018) explains the interaction between baseline vulnerability factors for delirium (i.e., factors present at the time of admission) and precipitating factors for delirium (i.e., things that happen to patients while hospitalized). This model has been used to refine screening instruments and to design hospital environments and systems that minimize delirium risk through a program called the Hospital Elder Life Program (HELP) (Hshieh et al., 2018). Predisposing risk factors and precipitating risk factors are listed in Box 21.2. Unrelieved or inadequately treated pain significantly increases the risk of delirium. Medications account for

22% to 39% of all deliriums, and all medications, particularly those with anticholinergic effects and any new medications, should be considered suspect. Invasive equipment such as nasogastric tubes, intravenous (IV) lines, catheters, and restraints also contribute to delirium by interfering with the normal feedback mechanisms of the body. Persons with multiple predisposing factors are more vulnerable to delirium—they may develop delirium on exposure to one precipitating event, such as a single dose of a sedative. Those with no predisposing factors and low vulnerability to delirium may not develop delirium, even in the face of several precipitating factors.

Most research on residents of LTC homes has focused on clinical factors that predict delirium (Lee, 2020). Predisposing factors may be more important, especially for residents with dementia. Environmental and clinical factors that are associated with worsening delirium symptoms among LTC residents are presented in Box 21.3.

BOX 21.2
PREDISPOSING AND PRECIPITATING RISK FACTORS FOR DELIRIUM

PREDISPOSING RISK FACTORS

- Demographic characteristics: age 65 years or older, male sex
- Cognitive status: dementia, cognitive impairment, history of delirium, depression
- Functional status: dependence, immobility, low level of activity, history of falls
- Sensory impairment: visual, hearing
- Decreased oral intake: dehydration, malnutrition
- Medications: multiple psychoactive medications, many medications, alcohol abuse
- Coexisting medical conditions: severe illness, multiple coexisting conditions, chronic renal or hepatic disease, history of stroke, neurological diseases, metabolic derangements, fracture or trauma, terminal illness, human immunodeficiency virus (HIV) infection

PRECIPITATING RISK FACTORS

- Medications: sedative–hypnotic, narcotic, anticholinergic medications; multiple medications; alcohol or medication withdrawal
- Primary neurological diseases: stroke, intracranial bleeding, meningitis or encephalitis
- Intercurrent illnesses: infections, iatrogenic complications, severe acute illness, hypoxia, shock, fever or hypothermia, anemia, dehydration, poor nutritional status, low serum albumin level, metabolic derangements (e.g., electrolyte or acid–base)
- Surgery: orthopedic, cardiac, prolonged cardiopulmonary bypass, noncardiac
- Environmental: admission to critical care unit, physical restraints, bladder catheter, multiple procedures
- Pain
- Emotional stress
- Prolonged sleep deprivation

Source: Adapted from Inouye, S. (2006). Delirium in older persons. *New England Journal of Medicine, 354*(11), 1157–1165. (Tables 2 and 3)

BOX 21.3
RISK FACTORS FOR DELIRIUM SEVERITY IN LONG-TERM CARE HOMES

Absence of the following:
- Adequate nutrition
- Aids to orientation
- Family member
- Glass of water
- Reading eyeglasses

Presence of the following:
- Antipsychotic prescription
- Bed rails and other restraints
- Dementia
- Depression
- Hearing impairment
- Pain

Sources: Adapted from Cheung, E. N. M., Benjamin, S., Heckman, G., et al. (2018). Clinical characteristics associated with the onset of delirium among long-term nursing home residents. *BMC Geriatrics, 8*, 39 doi:10.1186/s12877-018-0733-3; Lee, J. (2020). Risk factors for nursing home delirium: A systematic review. *Journal of Korean Gerontological Nursing, 22*(1), 75–83. doi:10.17079/jkgn.2020.22.1.75; McCusker, J., Cole, M. G., Voyer, P., et al. (2013). Environmental factors predict the severity of delirium symptoms in long-term care residents with and without delirium. *Journal of the American Geriatrics Society, 61*, 502–511. doi:10.1111/jgs.12164.

Clinical Subtypes of Delirium

Delirium is categorized into three clinical subtypes according to the level of the person's alertness and psychomotor activity—hyperactive, hypoactive, and mixed. *Hyperactive delirium* is characterized by agitation, vigilance, **hallucinations**, restlessness, and hyperactivity. *Hypoactive delirium* is characterized by lethargy and decreased motor activity. *Mixed delirium* comprises alternating features of hyperactive and hypoactive delirium. In settings other than critical care units (CCUs), approximately 30% of delirium is hyperactive, 24% is hypoactive, and 46% is mixed. Because of the increased severity of illness and the use of psychoactive medications, hypoactive delirium may be more prevalent in the CCU. Although the negative consequences of hyperactive delirium are serious, the hypoactive subtype is missed more often and is associated with a worse prognosis because of the development of complications such as aspiration, pulmonary embolism, pressure ulcers, and pneumonia. Hypoactive delirium is associated with increased hospital stays, a longer duration of delirium, and higher mortality.

Consequences of Delirium

Delirium has serious consequences, and nurses play a key role in preventing these (Blevins, 2020). Delirium results in significant distress for the person experiencing it, the person's family and significant others, and health care providers. Delirium during hospitalization is associated with high morbidity and mortality, functional decline, increased postoperative complications, increased length of hospital stay and hospital readmissions, increased services after discharge, long-term cognitive decline, and high rates of institutionalization (Hshieh et al., 2018; Blevins, 2020).

Although delirium is considered a reversible cause of altered mental status, a significant number of older adults with delirium never return to their baseline cognitive status, especially in the presence of pre-existing dementia (Goldberg et al., 2020).

IMPLICATIONS FOR GERONTOLOGICAL NURSING AND HEALTHY AGING

Assessment

To detect changes in cognition, it is important to determine the usual mental status. If the older adult cannot convey this information to the nurse, family members or other caregivers who are with the person can be asked to provide this information. In hospital, if the patient is alone, the responsible party or the institution transferring the patient can provide this information by phone. Nurses cannot assume that the person's current mental status represents their usual state and cannot attribute altered mental status to age or assume that dementia is present. All older adults, regardless of their current cognitive function, should have a formal assessment to identify possible delirium when admitted to hospital (see Box 21.1). Several instruments can be used to assess the presence and severity of delirium.

The Confusion Assessment Method (Inouye et al., 1990) is used to assess the presence and severity of delirium. The **R**ecognizing **A**cute **D**elirium **A**s part of your **R**outine (RADAR) is a brief screen to identify potential delirium as part of routine nursing assessment and care (Voyer et al., 2016; Voyer et al., 2017). If it is positive, then the Confusion Assessment Method should be completed. Persons with dementia are at higher risk for delirium superimposed on dementia and of having their delirium overlooked or misidentified by nurses. The "4 As" Test (4AT) is a validated screening instrument for patients who have dementia (Gagné et al., 2018). Training is necessary for the valid use of the Confusion Assessment Method. A video demonstrating its use is available at https://hign.org/.

The assessment of these patients must involve a person or persons who know the patient's baseline cognitive functioning, such as a family or staff member who has worked with the person at home or at an LTC home. In an LTC home, health care aides are often the first to identify subtle changes in a resident's behaviour that may indicate delirium; nurses in this setting must investigate any health care aide reports of changes in a person's behaviour. For all older patients who are at risk for delirium, assessment with the Confusion Assessment Method should be integrated into routine assessments, upon admission to hospital or an LTC home, in the first assessment by the home care nurse, and during every shift in hospital or routinely in LTC and community settings (Blevins, 2020). When a patient is identified as having delirium, a reassessment should be conducted as frequently as every 2 hours.

Documenting specific objective indicators of alterations in mental status rather than using the global nonspecific term "confusion" will lead to more appropriate prevention, detection, and management of delirium and its negative consequences. Findings from assessments using a validated instrument should be combined with observation, chart review, and physiological findings. Delirium often has a fluctuating course and can be difficult to recognize, so assessment must be ongoing and include multiple data sources.

Interventions

Effective care for delirium must include vigilant prevention efforts, as well as treatment to target the root cause of delirium that cannot be prevented. This care includes risk screening, ongoing assessment, and the implementation of prevention and treatment strategies (Fig. 21.1).

Nonpharmacological

Intervention for delirium begins with prevention. Prevention requires the identification of the person's risk factors for delirium and a formal assessment of the person's mental status. Nurses play a pivotal role in the identification of delirium, and it is imperative that they accurately report patients' mental status to the medical

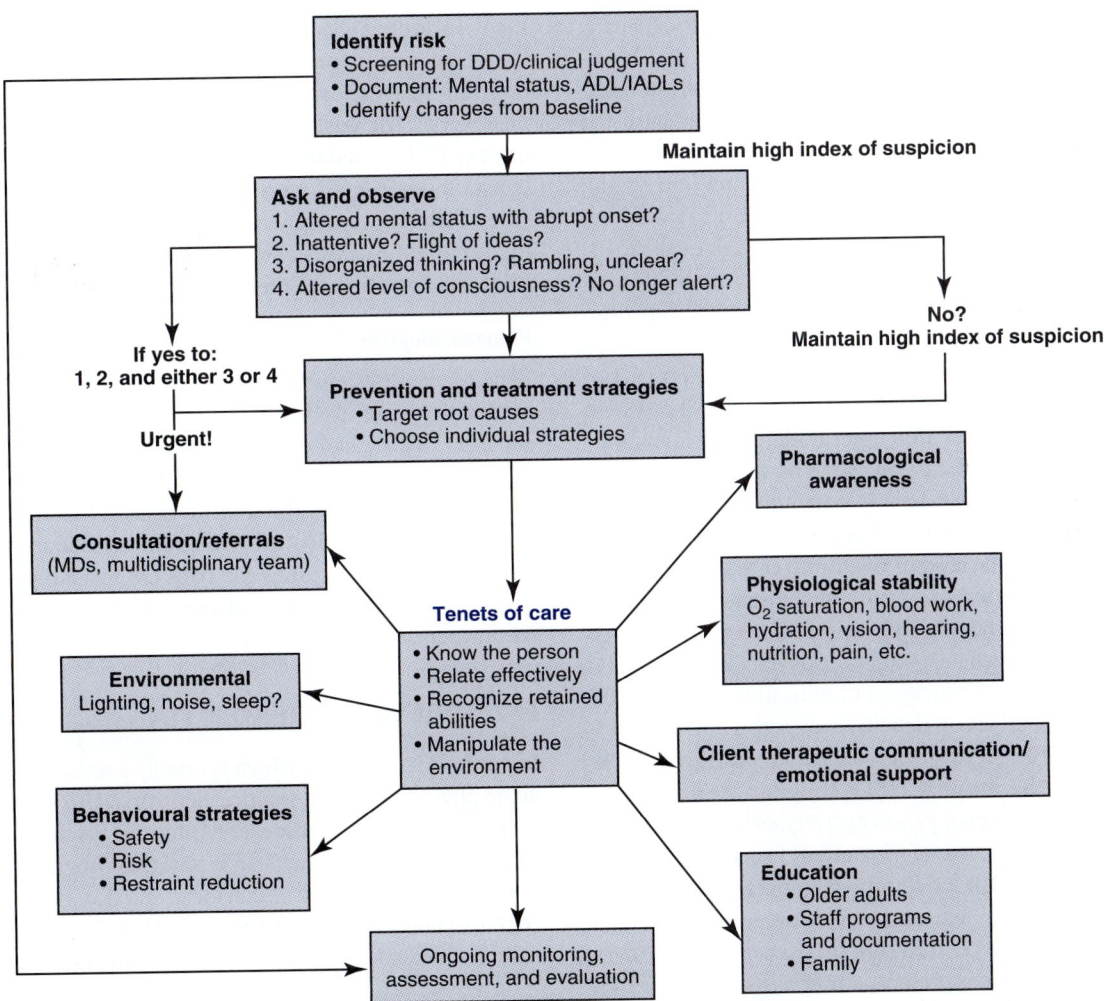

Fig. 21.1 ■ Flow-of-care diagram of caregiving strategies for delirium. *Source:* Registered Nurses' Association of Ontario. (2004). *Caregiving strategies for older persons with delirium, dementia, and depression* (p. 33, Fig. 2). Author.

team so that potential causative factors can be identified and treated (Blevins, 2020). Prevention should be targeted to the person's individual risk factors.

Interprofessional, multicomponent approaches to delirium prevention have the best evidence of effectiveness. One such approach, the well-researched Hospital Elder Life Program (AGS CoCare: HELP™; https://www.hospitalelderlifeprogram.org/), focuses on managing the following six risk factors for delirium: cognitive impairment, sleep deprivation, immobility, visual impairments, hearing impairments, and dehydration. Standardized intervention protocols target each risk factor (Inouye et al., 1999). The elements of the program are daily visitors, therapeutic activities, early mobilization, nonpharmacological sleep protocol, hearing and vision protocol, oral volume repletion and mealtime assistance, interdisciplinary care, transition assistance, and staff education. Patient outcomes with the use of this model include a 40% reduction in the incidence of delirium, a decrease in the number of days and episodes of delirium, and prevention of functional decline. The program is cost effective (Hshieh et al., 2018) and has been adapted and tested in LTC, rehabilitation, and home care settings (Huson et al., 2016; Simpson et al., 2019; Boockvar et al., 2020).

Most HELP interventions can be considered part of good nursing care. The interventions are at the system level (e.g., keeping the unit quiet at night by using vibrating beepers instead of paging systems, having volunteers be with restless patients, implementing fall risk reduction interventions such as low beds and bed and chair alarms) and at the level of the health care provider (e.g., offering herbal tea or warm milk instead of sleeping medications, removing catheters and other devices that hamper movement as soon as possible, assessing and managing pain, encouraging mobilization, and correcting hearing and vision deficits).

The family HELP program, an adaptation and extension of the original HELP program, trains family caregivers in selected protocols (e.g., orientation, therapeutic activities, use of vision and hearing aids). The active engagement of family members in preventive interventions for delirium is feasible and supports a culture of family-centred care (McKenzie & Joy, 2020).

When delirium is present, strategies used to prevent it should be maintained or implemented. In addition, identifying and treating the root cause of the delirium is vital. Because delirium is so complex, with multifactorial causes, effective treatment is often multifactorial and dependent on interprofessional collaboration. Caring for patients with delirium can be a challenging experience. They can be difficult to communicate with and can exhibit disturbing behaviours, such as pulling out IV lines or attempting to get out of bed. They may disrupt medical treatment and compromise safety. It is important for nurses to realize that the patient's behaviour is an attempt to communicate and express needs such as pain or anxiety. The patient with delirium feels frightened and out of control. The calmer and more reassuring the nurse is, the safer the patient will feel. Box 21.4 presents suggested interventions for delirium prevention and treatment, including effective communication strategies.

A commonly used intervention for older adults with delirium in acute care is the use of "sitters" or "constant observers." The costs associated with this practice can be very high, and data indicate that the use of sitters or constant observers does not consistently improve safety when delirium is present, nor does this practice assist in identifying the causes of delirium or identifying appropriate interventions (Colella et al., 2017).

Pharmacological

Benzodiazepines and (at times) other psychotropic medications are used in the treatment of delirium associated with alcohol withdrawal (Borgundvaag & Klaiman, 2020). Clinical trials of the use of sedatives and antipsychotics in the treatment of delirium due to causes other than alcohol withdrawal show either no effect or worse outcomes for patients receiving them. Thus, pharmacological treatment of delirium is not recommended (Oh et al., 2017).

OVERVIEW OF DEMENTIA

In contrast to delirium, which is usually a reflection of an acute physiological disturbance, dementia, also known as major neurocognitive disorder (American Psychiatric Association, 2013), is an irreversible state that progresses over years. It causes memory impairment and decline in other cognitive abilities that is severe enough to interfere with daily life. Other key features of dementia are the following:

- Aphasia—loss of the ability to express and understand spoken and written language

BOX 21.4
MULTICOMPONENT CARE STRATEGIES FOR DELIRIUM

CONSULTATION AND REFERRAL

- Initiate prompt consultation to specialized services when symptoms develop or worsen for assessment and possible treatment of a causative condition.

PHYSIOLOGICAL STABILITY/REVERSIBLE CAUSES

- Maintain ongoing assessment, interpretation, management, documentation, and communication of physiological status to interprofessional team.
- Ensure adequate hydration, nutrition, mobilization, and sleep.
- Avoid restraints.
- Provide hearing aids and eyeglasses.
- Assess and manage pain.
- Remove unnecessary catheters and IV lines (see Chapter 9).

PHARMACOLOGICAL

- Maintain—in collaboration with interprofessional team—an awareness of medications that contribute to delirium, and review patients' medication profiles for potential deliriogenic medications (see Beers Criteria for Potentially Inappropriate Medication Use in Older Adults at https://hign.org/).
- Limit use of psychoactive medication to the treatment of specific symptoms; use as a last resort.
- Discontinue nonessential medications when delirium is present.

ENVIRONMENTAL

- Identify, reduce, or eliminate environmental factors that may contribute to delirium.

- Ensure adequate sensory stimulation (provide light during the day, and reduce light at night).
- Introduce one task at a time; provide structure and predictable routine.
- Implement noise-reduction strategies.
- Foster a familiar environment (familiar objects are in sight of the patient; encourage family or friends to stay with the patient; consistent caregivers; minimal relocation).

EDUCATION

- Provide delirium education to the patient and family (see relevant Registered Nurses' Association of Ontario [RNAO] Health Education Fact Sheet at http://www.rnao.org/bestpractices).
- Provide postdelirium support and education.

COMMUNICATION AND EMOTIONAL SUPPORT

- Identify yourself.
- Establish and maintain a therapeutic relationship.
- Provide orientation and support.
- Communicate clearly and speak slowly.
- Tell the patient what you *want* them to do, not what you *do not want* them to do.
- Provide explanations.
- Provide one-step directions; use gestures and demonstrations.
- Allow time for responses.

BEHAVIOURAL INTERVENTIONS

- Avoid the use of restraints.
- Monitor safety regularly.

Sources: Adapted from Registered Nurses' Association of Ontario. (2016). *Delirium, dementia, and depression in older adults: Assessment and care* (2nd ed.). https://rnao.ca/bpg/guidelines/assessment-and-care-older-adults-delirium-dementia-and-depression. Author; Blevins, C. (2020). Delirium: Prevention, early recognition, and treatment. In M. Boltz, E. Capezuti, T. Fulmer, et al. (Eds.), *Evidence-based geriatric nursing protocols for best practice* (6th ed., pp. 317–330). Springer.

- Apraxia—inability to carry out purposeful movements, although motor and sensory abilities are intact
- Agnosia—inability to recognize common objects or faces of familiar people despite intact sensory abilities, and
- Disturbances in executive functioning—difficulty in planning, organizing, sequencing, and abstracting.

Types of Dementia

Degenerative dementias include Alzheimer's disease (AD), Parkinson's disease dementia, dementia with Lewy bodies, and frontotemporal dementias (FTD). AD accounts for 50% to 70% of all dementia cases. Vascular cognitive impairment encompasses several syndromes—vascular dementia; primary neurodegenerative disease mixed with vascular dementia; and cognitive impairment of vascular origin that does not meet the dementia criteria.

Less commonly occurring dementias are Creutzfeldt–Jakob disease (subacute spongiform encephalopathy), human immunodeficiency virus (HIV)–related dementia, and Korsakoff syndrome.

Many dementias in old age can be described as mixed dementia produced by a number of primary and secondary causes. For example, dementia can be caused by a combination of AD, vascular brain changes, and prior alcoholism (two primary causes and one secondary cause). Many dementias manifest symptoms of cognitive impairment. However, associated features and the age of onset vary among the different types of dementia syndromes (Table 21.2).

Incidence and Prevalence

Approximately 1% of the Canadian population and 47.6 million people worldwide have dementia (Public Health Agency of Canada, 2019b).

The prevalence of dementia increases with age, doubling approximately every 5 years for persons between the ages of 60 and 95 years. About 1% of Canadians between ages 65 and 69 have dementia, while the prevalence is 25% for those older than 85 years (Public Health Agency of Canada, 2019b). If current trends continue, then by the year 2030 the increasing prevalence of AD will mean that 912,000 Canadians will be affected (Alzheimer Society of Canada, 2020). The annual direct health care cost of dementia is over $8.3 billion (Public Health Agency of Canada, 2019b), not including the $1.4 billion in out-of-pocket expenses paid for by people

TABLE 21.2
Types of Dementia and Typical Characteristics

Type of Dementia	Characteristics
Alzheimer's disease (AD)	Most common type of dementia, accounting for 60%–80% of cases. Hallmark abnormalities are deposits of the protein fragment beta-amyloid (plaques) and twisted strands of the protein tau (tangles). Early symptoms often include difficulty remembering names and recent events; difficulty expressing oneself with words; spatial cognition problems; impaired reasoning and judgement; apathy; and depression. Language disturbances may also be a presenting symptom. Later symptoms include impaired judgement, disorientation, behaviour changes, and difficulty speaking, swallowing, and walking.
Vascular dementia (also known as multi-infarct or poststroke dementia or vascular cognitive impairment)	Second most common type of dementia. Impairment is caused by decreased blood flow to parts of the brain due to cerebrovascular events (stroke or transient ischemic episodes). Symptoms often overlap with those of AD, although memory may not be as seriously affected.
Mixed dementia	Characterized by the hallmark abnormalities of AD and another type of dementia (most commonly vascular dementia, but also other types, such as dementia with Lewy bodies).
Parkinson's disease dementia	Onset of dementia at least 1 year after onset of Parkinson's disease symptoms.
Dementia with Lewy bodies	Hallmark abnormality is Lewy bodies (abnormal deposits of the protein alpha-synuclein) that forms inside the nerve cells of the brain. Pattern of decline is similar to that of AD, including problems with memory and judgement as well as behaviour changes. Symptoms include fluctuating alertness, attention, and cognition; visual hallucinations; and parkinsonism (muscle rigidity and tremors). Severe sensitivity to neuroleptic drugs, and thus these medications should be avoided.
Dementia due to Creutzfeldt–Jakob disease and variant Creutzfeldt–Jakob disease (vCJD) (transmissible bovine spongiform encephalopathy [mad cow disease])	A rapidly fatal and rare form of dementia, characterized by tiny holes that give the brain a "spongy" appearance under microscope. May be hereditary, occur sporadically, or be transmitted from infected individuals. Failing memory, behavioural changes, lack of coordination, visual disturbances. vCJD occurs in younger patients; may be caused by contaminated cattle feed.
Frontotemporal dementia	Involves brain atrophy, especially in the frontal and temporal lobes. Symptoms of behavioural variant include disinhibition, repetitive behaviour, apathy, loss of empathy hyperorality, and impaired executive functioning and social cognition. The semantic variant involves decline in language ability.

Source: Adapted from American Psychiatric Association. (2013). *Diagnostic and statistical manual of mental disorders: DSM-5* (5th ed.). Author.

with dementia and their caregivers (Canadian Institute for Health Information [CIHI], 2018).

Women are more likely than men to have dementia. The prevalence of dementia is also higher among racial minorities. While most of the evidence for this comes from the United States (Mehta & Yeo, 2017), Canadian research has found that among older Canadians, members of a visible minority were more likely to report cognitive impairment (Haq & Penning, 2019).

Among Indigenous peoples in Canada, the prevalence of dementia is higher than in the general population, and there is also a younger age of onset. Furthermore, Indigenous men are more likely than Indigenous women to have dementia. These differences may be explained by the increased vulnerability associated with social determinants of health (Haq & Penning, 2019; Jacklin & Walker, 2020; MacDonald et al., 2018) (see Chapter 1).

Accurate diagnosis is important since treatment and prognosis vary. However, dementia is difficult to diagnose. The complexity of dementia, diagnostic uncertainty (there are no diagnostic tests, and the symptoms overlap those of other disorders), and a tendency to rely on specialists rather than family physicians for diagnosis mean that arriving at a diagnosis can take a long time (Drummond et al., 2016). A considerable length of time typically elapses between the moment a person first notices their symptoms to the moment they talk to a physician about their symptoms. More timely diagnoses and treatment requires educating the public and health care providers.

Culture and Ethnicity

A growing body of research is investigating the influence of culture and ethnicity on the recognition and interpretation of cognitive changes, help-seeking behaviours, and the assessment, diagnosis, and treatment of dementias. A cross-cultural comparison of the ways that dementia is understood and described by British, American, and Chinese people found many similarities—regardless of nationality, people associated dementia with aging, memory loss, disease, challenge, loss, and sadness (Calia et al., 2019). Differences in dementia representation were also identified. For example, Chinese participants described dementia in terms of observable behaviours, British participants described dementia from the perspective of the person with dementia, and in the United States, participants uniquely associated dementia with death, disability, and nursing homes.

Some minority ethnic groups are underrepresented with respect to seeking and receiving services for dementia. This underrepresentation may be related to specific cultural beliefs about mental illness and the causes of dementia. However, other factors also affect these persons' access to services, including the language of provision, stigmatization, lack of knowledge about dementia and available resources, hesitancy to use services viewed as culturally incongruent, and barriers to physically accessing services (Hossain & Khan, 2020; Koehn, 2020; Webkamigad et al., 2020a). A need for culturally and linguistically appropriate services and sources of information about dementia in Canada is identified in the national dementia strategy (Public Health Agency of Canada, 2019a). For instance, Webkamigad and colleagues (2020b) developed Indigenous-specific fact sheets about dementia. They engaged in extensive collaboration to create culturally appropriate resources.

Alzheimer's Disease

First described in 1906 by Dr. Alois Alzheimer, AD is a cerebral degenerative disorder of unknown origin. The disease destroys the proteins of nerve cells in the cerebral cortex by diffuse infiltration with nonfunctional tissue called neurofibrillary tangles and plaques. The tangles and plaques represent the death of nerve cells throughout the brain, which shrinks to about one-third of its normal weight. The tangles consist of a protein called tau protein, which "clogs" the insides of brain cells and their connections. Deposits of beta-amyloid accumulate abnormally in the brains of people with AD. The disease is progressive and is accompanied by increasing memory loss, inability to concentrate, personality deterioration, and impaired judgement.

There are two types of AD: early-onset dementia and late-onset dementia. Early-onset dementia is rare, affecting only 5% of all people who have AD, and develops between the ages of 30 and 60 years. It has a stronger genetic component than late-onset dementia does (Box 21.5).

The course of AD ranges from 1 to 20 years. The typical life expectancy is 8 to 9 years after the onset of symptoms; usually, death occurs as a result of pulmonary infections, urinary tract infections, pressure ulcers, or iatrogenic disorders. The most important risk factor is age.

The focus of AD research is on the interaction between risk-factor genes and lifestyle or environmental factors.

BOX 21.5
GENETICS IN ALZHEIMER'S DISEASE

GENETIC BASIS

Early Onset (Familial) (<60 Years Old at Onset)

- Autosomal dominant disorder
- Various mutations in the following genes:
  - Amyloid precursor protein (*APP*) gene on chromosome 21
  - Presenilin-1 (*PSEN1*) gene on chromosome 14
  - Presenilin-2 (*PSEN2*) gene on chromosome 1

Late Onset (Sporadic) (>60 Years Old at Onset)

- Genetically more complex than early-onset form
- Apolipoprotein E-4 (*ApoE-4*) allele on chromosome 19 increases likelihood of developing Alzheimer's disease (AD)
- Presence of *ApoE-2* allele associated with lower risk of AD

INCIDENCE

Early Onset

- Rare form of AD, accounting for <5% of cases
- 50% risk of disease for children of affected parents
- May occur in people as young as 30 years old

Late Onset

- *ApoE-4* present in ~40% of people with late-onset AD (present in 25%–30% of the normal population)
- Many *ApoE-4*-positive people do not develop AD, and many *ApoE-4*–negative people do

GENETIC TESTING

Early Onset

- Genetic screening available for mutations on chromosomes 1, 14, and 21

Late Onset

- Blood test can identify which *ApoE* allele a person has but cannot predict who will develop AD
- *ApoE* testing mainly used in research to identify people who may have increased risk of developing AD

CLINICAL IMPLICATIONS

- Genetic testing and counselling for family members of patients with early-onset AD may be appropriate.
- Positive test result for *ApoE-4* does not mean that person will develop AD

Source: Lewis, S. L., Dirksen, S. R., Heitkemper, M. M., et al. (2017). *Medical-surgical nursing: Assessment and management of clinical problems* (p. 1446). Mosby.

Increasing evidence strongly points to the potential risk roles of vascular disorders (e.g., obesity, dyslipidemia, hypertension, cigarette smoking, and cerebrovascular lesions) and the potential protective roles of psychosocial factors (e.g., higher education, regular exercise, healthy diet, intellectually challenging leisure activity, and active socially integrated lifestyles) (Peters et al., 2019). Head trauma is also a risk factor (Li et al., 2017). The intersecting risk factors associated with social and biological determinants of health are thought to explain the higher prevalence of AD and other dementias among ethnocultural minority groups (Haq & Penning, 2019; Henderson et al., 2019).

Diagnosis of Alzheimer's Disease

AD has three stages—the preclinical stage, mild cognitive impairment, and dementia due to AD pathology. The only way to confirm a diagnosis of AD is to perform a brain biopsy after the person dies. Clinically, the diagnosis of AD is based on the history of the affected person and their family and on testing to rule out other disorders that may mimic the disease. Neuroimaging using MRI is recommended in most cases where dementia is suspected (Ismail et al., 2020).

Preclinical Stage. In the preclinical stage, measurable changes in the brain, cerebrospinal fluid, or blood markers (or all three) are the earliest signs of the disease, but the person has not yet developed symptoms (such as memory loss). This preclinical, presymptomatic stage reflects the current view that AD begins causing changes in the brain up to 20 years before symptoms appear. Further research on biomarkers may make it possible to predict who is at risk for mild cognitive impairment and AD and who would benefit most from interventions (Aisen et al., 2017).

Mild Cognitive Impairment. A change in the level of cognition, in comparison to the prior level, signals mild cognitive impairment, also known as mild neurocognitive disorder (American Psychiatric Association, 2013). The cognitive changes at this stage are more than would be expected for the person's age and educational background. Cognitive performance problems are enough to be noticed and measured but do not compromise a person's functioning. People with mild cognitive impairment may or may not progress to AD.

Alzheimer's Disease. In addition to memory loss, the early symptoms of AD may include declines in other aspects of cognition such as word-finding problems, vision or spatial issues, and impaired reasoning or judgement. The symptoms of AD are often present several years before a diagnosis is made. Apathy and depression may be the first and earliest signs of AD, occurring up to 3 years before diagnosis. The history given by the affected person and the family is another important part of assessing and diagnosing probable AD. However, it often takes a long time for people who have dementia or their family members to recognize the early symptoms as something other than normal aging, and periods of up to 4 years from the emergence of the first symptom to the person's seeking of help are common (Perry-Young et al., 2018). Stigma associated with dementia also contributes to the delay in seeking help (Parker et al., 2020). A delayed diagnosis means that the affected person has been without critical support, resources, and treatment.

Pharmacological Treatment

Medication therapy with cholinesterase inhibitors (ChEIs) offers hope for enhanced function and reduction of the speed of decline associated with AD. ChEIs that are approved to treat AD include donepezil (Aricept), rivastigmine (Exelon), and galantamine (Reminyl). Memantine (Ebixa), an *N*-methyl-D-aspartate antagonist, is indicated for the treatment of moderate to severe AD. Unlike the ChEIs, which increase the amount of acetylcholine in the brain, memantine blocks the effect of abnormal glutamate activity that may lead to neuronal cell death and cognitive dysfunction. Memantine may be used alone or in combination with a ChEI. ChEIs are used for treatment of mild to severe AD, vascular dementia, mixed AD and vascular dementia, dementia associated with Parkinson's disease, and Lewy body dementia (LBD) (Ismail et al., 2020).

These medications may also be prescribed for mild cognitive impairment. Therapy should be long term, even if the person shows slight decline, if function is better than it would have been without treatment. These medications are usually well tolerated, but adverse effects include gastro-intestinal disturbances (nausea, vomiting, diarrhea, anorexia), sleep disturbances, and sedation (Singh & Sadiq, 2020). An initial low dose with slow titration is recommended to minimize side effects.

Rivastigmine (Exelon) is available in a patch that may be more convenient, has fewer adverse effects, and provides a consistent, daylong dose. There is no evidence that one ChEI is more effective than another. Because the medications work in similar ways, it is not expected that switching from one to another will produce significantly different results. However, a person may respond better to one medication than to another, and there is evidence that galantamine (Reminyl) may be better tolerated (Carney et al., 2019).

ChEIs are associated with increased risk of bradycardia and syncope (and associated falls) (Isik et al., 2018). The bradycardia may be transient and therefore difficult to detect in diagnostic investigations. The high mortality risk associated with falls for persons with dementia should be considered when making the decision regarding whether to initiate ChEI therapy. Cardiac evaluation and careful monitoring are necessary.

Medication therapy is directed toward the symptoms of AD and does not affect the neuronal decline that will eventually produce severe disability. However, medications are likely to produce a plateau of brain function and functional abilities and delay the progression of AD. Delaying both disease onset and progression would significantly reduce the burden of AD, particularly in the late stages of the disease. Therapy with ChEIs has positive effects on the behavioural manifestations of AD.

Vascular Dementia

Vascular dementia—also known as multi-infarct dementia, poststroke dementia, or vascular cognitive impairment—consists of a group of heterogeneous disorders arising from cerebrovascular insufficiency or ischemic or hemorrhagic brain damage. Vascular dementia often coexists with AD (a combination known as mixed dementia). Memory may not be impaired or may be more mildly impaired than in AD (Boltz, 2020). Apathy, mood changes, anxiety, and agitation are more common in vascular dementia than in AD (Boltz, 2020). Dementia after stroke is thought to occur in one-quarter to one-third of stroke cases. Hypertension, cardiac disease, diabetes, smoking, alcoholism, and dyslipidemia are risk factors for vascular dementia.

The management of diabetes, hypertension, and dyslipidemia is important for the primary prevention of vascular dementia. Secondary prevention includes treatments (e.g., the use of antihypertensives and anti-platelet medications) to prevent the recurrence of a vascular stroke.

Lewy Body Dementia

LBD, a widely underdiagnosed condition, is the second most common form of degenerative dementia. LBD is not a single disorder but rather a spectrum of disorders that includes dementia with Lewy bodies and Parkinson's disease dementia. Many individuals with LBD are erroneously diagnosed as having other types of dementia, most commonly AD, or Parkinson's disease if they present with movement problems. The presence of Lewy bodies, which are protein deposits in the nerve cells, characterizes LBD, and its presentation is different from that of AD; memory impairment is milder, and impaired executive function is common. Symptoms include cognitive fluctuations, unpredictable changes in concentration and attention, visual hallucinations, parkinsonian symptoms, rapid eye movement sleep behaviour disorder (see Chapter 10), and severe sensitivity to neuroleptics (McKeith, 2010).

No medications are approved specifically for the treatment of LBD, but ChEIs may offer symptomatic benefits. Early and accurate diagnosis of LBD is essential, as neuroleptics can cause a severe worsening of movement and a fatal condition known as neuroleptic malignant syndrome, which causes severe fever and muscle rigidity and can lead to kidney failure. Anti-cholinergics and some antiparkinsonian medications can worsen these symptoms.

Frontotemporal Dementia

FTD is a clinical syndrome associated with shrinkage of the frontal and temporal anterior lobes of the brain. FTD is linked to several chromosomal mutations, and 30% to 40% of people with FTD have family members with a neurodegenerative disease. Mean age at onset is between 52 and 56 years, but the disease has been found in younger and older adults as well. The disease progresses rapidly, and the prognosis is poor. As with LBD, FTD is often not accurately diagnosed. Its early symptoms are different from those of AD and are more often related to changes in personality and inappropriate or bizarre social behaviour. There are no approved medications that slow the progress of FTD. Medications for which there is some evidence of effectiveness for

depression and behaviours associated with FTD include trazodone (Desyrel) and selective serotonin reuptake inhibitors. However, evidence of their effectiveness is mixed (Young et al., 2018). Nonpharmacological interventions are aimed at managing behavioural symptoms, compensating for functional decline, and supporting family caregivers (Young et al., 2018).

IMPLICATIONS FOR GERONTOLOGICAL NURSING AND HEALTHY AGING

Person-Centred Care

Dementias such as AD have no cure, and although medications offer hope for improved function, the most important treatment for the disease is competent and compassionate person-centred care. Person-centred care looks beyond the disease and the tasks nurses must perform to the person within and the nurse's relationship with that person. The focus is not on what nurses need to "do to persons," but rather on the persons themselves and how to enhance their well-being and quality of life.

Gerontological nurses know that the person, not the disease, is the focus of care, and they practise in the belief that a person with dementia is still a whole person, someone who can think, feel, learn, grow, and be in a relationship. Person-centred care fosters abilities, supports limitations, ensures safety, enhances quality of life, prevents excess disability, and offers hope. The culture-change movement in dementia care is grounded in the concept of person-centred care and quality of life (de Witt & Fortune, 2019). There is good evidence that person-centred care approaches improve processes of care and outcomes for persons with dementia and their families (Weigel, 2017).

Quality of life, meaningful engagement, nutrition, activities of daily living (ADLs), maintenance of health and function, safety, communication, and caregiver needs and support are major care concerns for persons with dementia, their families, and the health care providers who care for them. The overriding goals in caring for older adults with dementia are to create a therapeutic **milieu** that nurtures the personhood of the individual and maintains quality of life, to maintain function and prevent excess disability, to structure the environment and relationships to maintain stability, and to compensate for the losses associated with the disease. Box 21.6 presents general nursing interventions in the care of persons with dementia.

BOX 21.6
GENERAL NURSING INTERVENTIONS IN CARE OF PERSONS WITH DEMENTIA

- Create meaningful moments and activities.
- Structure daily living to maximize remaining abilities.
- Monitor the general health and impact of dementia on the management of the person's acute and chronic medical conditions, paying careful attention to the person's experience of pain and mental health.
- Create opportunities for social engagement, freedom of choice, self-expression, spirituality, and creativity.
- Support advance care planning.
- Educate caregivers in the areas of problem solving, long-range planning, emotional support, and accessing resources and respite.

BOX 21.7
CONDITIONS PRECIPITATING RESPONSIVE BEHAVIOURS IN PERSONS WITH DEMENTIA

- Communication deficits
- Pain or discomfort
- Acute medical problems
- Sleep disturbances
- Perceptual deficits
- Depression
- Need for social contact
- Hunger, thirst, need to toilet
- Loss of control
- Misinterpretation of the situation or environment
- Crowded conditions
- Changes in environment or people
- Noise, disruption
- Being forced to do something
- Fear
- Loneliness
- Psychotic symptoms
- Fatigue
- Environmental overstimulation or understimulation
- Depersonalized, rushed care
- Restraints
- Psychoactive drugs

Three common care concerns for people with moderate- to late-stage dementia are behaviour, ADLs, and wandering. See Chapter 8 for a discussion of nutrition, Chapter 3 for a discussion of communication, and Chapter 23 for an in-depth discussion of family care for persons with dementia. The Hartford Institute for Geriatric Nursing's "Try This: Series" lists many excellent resources for the care of persons with dementia, as does the Resources section at the end of this chapter.

Behaviour Concerns and Nursing Models of Care for Persons With Dementia

Several nursing models of care are useful in guiding practice and assisting families and staff in providing care to people with dementia. The models share a common focus on understanding the meaning of the behaviour of the person with dementia. Using these models, nurses can avoid labelling the behaviour of persons with dementia as aggressive. The term "responsive behaviours" describes reactions that result from unmet needs or environmental stress (Dupuis et al., 2012). While responsive behaviours are disruptive and distressing to people with dementia and their caregivers, using terms such as "aggressive," "challenging behaviours," or the clinical term "behavioral and psychological symptoms (BPSD)" draws attention away from the perspective of the person (Cunningham et al., 2019).

Four models—the Progressively Lowered Stress Threshold (PLST) model, the Need-Driven Dementia-Compromised Behaviour Model, the recognition of retained abilities model, and the relating well model—describe the behaviour of the person with dementia as an interaction between the person's abilities and impairments and the physical and social environment. To understand these behaviours and provide care to a person with dementia, nurses and other care providers need to understand the person's experiences, abilities, and personality and how they align with the physical and social environment.

Progressively Lowered Stress Threshold Model

The PLST model was one of the first models used to plan and evaluate care for people with dementia (Hall, 1987, 1994). The person with dementia is seen to experience a progressive lowering of the stress threshold. Behavioural symptoms such as agitation are the result of a progressive loss of the person's ability to cope with demands and stimuli in the environment that exceed the person's stress threshold. Box 21.7 lists common stressors and conditions that may trigger these behavioural symptoms.

With the PLST model, the social and physical environment and nursing care are structured to reduce stressors and provide the person with a safe and predictable environment. Behaviours are monitored as an indicator of the patient's stress tolerance. Box 21.8 presents the principles of care derived from the PLST model in LTC settings. Reported outcomes include increased sleep, socialization, food intake, and caregiver satisfaction, along with reductions in night-time awakening, psychoactive medication use, psychotic symptoms, repetitive questions, wandering, agitation, and staff and family stress (Tyrrell, 2014; Isaac et al., 2020; Parajuli et al., 2021).

Need-Driven Dementia-Compromised Behaviour Model

The Need-Driven Dementia-Compromised Behaviour Model proposes that the behaviour of a person with dementia indicates a need that can be addressed appropriately if the person's history and habits, physiological status, and physical and social environment are carefully evaluated (Kolanowski, 1999). Behaviour is viewed as having meaning and expressing needs. Behaviour reflects the interaction between background factors (gender, ethnicity, culture, education, personality, response to stress, and cognitive changes resulting from dementia) and proximal factors (physiological needs [such as hunger or pain], mood, physical environment, and social environment) (Nolan, 2020).

Optimal care is provided by identifying the meaning of the behaviour, manipulating the proximal factors that precipitate that behaviour, and maximizing strengths and minimizing the limitations of the background factors. For instance, sleep disruptions are common. If the person with dementia is not getting adequate sleep at night, agitation during the day may signal the need for more rest. Interventions to modify proximal factors interfering with sleep, such as noise, frequent awakenings during the night, and daytime boredom, can help meet the need for rest and sleep and decrease agitation.

Developed and widely disseminated in Ontario, the Gentle Persuasive Approaches model trains health care providers to understand, minimize, accommodate, and manage responsive behaviours. It is based on the principles of person-centred care and the Need-Driven Dementia-Compromised Behaviour Model. Staff learn to reframe behaviours typically labelled as aggressive as self-protective and an attempt to exert control in a frightening situation (Pizzacalla et al., 2015). Staff training was shown to increase self-reported competence and to reduce responsive behaviours (Hung et al., 2019; see Box 21.9).

Recognition of Retained Abilities Approach

The recognition of retained abilities approach, developed by Canadian nurses, emphasizes the importance of focusing on abilities rather than disabilities (Dawson et al., 1993; Wells & Dawson, 2000). Careful assessment of the person's abilities allows the nurse to assist with care in ways that compensate for lost abilities and enhance remaining abilities. An environment that supports retained abilities is important. Education about this approach results in nurses' and health care aides' increased use of abilities-focused interventions and in

---

BOX 21.8

PRINCIPLES OF CARE DERIVED FROM THE PROGRESSIVELY LOWERED STRESS THRESHOLD MODEL

1. Maximize functional abilities by supporting all losses in an assistive manner.
2. Establish a caring relationship with the patient and provide unconditional positive regard.
3. Use the patient's behaviour (i.e., anxiety and avoidance) to determine the appropriate limits of activity and stimuli.
4. Teach caregivers to observe and listen to the person; try to determine the causes of behaviour.
5. Identify triggers related to discomfort or stress reactions (e.g., factors in the environment, caregiver communication).
6. Modify the environment to support losses and promote safe function.
7. Evaluate care routines and responses on a 24-hour basis, and adjust the plan of care accordingly.
8. Provide as much control as possible—encourage self-care, offer choices, explain all actions, and do not force the person to do something.
9. Keep the environment stable and predictable.
10. Provide ongoing education, support, care, and problem solving.

Source: Adapted from Hall, G. R., & Buckwalter, K. C. (1987). Progressively lowered stress threshold: A conceptual model for care of adults with Alzheimer's disease. *Archives of Psychiatric Nursing, 1*(6), 399–406.

BOX 21.9
RESEARCH FOR EVIDENCE-INFORMED PRACTICE: IMPROVING DEMENTIA CARE IN HOSPITALS

Problem: Gaps in knowledge about dementia and skills for dementia care are evidenced among nursing and interprofessional staff in acute care settings. This study described the experiences of health care providers who were learning and enacting Gentle Persuasive Approaches (GPA) in a hospital.

Method: This mixed-methods study consisted of a survey of 297 participants after they received training and education and a series of focus groups with 24 participants 1 year later.

Findings: Participants described their experiences enacting what they learned. Three themes were evident in their descriptions: (1) *changing attitudes*, including ability to have empathy, understanding the patient's perspective and increased value for teamwork and collaboration; (2) *changing practices* that recognized the complexity of dementia care and ability to focus on the person and provide person-centred care; and (3) *changing conditions to enable patient-centred care*, a recognition that supportive conditions are needed to enact the GPA training; this includes having sufficient staffing and time to enact person-centred care and meaningful recognition by leaders of what is required to change practice.

Implications for Nursing Practice: The GPA training and education contributed to improved person-centred dementia care in the hospital. This was supported by changes that included team huddles and support from a mental health nurse specialist. Clear and observable support from leaders is required to enable nurses to enact the learning, as is sufficient staffing.

Source: Hung, L., Son, C., & Hung, R. (2019). The experience of hospital staff in applying the Gentle Persuasive Approaches to dementia care. *Journal of Psychiatric and Mental Health Nursing, 26*(1–2), 19–28. doi:10.1111/jpm.12504.

patients' decreased agitation, increased engagement in morning care, and increased independence in dressing and grooming (Sidani et al., 2012). Excess disability is loss of ability that is not caused by the patient's illness and symptoms. It is not well recognized in dementia care; care providers may assume that a lack of capacity to perform ADLs means a lack of ability. Iatrogenic excess disability occurs when patients do not use existing abilities because of the way nursing care is provided; for example, when care providers "do for" rather than assist or facilitate participation in ADLs. A person-centred approach and environmental strategies may prevent or reduce excess disability (McGilton & Lemay, 2020).

Relating Well

In LTC homes, the relationship between the care provider and the resident enhances residents' quality of life and enriches the work experience of care providers. A therapeutic relationship is achieved when a care provider is reliable, empathetic, and consistent in interactions with the person who has dementia. Relating well involves staying close to the patient, using touch that is comfortable to the patient, focusing on care (not just the task) and the person's experience, and being flexible while adjusting to the patient's rhythm (McGilton & Lemay, 2020). These actions are associated with better outcomes for residents with dementia, including lower levels of anxiety, sadness, and agitation during care.

IMPLICATIONS FOR GERONTOLOGICAL NURSING AND HEALTHY AGING

Assessment

It is essential to view all behaviour as meaningful and an expression of needs. The focus must be on understanding that behavioural expressions communicate distress, and the response is to investigate the possible sources of distress and intervene appropriately. There are many possible reasons for behavioural and psychological symptoms of dementia. After medical problems (e.g., pneumonia, dehydration, impaction, infection, fractures, pain, and depression) are ruled out as causes of the behaviour, continued assessment is important in order to identify why distressing symptoms are occurring (Boltz, 2020). Conditions such as constipation or urinary tract infections can cause great distress that may not be readily communicated by the person with later-stage dementia. These conditions may lead to marked changes in behaviour (e.g., agitation or resistance to care), so careful assessment is important. Pain from comorbid musculoskeletal disorders is common among persons with dementia and is a frequent cause of agitation; after careful assessment of other possible causes, treatment with a trial of analgesics should be considered (Walaszek, 2020) (see Chapter 16).

Nurses must use appropriate assessment to understand the meaning of behaviours and determine what interventions would be most helpful to meet the needs being expressed. Yet, behaviours are frequently treated without appropriate assessment. Trying to see the world from the viewpoint of the person with dementia will help the nurse understand the person's behaviour. The questions *what, where, why, when, who,* and *what now* are important components of the assessment of behaviour. Box 21.10 presents a framework for asking questions about the possible meanings and messages behind observed behaviour. It is recommended that the nurse use a behavioural log for 2 to 3 days to track when the behaviour occurs, the circumstances under which it occurs, and the response to interventions.

Interventions

All evidence-informed guidelines endorse an approach that begins with the comprehensive assessment of the behaviour and its possible causes, followed by non-pharmacological interventions as the first line of treatment. Despite this recommendation, psychotropic medications are often the first-line treatment of the behavioural and psychological symptoms of dementia. In Canada, 20% of older adults living in LTC homes are prescribed an antipsychotic without a diagnosis of psychosis (CIHI, 2020). The overuse of antipsychotic medications to treat behavioural responses is of serious concern in light of the adverse drug events and risks associated with such medications, including sedation and associated orthostatic hypotension, falls and fractures, stroke, extrapyramidal symptoms, worsening cognition, and death (Ralph & Espinet, 2019).

Several factors contribute to inappropriate use of antipsychotics: insufficient staffing in LTC homes, time constraints, an emphasis on controlling residents rather than understanding them, lack of interdisciplinary team approaches and family involvement, inadequate training and education to apply person-centred and nonpharmacological approaches, and care providers' and managers' negative attitudes about dementia (Walsh et al., 2017). Successfully reducing inappropriate antipsychotic use requires a multi-pronged approach, including leadership and champions for practice change, staff and family education, establishing processes for reviewing and reducing inappropriate prescriptions, and increasing use of nonpharmacological approaches (BC Care Providers Association, 2018).

Pharmacological approaches may be considered in addition to nonpharmacological approaches if there

---

BOX 21.10

FRAMEWORK FOR ASKING QUESTIONS ABOUT THE MEANING OF THE BEHAVIOUR OF PERSONS WITH DEMENTIA

WHAT?

What is happening? Does the behaviour have a physical component, an emotional component, or both? What is the need? What is the behaviour saying? What emotion is being expressed? What are the risks to the person with dementia and others?

WHERE?

Where is the behaviour occurring? Are there environmental triggers such as noise, over- or under-stimulation, a change in routine, relocation?

WHEN?

When does the behaviour most frequently occur? For example, does it occur after performing activities of daily living, at mealtimes, or at a certain time of the day? A Dementia Observation System (DOS) assessment would be helpful to determine the answers to this question.

WHO?

Who is involved? (Other residents, caregivers, family?) Who else might know something about the person or the behaviour and approaches to it?

WHY?

What happened before the behaviour? Poor communication? Tasks too complicated? Physical or medical problems? Pain, discomfort? Lack of accommodation for a disability such as sensory or communication impairment? Change in medications? Being rushed or forced to do something? Has this happened before, and if so, why?

WHAT NOW?

Approaches and interventions (nonpharmacological or pharmacological)? Changes in staff behaviours and approaches needed? Implemented by whom? Is everyone who is involved communicated with and included in the plan of care? What is the plan for monitoring, evaluating, and reassessing?

Sources: Adapted from © PIECES Consult Group (2009). *PIECES Three question template.* http://pieceslearning. com/wp-content/uploads/2016/02/PIECES_Laminate_ Nov_09.pdf; Registered Nurses' Association of Ontario. (2016). *Delirium, dementia, and depression in older adults: Assessment and care* (2nd ed.). Author. http://rnao.ca/ sites/rnao-ca/files/3Ds_BPG_WEB_FINAL.pdf; brainX-change. (2020). *Behavioural Supports Ontario – Dementia Observation System (BSO-DOS).* https://brainxchange.ca/ BSODOS.

has been a comprehensive assessment of causes of behaviour, the person presents a danger to self or others, nonpharmacological interventions have not been effective, and the risk–benefit profiles of medications have been considered (Boltz, 2020). Risperidone is the only medication approved for this use in Canada (Health Canada, 2015). Appropriate medication must be carefully monitored and evaluated for tapering and discontinuation.

Nonpharmacological Approaches

The previously described approaches recommended in the PLST model, the Need-Driven Dementia-Compromised Behaviour Model, the recognition of retained abilities model, and the relating well model allow nurses to identify and address the underlying causes of behaviours. All health care providers who work in any setting with people with dementia need the knowledge and skills to effectively provide person-centred care and avoid the inappropriate use of medication. A team approach to care of persons with dementia is necessary.

In general, these interventions have shown promise for improving the quality of life for persons with dementia, despite a lack of rigorous evaluation. The most effective approaches are as follows: exercise (see Chapter 10), individualizing activities, music therapy, sensory interventions (e.g., touch, massage, and multisensory interventions), reminiscence, simplifying tasks, enhancing communication, group activities (e.g., animal-assisted therapy, dance, and cooking), and art therapy (Legere et al., 2018; Meyer & O'Keefe, 2018). Other interventions include environmental design (e.g., supportive care units, homelike environments, gardens, and safe walking areas), changes in mealtime and bathing environments, and consistent staffing assignments (Hebert & Scales, 2019; Boltz, 2020). Combining multiple interventions for the person with dementia is often more beneficial than using single interventions.

Activities of Daily Living

The cognitive changes associated with dementia interfere with the person's communication patterns and ability to understand and express thoughts and feelings. Perceptual disturbances and misinterpretations of reality often contribute to fear and misunderstanding. People with dementia sometimes struggle to understand the world and make their needs known. Often, bathing and the provision of other ADL care such as dressing, grooming, and toileting are the cause of much distress for both the person with dementia and the caregiver.

Bathing. Bathing and assistance with ADLs, particularly in LTC homes, can be perceived as attacks by persons with dementia, who may attempt to protect themselves by screaming or striking out. A rigid focus on tasks or institutional care routines (such as showering 2 days a week) can contribute to the person's distress and precipitate distressing behaviours. Being touched or bathed against one's will violates trust in the caregiver and can be a major affront. The resulting behaviours that may be exhibited by a person with dementia are not deliberate attacks by a violent person but efforts to protect the self (Pizzacalla et al., 2015).

Person-centred care is vital when persons with dementia are assisted with bathing. The *Bathing Without a Battle* approach results in reduced responsive behaviours such as hitting, agitation, distress, and crying or screaming (https://bathingwithoutabattle.unc.edu/; Barrick et al., 2008). Choices about approaches to bathing are made by answering the question "What is the easiest, most comfortable, least frightening way for me to bathe the person right now?" (Rader & Barrick, 2000, p. 42). It is important for the nurse who bathes a person with dementia to know the person's lifetime bathing routines and preferences; ensure the person's privacy and providing care only when the person is receptive; respect refusals to participate in care; explain all actions; recognize that a bath is not an essential intervention; encourage self-care to the extent possible; make bathrooms and shower areas warm, comfortable, and safe; keep the person warm with towels; be attentive to the person's pain and discomfort; reassure the person that they are safe; provide distractions; play preferred music; and use alternative bathing methods such as towel baths, thermal baths, and no-rinse cleaners. Individualized bathing care plans are helpful.

Wandering. Wandering associated with dementia is one of the most difficult management problems encountered in home and institutional settings. Three in five people with dementia wander (Neubauer et al., 2018). Wandering is a complex behaviour. Risk factors for wandering include visuospatial impairments, anxiety and depression, poor sleep patterns, unmet needs, delusions, depression, and more severe cognitive impairment (Barnard-Brak & Parmelee, 2020; Neubauer et al., 2018). Residents of LTC homes who wandered have reported that they walked for many different reasons: for enjoyment, to stay healthy, to be with their family, because it was a lifelong habit, to socialize, or to be with animals (Adekoya & Guse, 2019).

Wandering presents safety concerns in all settings. Wandering affects sleep, eating, safety, and the caregiver's ability to provide care; it also interferes with the privacy of others. It can lead to falls, elopement (i.e., leaving the home or LTC home), injury, and death (Barnard-Brak & Parmelee, 2020; Neubauer et al., 2018). The stimulus for wandering arises from many internal and external sources.

Wandering behaviours can be predicted through careful observation and knowing the person's patterns. For example, if the person with dementia starts wandering or trying to leave the home around dinnertime every day, meaningful activities such as music, exercise, and refreshment can be provided at this time. There are also several instruments with which to assess the person's risk for wandering. Guidelines for people with dementia, care partners in the community, and care homes (Neubauer, 2019) are available through the Alzheimer Society of Ontario (https://findingyourwayontario.ca).

Wandering may be less likely to occur when the person is involved in social interaction and activities. Music therapy and exercise programs may also reduce wandering behaviour (Neubauer et al., 2018). Environmental interventions include camouflaging doorways, providing enclosed outdoor gardens and paths for walking, and providing electronic bracelets that activate alarms at exits. GPS and radio frequency locating technologies are also available. Box 21.11 presents suggestions for strategies depending on the level of risk for wandering.

Wandering behaviour in a person with dementia may result in the person's going outside and getting lost. The Alzheimer Society of Canada's Medic Alert Safely Home program (https://www.medicalert.ca/safely-home) is designed to help identify, locate, and return people with dementia to safety. The Alzheimer Society of Ontario's website (https://findingyourwayontario.ca) has information for caregivers about wandering and how to manage it.

BOX 21.11
STRATEGIES TO ADDRESS WANDERING IN COMMUNITY-DWELLING PERSONS WITH DEMENTIA

LOW RISK
- Education about wandering
- Develop prevention plan
- Assess for increased risk
- Register in vulnerable persons registry
- Use identification products such as bracelets

MEDIUM RISK
- Redirection
- Exercise with a partner or location technology
- Make a list of previous places of employment and residences
- Increased supervision bracket such as day programs, friendly visitors

HIGH RISK
- Locating technologies and alarms
- Install locks and barriers
- Buddy system
- Home care support
- Relocate/move

Source: Adapted from Neubauer, N. (n.d.). *Wandering guideline for care partners in community settings.* http://findingyourwayontario.ca/wp-content/uploads/2019/03/Guidelines-Community-EN.pdf.

Advance Care Planning

The person with dementia, their family members, and the health care team should collaborate in making decisions related to care early in the disease. The patient and their family should be supported to discuss decision making for health care and advance care planning while the person still has the capacity to do so. Advance care planning contributes to better end-of-life experiences and positive outcomes for relatives after the person dies (Durepos et al., 2019). Resources to support advance care planning discussions with persons who have dementia are available online (Institute for Healthcare Improvement, 2020).

FAMILY CAREGIVING FOR PERSONS WITH DEMENTIA

Most Canadians with dementia live in the community; 85% of them rely on family and friends for assistance, and 41% rely solely on care from family and friends (Wong et al., 2016). Informal caregivers such as family and friends average 26 hours per week of caregiving and about $4,600 per year in out-of-pocket expenses, in addition to the lost income associated with reduced work hours or early retirement (Public Health Agency of Canada, 2019b). Family caregivers are usually women, most often wives or daughters (Stall et al., 2019).

These caregivers provide more hours of help than that provided by caregivers of persons who do not have dementia, and they experience more adverse consequences to their physical and mental health. Caregivers of persons with dementia have lower self-rated health scores; display fewer health-promoting behaviours; and have higher depression and anxiety rates, higher morbidity and mortality rates, higher numbers of illness-related symptoms, and sleep problems (Szabo et al., 2019). Higher levels of caregiver distress are associated with risk for elder abuse (Stall et al., 2019) (see Chapter 25). Factors that influence the stress of caregiving include grief over the multiple losses that occur, the physical demands and duration of caregiving (up to 20 years), and resource availability. The negative effects of caring for persons with dementia are intensified when the person with dementia experiences behavioural disturbances and impaired ability to perform ADLs and instrumental ADLs.

Most research on the care of persons with dementia has focused on the late stages of dementia and on the "burden" of caregiving. However, this is a simplification of the complex process of caregiving and a negation of the positive aspects and outcomes of family caregiving. Positive outcomes include role satisfaction (which is common among caregivers); emotional rewards; personal growth (such as increased self-awareness and humility); new skills; spiritual growth; strengthened family relationships; and the rewards of having a sense of duty and being able to give back to the person with dementia (Alcock, 2019; Quinn & Toms, 2019).

The most effective caregiver intervention programs include bundled interventions, such as individual and group interventions for both the person with dementia and the caregiver, as well as combined groups, education, counselling, support group participation, care management, and the continuous availability of telephone support. Teaching caregivers about AD and training them in the skills needed to manage behaviours, maintain social support, reframe negative emotions, manage stress, and enhance their own healthy behaviours appear to be most effective in reducing the caregiver's depression and burden and improving their quality of life (Abrahams et al., 2018). Web-based interventions for caregivers are associated with positive outcomes (Duggleby et al., 2019). It is important that caregiver support begin in the early stages of dementia.

Family caregiving continues after a person with dementia moves to an LTC home. Family caregiving in an LTC home involves not only providing personal care but also monitoring the quality of care; providing companionship; preserving the individuality, dignity, and self-esteem of the resident; and communicating the family member's unique knowledge of the resident to the staff (Puurveen et al., 2018). Positive relationships between staff in LTC homes and family caregivers of residents are important but not always supported by staff. Positive relationships depend on staff members establishing their trustworthiness; listening to family caregivers' views, including their complaints about care; and encouraging appropriate family involvement in the home and in care (Puurveen et al., 2018).

There is little research with Indigenous peoples about dementia caregiving. In her research with Indigenous female family caregivers in Ontario, Alcock (2019) found that obtaining support could be problematic because of lack of awareness of supports and services. Home care, nursing support, and respite care were important for caregivers, but not always geographically or culturally accessible. Homecare services from care providers who were members of the community, who spoke the local language, and who understood the culture was important for quality and continuity and led to improved wait times and coordination of care. (See Chapter 23 for additional information on caregiving.)

SUMMARY

Many of the interventions for preventing delirium and for caring for people with cognitive impairment are achieved by applying the principles of good gerontological nursing care. An understanding of these principles and how to adapt responses and the environment to older adults with cognitive impairment will ensure that basic needs are met and that quality of care and quality of life are enhanced. Some of these principles may seem straightforward, but too often they are not practised, leading to iatrogenesis, distress, and excess disability. Often, these consequences are more problematic than the illnesses themselves. Nursing care must not increase disability; care must be based on knowledge and research to be considered best practice.

KEY CONCEPTS

- Nurses must advocate for thorough assessment of any older adult who appears to be experiencing cognitive decline and a reduced ability to function in important aspects of life.
- *Delirium* is sometimes the result of physiological imbalances and may be caused by a variety of biological disturbances. Delirium is characterized by acute onset, inattention, disorganized thinking, and an altered level of consciousness. It often goes unrecognized or is falsely attributed to age or dementia. People with dementia are more susceptible to delirium. Knowledge of risk factors, preventive measures, and the treatment of underlying medical problems is essential to prevent serious consequences.
- Medications and pain are frequently the causes of delirium in older adults.
- Irreversible dementias follow a pattern of inevitable decline accompanied by decreased intellectual function, personality changes, and impaired judgement. The most common of these dementias is *Alzheimer's disease.*
- Alzheimer's disease has been the subject of an enormous amount of research aimed at understanding its causes. Research is continuing to discover ways to protect persons against AD or halt the progress of the disease. There is no known cure, but some medications seem to slow the progress of the dementia for a time.
- *Vascular dementia* is a group of heterogeneous disorders arising from cerebrovascular insufficiency or from ischemic or hemorrhagic brain damage. It is the second most prevalent type of dementia and often coexists with AD. Hypertension, cardiac disease, diabetes, smoking, and dyslipidemia are additional risk factors for vascular dementia. Prevention and treatment of risk factors are important.
- The assessment of cognitive impairment is complex. Nurses may do a screening assessment using any number of brief mental status examinations and must request a more thorough assessment when there is an indication of dementia.
- People with cognitive impairment respond best to calmness and patience, adaptations of communication techniques, and environments and relationships that support and enhance function, support limitations, ensure safety, and provide opportunities for a meaningful quality of life. Because persons with cognitive impairment may be unable to express their feelings and needs in ways that are easily understood, the gerontological nurse must always try to understand the world from their perspective.

ACTIVITIES AND DISCUSSION QUESTIONS

1. What are the differences between delirium, dementia, and depression?

2. What are some of the risk factors for the development of delirium?

3. Discuss communication strategies that are useful for the person experiencing delirium.

4. Why is it important to ensure that the person experiencing any change in mental status receive a thorough assessment and evaluation?

5. Brainstorm with fellow students about how it would feel to be bathed by a total stranger.

6. The health care aides in a long-term care home complain to you that Mr. G. hit them when they were trying to give him his required twice-weekly shower. How might you assist them in supporting Mr. G.'s care needs?

7. Describe how you would design a supportive care unit for individuals with dementia.

8. A family caregiver tells you that their loved one keeps trying to leave the house to find the children. What are some strategies you might share with the caregiver to help them deal with this situation?

HEALTHY AGING CARE PLAN

Caring for M.R.

Recall the *Lived Experience* testimonials and M.R.'s case presented at the beginning of the chapter.

1. M.R.'s cognitive changes appear to have worsened gradually over at least the last year. This is a sign of dementia. You should conduct a screening test for dementia such as the Montreal Cognitive Assessment and discuss the findings with the interprofessional team. He has several risk factors for delirium, so his mental status should be assessed regularly using a screening tool such as RADAR or the Confusion Assessment Method.

2. Priority nursing interventions include (1) promoting orientation and safety; (2) regular assessment of mental status; (3) delirium prevention, including review of medications, monitoring lab results, mobilization, adequate sleep, nutrition, and hydration, and screening for visual or hearing impairments; (4) health teaching for M.R. and his friend about delirium prevention.

3. Discharge planning should be guided by the results of investigations of the possible causes of M.R.'s mental status changes. If dementia is diagnosed, he should be referred to a memory disorder clinic and the local chapter of the Alzheimer Society. An occupational therapy assessment and social work assessment will help to determine the level of support M.R. needs at home and the extent to which his friend is able to continue supporting him.

RESOURCES

Alzheimer Society of Canada
https://alzheimer.ca/en
Alzheimer Society of Canada. *MedicAlert® Safely Home® program.*
https://alzheimer.ca/en/help-support/programs-services/medicalert-safely-home
BrainXchange
http://brainxchange.ca/
Gentle Persuasive Approaches
https://ageinc.ca/
Regional Geriatric Program (RGP) Central. *Resources.*
http://www.rgpc.ca/resources/

For additional resources, please visit *http://evolve.elsevier.com/Canada/Ebersole/gerontological/*

REFERENCES

Abrahams, R., Liu, K. P. Y., Bissett, M., et al. (2018). Effectiveness of interventions for co-residing family caregivers of people with dementia: Systematic review and meta-analysis. *Australian Occupational Therapy Journal*, 65(3), 208–224. doi:10.1111/1440-1630.12464.

Adekoya, A. A., & Guse, L. (2019). Wandering behavior from the perspectives of older adults with mild to moderate dementia in long-term care. *Research in Gerontological Nursing*, 12(5), 239–247. doi:10.3928/19404921-20190522-01.

Aisen, P. S., Cummings, J., Jack, C. R., et al. (2017). On the path to 2025: Understanding the Alzheimer's disease continuum. *Alzheimer's Research and Therapy*, 9(1), 1–10. doi:10.1186/s13195-017-0283-5.

Alcock, D. E. (2019). *"I honoured him until the end": Storytelling of Indigenous female caregivers and care poviders focused on Alzheimer's disease and other dementias (ADOD)* [Unpublished doctoral dissertation]. The University of Western Ontario.

Alzheimer Society of Canada. (2020). *Dementia numbers in Canada.* https://alzheimer.ca/en/about-dementia/what-dementia/dementia-numbers-canada.

American Psychiatric Association. (2013). *Diagnostic and statistical manual of mental disorders: DSM-5* (5th ed.). Author.

Barnard-Brak, L., & Parmelee, P. (2020). Measuring risk of wandering and symptoms of dementia via caregiver report. *Journal of Applied Gerontology*, 40(10), 1372–1376. doi:10.1177/0733464820947287.

Barrick, A. L., Rader, J., Hoeffer, B., et al. (Eds.) (2008). *Bathing without a battle: Person-directed care of individuals with dementia* (2nd ed.). Springer.

BC Care Providers Association. (2018). *A pathway to ensuring the appropriate use of antipsychotics in continuing care: Sharing success stories from BCCPA members.* https://bccare.ca/wp-content/uploads/2018/04/BCCPA-Antipsychotics-Guide-2018.pdf.

Blevins, C. (2020). Delirium: Prevention, early recognition, and treatment. In M. Boltz, L. Capezuti, T. Fulmer, et al. (Eds.), *Evidence-based geriatric nursing protocols for best practice* (6th ed., pp. 317–330). Springer.

Boltz, Marie. (2020). Dementia: Assessment and care strategies. In M. Boltz, E. A. Capezuti, D. Zwickler, et al. (Eds.), *Evidence-based geriatric nursing protocols for best practice* (6th ed., pp. 331–352). Springer.

Boockvar, K. S., Judon, K. M., Eimicke, J. P., et al. (2020). Hospital Elder Life Program in Long-Term Care (HELP-LTC): A cluster randomized controlled trial. *Journal of the American Geriatrics Society*, 68(10), 2329–2335. doi:10.1111/jgs.16695.

Borgundvaag, B., & Klaiman, M. (2020). Management of alcohol withdrawal: Time to "SHAKE" things up? *Canadian Journal of Emergency Medicine, 22*(2), 131–132. doi:10.1017/cem.2020.7.

Boucher, V., Lamontagne, M. E., Nadeau, A., et al. (2019). Unrecognized incident delirium in older emergency department patients. *Journal of Emergency Medicine, 57*(4), 535–542. doi:10.1016/j.jemermed.2019.05.024.

Brooke, J. (2018). Differentiation of delirium, dementia and delirium superimposed on dementia in the older person. *British Journal of Nursing, 27*(7), 363–367. doi:10.12968/bjon.2018.27.7.363.

Calia, C., Johnson, H., & Cristea, M. (2019). Cross-cultural representations of dementia: An exploratory study. *Journal of Global Health, 9*(1), 1–11. doi:10.7189/jogh.09.011001.

Canadian Institute for Health Information (CIHI). (2018). *Dementia in Canada*. https://www.cihi.ca/en/dementia-in-canada.

Canadian Institute for Health Information (CIHI). (2020). *Potentiallly inappropriate use of antipsychotics in long term care.* https://yourhealthsystem.cihi.ca/hsp/inbrief?lang=en#!/indicators/008/potentially-inappropriate-use-of-antipsychotics-in-long-term-care/.

Carney, G., Bassett, K., Wright, J. M., et al. (2019). Comparison of cholinesterase inhibitor safety in real-world practice. *Alzheimer's & Dementia (New York, N. Y.), 5*(1), 732–739. doi:10.1016/j.trci.2019.09.011.

Cheung, E. N. M., Benjamin, S., Heckman, G., et al. (2018). Clinical characteristics associated with the onset of delirium among long-term nursing home residents. *BMC Geriatrics, 18*(1), 1–7. doi:10.1186/s12877-018-0733-3.

Colella, J., Aroh, D., Douglas, C., et al. (2017). Managing delirium behaviors with one-to-one sitters. *Nursing Management, 48*(9), 1–6. doi:10.1097/01.NUMA.0000522172.15640.6b.

Cunningham, C., Macfarlane, S., & Brodaty, H. (2019). Language paradigms when behaviour changes with dementia: #BanBPSD. *International Journal of Geriatric Psychiatry, 34*(8), 1109–1113. doi:10.1002/gps.5122.

Dahlke, S., Hunter, K. F., Negrin, K., et al. (2019). The educational needs of nursing staff when working with hospitalised older people. *Journal of Clinical Nursing, 28*(1–2), 221–234. doi:10.1111/jocn.14631.

Dawson, P., Wells, D. L., & Kline, K. (1993). *Enhancing the abilities of persons with Alzheimer's and related dementias: A nursing perspective.* Springer.

de Witt, L., & Fortune, D. (2019). Relationship-centered dementia care: Insights from a community-based culture change coalition. *Dementia, 18*(3), 1146–1165. doi:10.1177/1471301217708814.

Drummond, N., Birtwhistle, R., Williamson, T., et al. (2016). Prevalence and management of dementia in primary care practices with electronic medical records: A report from the Canadian Primary Care Sentinel Surveillance Network. *CMAJ Open, 4*(2), E177–E184. doi:10.9778/cmajo.20150050.

Duggleby, W., Ploeg, J., McAiney, C., et al. (2019). A comparison of users and nonusers of a web-based intervention for carers of older persons with Alzheimer disease and related dementias: Mixed methods secondary analysis. *Journal of Medical Internet Research, 21*(10), 1–13. doi:10.2196/14254.

Dupuis, S. L., Wiersma, E., & Loiselle, L. (2012). Pathologizing behavior: Meanings of behaviors in dementia care. *Journal of Aging Studies, 26*(2), 162–173. doi:10.1016/j.jaging.2011.12.001.

Durepos, P., Sussman, T., Ploeg, J., et al. (2019). What does death preparedness mean for family caregivers of persons with dementia? *American Journal of Hospice and Palliative Medicine, 36*(5), 436–446. doi:10.1177/1049909118814240.

Émond, M., Boucher, V., Carmichael, P. H., et al. (2018). Incidence of delirium in the Canadian emergency department and its consequences on hospital length of stay: A prospective observational multicentre cohort study. *BMJ Open, 8*(3), 1–9. doi:10.1136/bmjopen-2017-018190.

Fick, D. M., Heeren, P., & Milisen, K. (2020). Assessing cognitive function in the older adult. In M. Boltz, L. Capezuti, T. T. Fulmer, et al. (Eds.), *Evidence-based geriatric nursing protocols for best practice* (6th ed., pp. 119–132). Springer.

Gagné, A. J., Voyer, P., Boucher, V., et al. (2018). Performance of the French version of the 4AT for screening the elderly for delirium in the emergency department. *Canadian Journal of Emergency Medicine, 20*(6), 903–910. doi:10.1017/cem.2018.367.

Goldberg, T. E., Chen, C., Wang, Y., et al. (2020). Association of delirium with long-term cognitive decline: A meta-analysis. *JAMA Neurology, 77*(11), 1373–1381. doi:10.1001/jamaneurol.2020.2273.

Hall, G. R. (1987). Progressively lowered stress threshold: A conceptual model for care of adults with Alzheimer's disease. *Archives of Psychiatric Nursing, 1*(6), 399–406.

Hall, G. R. (1994). Caring for people with Alzheimer's disease using the conceptual model of progressively lowered stress threshold in the clinical setting. *Nursing Clinics of North America, 29*(1), 129–141.

Haq, K. S., & Penning, M. J. (2019). Social determinants of racial disparities in cognitive functioning in later life in Canada. *Journal of Aging and Health, 32*(7–8), 817–829. doi:10.1177/0898264319853137.

Health Canada. (2015). *Recalls and safety alerts: Risperidone—Restriction of the dementia indication.* http://healthycanadians.gc.ca/recall-alert-rappel-avis/hc-sc/2015/43797a-eng.php.

Hebert, C. A., & Scales, K. (2019). Dementia friendly initiatives: A state of the science review. *Dementia, 18*(5), 1858–1895. doi:10.1177/1471301217731433.

Henderson, J. N., Carson, L. D., & King, K. (2019). Indigenous vascular dementia. In W. Hulko, D. Wilson, & J. E. Balestrery (Eds.), *Indigenous peoples and dementia: New understandings of memory loss and memory care* (pp. 41–60). UBC Press.

Hossain, M. Z., & Khan, H. T. A. (2020). Barriers to access and ways to improve dementia services for a minority ethnic group in England. *Journal of Evaluation in Clinical Practice, 26*(6), 1629–1637. doi:10.1111/jep.13361.

Hshieh, T. T., Yang, T., Gartaganis, S. L., et al. (2018). Hospital Elder Life Program: Systematic review and meta-analysis of effectiveness. *American Journal of Geriatric Psychiatry, 26*(10), 1015–1033. doi:10.1016/j.jagp.2018.06.007.

Hung, L., Son, C., & Hung, R. (2019). The experience of hospital staff in applying the Gentle Persuasive Approaches to dementia care. *Journal of Psychiatric and Mental Health Nursing, 26*(1–2), 19–28. doi:10.1111/jpm.12504.

Huson, K., Stolee, P., Pearce, N., et al. (2016). Examining the Hospital Elder Life Program in a rehabilitation setting: A pilot feasibility study. *BMC Geriatrics, 16*(1), 1–12. doi:10.1186/s12877-016-0313-3.

Inouye, S. K. (2018). Delirium—A framework to improve acute care for older persons. *Journal of the American Geriatrics Society*, 66(3), 446–451. doi:10.1111/jgs.15296.

Inouye, S. K., Bogardus, S. T., Charpentier, P. A., et al. (1999). A multicomponent intervention to prevent delirium in hospitalized older patients. *New England Journal of Medicine*, 340(9), 669–676. doi:10.1056/NEJM199903043400901.

Inouye, S., van Dyck, C. H., Alessi, C. et al. (1990). Clarifying confusion: The Confusion Assessment Method. *Annals of Internal Medicine*, 113, 941–948. doi:10.7326/0003-4819-113-12-941.

Institute for Healthcare Improvement. (2020). *Your conversation starter guide*. https://theconversationproject.org/wp-content/uploads/2020/12/ConversationStarterGuide.pdf.

Isaac, V., Kuot, A., Hamiduzzaman, M., et al. (2020). The outcomes of a person-centered, non-pharmacological intervention in reducing behavioral and psychiatric symptoms in residents with advanced dementia in Australian rural nursing homes. *BMC Geriatrics*, 21, 193. doi:10.21203/rs.3.rs-38968/v1.

Isik, A. T., Soysal, P., Stubbs, B., et al. (2018). Cardiovascular outcomes of cholinesterase inhibitors in individuals with dementia: A meta-analysis and systematic review. *Journal of the American Geriatrics Society*, 66(9), 1805–1811. doi:10.1111/jgs.15415.

Ismail, Z., Black, S. E., Camicioli, R., et al. (2020). Recommendations of the 5th Canadian Consensus Conference on the Diagnosis and Treatment of Dementia. *Alzheimer's and Dementia*, 16(8), 1182–1195. doi:10.1002/alz.12105.

Jacklin, K., & Walker, J. (2020). Cultural understandings of dementia in Indigenous peoples: A qualitative evidence synthesis. *Canadian Journal on Aging*, 39(2), 220–234. doi:10.1017/S071498081900028X.

Kagan, S. H. (2020). Ageisms, older people, and hospitalization: Walking a path through the past, looking to lead in the future. *Geriatric Nursing*, 41(5), 654–656. doi:10.1016/j.gerinurse.2020.08.012.

Koehn, S. (2020). "It is not a disease, only memory loss": Exploring the complexity of access to a diagnosis of dementia in a cross-cultural sample. In L. Garcia, L. McCleary, & N. Drummond (Eds.), *Evidence-informed approaches for managing dementia transitions* (pp. 29–52). Academic Press.

Kolanowski, A. M. (1999). An overview of the Need-Driven Dementia-Compromised Behavior Model. *Journal of Gerontological Nursing*, 25(9), 7–9. doi:10.3928/0098-9134-19990901-0.

Lau, T., Kozyra, E., & Cheng, C. (2019). Delirium: Risk factors, contributors, identification, work-up, and treatment. In H. Fenn, A. Hategan, & J. Bourgeois (Eds.), *Inpatient geriatric psychiatry* (pp. 219–235). Springer. doi:10.1007/978-3-030-10401-6_12.

Lee, J. (2020). Risk factors for nursing home delirium: A systematic review. *Journal of Korean Gerontological Nursing*, 22(1), 75–83. doi:10.17079/jkgn.2020.22.1.75.

Legere, L. E., McNeill, S., Schindel Martin, L., et al. (2018). Nonpharmacological approaches for behavioural and psychological symptoms of dementia in older adults: A systematic review of reviews. *Journal of Clinical Nursing*, 27(7–8), e1360–e1376. doi:10.1111/jocn.14007.

Li, Y., Li, Y., Li, X., et al. (2017). Head injury as a risk factor for dementia and Alzheimer's disease: A systematic review and meta-analysis of 32 observational studies. *PLOS One*, 12(1), e0169650. doi:10.1371/journal.pone.0169650.

MacDonald, J. P., Ward, V., & Halseth, R. (2018). *Alzheimer's disease and related dementias in Indigenous populations in Canada: Prevalence and risk factors*. National Collaborating Centre for Aboriginal Health. https://www.nccih.ca/docs/emerging/RPT-Alzheimer-Dementia-MacDonald-Ward-Halseth-EN.pdf.

McGilton, K. S., & Lemay, G. (2020). Hospitalization of persons with dementia. In L. Garcia, L. McCleary, & N. Drummond (Eds.), *Evidence-informed approaches for managing dementia transitions* (pp. 109–135). Elsevier.

McKeith, I. G. (2010). Dementia with Lewy bodies. In K. Miyoshi, Y. Morimura, & K. Maeda (Eds.), *Neuropsychiatric disorders* (pp. 247–254). doi:10.1007/978-4-431-53871-4_18.

McKenzie, J., & Joy, A. (2020). Family intervention improves outcomes for patients with delirium: Systematic review and meta-analysis. *Australasian Journal on Ageing*, 39(1), 21–30. doi:10.1111/ajag.12688.

Mehta, K. M., & Yeo, G. W. (2017). Systematic review of dementia prevalence and incidence in United States race/ethnic populations. *Alzheimer's and Dementia*, 13(1), 72–83. doi:10.1016/j.jalz.2016.06.2360.

Meyer, C., & O'Keefe, F. (2018). Non-pharmacological interventions for people with dementia: A review of reviews. *Dementia*, 19(6), 1927–1954. doi:10.1177/1471301218813234.

Morandi, A., Davis, D., Bellelli, G., et al. (2017). The diagnosis of delirium superimposed on dementia: An emerging challenge. *Journal of the American Medical Directors Association*, 18(1), 12–18. doi:10.1016/j.jamda.2016.07.014.

Mukaetova-Ladinska, E. B., Cosker, G., Chan, M., et al. (2019). Delirium stigma among healthcare staff. *Geriatrics*, 4(1), 1–14. doi:10.3390/geriatrics4010006.

Neubauer, N. (2019). *A framework to describe the levels of risk associated with dementia-related wandering* [Unpublished doctoral dissertation]. University of Alberta. doi:10.7939/r3-z0nz-0p16.

Neubauer, N. A., Azad-Khaneghah, P., Miguel-Cruz, A., et al. (2018). What do we know about strategies to manage dementia-related wandering? A scoping review. *Alzheimer's and Dementia: Diagnosis, Assessment and Disease Monitoring*, 10, 615–628. doi:10.1016/j.dadm.2018.08.001.

Nolan, A. M. (2020). *Development of practice guidelines based on need-driven dementia-compromised behavior model* (Publication No. 8567) [Doctoral dissertation, Walden University]. Walden Dissertations and Doctoral Studies. https://scholarworks.waldenu.edu/cgi/viewcontent.cgi?article=9839&context=dissertations.

O'Driscoll, C., & Shaikh, M. (2017). Cross-cultural applicability of the Montreal Cognitive Assessment (MoCA): A systematic review. *Journal of Alzheimer's Disease*, 58(3), 789–801. doi:10.3233/JAD-161042.

Oh, E. S., Fong, T. G., Hshieh, T. T., et al. (2017). Delirium in older persons: Advances in diagnosis and treatment. *Journal of the American Medical Association*, 318(12), 1161–1174. doi:10.1001/jama.2017.12067.

Oldham, M. A., Flaherty, J. H., & Maldonado, J. R. (2018). Refining delirium: A transtheoretical model of delirium disorder with preliminary neurophysiologic subtypes. *American Journal of Geriatric Psychiatry*, 26(9), 913–924. doi:10.1016/j.jagp.2018.04.002.

Parajuli, D. R., Kuot, A., Hamiduzzaman, M., et al. (2021). Person-centered, non-pharmacological intervention in reducing psychotropic medication use among residents with dementia in Australian rural aged care homes. *BMB Psychiatry, 21*, 36. doi:10.1186/s12888-020-03033-w.

Parker, M., Barlow, S., Hoe, J., et al. (2020). Persistent barriers and facilitators to seeking help for a dementia diagnosis: A systematic review of 30 years of the perspectives of carers and people with dementia. *International Psychogeriatrics*, 1–24. doi:10.1017/s1041610219002229.

Perry-Young, L., Owen, G., Kelly, S., et al. (2018). How people come to recognise a problem and seek medical help for a person showing early signs of dementia: A systematic review and meta-ethnography. *Dementia, 17*(1), 34–60. doi:10.1177/1471301215626889.

Peters, R., Booth, A., Rockwood, K., et al. (2019). Combining modifiable risk factors and risk of dementia: A systematic review and meta-analysis. *BMJ Open, 9*(1). doi:10.1136/bmjopen-2018-022846.

Pizzacalla, A., Montemuro, M., Coker, E., et al. (2015). Gentle Persuasive Approaches: Introducing an educational program on an orthopaedic unit for staff caring for patients with dementia and delirium. *Orthopaedic Nursing, 34*(2), 101–107. doi:10.1097/NOR.0000000000000127.

Public Health Agency of Canada. (2019a). *A Dementia Strategy for Canada: Together we aspire.* https://www.canada.ca/en/public-health/services/publications/diseases-conditions/dementia-strategy.html.

Public Health Agency of Canada. (2019b). *Dementia.* https://www.canada.ca/en/public-health/services/diseases/dementia.html.

Puurveen, G., Baumbusch, J., & Gandhi, P. (2018). From family involvement to family inclusion in nursing home settings: A critical interpretive synthesis. *Journal of Family Nursing, 24*(1), 60–85. doi:10.1177/1074840718754314.

Quinn, C., & Toms, G. (2019). Influence of positive aspects of dementia caregiving on caregivers' well-being: A systematic review. *The Gerontologist, 59*(5), e584–e596. doi:10.1093/geront/gny168.

Rader, J., & Barrick, A. (2000). Ways that work: Bathing without a battle. *Alzheimers Care Quarterly, 1*(4), 35–49.

Ralph, S. J., & Espinet, A. J. (2019). Use of antipsychotics and benzodiazepines for dementia: Time for action? What will be required before global de-prescribing? *Dementia, 18*(6), 2322–2339. doi:10.1177/1471301217746769.

Schnitker, L., Nović, A., Arendts, G., et al. (2020). Prevention of delirium in older adults with dementia: A systematic literature review. *Journal of Gerontological Nursing, 46*(10). doi:10.3928/00989134-20200820-02.

Sidani, S., Streiner, D., & Leclerc, C. (2012). Evaluating the effectiveness of the abilities-focused approach to morning care of people with dementia. *International Journal of Older People Nursing, 7*(1), 37–45. doi:10.1111/j.1748-3743.2011.00273.x.

Simpson, M., Macias Tejada, J., Driscoll, A., et al. (2019). The bundled Hospital Elder Life Program—HELP and HELP in Home Care—and its association with clinical outcomes among older adults discharged to home healthcare. *Journal of the American Geriatrics Society, 67*(8), 1730–1736. doi:10.1111/jgs.15979.

Singh, R., & Sadiq, N. M. (2020). *Cholinesterase inhibitors.* StatPearls. https://www.ncbi.nlm.nih.gov/books/NBK544336/.

Stall, N. M., Kim, S. J., Hardacre, K. A., et al. (2019). Association of informal caregiver distress with health outcomes of community-dwelling dementia care recipients: A systematic review. *Journal of the American Geriatrics Society, 67*(3), 609–617. doi:10.1111/jgs.15690.

Szabo, S., Lakzadeh, P., Cline, S., et al. (2019). The clinical and economic burden among caregivers of patients with Alzheimer's disease in Canada. *International Journal of Geriatric Psychiatry, 34*(11), 1677–1688. doi:10.1002/gps.5182.

Tyrrell, M. P. (2014). The progressively lowered stress threshold model. In J. J. Fitzpatrick & G. McCarthy (Eds.), *Theories guiding nursing research and practice: Making nursing knowledge development explicit* (pp. 141–158). Springer.

Voyer, P., Champoux, N., Desrosiers, J., et al. (2016). RADAR: A measure of the sixth vital sign? *Clinical Nursing Research, 25*(1), 9–29. doi:10.1177/1054773815603346.

Voyer, P., Émond, M., Boucher, V., et al. (2017). RADAR: A rapid detection tool for signs of delirium (6th vital sign) in emergency departments. *Canadian Journal of Emergency Nursing, 40*(2), 37–43. doi:10.29173/cjen79.

Walaszek, A. (2020). *Behavioral and psychological symptoms of dementia.* American Psychiatric Association Publishing.

Walsh, K. A., Dennehy, R., Sinnott, C., et al. (2017). Influences on decision-making regarding antipsychotic prescribing in nursing home residents with dementia: A systematic review and synthesis of qualitative evidence. *Journal of the American Medical Directors Association, 18*(10), 897.e1–897.e12. doi:10.1016/j.jamda.2017.06.032.

Webkamigad, S., Cote-Meek, S., Pianosi, B., et al. (2020a). Exploring the appropriateness of culturally safe dementia information with Indigenous people in an urban northern Ontario community. *Canadian Journal on Aging, 39*(2), 235–246. doi:10.1017/S0714980819000606.

Webkamigad, S., Warry, W., Blind, M., et al. (2020b). An approach to improve dementia health literacy in Indigenous communities. *Journal of Cross-Cultural Gerontology, 35*(1), 69–83. doi:10.1007/s10823-019-09388-2.

Weigel, K. A. (2017). Patient-/person-centred care. In S. Schüssler & C. Lohrmann (Eds.), *Dementia in nursing homes* (pp. 1–248). Springer.

Wells, D. L., & Dawson, P. (2000). Description of retained abilities in older persons with dementia. *Research in Nursing and Health, 23*(2), 158–166. doi:10.1002/(SICI)1098-240X(200004)23:2<158::AID-NUR8>3.0.CO;2-L.

Wong, S. L., Gilmour, H., & Ramage-Morin, P. L. (2016). Alzheimer's disease and other dementias in Canada. *Health Reports, 27*(5), 11–16.

Young, J. J., Lavakumar, M., Tampi, D., et al. (2018). Frontotemporal dementia: Latest evidence and clinical implications. *Therapeutic Advances in Psychopharmacology, 8*(1), 33–48. doi:10.1177/2045125317739818.

22

NEUROLOGICAL DISORDERS

■ ■ ■ ■ ■ ■ ■ ■ ■ ■ ■ ■ ■ ■ ■ ■ ■ ■ ■ ■

LEARNING OBJECTIVES

Upon completion of this chapter, the reader will be able to:

- Explain the differences between hemorrhagic stroke, ischemic stroke, and transient ischemic attack.
- Identify strategies to decrease the risk of having a transient ischemic attack or stroke.
- Develop a nursing care plan for a patient with cerebrovascular disease.
- Describe the effects of Parkinson's disease.
- Develop a nursing care plan for a patient with Parkinson's disease.

GLOSSARY

Dysarthria A speech disorder caused by a weakness or incoordination of the muscles used for speech.

Subarachnoid space The space under the arachnoid membrane and above the pia mater; it may fill with blood during a cerebral hemorrhage.

THE LIVED EXPERIENCE

"I thank God that it (my hand) has come back. I picked up a glass, and said "I'm going to drink" (shows how she drinks). I had to put the glass back down again. And I tried the whole time, and talked to my hand. "Come on, come on" and in the end I saw two fingers move. On the Friday I had a ball in my hand and I could throw it away . . . So I screamed (of joy), and the physiotherapist screamed, because it was so fantastic!" (Woman, 63 years old)

Törnbom, K., Lundälv, J., Palstam, A., et al. (2019). "My life after stroke through a camera lens"—A photovoice study on participation in Sweden. *PLOS One, 14*(9), e0222099. doi:10.1371/journal.pone.0222099.

HEALTHY AGING CARE PLAN

About R.P.

R.P. (pronouns they/them), 63 years old, lives with their daughter and her family. R.P.'s diabetes is controlled with diet. They enjoy spending time with their friends and family, especially their grandchildren. One afternoon, R.P.'s grandson noticed that R.P.'s speech was slurred and there was weakness in their right hand. The grandson called 911. Most of R.P.'s symptoms resolved within a few hours while at the emergency department. R.P. was diagnosed as having had a transient ischemic attack. They were referred to the stroke clinic and physiotherapy in the next couple of days. R.P. tells the nurse at the stroke clinic that they are relieved that they recovered so quickly. They're not sure that they need to come back to the clinic, but R.P.'s daughter and family are worried about R.P. and want them to continue the regular check-in appointments.

QUESTIONS TO CONSIDER

1. How do you respond to R.P.'s uncertainty about attending follow-up appointments at the clinic?
2. What are the priority health teaching needs for R.P. and their family?

Neurological disorders are seen in older adults more than any other age group. The dementias, described in Chapter 21, are among the most common neurological disorders affecting older adults. In this chapter, we discuss Parkinson's disease (PD), another common neurological disorder. We also include the cerebrovascular conditions of the transient ischemic attack (TIA) and stroke. Although these are cardiovascular in origin, their effects are neurological. These disorders have the potential to significantly impair a person's function and affect every aspect of life at some point. Like dementia, PD is neurodegenerative in nature in that it is a terminal condition characterized by a progressive decline in function leading to death.

The nurse plays an active role in helping the patient and family navigate the health care system, with care focused on rehabilitation whenever possible and always on comfort. The goal is to minimize the loss of function for a long as possible. Care may occur in the acute care, long-term care, and rehabilitation settings and in the person's home. In the case of cerebrovascular disease, the nurse is active in health promotion and disease prevention by promoting strategies to decrease risk of disease and in secondary prevention by ensuring a prompt diagnosis and treatment at the time of the acute event. Finally, the gerontological nurse helps patients and those who love them cope with the changes inherent in these disorders, including grief support (see Chapters 25 and 27).

CEREBROVASCULAR DISEASE

Cerebrovascular disease, a group of pathological processes in cerebral blood vessels that results in brain injury, is the most commonly occurring neurological disorder. Cerebrovascular disease is either ischemic or hemorrhagic and manifests as either a stroke or a TIA. The initial signs and symptoms of different kinds of stroke and TIA are similar, but the underlying pathology is different. Diagnosis is therefore geared toward identifying the specific cause of the symptoms and the location of the brain injury. Only when the cause is known can appropriate therapy be implemented.

Although the rate of stroke and death from stroke is decreasing, the aging population means that the number of people who will experience a stroke is increasing. Stroke is the third most common cause of death (Public Health Agency of Canada, 2019). Each year in Canada, about 62,000 people have a stroke (Heart and Stroke Foundation of Canada, 2018). One in 10 Canadians aged 65 and older are affected by stroke, with more than 75% of all strokes occurring in that age group. Premenopausal women are at lower risk than men are, and people with a family history of stroke are at higher risk. Indigenous peoples and people of African or South Asian descent are at higher risk because they are more likely to have high blood pressure and diabetes (Heart and Stroke Foundation of Canada, 2018). Among older adults, men are more likely than women to have a stroke (Public Health Agency of Canada, 2019). However, women are more likely than men to die following a stroke—they tend to have worse outcomes, are less likely to participate in rehabilitation, and are less likely than men to go home after a stroke (Heart and Stroke Foundation of Canada, 2018). People who have had a stroke or TIA are at increased risk of having another. In Canada, about 405,000 people are living with the effects of a stroke (Heart and Stroke Foundation of Canada, 2018).

Etiology

Ischemic Events

Ischemic stroke occurs when arterial blood flow is blocked, resulting in insufficient supply of blood and oxygen and the death of brain cells. The three most common causes of ischemic strokes are arterial disease, thromboembolism, and intracranial small-vessel disease (lacunar strokes). Ischemic strokes can also be associated with hematological disorders and systemic hypoperfusion. Arterial disease in the form of atherosclerosis is the most common cause. About one-third of ischemic strokes are caused by cardioembolism (Norrving, 2014). Cardioembolism includes events caused by a dysrhythmia such as atrial fibrillation, which is frequently seen in coronary heart disease (see Chapter 20). Lacunar strokes are rare. They result from blockage of a single deep penetrating artery—for example, in the basal ganglia, thalamus, or brainstem (Norrving, 2014). Hematological disorders include coagulation disorders and hyperviscosity syndromes. Systemic hypoperfusion can occur with cardiac failure, pulmonary embolism, or reduced blood supply due to bleeding (Boss et al., 2018a).

TIAs share the same underlying disease processes as atherosclerotic stroke. They have different clinical presentations, as the symptoms of a TIA begin to resolve within minutes, and all neurological deficits caused by it resolve within 24 hours. A person who has a TIA is at risk for stroke or another TIA; 2% to 4% have a stroke within the next 1 to 3 months, and about 10% have a stroke within the next year (Boulanger et al., 2018). In some cases, a TIA is followed by a stroke, yet most strokes are not preceded by TIAs. Clinical characteristics of the TIA, age of the patient, and presence of comorbid diabetes have been used to predict a subsequent stroke. However, there are no validated predictor tools. Urgent clinical assessment by a stroke specialist is required, including assessment for possible atrial fibrillation or carotid stenosis, conditions that significantly increase the risk of subsequent stroke (Boulanger et al., 2018). TIA is more prevalent in men than in women, and more prevalent in older adults.

Hemorrhagic Events

Hemorrhagic strokes are less frequent than ischemic strokes but are more life-threatening. They are primarily caused by uncontrolled hypertension and less often by malformations of the blood vessels (e.g., aneurysms). Although the exact mechanism is not fully understood, it appears that chronic hypertension causes thickening of the vessel wall, microaneurysms, and necrosis. When enough damage to the vessel accumulates, it is at risk for rupture. The rupture may be large and acute, or it may be small, with a slow leakage of blood into the adjacent brain tissue. In many cases, there is a rupture or seepage of blood into the ventricular system of the brain and damage to the affected tissue through necrosis (Boss et al., 2018a). Resolution of the event can occur only with the resorption of excess blood and damaged tissue. Hemorrhagic strokes are more life-threatening than ischemic strokes but are much less frequent.

Signs and Symptoms of Cerebrovascular Disease

The first signs of both strokes and TIAs are acute neurological deficits consistent with the part of the brain affected. Hemorrhagic strokes are often heralded by a severe headache. In **subarachnoid** hemorrhage, which usually results from a cerebral aneurysm, headache may be the main symptom, without other neurological manifestations (Boss et al., 2018a).

Clinical signs and symptoms of ischemic and hemorrhagic stroke are similar, making it difficult to distinguish the type of stroke based on symptoms. Persons with hemorrhage have more focal neurological changes, including seizures and a more depressed level of consciousness, than persons who have an ischemic stroke. If a deep unresponsive state occurs, the person is unlikely to survive (Boss et al., 2018a). Nausea and vomiting are suggestions of increased cerebral edema in response to an event of either type. Clinical effects of stroke depend on the location of the stroke, which artery is affected, and which side of the brain it affects. Neurological deficits include alterations in coordination, cognition, language, and motor, sensory, and visual function (see Table 22.1)

TABLE 22.1
Stroke Manifestations Related to Artery Involvement

Artery	Deficit or Syndrome
Anterior cerebral	Motor or sensory deficit (contralateral), or both; sucking or rooting reflex; rigidity; gait problems; loss of proprioception, fine touch
Middle cerebral	*Dominant side:* Aphasia, motor or sensory deficit, hemianopia (blindness of half of the field of vision) *Nondominant side:* Neglect, motor and sensory deficit, hemianopia
Posterior cerebral	Hemianopia, visual hallucination, spontaneous pain, motor deficit
Vertebral	Cranial nerve deficits, diplopia, dizziness, nausea, vomiting, dysarthria, dysphagia, coma

Source: Zomorodi, M., & Elliott, D. (2019). Stroke. In S. L. Lewis, L. Bucher, M. McLean Heitkemper, et al. (Eds.), *Medical-surgical nursing in Canada* (4th Canadian ed., pp. 1507–1533). Elsevier.

Diagnosis

Diagnosis includes the determination of possible extra-cerebral causes (e.g., infection or hypoglycemia), the confirmation of stroke and identification of the exact location of the damage in the brain through computed tomography (CT) or magnetic resonance imaging (MRI), and additional diagnostic investigations to identify risk for another stroke or TIA. These include vascular imaging of the carotid artery, electrocardio-gram (ECG) to identify atrial fibrillation or heart disease, and bloodwork (Boulanger et al., 2018).

Complications

After a TIA resolves, there should be no residual effect other than an increased chance of recurrence and in-creased risk for stroke. Early complications of a simple stroke include extension of the amount of damage and recurrence. Brain edema, which occurs in 10% to 15% of strokes, is associated with increased mortality. Signs include nausea, vomiting, dizziness, headache, worsening neurological deficits, and declining level of consciousness (Arora & O'Phelan, 2019).

Although the potential long-term effects of a stroke may be minimal, they may include paralysis and hemipa-resis, **dysarthria**, dysphagia, and aphasia. Effects depend on type, extent, and area affected. Poststroke depression negatively affects rehabilitation (see Chapter 23).

Whenever paralysis results from a stroke, there is a risk of the development of spasticity in the affected limb or limbs. Spasticity can lead to contractures if it is not managed. Pain in the affected side is common and may be treated with muscle relaxants or medications specific for neuropathic pain. (See Chapter 3 for a dis-cussion of aphasia, and Chapter 8 for a discussion of dysphagia.) Iatrogenic complications include deep vein thrombosis, aspiration pneumonia, urinary tract infec-tions, and medication toxicity (Behrouz & Birnbaum, 2019). Vascular dementia is more common in people who have a history of hypertension, TIAs, or stroke (see Chapter 21). Delirium occurs in 25% of patients post-stroke and is associated with worse outcomes (Shaw et al., 2019) (see Chapter 21).

Management

All actual or potential cerebrovascular events should be treated as emergencies. However, because TIAs are highly transient, they often resolve on their own before the affected person is seen by a health care provider. Instead, the person reports, "I think I had a small stroke last week," or they do not seek care at all. If the deficits and symptoms were fleeting, the diagnosis is made through the clinical interview. Management of TIA is considered preventive; its aim is to prevent recurrences and to reduce the risk factors for strokes (Boulanger et al., 2018) (Box 22.1). The person and family are also instructed in the appropriate emer-gency response to the return of any signs or symptoms of a stroke or another TIA. Anticoagulant therapy pre-vents recurrent embolic strokes and TIAs. Acetylsali-cylic acid (Aspirin; 81–325 mg per day) is the mainstay of therapy for persons with TIAs, and clopidogrel (Plavix) may be used for persons who are Aspirin sensitive (Boulanger et al., 2018). Oral anticoagulants are usually used to prevent another stroke, and for those with atrial fibrillation, they are used to prevent the occurrence of the first stroke (Ying et al., 2017).

Acute management is usually accomplished in emergency departments, critical care units, and spe-cialize acute stroke units. Acute stroke units are associ-ated with better outcomes and are the recommended site for treatment (Boulanger et al., 2018). However, 15% of Canadians do not have access to these units owing to geographic barriers (Heart and Stroke Foun-dation of Canada, 2020a). The acute management of the stroke requires careful attention to the accuracy of the diagnosis. Reperfusion therapy with recombinant tissue–type plasminogen activator (rt-PA) is used to

---

BOX 22.1
RISK FACTORS FOR STROKE

Heart disease and risk factors for heart disease
Hypertension
Arrhythmias
Hypercholesterolemia
Diabetes
Smoking
Heavy alcohol use
Physical inactivity
Diet low in fruit and vegetables
Self-perceived stress
Coagulopathies
Brain tumours
Family history

dissolve an occlusion. It is used for ischemic strokes if a CT scan confirms the absence of hemorrhage. It should be started within 4.5 hours of the first symptoms of stroke (Boulanger et al., 2018). The sooner rt-PA or other appropriate treatment is begun, the better the chances for recovery. The initial response to a hemorrhagic stroke is to find a means to stop the bleeding rather than dissolve an occlusion (Box 22.2).

Most recovery occurs during the first 3 months after a stroke. Recovery can continue for years at a slower pace (Bowker, 2018). The inverse relationship between functional improvement and advanced age, social isolation, and emotional distress is clear. Recovery from a stroke is affected by the location and extent of the brain damage. Between 40% and 50% of stroke survivors are independent 1 year poststroke (Bowker, 2018). Difficulties and handicaps after stroke often involve neurological and functional deficits.

The interprofessional team is essential to the care of the person after a stroke. The needs assessment after a stroke is extremely complex and requires a team coordinated by a nurse that includes a neurologist, a physiatrist, a speech pathologist, an occupational therapist, a physiotherapist, an ophthalmologist, a rehabilitation specialist, a psychologist, a social worker, and a spiritual advisor. The older adult's family members, who may be involved with the day-to-day life and needs of the person after a stroke, are also included. The Canadian Heart and Stroke Foundation provides excellent educational resources, as well as support groups, for persons affected by stroke and their families. (See Resources at the end of this chapter.)

IMPLICATIONS FOR GERONTOLOGICAL NURSING AND HEALTHY AGING

The best approach to stroke is prevention and prompt intervention. Identifying high-risk or stroke-prone persons is something nurses can do in their patient's homes, in the community, or at the health facilities where they work. Following an assessment of risk factors (see Box 22.1), the nurse can work with individuals to reduce their risk for stroke or stroke recurrence.

Smoking cessation and control of blood pressure may be the most important strategies for reducing modifiable risk factors. Maintaining a blood pressure equal to or less than 130/85 mm Hg is recommended. Additional prevention includes a healthy diet, limited salt and alcohol intake, and acetylsalicylic acid therapy unless contraindicated. Controlling lipids and diabetes and preventing atrial fibrillation are helpful, as well as regular exercise and weight-management programs. Nurse-led atrial fibrillation clinics increase accessibility, are cost effective, and have positive patient outcomes (Rush et al., 2019).

It is imperative that treatment start within hours of first stroke symptoms, yet many people do not know the signs of stroke. Health teaching about how to recognize and respond to symptoms of TIA and stroke is important. This should include recommendations to call 911 if the person experiences the FAST signs (Fig. 22.1) or sudden onset of vision changes, severe headache, numbness, or problems with balance (Heart and Stroke Foundation of Canada, 2020b). Culturally appropriate health education for stroke recognition and prevention is needed (Box 22.3). For example, educating children about stroke is a way to transfer knowledge to their parents and families. A Canadian participatory community-based study arose from Indigenous Elders' identifying the education of children about stroke as a way to improve stroke outcomes (Hill et al., 2017). It resulted in the creation of a culturally responsive educational DVD for children called F-A-S-T-1-2-3.

Nursing assessment during the acute period includes general and neurological assessments (Table 22.2; also see Chapter 21). Aspiration and sepsis precautions, maintaining cardiovascular homeostasis, safety precautions,

---

BOX 22.2
SAFETY ALERT

REPERFUSION THERAPY WITH RECOMBINANT TISSUE–TYPE PLASMINOGEN ACTIVATOR

Reperfusion therapy (using recombinant tissue plasminogen activator) can be used only for ischemic strokes and only if a CT scan confirms the absence of hemorrhage and is performed within 4.5 hours of the onset of the event.

Source: Boulanger, J. M., Butcher, K., Gubitz, G., et al. (2018). *Canadian stroke best practice recommendations. Acute stroke management: Prehospital, emergency department, and acute inpatient stroke care.* Heart and Stroke Foundation. https://www.heartandstroke.ca/-/media/1-stroke-best-practices/acute-stroke-management/csbpr2018-acute-stroke-module-final-17jul2018-en.ashx.

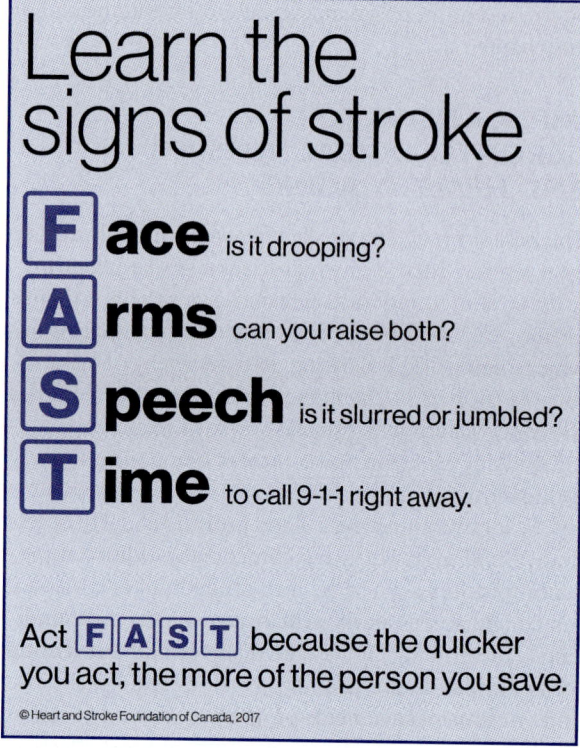

Fig. 22.1 ■ FAST signs of stroke. ***Source:*** © 2017 Heart and Stroke Foundation of Canada. Reproduced with permission of the Heart and Stroke Foundation of Canada. https://www.heartandstroke.ca.

preventing skin breakdown, attention to bowel function, and optimizing musculo-skeletal function are necessary. Delirium prevention should be instituted (see Chapter 21). Dysphagia is common. Swallowing assessment is required prior to oral intake. Depending on severity of the stroke, eating may be a problem; a nasogastric or semipermanent percutaneous endoscopic gastrostomy (PEG) tube may be needed. Bladder retraining may be needed. Rehabilitation begins as soon as possible in the acute care setting, beginning with mobilization within a day or two after the stroke, depending on the stroke's severity (Mehroholz, 2019).

The goals of nursing care include maximizing the person's capacity for self-care, improving the person's quality of life, and preventing iatrogenic complications. A period of intense rehabilitation often takes place in a rehabilitation or complex continuing care facility setting and continues long after the person returns home

BOX 22.3
RESEARCH FOR EVIDENCE-INFORMED PRACTICE: STROKE PREVENTION IN ARAB MUSLIM IMMIGRANT WOMEN IN CANADA

Problem: Risk factors for stroke are higher among Arab immigrants in Western countries and stroke outcomes are worse. Arab immigrants experience barriers to accessing health services. Many women do not know the signs of stroke. There is a need for culturally appropriate stroke prevention policy and practice. This study examined stroke prevention practices among Arab immigrant women.

Method: Interpretive description using an intersectionality perspective. Sixteen middle-aged and older women who live in Edmonton, Alberta, and self-identify as Arab immigrants were interviewed.

Findings: Five themes were identified: (1) Women identified life stressors as precipitants of chronic illness conditions. (2) Women at high risk for stroke did not know the signs of stroke, even when they knew that they were at risk for stroke. (3) Participants had negative views of taking and continuing to take medications. This was associated with their personal beliefs and with limited health coverage for the cost of medications and treatments. (4) Participants made efforts to eat healthy and exercise. Barriers to exercise included efficacy beliefs, household obligations, transportation, and access to culturally appropriate facilities. (5) Participants identified three elements that empowered them. English-language competence and being able to drive were associated with viewing themselves as healthy. However, access to language classes was problematic. Religious practices and faith were connected to views of health and stress management.

Implications for Nursing Practice: Stress management and faith-based approaches were identified as potential ways to reach these women. Structural barriers to health-promoting behaviours, including transportation, cost, and language of services, need to be addressed.

Source: Salma, J., Hunter, K. F., Ogilvie, L., et al. (2018). An intersectional exploration: Experiences of stroke prevention in middle-aged and older Arab Muslim immigrant women in Canada. *Canadian Journal of Nursing Research, 50*(3), 110–119. doi:10.1177/0844562118760076.

or to an assisted-living setting. Important roles for the nurse include documenting clearly and in detail the functional capacities that are retained and those that are impaired, assessing and supporting the coping abilities of the patient and family, and evaluating mental status (see Chapter 23). For family members, adjusting

TABLE 22.2	
Assessment of Person After Stroke or TIA	
General	**Neurological**
Vital signs	Level of arousal, orientation, attention
Cardiovascular	Speech (dysarthria, dysphasia)
Respiratory	Cranial nerves
Gastrointestinal	Motor function and response
Urinary	Proprioception
	Sensation
	Gait (if possible)
	Reflexes

to changes in the patient's functioning and relationship changes, grieving lost expectations, and coping with the caregiving demands can be overwhelming (Kokorelias et al., 2020). Psychoeducational programs for family caregivers may reduce caregiver burden (Mores et al., 2018) (see Chapter 25).

PARKINSON'S DISEASE

PD is one of the most common neurodegenerative diseases. It was first described in 1817 by Dr. James Parkinson, a British physician, who described "the shaking palsy" and major symptoms of the disease.

Etiology

PD is a slowly progressing disease that results from the destruction of the cells in the substantia nigra in the brain. As the nigrostriatal pathway deteriorates, it is no longer able to produce the neurotransmitter dopamine. Dopamine loss also occurs in the brainstem, thalamus, and cortex. Dopamine plays a major role in regulating movement; thus, PD is considered a movement disorder. Changes in dopamine neurons begin at least 3 to 6 years before symptom onset. The average age of onset is 60 years (Boss et al., 2018b).

The exact cause of PD is unknown. PD is more common in men than in women (Boss et al., 2018b). There is conflicting evidence about other possible risk factors. Tobacco and caffeine use may be associated with lower risk for PD. Environmental exposures (for example, exposure to pesticides) may interact with genetic factors, but evidence of causal associations is limited (Hu et al., 2019).

PD is classified as either primary or secondary parkinsonism. Primary parkinsonism is either idiopathic or genetic. In about 10% of people who have primary PD, the disorder appears to have a familial component (Boss et al., 2018b). Secondary parkinsonism occurs as a secondary effect of another disorder that causes loss of or interference with the action of dopamine in the basal ganglia (e.g., head trauma, postencephalitic parkinsonism, stroke, tumours, and toxin- and medication-induced parkinsonian syndrome).

Signs and Symptoms

PD has an insidious onset and usually progresses very slowly, making it difficult to diagnose, particularly in the early stages. Diagnosis consists of ruling out other possible causes of symptoms. When there is no other explanation, a diagnosis is made based on the presence of two of the four classic symptoms (Box 22.4). One of these symptoms must be either a resting tremor or bradykinesia ("paucity of movement") (Soileau, 2017). Diagnosis is supported by a challenge test in which a person with symptoms is given a dose of levodopa; if there is significant and rapid improvement, the diagnosis is thought to be confirmed. Falls early in the course of the illness, poor response to levodopa, symmetry of motor symptoms, lack of tremor, and early autonomic dysfunction (e.g., incontinence) are conditions that may be useful in distinguishing PD from other motor disorders (Soileau, 2017).

The most conspicuous sign of PD is an asymmetrical, regular, rhythmic, low-amplitude tremor. It disappears briefly during voluntary movement and increases with stress and anxiety. Tremor, however, is a minor part of the clinical picture. Other symptoms that can cause disability include rigidity and postural instability. The characteristic gait is called "festination" and consists of very short steps and minimal arm movement. Postural reflexes are lost. The person has difficulty initiating movement. "Freezing" is a common problem and may be precipitated by trying to move, by turning, or by initiating tactile and visual contact. The person will have involuntary flexion of the head and neck, a stooped posture, and a tendency to fall backward. If the person is off balance, correction is very slow, so falls are common. A person with moderately advanced PD will

BOX 22.4
SIGNS AND SYMPTOMS OF PARKINSON'S DISEASE

CLASSIC SIGNS AND SYMPTOMS

Bradykinesia (slowness of movement)
Tremor at rest (trembling in hands, arms, legs, jaw, or face)
Cogwheel rigidity (resistance of the limbs and trunk in a jerking manner)
Postural instability (impaired balance and coordination)

OTHER SIGNS

Disordered sleep
Constipation
Fatigue
Excessive salivation
Pain
Depression
Visual disturbances
Psychosis
Seborrhea
Excessive sweating
Hypertension
Soft-spoken voice
Little facial animation
Infrequent blinking
Restless legs

Nonmotor symptoms become more common as PD progresses. One-third of persons with PD have symptoms of depression, which is associated with worse outcomes (Goodarzi & Ismail, 2017). Anxiety and apathy are common, and in later stages over one-third of patients experience psychosis (Armstrong & Okun, 2020). About one-quarter of patients with PD have mild cognitive impairment at the time of diagnosis. Between 15% and 20% have dementia by 5 years after diagnosis, with prevalence increasing to close to 50% by 10 years (Aarsland et al., 2017).

The symptoms of PD worsen over time. The symptoms vary, and their intensity also varies from person to person; some persons become severely disabled, but others experience only minor motor disturbances. The progression of symptoms may take 20 years or more. In the late stages of the disease, complications such as pressure ulcers, pneumonia, aspiration, and falls can lead to death.

Management

The management of PD focuses on relieving symptoms with medication, increasing functional ability, preventing excess disability, and reducing the risk of injury.

Medication therapy focuses on dopamine replacement, mimicking, or slowing dopamine breakdown. The choice of medication is based on specific symptoms, the person's age, potential benefits and risks of adverse effects, and disease progression (Armstrong & Okun, 2020). First-line approaches include a combination of carbidopa and levodopa (Sinemet) or other dopamine agonists (pramipexole [Miraplex] or ropinirole [Requip]). Monoamine oxidase inhibitors (MAIOs) such as selegiline (Eldepryl) and rasagiline (Azitect) are also used in initial treatment (Armstrong & Okun, 2020). People who are taking MAOIs must avoid food or drink containing tyramine because of interactions that cause sudden and severe rises in blood pressure, leading to stroke or death (Box 22.5). Sinemet loses effectiveness since the amino acid levodopa competes with other amino acids for absorption at both the intestinal wall and the blood–brain barrier. It also poses a higher risk for the adverse effect dyskinesia (involuntary movement).

Other medications useful in PD management are the dopamine agonists catechol-*O*-methyltransferase

typically be bent forward from the waist but with the head up, standing still, and then suddenly moving forward relatively rapidly but in a shuffling manner and with small steps. The person may come to a sudden halt, only to start all over again, clearly with effort. The necessity of high-back wheelchairs is common sometime during the course of the illness.

Rigidity, a state of involuntary contractions of all striated muscles, impedes both passive and active movement. Severe muscle cramps may occur in the toes or hands. When examined, a limb may exhibit either "lead pipe" or "cogwheel" (intermittent) resistance during passive movement. All the striated muscles in the extremities, trunk, ocular area, and face are affected, including the muscles of mastication (chewing), deglutition (swallowing), and articulation. Handwriting is small (micrographia). The person with PD will sit for long periods or lie motionless with few shifts in position and few changes in facial expression (Boss et al., 2018b). This lack of movement puts the person at high risk for pressure ulcers.

(COMT) inhibitors, antihistamines, and anticholinergics (for tremor relief) (Armstrong & Okun, 2020). Although anticholinergics are not usually recommended for use in older adults because of their high association with falls, they are sometimes necessary for the person with PD. Amantadine may be used to reduce dyskinesia. Many of the medications may be used in combination for specific effects.

Persons who are stable on Sinemet are often followed by their primary care providers (Box 22.6). However, when this treatment is no longer effective, such persons are more often cared for by neurologists specializing in PD.

Medication therapy is complicated and should be closely supervised. The medications used to treat PD are not without serious side effects. Hypotension, dyskinesia (involuntary movement), dystonia (lack of control of movement), hallucinations, sleep disorders, and depression are common effects of the disease and side effects of the medications used to treat it. The medications of choice for depression are the selective serotonin reuptake inhibitors (SSRIs), such as sertraline and paroxetine, and the serotonin–norepinephrine reuptake inhibitors (SNRIs), such as venlafaxine. Bupropion, which is neither an SSRI nor an SNRI, is also used. Tricyclic antidepressants may be used but have a higher risk of adverse effects (Armstrong & Okun, 2020).

Cholinesterase inhibitors may be used for the cognitive impairment and dementia associated with PD.

However, many patients do not benefit, and the gastrointestinal side effects may be significant (Seppi et al., 2019). Deep-brain stimulation or MRI-guided focused ultrasound may be used in patients who have not responded to drug therapy or who have intractable motor fluctuations, dyskinesias, or tremor (Armstrong & Okun, 2020).

Nonpharmacological interventions such as exercise therapy, speech therapy (for those with dysarthria), relaxation, stress management, education, self-care management, and caregiver support should be considered.

IMPLICATIONS FOR GERONTOLOGICAL NURSING AND HEALTHY AGING

Ongoing nursing care focuses on enhancing quality of life, increasing functional ability, preventing excess disability, and decreasing the risk of injury. Persons with PD experience great functional problems in mobility, communication, and performance of activities of daily living (ADLs). Collaboration with and between health care providers is important to people with PD (Box 22.7). Integrated team care models result in better quality-of-life outcomes (Rajan et al., 2020). Within these teams, nurses provide direct care and act as care coordinators. The teams may include movement disorders neurologists, rehabilitation professionals (physiotherapists, occupational therapists, speech therapists), PD specialist nurses, social workers, psychologists, and dietitians.

The goal of treatment is to preserve self-care abilities and prevent complications. Comprehensive functional assessments with attention to self-care abilities in ADLs and nutritional assessment are important (see Chapter 8), as well as fall assessment and risk-reduction interventions. Nursing interventions can contribute to quality of life and functional ability. Information about the disease, support for self-management, and opportunity to discuss the future are important for patients and family caregivers to cope and to plan for the future (see Box 22.7). The Sickness Impact Profile is a helpful tool that can be used by nurses to determine the issues that are most troublesome from the person's perspective. Many resources are available for people with PD that provide practical information about living with the disease, as well as information about new developments and treatments. (See the Resources section at the end of this chapter for more information.)

BOX 22.7
HEALTH CARE NEEDS OF PATIENTS WITH PARKINSON'S DISEASE

1. Support for self-management.
2. Effective collaboration between health care providers.
3. Time to discuss the future.
4. Effective case management with a single point of access.

Source: Adapted from Vlaanderen, F. P., Rompen, L., Munneke, M., et al. (2019). The voice of the Parkinson customer. *Journal of Parkinson's Disease, 9*(1), 197–201. doi:10.3233/JPD-181431.

People in the patient's support network, including family and friends, need information and guidance as the disease progresses. Family caregivers initially support deficits in ADLs. As the disease progresses and if the person develops dementia, their caregiving needs increase. Caregivers of those with dementia and PD experience more burden, distress, and dissatisfaction than do caregivers of patients with either PD or dementia (Roland & Chappell, 2019) (see Chapter 23).

Exercise—including walking, moving all the joints, and improving balance—needs to be included early in the course of PD; physical therapy evaluation and treatment are important. Rigidity of facial muscles and bradykinesia can affect eating ability, nutrition, swallowing, and communicating. Occupational therapy can assist the person in using adaptive equipment such as weighted utensils, nonslip dinnerware, and other self-care aids. Speech therapy is beneficial for dysarthria and dysphagia (swallowing difficulty). Patients can be taught facial exercises and swallowing techniques.

Regular pain assessments and appropriate pain management are also essential to address the often-unnoticed problem of pain related to rigidity, contractures, dystonia, and central-pain syndromes of the disease itself (see Chapter 16). Other important interventions are the treatments of postural hypotension, incontinence (see Chapter 9), gastro-intestinal distress, depression and anxiety (see Chapter 23), sleep disturbances (see Chapter 10), and constipation (see Chapter 9).

Because of the usually slow progression of the disease and the disability that accompanies PD, affected persons experience changes in roles, activities, and social participation. Tremors may produce embarrassing moments. The expressionless face, slowed movement, and soft, monotone speech may give the impression of apathy, depression, or disinterest and might discourage others from socializing with affected individuals. Observing these symptoms, others may think that the person is unable to participate in activities and relationships and may even think the person is cognitively impaired. A sensitive nurse is aware that the visible symptoms produce an undesired facade that may hide an alert and responsive individual who wishes to interact but is trapped in a body that no longer responds. It is important to see beyond the disease to the person and provide nursing interventions that enhance the person's hope and promote the highest quality of life despite the disease.

KEY CONCEPTS

- Ischemic stroke is caused by a temporary loss of oxygen to the brain, resulting in damage to the tissue. Symptoms persist for at least 24 hours.
- Transient ischemic attack has the same cause as ischemic stroke but symptoms resolve within hours.
- Hemorrhagic stroke results from a ruptured blood vessel in the brain. It is less common than ischemic stroke but much more deadly.
- For the best possible outcome, immediate treatment is required for the person having a transient ischemic attack or stroke. People need to know the signs and symptoms of stroke and how to activate the emergency response system.
- Correct diagnosis of the type of stroke is necessary before treatment can begin.
- Nursing care for patients with stroke varies depending on the effect of the stroke on functioning and the stage of treatment.
- Nursing care for patients with stroke is focused on maximizing capabilities, functioning, and quality of life and preventing iatrogenic complications.
- Parkinson's disease is a progressive, incurable disorder that affects voluntary control of movement and cognition.
- Collaborative care of Parkinson's disease focuses on symptom relief, maximizing functioning, promoting safety, preventing complications, and supporting the coping of the patient and family.

ACTIVITIES AND DISCUSSION QUESTIONS

1. What would you say to a person who reports to you that they have had symptoms of a transient ischemic attack?

2. What safety considerations would be important in planning nursing care for a person who has experienced a stroke?

3. How do the symptoms of Parkinson's disease affect functional abilities? What nursing interventions would be important when caring for a person with Parkinson's disease?

HEALTHY AGING CARE PLAN

Caring for R.P.

Recall the *Lived Experience* testimonials and R.P.'s case presented at the beginning of the chapter.

1. As R.P.'s nurse in the stroke clinic, you inquire about their comfort with attending the clinic, empathizing with their perspective that it may not seem important to attend a clinic now that they are feeling better. You explain that people who experience TIAs are at increased risk for stroke and that attending the clinic means that R.P.'s symptoms will be thoroughly assessed to find out what caused them. You explain that there are things R.P. can do to help decrease their chance of having another TIA or stroke and that you will help R.P. with that.

2. You meet with R.P. and their daughter. First, you assess their knowledge about signs and symptoms of stroke and what to do if R.P. experiences symptoms. You explain and clarify their understanding of signs and symptoms. You reinforce that the grandson was correct to call 911. Second, you assess R.P. and their daughters' understanding of modifiable risks for stroke. Learning that the family adheres to a healthy diet, you reinforce the importance of maintaining it. You explore opportunities to increase R.P.'s activity level—for example, through activities with R.P.'s friends or grandchildren.

RESOURCES

Canadian Stroke Best Practices
http://www.strokebestpractices.ca/
Heart and Stroke Foundation of Canada
https://www.heartandstroke.ca/
Parkinson Canada
http://www.parkinson.ca
Regional Geriatric Program (RGP) Central. *Resources.*
http://www.rgpc.ca/resources/

For additional resources, please visit *http://evolve.elsevier.com/Canada/Ebersole/gerontological/*

REFERENCES

Aarsland, D., Cresse, B., Politis, M., et al. (2017). Cognitive decline in Parkinson disease. *Nature Reviews Neurology, 13*(4), 217–231. doi:110.1038/nrneurol.2017.27.

Armstrong, M. J., & Okun, M. S. (2020). Diagnosis and treatment of Parkinson disease: A review. *Journal of the American Medical Association, 323*(6), 548–560. doi:10.1001/jama.2019.22360.

Arora, N. A., & O'Phelan, K. H. (2019). Cerebral edema in stroke. In R. Behrouz & L. Birnbaum (Eds.), *Complications of acute stroke: A concise guide to prevention, recognition, and management* (pp. 59–78). Springer.

Behrouz, R., & Birnbaum, L. A. (2019). Complications of acute stroke: An introduction. In R. Behrouz & L. Birnbaum (Eds.), *Complications of acute stroke: A concise guide to prevention, recognition, and management* (pp. 1–8). Springer.

Boss, B. J., Huether, S. E., & Power-Kean, K. (2018a). Alterations in cognitive systems, cerebral hemodynamics, and motor function. In S. E. Huether, K. L. McCance, M. T. El-Hussein, et al. (Eds.), *Understanding pathophysiology, Canadian edition* (1st ed., pp. 363–393). Elsevier Health Sciences.

Boss, B. J., Heuther, S. E., & Power-Kean, K. (2018b). Disorders of the central and peripheral nervous systems and neuromuscular junction. In S. E. Huether, K. L. McCance, M. T. El-Hussein, K. Power-Kean, & S. Zettel (Eds.), *Understanding pathophysiology, Canadian Edition* (1st ed., pp. 394–425). Elsevier Health Sciences.

Boulanger, J. M., Butcher, K., Gubitz, G., et al. (2018). *Canadian stroke best practice recommendations. Acute stroke management: Prehospital, emergency department, and acute inpatient stroke care.*

https://www.heartandstroke.ca/-/media/1-stroke-best-practices/acute-stroke-management/csbpr2018-acute-stroke-module-final-17jul2018-en.ashx.

Bowker, L. K. (2018). Stroke. In L. K. Bowker, J. D. Price, K. S. Shah, et al. (Eds.), *Oxford handbook of geriatric medicine* (pp. 177–200). Oxford University Press.

Goodarzi, Z., & Ismail, Z. (2017). A practical approach to detection and treatment of depression in Parkinson disease and dementia. *Neurology: Clinical Practice, 7*(2), 128–140. doi:10.1212/CPJ.0000000000000351.

Heart and Stroke Foundation of Canada. (2018). *Lives disrupted: The impact of stroke on women.* https://www.heartandstroke.ca/-/media/pdf-files/canada/stroke-report/strokereport2018.ashx?la=en.

Heart and Stroke Foundation of Canada. (2020a). *Can Canadians get to stroke treatment in time?* https://www.heartandstroke.ca/articles/can-canadians-get-to-stroke-treatment-in-time.

Heart and Stroke Foundation of Canada. (2020b). *FAST signs of stroke . . . what are the other signs?* https://www.heartandstroke.ca/stroke/signs-of-stroke/fast-signs-of-stroke-are-there-other-signs.

Hill, M. E., Bodnar, P., Fenton, R., et al. (2017). Teach our children: Stroke education for Indigenous children, First Nations, Ontario, Canada, 2009–2012. *Preventing Chronic Disease, 14*, E68. doi:10.5888/pcd14.160506.

Hu, C. Y., Fang, Y., Li, F. L., et al. (2019). Association between ambient air pollution and Parkinson's disease: Systematic review and meta-analysis. *Environmental Research, 168*, 448–459. doi:10.1016/j.envres.2018.10.008.

Kokorelias, K. M., Lu, F. K. T., Santos, J. R., et al. (2020). "Caregiving is a full-time job" impacting stroke caregivers' health and well-being: A qualitative meta-synthesis. *Health & Social Care in the Community, 28*(2), 325–340. doi:10.1111/hsc.12895.

Mehroholz, J. (2019). Neurorehabilitation practice for stroke patients. In M. Brainin & W. Heiss (Eds.), *Textbook of stroke medicine* (pp. 426–448). Cambridge University Press. doi:10.1017/9781108659574.026.

Mores, G., Whiteman, R. M. N., Ploeg, J., et al. (2018). An evaluation of the family informal daregiver stroke self-management program.

Canadian Journal of Neurological Sciences, 45(6), 660–668. doi:10.1017/cjn.2018.335.

Norrving, B. (2014). Common causes of ischemic stroke. In M. Brainin & W.-D. Heiss (Eds.), *Textbook of stroke medicine* (pp. 33–44). Cambridge University Press. doi:10.1017/cbo9781107239340.003.

Public Health Agency of Canada. (2019). *Stroke in Canada: Highlights from the Canadian Chronic Disease Surveillance System.* https://www.canada.ca/content/dam/phac-aspc/documents/services/publications/diseases-conditions/stroke-vascularies/stroke-vascularies-canada-eng.pdf.

Rajan, R., Brennan, L., Bloem, B. R., et al. (2020). Integrated care in Parkinson's disease: A systematic review and meta-analysis. *Movement Disorders, 35*(9), 1509–1531. doi:10.1002/mds.28097.

Roland, K. P., & Chappell, N. L. (2019). Caregiver experiences across three neurodegenerative diseases: Alzheimer's, Parkinson's, and Parkinson's with dementia. *Journal of Aging and Health, 31*(2), 256–279. doi:10.1177/0898264317729980.

Rush, K. L., Burton, L., Schaab, K., et al. (2019). The impact of nurse-led atrial fibrillation clinics on patient and healthcare outcomes: A systematic mixed studies review. *European Journal of Cardiovascular Nursing, 18*(7), 526–533. doi:10.1177/1474515119845198.

Seppi, K., Ray Chaudhuri, K., Coelho, M., et al.. (2019). Update on treatments for nonmotor symptoms of Parkinson's disease—An evidence-based medicine review. *Movement Disorders, 34*(2), 180–198. doi:10.1002/mds.27602.

Shaw, R. C., Walker, G., Elliott, E., et al. (2019). Occurrence rate of delirium in acute stroke settings: Systematic review and meta-analysis. *Stroke, 50*(11), 3028–3036. doi:10.1161/STROKEAHA.119.025015.

Soileau, M. J. (2017). Defining idiopathic Parkinson's disease. In A. Armitage (Ed.), *A practical guide to Parkinson's disease: Diagnosis and management* (pp. 39–49). Springer.

Ying, B., Hai, D., Alena, S., et al. (2017). Rivaroxaban versus Dabigatran or Warfarin in real-world studies of stroke prevention in atrial fibrillation. *Stroke, 48*(4), 970–976. doi:10.1161/STROKEAHA.116.016275.

23

MENTAL HEALTH AND WELLNESS IN LATER LIFE

LEARNING OBJECTIVES

Upon completion of this chapter, the reader will be able to:

- Discuss factors contributing to mental health and wellness in later life.

- List symptoms of late-life anxiety and depression, and discuss assessment, treatment, and nursing interventions.

- Recognize older adults who are at risk for suicide, and use appropriate techniques for suicide prevention, assessment, and intervention.

- Specify several indications of substance abuse disorder in older adults, and discuss appropriate nursing responses.

- Recognize signs of problem gambling and use appropriate techniques to screen for it.

- Provide culturally safe and competent mental health care to older adults.

- Evaluate interventions aimed at promoting mental health and wellness in older adults.

GLOSSARY

Delusion   A fixed, false belief.

Hallucination   The perception of a sensory experience with no external stimulus (e.g., hearing voices that no one else can hear).

Illusion   Misinterpretation of a real experience (e.g., thinking a curled rope is a snake).

Insight   Recognition that one has a (health) problem or illness.

Mental disorder   Mental illness diagnosed based on the criteria from the American Psychiatric Association *Diagnostic and Statistical Manual of Mental Disorders*.

Mood   A person's internal, self-reported emotional state.

Paranoia   An intense and strongly defended irrational suspicion.

Persistent depressive disorder   This disorder, previously called dysthymia, describes a state of at least 2 years of depressed mood for more days than not, accompanied by additional depressive symptoms that do not meet the criteria for a major depressive episode.

Suicidal behaviour   Potentially self-injurious behaviour with a nonfatal outcome, but for which there is evidence of the person's intention to die.

THE LIVED EXPERIENCE

"During those bad times, I didn't get along with my family at all. I didn't know if they felt I [was] not doing a good job, like maybe they weren't sympathetic enough, but I think they just didn't know how people can feel when things like this [not working, being sick] happen . . . I didn't get along with them for a long time. I had to, but I didn't. Just like that. That was tough.
A 68-year-old man

Apesoa-Varano, E. C., Barker, J. C., & Hinton, L. (2015). Shards of sorrow: Older men's accounts of their depression experience. *Social Science & Medicine, 124,* 1–8. doi:10.1016/j.socscimed.2014.10.054.

Mental health in later life is not different from mental health earlier in life, but the challenges of maintaining mental health may be different in later life. Developmental transitions, life events, physical illness, cognitive impairment, and situations calling for energy may interfere with mental health in older adults. These factors, although not unique to older adults, often influence adaptation. However, anyone who has survived for 80 years or so has been exposed to many stressors and crises and has developed resilience. Most older adults face life's challenges with equanimity and courage. It is up to the nurse to discover the strengths and adaptive mechanisms that will help the person cope with the challenges.

This chapter focuses on the different presentations of mental disorders that may occur in older adults and the appropriate assessments and interventions. Readers should refer to a comprehensive psychiatric – mental health text for more in-depth discussion of mental disorders.

MENTAL HEALTH AND MENTAL DISORDER IN LATER LIFE

The meaning of mental health is subject to many interpretations and many familial and cultural influences. According to the World Health Organization (WHO), mental health is "a state of well-being in which an individual realizes his or her own abilities, can cope with the normal stresses of life, can work productively, and is able to make a contribution to his or her community" (World Health Organization [WHO], 2018, para. 1). Erikson et al. (1986) proposed that autonomy, intimacy, integrity, and generativity are all aspects of mentally healthy adult adaptation (see Chapter 7).

These definitions of mental health do not mention psychiatric symptoms or symptoms of mental disorder. Mental health is conceptually distinct from **mental disorder**. A mental disorder, or diagnosable mental illness, is a health condition "generally characterized by a combination of abnormal thoughts, perceptions, emotions, behaviour and relationships with others. Mental disorders include depression, bipolar disorder, schizophrenia and other psychoses, dementia, and developmental disorders including autism" (WHO, 2019). There are many causes of mental disorders, including genetic and biological factors, as well as their interaction with social, psychological, and economic factors.

The Mental Health Commission of Canada (MHCC) (2012) distinguishes four groups of people who live with mental illness in older age. The first group consists of people who have had a recurrent or persistent mental illness for many years. Because most mental illnesses have their initial onset in young adulthood, the most common experience of mental illness in older age is this recurrent or persistent illness. The second population consists of people who have a mental illness with an onset in older age. The third group is made up of those living with dementia (see Chapter 21). The fourth population consists of older adults who experience mental illness in conjunction with a medical condition that presents with mental health symptoms, such as Parkinson's disease or cerebrovascular disease (see Chapter 22).

People can achieve mental health, as defined by the WHO, despite the presence of a mental disorder or symptoms of a mental illness. Likewise, the absence of symptoms of mental illness does not guarantee mental health. The Canadian framework for a national mental health strategy builds on the WHO definition of mental health and explains the interaction between mental health and mental disorder as follows:

> People can have varying degrees of mental health, regardless of whether or not they have a mental illness. For example, some people, whether they have a mental illness or not, have tremendous resilience, strength, healthy relationships, and a positive outlook. Others, whether they have a mental illness or not, may feel that day-to-day life is a struggle, that they have limited prospects, few friends, and are more easily set back by life's challenges. (MHCC, 2009, p. 10)

It is important for nurses who work with older adults to create relationships and environments that contribute to mental health and wellness, happiness, and meaning throughout life, even at the end of life, regardless of whether the older adult experiences a mental disorder.

Mental Health Care

One in three Canadians experiences mental illness at some time in their lives (Government of Canada, 2017). Up to 30% of older adults experience a mental health issue or illness (Canadian Mental Health Association [CMHA] Ontario, 2021). The most prevalent mental disorders in later life are anxiety, dementia, and mood disorders such as depression. Addictions and substance use disorders among older adults are also concerning.

The stigma of having a mental illness discourages many people from seeking treatment. The rate of use of mental health services by older adults, even when such services are available, is less than that by any other age group. Some of the reasons for this may be a stoic acceptance of difficulty, an unawareness of resources, a reluctance to seek help because of pride of independence, and the fear of being "put away." Ageism also affects the identification and treatment of mental health disorders in older adults.

Symptoms of mental health issues may be overlooked, mistakenly seen as normal consequences of aging, or blamed on dementia by both older adults and health care providers. Furthermore, the presence of comorbid medical conditions in older adults complicates the recognition and diagnosis of mental disorders. Also, the myth that older adults do not respond well to treatment is still prevalent. Other factors—including health care providers' knowledge deficits; inadequate numbers of mental health care providers; and limited availability of specialized mental health services for older adults—are all barriers (Adams et al., 2015).

Older adults can receive psychiatric services across a wide range of settings, including acute and long-term inpatient psychiatric units, primary care, community and home care, and long-term care (LTC) homes. Nurses will encounter older adults with mental illness in all these settings. Acute care admissions for medical problems are often exacerbated by depression, anxiety, cognitive impairment, substance abuse, or chronic mental illness.

Cultural and Ethnic Disparities in Mental Health

Recent research suggests that the mental health of young Canadians, women, Indigenous peoples, immigrants, persons living with disabilities, and health care workers have been significantly affected by the COVID-19 pandemic (Moyser, 2020; Havaei et al., 2021; Jenkins et al., 2021). Yet, a lack of knowledge and awareness of cultural differences in regard to the meaning of mental health and well-being, differences in the way concerns may become apparent, limited access to culturally competent mental health treatment, and insufficient research in this area will need to be addressed in light of the ethnocultural diversity among older

adults in Canada. Culturally and ethnically diverse older people have less access to mental health services and are at risk of receiving poorer-quality mental health care. Some barriers to the use of services are cultural beliefs, lack of culturally appropriate services, lack of services in the older adult's language, lack of awareness of services, and ageism (Guruge et al., 2015).

"Aging out of place" refers to spending one's later years in a foreign land (Government of Canada, 2018a). Immigrating to another country later in life poses a risk for social isolation and feelings of unfamiliarity and loss. Older adults who identify as immigrants and refugees experience higher rates of depression and social anxiety, among other health issues (Government of Canada, 2018a).

For nurses, it is important to include a cultural assessment and a discussion of what culturally and ethnically diverse older adults believe about their mental health issues. Box 23.1 describes a study of older Chinese Canadian immigrants who sought mental health assistance. In addition, culturally appropriate education about mental health concerns is important. (See Chapter 4 for an in-depth discussion of culture and aging.).

LGBTQ2 Older Adults and Mental Health

Approximately 400,000 older adults self-identify as members of the lesbian, gay, bisexual, transgender, queer or questioning, and Two-Spirit (LGBTQ2) community (Wilson et al., 2016; Wilson & Stinchcombe, 2019). Sexual identities other than heterosexuality have not always been accepted in society, and many older adults who identify as LGBTQ2 were stigmatized or felt the need to hide their sexual orientation to prevent discrimination. Sexual orientation was thought of as a mental illness and was not protected under the Canadian Charter of Rights and Freedoms until 1996 (Government of Canada, 2018b). These experiences could bring forth feelings of trauma, anxiety, and depression. One study by Stinchcombe and colleagues (2018) used data on participants aged 45 years and older from the Canadian Longitudinal Study on Aging to compare self-reported physical and mental health by sex and sexual orientation. Compared to heterosexual female peers, lesbian and bisexual females had greater odds of heavy drinking and anxiety disorders. Compared to heterosexual males, gay and bisexual

BOX 23.1

RESEARCH FOR EVIDENCE-INFORMED PRACTICE: HELP SEEKING FOR MENTAL HEALTH ISSUES AMONG OLDER CHINESE CANADIAN IMMIGRANTS

Problem: Older adults are less likely than younger adults to seek help for mental disorders and mental health issues. Older adults who are members of minority ethnic groups are even less likely to seek help, even though their rates of mental disorder are higher. This study examined whether seeking help for mental health issues was associated with demographic and health factors, social support, and cultural values.

Method: Data were collected through a survey and semi-structured interviews with Chinese Canadians 55 years and older who lived in the community or in assisted-living residences. A convenience sample of 149 participants participated in the study and were asked questions related to social support, health-related quality of life, mental health care use, help-seeking attitudes, intentions to seek help, and Chinese cultural beliefs and values.

Findings: Sixteen percent of the participants sought help for mental health issues in the previous year, more often from other types of practitioners than from health care providers. Positive help-seeking attitudes were associated with higher social support, better physical health, and lower levels of influence of Chinese cultural beliefs and values.

Implications for Nursing Practice: Attitudes toward seeking help were less positive than those in the general population. Older individuals from cultures that stigmatize mental illness, distress, and help seeking are less likely to seek help. Outreach to immigrant communities may increase awareness of resources and reduce stigmatization. When discussing mental health, nurses should consider the person's cultural values and beliefs about mental illness.

Source: Tieu, U., & Konnert, C. A. (2014). Mental health help-seeking attitudes, utilization and intentions among older Chinese immigrants in Canada. *Aging & Mental Health*, *18*(2), 140–147. doi:10.1080/13607863.2013.814104.

men had greater odds of reporting a mood disorder and of seeing a psychologist within the past year (Stinchcombe et al., 2018).

Indigenous Older Adults and Mental Health

Most Indigenous older adults have experienced severe trauma in their lives. The residential school experience built on previous trauma of injustice and oppression for older adults (Government of Canada, 2018c) (see Chapter 4). Feelings of anxiety and depression can stem from these experiences for Indigenous peoples. There are many resources and stories available that acknowledge the detrimental impact of colonization and Western assimilation on the well-being of Indigenous peoples in Canada (MacDonald & Steenbeek, 2015; Battiste, 2005; King et al., 2005; Knockwood, 1992). It is vital for nurses to understand the lived experiences of Indigenous older adults in order to provide person-centred care to Indigenous peoples and communities and to support healing (Hill, 2021).

Many Indigenous peoples are cared for in the community and do not move into LTC homes owing to Indigenous beliefs about Elders and Elder care. Those who do move into LTC homes away from their community may experience social isolation (Government of Canada, 2018c).

Risk factors of social isolation could result from past traumatic experiences, as well as racism, cultural differences, moving into the city or town to access health and community services, and lack of culturally appropriate activities (Government of Canada, 2018c).

Assessment and Mental Illness

Accurate and appropriate assessment is critical. Chapter 13 presents a discussion about assessment tools for gerontological nursing. Specific information on instruments for assessment of depression, suicide, and substance abuse are described in this chapter. Mental status is assessed through careful observation and interviewing, as well by using standardized assessments. Psychosocial functioning and biological factors, such as medical conditions and medication side effects that may result in symptoms of mental disorders, must be considered. Mental health assessment is best done during short sessions after rapport has been established. Performing repeated assessments at various times of the day and in different situations will lead to a more complete and accurate assessment. The assessment should focus on the person's resilience, culture, strengths, and skills, as well as their challenges. Assessment should include past experiences of mental illness and treatment.

Anxiety Disorders

Anxiety is defined as unpleasant and unwarranted feelings of apprehension that may be accompanied by physical symptoms. Anxiety itself is a normal human reaction and part of a fear response; it is rational, within reason. When a person experiences problematic anxiety, called an *anxiety disorder*, the anxiety is prolonged and exaggerated and interferes with function. Anxiety disorders are not considered part of the normal aging process, but the changes and challenges that older adults often face may contribute to the development of anxiety symptoms and disorders. Many older adults with anxiety disorders had an anxiety disorder earlier in their lives; however, late-onset anxiety is common. Anxiety disorders that may occur in older adults include generalized anxiety disorder (GAD), phobic disorder, obsessive-compulsive disorder (OCD), panic disorder, and post-traumatic stress disorder (PTSD). Anxiety disorders are frequently comorbid with depression.

Prevalence

Epidemiological studies indicate that anxiety disorders are common in older adults; about 11% of older adults experience an anxiety disorder in any given year (Bower & Wetherell, 2015). However, relatively few people are diagnosed with these disorders. GAD and specific phobias are the most common anxiety disorders in older adults (Canuto et al., 2018). In addition to unwarranted worries and feelings of apprehension that interfere with functioning, the symptoms of GAD include excessive worries; restlessness or a feeling of being keyed up or on edge; fatigue that develops readily; difficulty concentrating, or the mind's going blank; irritability; muscle tension; and sleep disturbance (Munir & Takov, 2020).

Phobia is an unrealistic or irrational fear that interferes with a person's life. Between 2% and 10% of older adults experience phobias. This may be an underestimate, because older adults tend to have less **insight** into the extent to which phobias and associated avoidance affect their lives (Bower & Wetherell, 2015). Fear of falling is likely the most common phobia among older adults (Pary et al., 2019).

Some of the risk factors for anxiety disorders in older adults are female gender, a history of worry or rumination, poor physical health or physical illness, low socioeconomic status, high-stress life events, early childhood abuse, depression, cognitive impairment, a family history of anxiety disorder, and alcohol or drug misuse. Protective factors that decrease the risk for anxiety disorders include receiving social support from family, having a spouse or living with someone, and being physically active (Bower & Wetherell, 2015).

Anxiety in older adults is associated with more visits to primary care providers and an increase in the average length of visits. Some of the negative consequences of anxiety symptoms and disorders are decreases in physical activity, functional status, and satisfaction with life and an increased risk of mortality (Bower & Wetherell, 2015). Unidentified or untreated anxiety disorders in older adults adversely affect well-being and quality of life.

IMPLICATIONS FOR GERONTOLOGICAL NURSING AND HEALTHY AGING

Assessment

Nurses often encounter anxious older adults and can identify anxiety-related symptoms and initiate assessments that will lead to appropriate treatment and management. When assessing older adults, nurses should be aware of factors that can reduce the chance of recognizing anxiety (Box 23.2).

Older adults are less likely to report psychiatric symptoms or acknowledge anxiety, often attribute their symptoms to physical health problems, and are likely to

---

BOX 23.2

FACTORS THAT REDUCE THE CHANCES OF SEEKING HELP FOR AND RECOGNIZING ANXIETY

1. Stigmatization of mental illness; discomfort when talking to health care providers about anxiety
2. Attribution of psychological symptoms to physical causes
3. Nonrecognition of the impact of symptoms on daily life and functioning
4. Labels and words that are used to describe anxiety (e.g., "worry," as opposed to "concerns" or "issues")
5. Ageist attitudes and beliefs
6. Pessimism about treatment effectiveness
7. Diagnostic difficulties
8. Time constraints in primary care settings

Source: Adapted from Bower, E. S., & Wetherell, J. L. (2015). Late-life anxiety disorders. In P. A. Lichtenberg, B. T. Mast, B. D. Carpenter, et al. (Eds.), *APA handbook of clinical gero-psychology, Vol. 2: Assessment, treatment, and issues in later life* (pp. 49–77). American Psychological Association.

have coexistent medical conditions that mimic the symptoms of anxiety. Some of the medical disorders that cause anxiety symptoms are cardiac arrhythmias, delirium, dementia, chronic obstructive pulmonary disease, heart failure, hyperthyroidism, hypoglycemia, postural hypotension, pulmonary edema, and pulmonary embolism. Distinguishing a medical condition from the physical symptoms of an anxiety disorder may be difficult.

Anxiety is also a common adverse effect of many drugs, including anticholinergics, digitalis, theophylline, antihypertensives, beta-blockers, beta-adrenergic stimulators, corticosteroids, and over-the-counter (OTC) medications such as appetite suppressants and cough and cold preparations. Caffeine; nicotine; and withdrawal from alcohol, sedatives, and hypnotics also cause symptoms of anxiety.

Assessment of anxiety in older adults focuses on physical, social, and environmental factors, as well as past life history and recent events. Older adults more often report somatic complaints such as gastro-intestinal symptoms, headaches, dizziness, pain, dyspnea, and palpitations rather than cognitive symptoms such as excessive worrying. It is important to remember that expressed fears and worries may be realistic or unrealistic, so the nurse must investigate and obtain collateral information from family or caregivers. For example, fear of leaving the home may be related to falling or to crime in the neighbourhood. Worries about financial stability may be related to the economy or financial abuse by others.

The nurse should also be sure to investigate other possible causes of anxiety, such as medical conditions and depression. Diagnostic and laboratory tests may be ordered as indicated to rule out medical conditions. Cognitive assessment, brain imaging, and neuropsychological evaluation are included if cognitive impairment is suspected (see Chapter 21). A review of medications, including OTC medications and herbal or home remedies, is essential, as is the elimination of those that cause anxiety symptoms.

Scales may be used to supplement the clinical assessment. Numerous self-report rating scales are available, but few have been adequately tested with older adults. Rating scales developed for use with older adults include the Geriatric Anxiety Inventory (Pachana et al., 2007), the Worry Scale (Wisocki et al., 1986), and the

---

BOX 23.3

SUGGESTED QUESTIONS FOR IDENTIFYING ANXIETY IN OLDER ADULTS

1. Can you say what triggers your feeling anxious?
2. Have you been concerned about or fretted over a number of things?
3. Is there anything going on in your life that is causing you concern?
4. Do you find that you have a hard time putting things out of your mind?

The following questions are useful in identifying how and when physical symptoms began:
1. What were you doing when you noticed the chest pain?
2. What were you thinking about when you felt your heart starting to race?
3. When you can't sleep, what is usually going through your head?

Source: The Anxiety Disorder Association of America. (2010–2020). *Symptoms—Generalized anxiety disorder (GAD).* https://adaa.org/understanding-anxiety/generalized-anxiety-disorder-gad/symptoms.

Geriatric Anxiety Scale (Segal et al., 2010). Box 23.3 lists suggested questions to identify anxiety disorders in older adults.

Interventions

Anxiety disorders in older adults can be treated effectively. Treatment choices depend on the preference of the older adult, symptoms, the specific anxiety diagnosis, comorbid medical conditions, and any current medication regimen. Pharmacological and nonpharmacological interventions are effective and may be used conjointly (Dyer et al., 2018). Many older adults prefer nonpharmacological treatments.

Nonpharmacological Interventions

The therapeutic relationship is the foundation for any intervention. Family support, community resources and therapists, support groups, ethnic and cultural traditions and practices (healers, smudging, etc.) and the provision of information are all important.

Cognitive behavioural therapy (CBT), relaxation training, mindfulness meditation, acceptance and commitment therapy, supportive therapy, and psychoeducation can be used to treat anxiety disorders. Many of these approaches can be provided individually or in groups, and some may also be provided via the Internet. CBT is a widely used approach for the treatment of both anxiety and depression. It is designed to modify thought patterns, improve skills, and alter the environmental states that contribute to anxiety. This therapy may involve relaxation training, cognitive restructuring (i.e., replacing anxiety-producing thoughts with more realistic, less catastrophic ones), and education about signs and symptoms of anxiety. It is moderately effective for older adults but less effective than it is for younger people (Ayers et al., 2015). CBT is time consuming and requires a commitment to daily homework and practice. Given that other approaches such as mindfulness and supportive therapy may be equally as effective for older adults, CBT may not be the first-line nonpharmacological approach (Ayers et al., 2015).

Mindfulness approaches encourage the person to have a focused nonjudgemental awareness of the present instead of worrying. The training involves practising mindfulness, meditation, yoga, and awareness of breathing (Lenze et al., 2014). Some studies show positive results for older adults with anxiety symptoms or disorders (Franco et al., 2017).

Pharmacological Interventions

Issues of polypharmacy and age-related changes in pharmacodynamics make prescribing and monitoring medications in older adults a complex undertaking (see Chapter 14). Antidepressants in the form of selective serotonin reuptake inhibitors (SSRIs) and serotonin–norepinephrine reuptake inhibitors (SNRIs) have been found to be effective for the treatment of GAD and panic disorder. Within these classes of medications, those with sedating rather than stimulating properties are preferred (e.g., citalopram, paroxetine, and sertraline). When SSRIs are prescribed, it is important to educate the person about (and to watch for) potential side effects, such as initial increased nervousness, insomnia, nausea, and sexual dysfunction. A discontinuation syndrome of dizziness, insomnia, and flu-like symptoms is common when SSRIs are stopped.

Second-line treatment may include short-acting benzodiazepines, such as alprazolam (Xanax) and lorazepam (Ativan). Treatment with benzodiazepines should be used only for short-term therapy (less than 6 months) and for relief of immediate symptoms; these medications must be used carefully in older adults. Older medications, such as diazepam (Valium), should be avoided because of their long half-lives and the increased risk of accumulation and toxicity in older adults. All of these medications can have problematic side effects such as sedation, falls, cognitive impairment, and dependence (see Chapter 14). Nonbenzodiazepine anxiolytic agents, such as buspirone, may also be used. Buspirone has fewer side effects but requires a longer period of administration (up to 4 weeks) for effectiveness.

Obsessive-Compulsive Disorders

OCD is characterized by recurrent and persistent thoughts, impulses, or images (obsessions) that are repetitive and purposeful and by intentional ritualistic behaviours (compulsions) that improve the person's comfort level. The person cannot control their compulsions even when they recognize that these behaviours are excessive and unreasonable. OCD significantly impairs function for more than an hour each day (American Psychiatric Association, 2020a). Symptoms in older adults are often not sufficient to disrupt function seriously and thus may not be considered symptoms of a true disorder but rather a coping strategy. If symptoms progress to the point at which they disrupt function, the older adult will need clinical attention. Recommended treatments include exercise and CBT combined with pharmacological treatment (i.e., SSRIs) if indicated.

Post-Traumatic Stress Disorder

PTSD is a disorder that may affect "people who have experienced or witnessed a traumatic event such as a natural disaster, a serious accident, a terrorist act, war/combat, or rape or who have been threatened with death, sexual violence or serious injury (American Psychiatric Association, 2020b). Most older adults have experienced a potentially traumatic event at some time, and some of them develop PTSD as a consequence (Bower & Wetherell, 2015). The *Diagnostic and Statistical Manual of Mental Disorders* (5th ed.; DSM-5) changed the classification of PTSD from an anxiety disorder to a new disorder called *trauma and stress-related disorder* (American Psychiatric Association, 2020b).

Individuals with PTSD often re-experience the traumatic event in episodes of fear, and they experience symptoms such as helplessness, flashbacks, intrusive thoughts, memories, images, emotional numbing, loss of interest, avoidance of any place that reminds the person of the traumatic event, poor concentration, irritability, startle reactions, jumpiness, and hypervigilance. They may experience ongoing sleep problems, somatic disturbances, anxiety, depression, and restlessness. The severity of the symptoms may decline over time. Older adults with a history of PTSD have high rates of several physical health conditions, as well as worse physical functioning and cognitive performance (Bower & Wetherell, 2015).

The lifetime prevalence of PTSD among Canadian adults is 9.2% (Katzman et al., 2014). A study of older adults attending primary care clinics in Quebec found that 11% had significant PTSD symptoms in the previous 6 months (Lamoureux-Lamarche et al., 2016). The disorder is more common in women. Sexual assault is the most common cause of PTSD in women, followed by being physically abused as a child, being threatened with a weapon, being molested, being neglected as a child, and being subjected to physical violence. For men, the most common cause is also sexual assault, followed by abuse as a child, combat (war), and molestation.

In older adults, PTSD may develop as a new disorder in response to a recent trauma, or it may be related to trauma long past. Compared to younger adults, older adults are more likely to experience PTSD after natural disasters and human-induced disasters (Parker et al., 2016; Siskind et al., 2016). Older adults who are at greatest risk for PTSD after a disaster are those with lower socioeconomic status; poor subjective health and functioning; a mental illness; chronic medical conditions; or low levels of social support (Heid et al., 2016).

Although trauma has long been associated with PTSD symptoms (e.g., First World War soldiers with these symptoms were labelled as having "shell shock"), it was first recognized as a psychiatric diagnosis in 1980. At that time, attention to PTSD symptoms was an outcome of the overwhelmingly stressful experiences of combatants in the American war in Vietnam. Many Second World War veterans have lived most of their lives under the shadow of PTSD without its being recognized. Older adults have also experienced the Great Depression, the Holocaust and other genocides, residential schools (see Chapter 4), racism, and the COVID-19 pandemic—all events

that may have precipitated PTSD. Mental health resources for veterans can be found on the National Association of Federal Retirees website (https://www.federalretirees.ca/en/my-health/for-veterans/mental-health-resources).

IMPLICATIONS FOR GERONTOLOGICAL NURSING AND HEALTHY AGING

Assessment

The care of the person with PTSD involves an awareness that certain events may trigger PTSD reactions; the pattern of these reactions should be identified when possible. Provision of intimate bodily care can trigger a traumatic response among older adults with a history of sexual assault or abuse as a child. Knowing the person's past history and life experiences is essential to understanding the person's behaviour and implementing appropriate interventions. However, the person's history of trauma may be unknown, and if the person has dementia, the history may be difficult to ascertain. Self-protective behaviours of individuals who live with dementia may be linked to their past experiences of trauma (see Chapter 21). Nurses who work in hospitals and LTC homes should be aware of potential environmental triggers of traumatic memories for older adults living with dementia who have a history of trauma. The Hartford Institute for Geriatric Nursing website describes a tool for assessing the impact of trauma on older adults (Weiss & Marmar, 1997).

Interventions

The capacity to effectively cope with traumatic events seems to be associated with adults who have secure and supportive relationships; the ability to freely express or fully suppress the experience; favourable circumstances immediately following the trauma; a productive and active lifestyle; strong faith, religion, and hope; and biological integrity. CBT with prolonged exposure involves psychoeducation, breath retraining, imagining the past traumatic event, and exposure to situations that have been avoided since the traumatic event. CBT is effective for PTSD, and there is some evidence of its effectiveness with older adults (Cook & Dinnen, 2015). Pharmacological treatment with antidepressants (i.e., SSRIs and

SNRIs) may be helpful. Paroxetine (Paxil) and venlafax-ine (Effexor) are recommended as first-line treatments for PTSD in adults (Katzman et al., 2014). However, older adults have not been included in most clinical trials of medications for PTSD.

Psychosis and Psychotic Symptoms in Late Life

Psychosis is a syndrome or constellation of psychiatric symptoms that occurs in a number of physical and mental disorders. The predominating symptoms are hallucinations and delusions. Older adults may experience psychosis from a persistent, recurrent mental illness such as schizophrenia, delusional disorder, depression, or bipolar affective disorder. In older adults, a new onset of psychosis may occur as a secondary syndrome in a variety of disorders, the most common being dementia and Parkinson's disease. Temporal lobe epilepsy, untreated endocrine disorders, tumours, and the use of some medications and illicit drugs also may result in psychosis (Ngo et al., 2019; Tamminga, 2020). Risk factors for psychosis in older adults are social isolation, sensory deficits, physical illness, cognitive impairment, and polypharmacy (Ceglowski et al., 2015).

Paranoia

Paranoia is best described as an intense and strongly defended irrational suspicion. Symptoms of **paranoia** can signify an acute change in mental status as a result of a medical emergency, illness, or delirium (see Chapter 21), or they can be caused by an underlying mental disorder such as depression, PTSD, or substance use disorder. Paranoia is also an early symptom of Alzheimer's disease. Medications, vision and hearing loss, social isolation, negative life events, financial strain, and PTSD can also precipitate symptoms of paranoia. The dynamics of paranoia seem to be loss of control, the inability to evaluate the social milieu appropriately, and the feeling that external forces are controlling life (which in many instances may be true).

Delusions

A **delusion** is a fixed, false belief that guides a person's interpretation of events but is not shared by others. Delusions may be comforting or threatening, but they always form a structure for understanding situations that otherwise might seem unmanageable. A delusional disorder is one in which conceivable ideas that are without factual foundation persist for more than 1 month (Center for Behavioral Health Statistics and Quality, 2016).

Those living with Alzheimer's disease and other dementias may experience delusions (Alzheimer Society of Canada, 2021). Common delusions are those in which a person believes they are being poisoned, children are taking assets, they are being held prisoner, or they are being deceived by a spouse or lover. The delusions of older adults often incorporate significant persons. Fear and a lack of trust originating from a basis in reality may become magnified, especially when the person is isolated from others and does not receive reality feedback. Delusions related to family members or care partners and their actions or intentions may occur among older adults. Some delusions may aid in coping, but most are troubling to the person. It is always important to determine whether what "appears" to be a delusion is in fact based in reality. For example, many older adults living in a LTC home during COVID-19 may voice feelings of being forgotten or held prisoner and children having deserted them. Unfortunately, the reality of outbreak protocols and strict visiting policies are causing these situations and are of great concern to the mental health of older adults.

Hallucinations

A **hallucination** is the sensory perception of a nonexistent object. Any of the five senses can be subject to hallucinations. Although not attributable to environmental stimuli, hallucinations may occur as the result of a combination of environmental factors. Among older adults, hallucinations that arise from psychotic disorders (e.g., schizophrenia) are less common than hallucinations that arise from other causes.

The character and stages of hallucinatory experiences in later life have not been adequately defined. Many hallucinations are associated with medications, neurological disorders such as dementia and Parkinson's disease, and physiological and sensory disorders. The hallucinations of older adults most often appear along with disorientation, illusion, intense grief, or immersion in retrospection, the origins being difficult to separate. Older adults with hearing and vision deficits may also hear voices or see people and objects that are not actually present (**illusions**). Some researchers have explained these illusions as the brain's attempt to create stimulation in the absence of adequate sensory input. Illusions and hallucinations that are not disturbing to the person may not necessitate treatment.

IMPLICATIONS FOR GERONTOLOGICAL NURSING AND HEALTHY AGING

Assessment

Determining whether a person's psychotic symptoms (paranoia, delusions, and hallucinations) are the result of medical illnesses, medications, dementia, psychoses, deprivations, or overload is challenging because the treatment will vary accordingly. Treatment must be based on a comprehensive assessment and a determination of the nature of the psychotic behaviour (primary or secondary psychosis) and the time of onset of first symptoms. Treating the underlying cause of a secondary psychosis brought on by medical illnesses, head trauma, dementia, illicit substances, medication misuse, or delirium is a priority (Ceglowski et al., 2015).

An assessment of vision and hearing is important, as these impairments may predispose a person to paranoia and suspiciousness. Screening for depression should be conducted. Assessment of suicide potential is also indicated because individuals experiencing paranoid symptoms are at significant risk for self-harm.

It is never safe to conclude that someone is delusional or paranoid or experiencing hallucinations unless the claims have been thoroughly investigated, physical and cognitive status evaluated, and the environment assessed for contributing factors to the behaviours.

Interventions

Frightening hallucinations or delusions (e.g., that the person is being poisoned) usually arise in response to anxiety-provoking situations. Caregivers may best manage these symptoms by reducing the situational stress, being available to the person, providing a safe and nonjudgemental environment, and attending to the person's fears more than to the content of the delusion or hallucination. Direct confrontation is likely to increase the person's anxiety, agitation, and sense of vulnerability; it also may disrupt the relationship with

the caregiver. A more useful approach is to establish a trusting relationship that is not demanding and not too intense.

It is important to identify the person's strengths and build on them. Demonstrating respect and a willingness to listen to complaints and fears is important. The nurse must be trustworthy, give clear information, and present clear choices. The nurse should not pretend to agree with paranoid beliefs or delusions but rather should ask what is troubling to the person and provide reassurance of safety. The nurse should try to understand what the experience is like for the person and how distressing it is. Other suggestions are to avoid television, which can be confusing, especially if the person has a hearing or vision impairment and awakens with the television on. In addition, clutter in the person's room should be reduced, large mirrors should be removed, and shadows that can appear threatening should be eliminated. Eyeglasses and hearing aids need to be provided to maximize sensory input and reduce misinterpretations.

If symptoms are interfering with function and environmental strategies and if nonpharmacological approaches are not effective, antipsychotic medications may be used. The newer atypical antipsychotics such as risperidone (Risperdal) and olanzapine (Zyprexa) are preferred but must be used judiciously, with careful attention to side effects and monitoring response. Antipsychotic medications are not recommended as a first-line treatment of psychotic symptoms associated with dementia, except in cases of severe agitation or psychosis (see Chapter 21).

Schizophrenia

Schizophrenia is a severe mental disorder characterized by two or more of the following symptoms (one of which must be hallucinations, delusions, or disorganized speech for at least 1 month): delusions, hallucinations, disorganized thinking, disorganized or catatonic behaviour, affective flattening, poverty of speech, or apathy. These symptoms cause significant social or occupational dysfunction and are not accompanied by prominent mood symptoms or substance use or attributed to medical causes (American Psychiatric Association, 2020c).

The prevalence of schizophrenia in older adults is approximately 0.5%, about half of its prevalence in younger adults (Ceglowski et al., 2015). Most people diagnosed with schizophrenia are diagnosed in early adulthood. However, a substantial minority of patients have onset of a first episode after the age of 40 years. There is also a very late-onset group (onset after the age of 60 years), which is classified as *schizophrenia-like* psychosis based on clinical, epidemiological, neuroimaging, and neuropsychological data (Sachdev et al., 2016).

Cognitive impairment is common in schizophrenia. It affects memory, verbal and language functioning, attention, concentration, and executive functioning. These impairments persist even with effective treatment. Cognitive impairment is worse for people whose schizophrenia began when they were young adults (Ceglowski et al., 2015; Mausbach & Ho, 2015).

Metabolic syndrome, common in schizophrenia, is a constellation of clinical and metabolic risk factors for cardiovascular disease, including elevated blood pressure and cholesterol, insulin resistance and diabetes, and abdominal obesity. Metabolic syndrome is partly attributed to the effects of antipsychotic medications. The prevalence of metabolic syndrome associated with schizophrenia is about 40%, and the condition is more common among older adults with a longer history of schizophrenia (Ceglowski et al., 2015). Individuals with schizophrenia have a 20% lower life expectancy and a higher prevalence of many physical illnesses, especially diabetes. These health disparities are the result of limited access to adequate preventive and primary health care as well as the health risks associated with antipsychotic medications (Kredenster et al., 2014).

IMPLICATIONS FOR GERONTOLOGICAL NURSING AND HEALTHY AGING

Assessment

Holistic and culturally safe assessments should include a review of the person's social skills, social functioning, and social support. Monitoring for metabolic syndrome is important. Care partners and families of older adults living with schizophrenia may have been providing care for years and into very old age. Caregiver needs and resources should be assessed. In addition, trauma history should be considered, since people with schizophrenia are vulnerable to housing insecurity, assault, and mistreatment.

Treatment

Nursing interventions with people living with schizophrenia focus on recovery and well-being. This means supporting the person in an authentic, empathetic, nonstigmatized manner to help them live a meaningful life, contribute to their community, and achieve their potential regardless of their age or the effects of their schizophrenia (de Pinho et al., 2017). Hope, choice, self-care, and self-determination are important within a recovery approach. Nurses must support both pharmacological and nonpharmacological treatment. Conventional neuroleptic medications such as haloperidol (Haldol) have been effective in managing the positive symptoms but are problematic with older adults and carry a high risk of disabling and persistent adverse effects such as tardive dyskinesia (see Chapter 14). When given in low doses, the newer atypical antipsychotic medications—such as risperidone (Risperdal), olanzapine (Zyprexa), and quetiapine (Seroquel)—are associated with a lower risk for extrapyramidal symptoms and tardive dyskinesia. Psychosocial treatments include CBT, family psychoeducation, social skills therapy, cognitive remediation therapy, and a combination of these approaches. Some of these treatments have been modified and tested with older adults, and the results for social skills training and cognitive behaviour social skills training are promising (Mausbach & Ho, 2015). Other important interventions include case management, weight management, and support for the self-care of chronic physical illnesses.

Bipolar Disorder and Mania

Although bipolar disorder is not common in later life, more cases will be seen as the number of older adults grows. Ten percent of inpatient psychiatric admissions of older adults are for bipolar disorder. Bipolar disorders, characterized by periods of mania and depression, often level out in later life, and bipolar individuals tend to have longer periods of depression. Mania is a more frequent cause of hospitalization than depression, but depression may account for more disability. New episodes of mania in older age are often due to underlying medical conditions that must be identified and treated (Valiengo et al., 2016). Metabolic syndrome is common among older adults with bipolar disorder (Chen et al., 2018).

IMPLICATIONS FOR GERONTOLOGICAL NURSING AND HEALTHY AGING

Recommended treatment consists of a combination of one or more mood stabilizers and intensive psychosocial intervention. Lithium is a mood stabilizer and the first-line pharmacological treatment for bipolar disorder. Lithium's side effects of fine hand tremor, polyuria, mild thirst, mild nausea, and weight gain make it difficult for older adults to tolerate this medication. However, most older adults who use lithium are positive about it, despite the side effects (Rej et al., 2016). Lithium has a long half-life (more than 36 hours) and a narrow therapeutic window, meaning that there is a small difference between a therapeutic level and a toxic level. Serum lithium levels must be monitored regularly. Lithium is excreted by the kidneys, so adequate kidney function and salt and fluid intake are necessary to maintain a therapeutic level. Signs of toxicity include nausea, vomiting, diarrhea, thirst, polyuria, lethargy, slurred speech, muscle weakness, and coarse hand tremors. Confusion and other neurological changes are signs of severe toxicity. Antidepressants (i.e., SSRIs) may be used for individuals who have little or no history of mania.

Education and support are essential, and the family and care partners must understand that the individual is unable to control mania and irritating behaviours. Education about lithium therapy should include information about the importance of a maintaining a normal diet, maintaining hydration, taking lithium with meals to avoid nausea, and knowing what to do if signs of toxicity develop. Other resources for bipolar disorder can be found in the Resources section at the end of this chapter.

Depression

Depression is not a normal part of aging, and studies show that most older adults are satisfied with their lives, despite physical problems. To understand depression, nurses must comprehend the influence of late-life stressors, culture, and the beliefs that older adults, society, and health care providers may have about depression and its treatment.

Prevalence and Consequences

Depression is the most common mental health issue in later life. The estimated prevalence of major depressive disorder in later life is between 1.5% and 3.3% (Statistics Canada, 2016). Estimates of prevalence vary depending on how depression is measured and the clinical setting. Major depression is more prevalent in hospitalized older adults (13% to 22%) and those in LTC homes (6% to 16%) (DiNapoli & Scogin, 2015).

The prevalence of milder forms of depression is much higher, between 4% and 18% (DiNapoli & Scogin, 2015). Depression symptoms are present in 10% to 15% of older adults living in the community and about 44% of those living in LTC homes (Government of Canada, 2016). More than 15% of older adults with persistent physical conditions are depressed, and depression has been called "the unwanted co-traveler" accompanying many medical illnesses (Byrd, 2005). Many medications that older adults take can also cause depression.

Depression and depressive symptoms are associated with negative consequences, such as increased disability and functional decline, delayed recovery from illness and surgery, increased use of health services, cognitive impairment, malnutrition, decreased quality of life, substance use, and an elevated risk of suicide and non–suicide-related death (DiNapoli & Scogin, 2015; McKenzie & Harvath, 2016).

Depression remains underdiagnosed and undertreated, which may be explained by the attitudes and beliefs of older adults, society, and health care providers and by how difficult it is to differentiate the symptoms of depression from those of other illnesses. Although public attitudes about mental illness and depression are improving, the stigma associated with depression may be more prevalent for older adults, and they themselves may not acknowledge depressive symptoms or seek treatment. Some older adults, particularly those who have survived abuse or tragedies, may see depression as shameful, evidence of flawed character, being self-centred, a spiritual weakness, sin, or retribution.

Health care providers may mistakenly believe that depression is normal in aging and may not take appropriate action to assess and treat depression in older adults. The differing presentation of depression in older adults, as well as the high prevalence of medical problems that may cause depressive symptoms, also contributes to inadequate recognition and treatment.

Older adults of various ethnic and cultural groups have different risk factors for depression. For example, older visible minority Canadian immigrants have a higher prevalence of depression symptoms, owing to their experiences of discrimination (Davison et al., 2019). They also face additional barriers to accessing depression treatment. Culturally based beliefs may contribute to a reluctance to seek help for depression (AlAteeq et al., 2018; Lopez et al., 2018; Park et al., 2018). However, there is considerable variability between and among ethnic and cultural groups (Kim et al., 2015), and the lack of accessible services is problematic (Guruge et al., 2015).

Failure to treat depression increases morbidity and mortality. Yet, treatments for depression are as effective for older adults as they are for the general population. It is highly likely that nurses in all settings will encounter a large number of older adults with depressive symptoms. The nurse's recognition of depression and role in enhancing the access to appropriate mental health care are important to improve outcomes for older adults.

Etiology and Risk Factors

The causes of depression in older adults are complex and must be examined within a biopsychosocial framework. It is thought that an interaction of biological and psychosocial vulnerabilities and stressful life events explain risk for depression in older age (Edelstein et al., 2015).

Genetic risk is linked with depression onset in younger adulthood and is thus more relevant to older adults with recurrent depression (Edelstein et al., 2015). Medical illnesses are commonly comorbid. Some of the medical conditions that contribute to depression are cardiovascular disorders, chronic lung diseases, end-stage renal disease, arthritis, endocrine disorders (such as thyroid problems and diabetes mellitus), and insomnia (Gold et al., 2020). Medications used to treat medical disorders can also result in depressive symptoms. Psychosocial and environmental risk factors for depression in older age include lack of social support; financial strain; neurotic personality; low self-efficacy; stressful life events and losses; and family caregiving (DiNapoli & Scogin, 2015; McKenzie & Harvath, 2016). Depression in older adults is commonly comorbid with other mental illnesses, particularly anxiety disorder, personality disorder, dementia, and alcohol use disorder (DiNapoli & Scogin, 2015). Some common risk factors for depression are presented in Box 23.4.

Factors that protect older adults who have these risks for depression include socioeconomic and health

---

> **BOX 23.4**
> ## COMMON RISK FACTORS FOR DEPRESSION IN OLDER ADULTS
>
> **PREDISPOSING FACTORS**
> - Female
> - Widowed or divorced
> - History of depression
> - Vascular brain changes
> - Neurotic personality characteristics
> - Major physical and chronic illnesses
> - Medications—antihypertensives, narcotic analgesics, indomethacin, steroids, L-dopa, antimicrobials, benzodiazepines, digoxin, cimetidine, cancer chemotherapeutics
> - Excessive alcohol consumption
> - Social disadvantages and low social support or isolation
> - Family caregiving
>
> **PRECIPITATING FACTORS**
> - Recent bereavement
> - Moving to a long-term care home
> - Adverse life events
> - Long-term stress
> - Persistent sleep difficulties
>
> ---
>
> **Sources:** Adapted from National Institute of Mental Health. (2019). *Older adults and depression.* https://www.nimh.nih.gov/health/publications/older-adults-and-depression/; McKenzie, G. L., & Harvath, T. A. (2016). Late-life depression. In M. Boltz, E. Capezuti, T. Fulmer, et al. (Eds.), *Evidenced-based geriatric nursing protocols for best practice* (5th ed., pp. 211–232). Springer.

resources, coping, and engagement in meaningful activities. Through life experience, most older adults learn coping strategies that work for them. Many stressful events in older age can be anticipated and may thus be viewed as somewhat manageable. Lastly, older adults who remain engaged in activities and relationships despite their physical limitations are less likely to experience depression (Kok & Reynolds, 2017).

Differing Presentation of Depression in Older Adults

The DSM-5 provides criteria for the diagnosis of major depression and **persistent depressive disorder** (previously called "dysthymia") (American Psychiatric Association, 2020d). Depression is a syndrome consisting of an array of affective, cognitive, and somatic or physiological symptoms. Affective symptoms include depressed, sad, or irritable mood; loss of pleasure in usual activities; and feelings of worthlessness or guilt. Two cognitive symptoms are decreased concentration and suicidal thoughts or behaviour. Some of the somatic and physiological symptoms are fatigue and decreased energy, increased or decreased appetite or weight, sleep disturbance, and psychomotor agitation or retardation (American Psychiatric Association, 2020d). Depression may result in dependency, poor grooming, difficulty completing activities of daily living, decreased motivation, and decreased sexual interest. Depression may range in severity from mild symptoms to more severe forms, both of which can persist over long periods. Suicidal ideation and psychotic features (e.g., delusional thinking) accompany more severe depression (Zimmerman et al., 2018).

The symptoms of depression in older adults are different from those in people in other age groups. Older adults report more somatic complaints, such as physical symptoms, insomnia, loss of appetite and weight loss, memory problems, and persistent pain. They are less likely to have the feelings of guilt and worthlessness seen in younger individuals. Oftentimes, somatic complaints can be difficult to distinguish from symptoms associated with a physical illnesses (McKenzie & Harvath, 2016). Compared to younger adults with depression, people with late-life depression are also less likely to have a family history of depression (Edelstein et al., 2015).

Hypochondriasis, complaining, and criticism may actually be expressions of depression. Depression may be an early symptom of dementia, but it is unclear whether it is a prodrome for the onset of dementia, a risk factor for dementia, or an independent event (Edelstein et al., 2015). Symptoms such as agitation and repetitive verbalizations in people with dementia may be symptoms of depression. It is very important that older adults with memory impairment be evaluated for depression (see Chapters 7 and 21).

IMPLICATIONS FOR GERONTOLOGICAL NURSING AND HEALTHY AGING

Assessment

Assessment involves a systematic and thorough evaluation with a depression screening instrument, interview, history and physical assessment, functional assessment, cognitive assessment, laboratory tests, medication review, determination of iatrogenic or medical causes, and family or care partner interview, as indicated. Assessment for depressogenic medications and for related comorbid conditions that may contribute to or complicate treatment of depression must also be included. A comprehensive guide to the assessment and treatment of depression in older adults is included in the Registered Nurses' Association of Ontario's (RNAO's) best practice guideline entitled *Delirium, Dementia, and Depression in Older Adults: Assessment and Care* (2nd ed.) (Registered Nurses' Association of Ontario [RNAO], 2016).

Screening of all older adults for depression should be incorporated into routine health assessments across the continuum of care—in hospitals, primary care, LTC and retirement homes, home care, and community-based settings (McKenzie & Harvath, 2016). The Geriatric Depression Scale Short Form (GDS-SF) has been validated and used extensively with older adults (see Chapter 13). The GDS-SF takes approximately 5 minutes to administer, and although it is not a substitute for individualized assessment, it is an effective screening tool for older adults. A video demonstrating use of the GDS-SF is available at https://hign.org/consultgeri/try-this-series/geriatric-depression-scale-gds. The Cornell Scale for Depression in Dementia, a caregiver reporting tool, is used to screen for depression in older adults with dementia (Alexopoulos et al., 1988).

Interventions

When a depression is diagnosed, treatment should begin as soon as possible, and appropriate follow-up should be provided. People living with depression are often unable to follow through on their own; without appropriate treatment and monitoring, they may develop deeper depression or die by suicide. People with severe depression or high suicide risk are often admitted to a health care setting for initial treatment.

The major treatment options for depression are pharmacotherapy and electroconvulsive therapy (ECT), psychotherapy, and psychosocial interventions. The most effective treatment is a combination of pharmacological therapy and psychosocial interventions or psychotherapy. Older adults tend to prefer psychosocial interventions. Interventions are individualized and are based on history, severity of symptoms, concomitant illnesses, and level of disability.

Effective psychosocial treatments include behavioural therapy, CBT, problem-solving therapy, cognitive bibliotherapy, reminiscence therapy, and brief dynamic psychotherapy (Edelstein et al., 2015). Behavioural therapy addresses the link between mood and behaviour. The person learns to monitor mood and activity, increase engagement in activities that improve mood, decrease involvement in unpleasant activities, and develop problem-solving skills to overcome barriers to engaging in activities (Edelstein et al., 2015). Problem-solving therapy teaches people to manage and cope with stressors; it is effective in primary care settings and for medically ill people living at home (Cuijpers et al., 2018). Cognitive bibliotherapy is structured, self-administered CBT in which a person follows written directions with minimal input from a therapist (Gualano et al., 2017). Reminiscence and life review therapy (see Chapter 3) is an effective treatment for depression in older adults and also improves depression symptoms of people living with dementia (Bohlken et al., 2017). One study has found that exercise can assist in the treatment for major depression (Calisgan et al., 2020). In addition, family and social support, education, grief management, and reminiscence and life-review therapy (see Chapter 3) have been helpful for depression. Box 23.5 lists suggestions for families and providers who are caring for older adults living with depression.

A collaborative-care approach in primary care, home care, and LTC homes is recommended. This model involves an interprofessional approach whereby team members, including nurses, are trained in geropsychiatry. Nurses often function as case managers. Nurse-led collaborative care for older adults with persistent illness results in improved depression symptoms (McKenzie & Harvath, 2016). (See Chapter 15 for an in-depth discussion of care models.)

Nursing care of a person with depression should consider the person's comorbid medical conditions and abilities. Priorities for nursing care are outlined in Box 23.6.

Somatic Therapies and Medications

ECT is considered a somatic therapy. It is more often used for older adults with psychotic depression, those who do not respond to antidepressant medications,

---

BOX 23.5

SUGGESTIONS FOR FAMILY AND PROVIDERS OF INTERPERSONAL SUPPORT

- Provide relief from the discomfort of physical illness.
- Enhance physical function (i.e., regular exercise or activity; physical, occupational, and recreational therapies).
- Develop a daily activity schedule that includes pleasant activities.
- Increase opportunities for socialization and enhance social support.
- Provide opportunities for decision making and exercising control.
- Focus on spiritual renewal and rediscovery of meaning.
- Reactivate latent interests, or help develop new ones.
- Validate depressed feelings as a means of aiding recovery (i.e., do not try to bolster the person's mood or deny their despair).
- Help the person become aware of the presence of depression, the nature of the symptoms, and the time-limited nature of depression.
- Provide an accepting atmosphere and an empathic response.
- Share yourself with the person.
- Demonstrate faith in the person's strengths.
- Praise any and all efforts at recovery, no matter how small.
- Assist the person in expressing and dealing with anger.
- Avoid stifling the grief process; grief cannot be hurried.
- Create a hopeful environment where self-esteem is fostered and life is meaningful.
- Assist the person in dealing with guilt.
- Foster the development of connections with others.

---

and those who have a high suicide risk (Rönnqvst et al., 2021). People who have received no treatment, treatment of short duration, or treatment with inadequate doses of medication may respond quite well to ECT. The advantage of ECT as compared to medications is its rapid treatment response with minimal side effects (McKenzie & Harvath, 2016).

Medication therapies are often effective in managing depression. The most commonly prescribed are SSRIs and SNRIs. Tricyclic antidepressants are rarely used for older adults because of significant side effects and risks. The SSRIs are generally well tolerated in older adults; common side effects include nausea, vomiting, dizziness, drowsiness, and hyponatremia (see Chapter 14).

BOX 23.6
NURSING INTERVENTIONS FOR
PEOPLE WITH DEPRESSION

- Provide a therapeutic relationship with the person.
- Ensure a suicidal person's safety.
- Promote adequate nutrition, elimination, and sleep and rest.
- Provide adequate pain control, including the use of adjunctive relaxation strategies.
- Encourage daily exercise.
- Facilitate support from family and friends.
- Facilitate engagement in pleasant activities.
- Maximize the person's control and autonomy.
- Acknowledge and support strengths, capabilities, and hope.

Source: Adapted from McKenzie, G. L., & Harvath, T. A. (2016). Late-life depression. In M. Boltz, E. Capezuti, T. T. Fulmer, et al. (Eds.), *Evidenced-based geriatric nursing protocols for best practice* (5th ed., pp. 211–232). Springer.

Medications must be closely monitored for side effects and therapeutic response. Doses should be lower at first and titrated as indicated (McKenzie & Harvath, 2016). Most antidepressants take about 6 weeks to have a therapeutic effect. The response rate in older adults is similar to that in younger adults, and about half of the people who are prescribed a given antidepressant respond to it. Even with therapeutic doses, many people do not experience complete symptom resolution and may have to try several different antidepressants before finding one that is effective (McKenzie & Harvath, 2016). Therapy is continued for 4 to 6 months. For those with more severe or recurring depression, it is recommended that medication be continued for up to 3 years (Edelstein et al., 2015).

SUICIDE

In 2019, approximately 57.8 per 100,000 people aged 65 years or older were known to have died by suicide (Statistics Canada, 2021). Suicide rates are believed to underestimate the true number of suicides, because suicide is often mistaken for accidental death, and stigmatization leads to a reluctance to label a death suicide. Rates of **suicidal behaviour** are thought to be lower for older adults than for younger adults. However, older adults who have suicidal behaviour are more likely to use lethal methods such as hanging, poisoning, and firearms.

One of the most significant risk factors for suicide is depressive disorder. Other mental disorders (including anxiety, schizophrenia, and substance use disorders) are also important risk factors for suicide in older adults (Vasiliadis et al., 2017). As many as 97% of older adults who die of suicide have a mental illness (Fiske et al., 2015). Hopelessness, a symptom of depression, is also an indicator of suicide risk. Physical health problems such as disability, pain, or multiple serious illnesses—particularly when they are accompanied by depression—confer risk for suicide (McKenzie & Harvath, 2016). Social isolation, loneliness, family discord, and the perception of oneself as a burden are associated with suicidal thoughts (Fiske et al., 2015). Research has shown a link between residential school survivors and suicide (McQuaid et al., 2017; Kitson & Berglund, 2020). Suicide risk is higher for people who have access to lethal means.

As many as half of older adults who die by suicide visited a physician within a month before death, but their depression symptoms and suicidal ideation often go unrecognized (McKenzie & Harvath, 2016). Older adults who are depressed or suicidal often present to their primary care providers with somatic rather than psychological symptoms, which suggests that opportunities for assessing suicidal risk may be missed.

Warning signs of suicidal risk are presented in Box 23.7. Having a purpose in life and feeling that life is meaningful are important resiliency factors for older adults (Heisel & Flett, 2016). Of importance is that risk factors interact with one another.

IMPLICATIONS FOR GERONTOLOGICAL NURSING AND HEALTHY AGING

Assessment

Older adults with suicidal ideas and intent are encountered in many settings. It is the nurse's obligation to prevent suicide whenever possible. Nurses should be vigilant in recognizing suicide risk factors and assessing suicide potential, not only among people who experience mood disorders, but also among those with no apparent mental disorder. The major risk factors

BOX 23.7
SUICIDE WARNING SIGNS FOR OLDER ADULTS

- History of depression or sadness
- Trouble sleeping and eating
- Isolated or withdrawn from social supports
- Feelings of hopelessness, helplessness, anxiousness, or worthlessness
- Lost interest in things they once cared about
- Lost independence or feeling like a burden to others
- See no reason for living or lost sense of purpose in life
- Switching suddenly from deep sadness to calmness or happiness
- Feelings of being "trapped" or that there is no way out of a situation
- Overwhelming feelings or inability to cope
- Experienced trauma or past suicide attempt

Source: Adapted from Canadian Coalition for Seniors' Mental Health. (2016). *Prevention of suicide in older adults.* Author. https://ccsmh.ca/projects/suicide/.

for suicide are detectable, and any direct, indirect, or enigmatic references to the ending of life must be taken seriously and discussed with the person. Putting affairs in order in preparation for death (e.g., giving away possessions and making wills and funeral plans) is a warning sign of suicide. However, this behaviour may be difficult to interpret among older adults, as such behaviours are typically indications of maturity.

The most important task for the nurse is to establish a trusting and respectful relationship with the person. Since many older adults grew up in an era when suicide bore stigma and even criminal implications, they may not bring up their suicidal thoughts. It is important to accept and validate the person's suicidal symptoms. Self-awareness on the part of the nurse is important. Nurses should be careful to avoid statements that normalize thoughts of suicide and should avoid statements that could be perceived as judgemental.

Nurses may be reluctant to ask questions about suicide because of a myth that talking about suicide will incite suicidal ideation. This is not true. Talking about suicide does not increase suicide risk. Rather, in the context of assessment and discussion about the meaning of stressors in life, the person may experience being asked about suicide as a validation of the person's feelings and,

therefore, may experience relief. By talking about suicide, nurses demonstrate interest in the individual and open the door to honest interaction and connection at deep levels of psychological need. Superficial interest and mechanical questioning will not be meaningful. What will make a difference is the nature of the nurse's concern and the nurse's ability to connect with the alienation and desperation of the individual.

If there is suspicion that the older adult is suicidal, the use of direct and straightforward questions, such as the following, is most helpful:

- How often have you thought about dying or killing yourself?
- How often do you feel like life isn't worth living?
- How would you kill yourself if you decided to do it?

In addition to examining risk factors and suicidal intent, the assessment should also include lethality, access to means, and the presence of protective factors. It is important to obtain collateral information from family, friends, care partners, and other care providers who know the older adult. Detailed interview questions for assessing suicidal ideation and plans are available in the RNAO's best practice guideline *Assessment and Care of Adults at Risk for Suicidal Ideation and Behaviour* (2nd ed.) (RNAO, 2009) as well as Sadek's (2019) *A Clinician's Guide to Suicide Risk Assessment and Management*.

Interventions

It is important to have in place a suicide protocol that clearly defines how the nurse will intervene if a positive response is obtained from the suicide assessment. The person should not be left alone until help arrives to assist and care for them. If a person is at risk of suicide, access to lethal means of suicide should be limited. People at high risk should be hospitalized, especially if they have current psychological stressors, access to lethal means of suicide, or both. People at moderate risk may be treated as outpatients, provided they have adequate social support and no access to lethal means. People at lower risk should have a full psychiatric evaluation and receive careful follow-up. Box 23.8 presents interventions to perform if suicidal intent has been established. Interventions should address underlying mental disorders and risk factors such as isolation, hopelessness, pain, and loss.

BOX 23.8
INTERVENTIONS FOR AN OLDER ADULT WITH SUICIDAL INTENT

If suicidal intent has been established, the following interventions, arranged in order of immediacy, are necessary:

1. Reduce immediate danger by removing hazardous articles.
2. Do not leave the person alone; evaluate the need for constant attendance; and arrange for a family member, a friend, or a health care provider to be present during the period of immediate danger.
3. Provide an honest expression of concern, such as "I do not want you to take your life. I will help you with this troubling situation."
4. Consult with a mental health professional and evaluate the person for possible hospitalization.
5. Find out whether a "no-suicide contract" can be drawn up with the person; however, there is no evidence that such an agreement is effective in preventing suicide.
6. Evaluate the need for medication.
7. Focus on the hazard or crisis that is currently causing the most stress for the person.
8. Mobilize internal and external resources by getting the person reinvolved with external supports and reconnected with their internal capabilities. The health care provider, family, or caregiver may have to take the initiative to find activities, support systems, transportation, and other resources for the person.
9. Implement a specific plan of action with an ongoing structured program. Develop a lifeline of individuals who can be called on at any hour of distress, and plan regular calls and follow-up for the person.

BOX 23.9
RISK FACTORS FOR SUBSTANCE USE DISORDERS

1. Male sex (for alcohol), female sex (for prescription drugs)
2. Family history of dependence on alcohol, tobacco, or prescription or illicit drugs
3. Co-occurrence of addiction with dependence on or abuse of another substance (e.g., alcohol and tobacco)
4. Lifelong pattern of substance use, including heavy drinking
5. Social isolation
6. Recent and multiple losses
7. Persistent pain or health issues
8. Physical disabilities or reduced mobility
9. Previous and/or concurrent psychiatric illness
10. Living alone

Sources: Extracted from Kuerbis, A., Sacco, P., Blazer, D. G., et al. (2014). Substance abuse among older adults. *Clinical Geriatric Medicine, 30*(3), 629–654. doi:10.1016/j.cger.2014.04.008; Naegle, M. (2012). *Nursing standard of practice protocol: Substance abuse in older adults.* https://consultgeri.org/geriatric-topics/substance-abuse.

SUBSTANCE USE DISORDERS

Substance use disorders in older adults can be a continuation of long-term problems or they can arise in older age, often in the context of stressful life events or other stressors. This section discusses substance use disorders and substance use, focusing on alcohol, prescription medication, and illicit drugs. (See Chapter 6 for information about smoking cessation.) Risk factors for substance use disorders in older adults are presented in Box 23.9. Terms used to describe substance use disorder are defined in Table 23.1.

Alcohol

The most common type of substance use disorder is problem drinking (Naegle & McCabe, 2016).

TABLE 23.1
Definitions of Substance Use Terms

Term	Definition
Substance use disorder	A disorder affecting a person's brain and behaviour, which leads to the inability to control the use of legal or illegal substances such as alcohol, tobacco, prescription or illicit drugs.
Substance abuse	A maladaptive pattern of using a substance that causes significant consequences, problems or distress.
Substance dependence	A pattern of using a substance that results in the development of tolerance, withdrawal, and compulsive drug-taking behaviour. Dependence can be both physiological and psychological.

Sources: National Institute of Mental Health. (2022). Substance use and co-occurring mental disorders. https://www.nimh.nih.gov/health/topics/substance-use-and-mental-health; John Hopkins Medicine. (2022). Substance abuse/chemical dependency. https://www.hopkinsmedicine.org/health/conditions-and-diseases/substance-abuse-chemical-dependency.

Alcohol-related problems in the older population often go unrecognized, although the long-term effects of alcohol misuse complicate the presentation and treatment of many persistent disorders in older adults. About 75% of older men and 66% of older women drink alcohol occasionally or regularly; for the majority of them, this is not a problem. However, 10% to 13% of older adults have a problem with alcohol use, and the prevalence of unhealthy drinking among men is higher than that among women (Satre & Wolf, 2015). Alcohol use disorders are more likely to emerge in adulthood than in older age, and many people reduce their drinking as they age. For some people, however, the problem emerges or recurs in older age. Late-onset problem drinking may be related to situational events such as illness, retirement, or the death of a spouse and is more common among women than among men (Satre & Wolf, 2015).

Gender Issues

Men (particularly older widowers) are four times more likely than women to misuse alcohol, but the prevalence of alcohol misuse in women may be underestimated. Women of all ages are significantly more vulnerable to the effects of alcohol misuse, including drug interactions, physical injury from alcohol-related falls and accidents, cognitive impairment, and liver and heart disease. Health care providers may assume that older women do not drink problematically and therefore not screen for alcohol misuse. Often, alcohol misuse among women is undetected until the consequences are severe.

Medication Effects

Many medications that older adults use for persistent illnesses have adverse effects when combined with alcohol. Alcohol interacts with at least 50% of prescription medications (Naegle & McCabe, 2016). Medications that interact with alcohol include analgesics, antibiotics, antidepressants, benzodiazepines, H_2 receptor antagonists, nonsteroidal anti-inflammatory drugs, and herbal medications (e.g., echinacea and valerian). When combined with alcohol, acetaminophen taken on a regular basis may lead to liver failure. Alcohol diminishes the effects of oral hypoglycemics, anticoagulants, and anticonvulsants. All older adults should be given precise information about the interaction of alcohol with their medications.

Other effects of alcohol use disorder in older adults include urinary incontinence, which results from rapid bladder filling and diminished neuromuscular control of the bladder; gait disturbances from alcohol-induced cerebellar degeneration and peripheral neuropathy; depression and suicide; sleep disturbances and insomnia; dementia; and delirium. Older adults with alcohol use disorder are also susceptible to cognitive, physical, and functional decline and have increased risk for injury.

Physiology

Normal physiological changes of aging may make older adults more susceptible to health problems when they drink alcohol. Increased body fat, decreased lean body mass, and decreased total body water content can result in a higher blood alcohol level for a given dose of alcohol and alter the absorption and distribution of alcohol (Satre & Wolf, 2015). Reduced liver and kidney functioning result in slower alcohol metabolism and elimination. A decrease in the gastric enzyme alcohol dehydrogenase results in slower metabolism of alcohol and higher blood levels for a longer time.

Because of the high risk of adverse effects from alcohol use, the US National Institute on Alcohol Abuse and Alcoholism recommends that individuals over the age of 65 years limit alcohol consumption to no more than one standard drink per day (that is, 12 ounces of beer, 5 ounces of wine, or 1.5 ounces of liquor) (US National Institute on Alcohol Abuse and Alcoholism, 2021).

Other Substances
Illicit Drugs

Historically, the use of illicit drugs was rare among older adults. However, this is changing rapidly as the "baby boomers" age. Those between the ages of 50 and 64 years report that they use more illicit drugs that are considered "nonmedical" than those in the 65 years and older cohort (Flint et al., 2018). A person's use of an illicit substance does not necessarily mean that the person has a substance use disorder; the use of illicit drugs is problematic when it interferes with the person's health, functioning, relationships, responsibilities, or safety. Supervised consumption and treatment sites in Canada offer services such as safe consumption and overdose prevention services, harm reduction supply distribution, sharps disposal, mental health support and access to social services, primary care, and treatment supports (Region of Waterloo, 2021).

Although few older adults visit these sites, they offer a safe place for authorized use of illicit drugs.

Prescription and Over-the-Counter Medications

Licit substances such as alcohol, opioids, benzodiazepines, and cannabis can cause more harm to older adults than illicit drugs, whether prescribed or misused (Flint et al., 2018). Among older adults, the misuse of prescription and OTC medications is more common than illicit drug use. Medication misuse is defined as using a medication for reasons other than those for which it was prescribed. (More information on prescribed medications and the legalization of marijuana can be found in Chapter 14.)

One-quarter of older adults are prescribed a medication that can potentially be misused, such as benzodiazepines and opioid analgesics (Naegle & McCabe, 2016). The World Health Organization states that, in 2015, 39% of drug use–related deaths were in people over the age of 50; of those, 75% of deaths were due to opioid misuse (Canadian Coalition for Seniors Mental Health, 2021). Even with prescribed opioids, addiction and drug use disorders can occur. Taking opioids for a prolonged period of time can cause the body to get used to the effect and may make people feel like they require a higher dose of the medication (Canadian Coalition for Seniors' Mental Health, 2021). This may result in misuse, overdose, and addiction (Canadian Coalition for Seniors' Mental Health, 2020).

Most older adults who misuse medications do so unintentionally by not taking the medication as directed; using a medication for reasons other than those for which it was intended (e.g., taking dimenhydrinate [Gravol] for sleep); using old medications to treat new symptoms; taking herbal remedies without consulting a pharmacist; sharing medications with others; obtaining prescriptions from multiple physicians; drinking alcohol while taking medication; and taking prescription and OTC medications that interact. Some reasons for misuse of psychoactive prescription medications may be inappropriate prescribing, inadequate health teaching, ineffective monitoring of response, and ineffective follow-up. In many instances, older adults are given prescriptions for benzodiazepines or sedatives because of complaints of insomnia or nervousness, without adequate assessment for depression, anxiety, or other conditions that may be causing the symptoms.

Misuse of benzodiazepines and barbiturates increases risks for sedation, balance problems, falls, and delirium (see Chapter 21). These risks increase with concurrent use of alcohol. Withdrawal from benzodiazepines in older adults is complex and requires careful monitoring.

IMPLICATIONS FOR GERONTOLOGICAL NURSING AND HEALTHY AGING

Assessment

Routine screening for misuse of alcohol, prescription drugs, and illicit drugs is recommended. It is important to establish rapport and explain the reasons for the questions. The questions should be easy to understand and presented in a manner similar to questions asked in a routine assessment. Screening may include short self-report questionnaires or may be part of an assessment interview (Han & Moore, 2018). A caring and supportive approach that provides a culturally safe and open atmosphere is the foundation of a therapeutic relationship. It may also be helpful to discuss the issue factually. For example, the nurse might offer the following explanation: "Many older adults find that the stresses, loneliness, and losses of aging are very hard to bear. Some retreat into alcohol or medication as a way of coping. There are treatments and groups that help people make these difficult adjustments. If this is a problem for you, or if it becomes a problem, please let us know so we may provide resources or referrals for you."

Box 23.10 lists prescreening questions whose answers may alert the nurse to the need for additional assessment, including medical history, physical examination, cognitive and functional assessment, and review of medications. Diagnostic tests should include a complete blood count, liver function tests, chemistries, and an electrocardiogram when appropriate.

As is the case with the previously described mental disorders, many health care providers do not routinely screen for alcohol or other substance use in older adults. This may be related to poor symptom recognition, inadequate knowledge about screening instruments, lack of age-appropriate diagnostic criteria for misuse by older adults, and ageism. The signs of substance use disorders and misuse among older adults may be mistaken for dementia or depression. Furthermore, health

BOX 23.10

PRESCREENING QUESTIONS FOR ALCOHOL AND PRESCRIPTION DRUG MISUSE

ALCOHOL MISUSE

Prescreening question: "Do you drink beer, wine, or other alcoholic beverages?"

Follow-up (if yes): "How many times in the [past year; past 3 months; past week] have you had five or more drinks in a day (for men)/four or more drinks in a day (for women)?"

"On average, how many days per week do you drink alcoholic beverages?"

If weekly or more: "On a day when you drink alcohol, how many drinks do you have?"

PRESCRIPTION DRUG MISUSE

Prescreening questions: "Do you use prescription medicines for pain? Anxiety? Sleep? Do you use any of these prescription drugs in a way that is different from how they were prescribed?"

Follow-up (if yes): Follow up with additional questions regarding which substances, frequency, and quantity of use.

Source: Extracted from Barry, K. L., & Blow, F. C. (2015). Substance use, misuse, and abuse: Special issues for older adults. In N. A. Pachana & K. Laidlaw (Eds.), *The Oxford handbook of clinical geropsychology* (p. 10). Oxford University Press. Reprinted by permission of Oxford University Press. doi:10.1093/oxfordhb/9780199663170.013.015.

BOX 23.11

SIGNS AND SYMPTOMS OF POTENTIAL ALCOHOL USE PROBLEMS IN OLDER ADULTS

- Loss of coordination, falls, slurred speech
- Problems sleeping
- Poor personal care, such as not bathing, not eating (or not eating well), or not taking care of health problems
- Irritability, depression, or confusion
- Stomach problems, lack of desire to eat
- Making excuses or making up stories to cover up the truth about drinking
- Tension in relationships, losing touch with friends or family
- Lack of interest in usual activities, desire to stay alone much of the time
- Signs of alcohol withdrawal, such as a racing pulse, tremors, and agitation

---

Source: Extracted from Centre for Addiction and Mental Health. (2021). *Alcohol use in older adults.* https://www.camh.ca/en/health-info/guides-and-publications/alcohol-use-in-older-adults.

care providers may be pessimistic about the ability of older adults to change longstanding habits (Naegle & McCabe, 2016).

Alcohol

People with alcohol use disorders often reject or deny the diagnosis, or may take offense at the suggestion of it. Feelings of shame may make older adults reluctant to disclose a drinking problem. Family or care partners of older adults with substance use disorders (particularly adult children) may be ashamed of the problem and may choose not to address it. Box 23.11 lists signs and symptoms that may indicate alcohol problems in older adults.

Positive responses to prescreening questions about alcohol use may be followed by using the Michigan Alcoholism Screening Test, Geriatric Version (MAST-G) (available at https://hign.org/consultgeri/try-this-series/alcohol-use-screening-and-assessment-older-adults) or the Alcohol Use Disorders Identification Test (AUDIT) to identify problem drinking or dependence. The AUDIT has good validity for ethnically mixed groups and for older adults (Naegle & McCabe, 2016).

Because of the high risk for depression among heavy drinkers, assessment and screening for depression is important when alcohol misuse is suspected. Screening should also be done before any new medications are prescribed that may interact with alcohol and as needed after life-changing events.

Other Substances

The signs and symptoms of disordered use of illicit drugs or prescription medication are feelings of anxiety, irritability or depression, trouble thinking clearly, problems with relationships, spending money on substances rather than on food, rent, and other essentials, and a loss of hope or feelings of emptiness (Centre for Addiction and Mental Health [CAMH], 2021). For information about signs of problems specific to particular drugs, see the Centre for Addiction and Mental Health (CAMH) website at https://www.camh.ca.

BOX 23.12

QUESTIONS TO ASK ABOUT POTENTIAL MEDICATION MISUSE

- Do you take your medication regularly?
- How often do you skip or forget to take your medication?
- Do you ever have difficulty remembering when to take your medication?
- Do you ever take medication that belongs to someone else?
- Which doctor knows all the medications you are taking?
- Do you ever drink alcohol while you are also taking medication, without first checking with a doctor or pharmacist?
- What do you do with old unused medications that are no longer prescribed?

Source: Extracted from Centre for Addiction and Mental Health. (2008). *Improving our response to older adults with substance use, mental health and gambling problems: A guide for supervisors, managers and clinical staff* (pp. 72–73). Author.

When assessing potential misuse of prescription and OTC medications, assessment should include obtaining a comprehensive list of all medications and determining whether these are used as directed. Some questions to ask as part of this assessment are listed in Box 23.12.

Interventions

Nurses should share information with older adults about safe drinking and the deleterious effects of alcohol. Alcohol and substance use problems affect one's physical, mental, spiritual, and emotional health. Nurses should use nonjudgemental approaches. Interventions must address quality of life and be adapted to meet the unique needs of the older adult (Box 23.13). Older adults may refuse addiction treatment that requires abstinence, and a harm-reduction approach may be more appropriate (Han, 2018):

> *Harm reduction is an evidence-based, client-centred approach that seeks to reduce the health and social harms associated with addiction and substance use, without necessarily requiring people who use substances from abstaining or stopping. Included in the harm reduction approach to substance use is a series of programs, services and practices.* (CMHA, 2021, para. 1)

BOX 23.13

ADAPTING ALCOHOL TREATMENT INTERVENTIONS FOR OLDER ADULTS

- Use supportive, nonconfrontational approaches rather than more assertive styles of assessment.
- Focus on cognitive behavioural approaches.
- Recruit personnel trained to work with older adults.
- Use age-appropriate pace and content. Take into account vision, hearing, and other functional impairments.
- Consider and address issues such as trauma, loss, grief, and health problems.
- Include relevant topics such as worries about the future, including worries about independent living, grandparenting, being retired, and having a fixed income.
- Consider using life review and reminiscence techniques.
- Use a respectful rather than confrontational approach.
- Slow the pace of treatment.
- Use case management and interprofessional approaches.
- Address spiritual needs.
- Tailor treatment to the level of cognitive function.
- Provide opportunities for interesting activities and socialization opportunities that do not involve drinking.
- Focus on strengths and past coping skills used during difficult times.
- Demonstrate faith in the person's ability to change, and avoid ageist attitudes.
- Consider groups designed for women only, as their needs are different.

Sources: Adapted from Lal, R., & Pattanayak, R. D. (2017). Alcohol use among the elderly: Issues and considerations. *Journal of Geriatric Mental Health, 4*(1), 4–10. doi:10.4103/jgmh.jgmh_34_16; Epstein, E., Fischer-Elber, K., & Al-Otaiba, Z. (2007). Women, aging, and alcohol use disorders. *Journal of Women & Aging, 19*(1–2), 31–48; Malatesta, V. (Ed.). (2007). *Mental health issues of older women: A comprehensive review for health care professionals.* Routledge.

Increasing the awareness of older adults about the risks and benefits of consuming alcohol and other substances in the context of their own situation is an important goal. Treatment and intervention strategies include cognitive behavioural approaches, individual and group counselling, medical and psychiatric approaches, referral to Alcoholics Anonymous where appropriate, family or partner therapy, case management and community and home care services, and formalized substance abuse treatment. Treatment outcomes for older adults are similar to or better than outcomes for younger people (Naegle & McCabe, 2016).

Unless the person is in immediate danger, a stepped-care approach should be used, beginning with brief interventions followed by more intensive therapies if necessary. The goals of brief intervention are to (1) reduce or stop consumption of the substance and (2) facilitate entry into formalized treatment if needed. Research results indicate that this type of intervention has positive outcomes for older adults with alcohol use disorders (Han & Moore, 2018).

Long-term self-help treatment programs for older adults show high rates of success, especially when social outlets are emphasized and cohort supports are available. A significant concern is the lack of programs designed specifically for older adults, particularly older women, whose concerns are very different from those of younger people who use drugs or alcohol. Health status, availability of transportation, or impaired mobility may further limit access to treatment. Accessibility can be improved by locating treatment programs in more accessible settings, such as community health centres, senior centres, and assisted-living residences.

Acute Alcohol Withdrawal

When there is significant physical dependence, withdrawal from alcohol can become a life-threatening emergency. Detoxification should be done in a specialized care setting because of the potential medical complications and because withdrawal symptoms in older adults can be prolonged.

Older adults who drink heavily are at risk of experiencing acute alcohol withdrawal if they are admitted to the hospital for treatment of acute illnesses or emergencies. Those with a long history of consuming excess alcohol, previous episodes of acute withdrawal, or a history of prior detoxification are at increased risk for acute alcohol withdrawal (Naegle & McCabe, 2016). Symptoms of acute alcohol withdrawal vary, but may be more severe and last longer in older adults. Minor withdrawal (withdrawal tremulousness) begins 6 to 12 hours after a person has consumed the last drink. Symptoms include tremor, anxiety, nausea, insomnia, tachycardia, and increased blood pressure, and withdrawal may frequently be mistaken for common problems

in older adults. Major withdrawal is seen 10 to 72 hours after cessation of alcohol intake, and the symptoms include vomiting, diaphoresis, hallucinations, tremors, and seizures (Naegle & McCabe, 2016).

Delirium tremens (DT) is alcohol withdrawal delirium; it usually occurs 24 to 72 hours after the last drink but may occur up to 10 days later. Delirium tremens occurs in 5% of people in acute alcohol withdrawal and is considered a medical emergency; the mortality rate is as high as 15% from respiratory failure and cardiac arrhythmia. Other signs and symptoms include confusion, disorientation, hallucinations, hyperthermia, and hypertension. The Clinical Institute Withdrawal Assessment (CIWA) scale is a valid and reliable screening instrument (Larose & Renner, 2016).

Recommended treatment is the use of short-acting benzodiazepines at one-half to one-third the normal dose around the clock, or as needed, during withdrawal. Disulfiram (Antabuse) use in older adults to promote abstinence is not recommended because of the potential for serious cardiovascular complications.

The CIWA scale aids the adjustment of medication. Other interventions are assessing mental status, monitoring vital signs, and maintaining fluid balance without overhydrating the person. Calm and quiet surroundings, no unnecessary stimuli, consistent caregivers, frequent reorientation, prevention of injury, and support and caring are additional interventions. Nutritional assessment is indicated, as well as the addition of thiamine and multivitamins (Naegle & McCabe, 2016).

PROBLEM GAMBLING

Up to 66% of Canadians 18 years of age and older participate in some form of gambling, be it through lotteries, bingo, casinos, or race tracks (Williams et al., 2020). One study found that 2% of Ontarians over 55 years of age experienced a moderate to severe gambling problem (van der Maas et al., 2018). When asked why they gamble, older adults indicate that they gamble for entertainment or fun, to socialize, to support charitable causes, to relieve boredom or loneliness, to make money, and to take advantage of promotions offered to older adults at casinos and race tracks (Community Links, 2010).

Problem gambling is gambling that (1) interferes with work, school, or other activities; (2) harms the person's mental or physical health; (3) hurts the person financially; (4) damages the person's reputation; or (5) causes problems with family or social relationships (CAMH, 2008). Problem gambling can cause anxiety and depression and is a risk factor for suicide. It is more common among those with a history of mental illness or substance abuse. When problem gambling emerges in older adults, it is often related to emotional distress (Tira et al., 2014). The negative effects of problem gambling include financial loss for the person and family, strained family or care partner relationships, a higher risk of experiencing physical and emotional abuse, and a higher risk for physical and mental illnesses, both for the person and for the family.

IMPLICATIONS FOR GERONTOLOGICAL NURSING AND HEALTHY AGING

Assessment

Assessment is often complicated, as people who are affected by problem gambling may hide or deny the problem (possibly owing to shame, embarrassment, fear of the consequences of disclosure, or hopelessness). A nonjudgemental approach is important. Screening for problem gambling can be integrated into the assessment of recreation activities and the assessment of financial well-being. Nurses should be aware of the signs of problem gambling (Box 23.14). A detailed list of behavioural, emotional, financial, and health signs of problem gambling, as well as screening tools for problem gambling, are available from CAMH (https://www.problemgambling.ca). The CAMH gambling screen is a short self-assessment and screening tool (Box 23.15). If problem gambling is suspected, the Problem Gambling Severity Index can be used (available at https://www.problemgambling.ca).

Interventions

Public education and increased public awareness of problem gambling contribute to prevention, early identification, and earlier treatment of gambling. A good educational tool is *Betting on Older Adults: A Problem Gambling Awareness Kit*, which includes a video, interactive activities, and a facilitator's guide (https://www.problemgambling.ca). All provinces and

---

BOX 23.14
SIGNS OF PROBLEM GAMBLING

- Spending more money on gambling than intended.
- Feeling bad, sad, or guilty about gambling.
- Placing larger, more frequent bets.
- Not having enough money for food, rent, or bills after gambling.
- Loss of interest and participation in normal activities with friends and family.
- Placing a high priority on gambling.
- Being secretive about the amount of time and money spent gambling.

Source: Extracted from Centre for Addiction and Mental Health. (2021). *Gambling in older adults.* https://www.camh.ca/en/health-info/guides-and-publications/gambling-in-older-adults.

BOX 23.15
CENTRE FOR ADDICTION AND MENTAL HEALTH GAMBLING SCREEN

1. In the past 12 months, have you gambled more than you intended to?
2. In the past 12 months, have you claimed to be winning money when you were not?
3. In the past 12 months, have you felt guilty about the way you gamble or about what happens when you gamble?
4. In the past 12 months, have people criticized you for your gambling?
5. In the past 12 months, have you had money arguments centred on gambling?
6. In the past 12 months, did you feel you had to persist until you won?
7. If you answered "yes" to two or more of these questions, how often has it happened? Once, only sometimes, or often?

Source: Centre for Addition and Mental Health. (2011). *CAMH Gambling Screen.* http://www.insightcounsellingservices.ca/files/documents/CAMH-Gambling-Screen-new.pdf.

---

territories have gambling help lines and websites with information about accessing services. When problem gambling is identified, the person should be referred to a mental health provider. Specialized gambling counselling is available through addiction treatment services. Peer support may be especially important for reaching and helping older adults who are at risk for or are experiencing problem gambling (Matheson et al., 2018). Therapeutic approaches include CBT, motivational interviewing, psychotherapy, aversion therapy, the 12-step program, and self-exclusion. The evidence of effectiveness is greatest for CBT and motivational interviewing (Merkouris et al., 2016). Although older adults may be more likely to drop out of treatment, older age is associated with better treatment outcomes (Merkouris et al., 2016). It is important to address the comorbid medical and mental health conditions of people who have problem gambling. Self-help tools and resources for families are available in 22 languages at https://www.problemgambling.ca.

IMPLICATIONS FOR GERONTOLOGICAL NURSING AND HEALTHY AGING

The development of holistic and humanistic models of care for older adults experiencing mental health disturbances is critically important in gerontological nursing. Much of the distress associated with mental disorders in late life can be relieved through competent and compassionate gerontological nursing care. An awareness of appropriate assessment and treatment of the mental illnesses that can occur in later life is a very important component of care.

Knowing and appreciating each older adult's uniqueness, their past and present experiences, and how these experiences influence the present are important to promoting mental health and wellness. Believing in and supporting the strength and wisdom of older adults supports their self-confidence and feelings of worth, important components of mental health and wellness. To appreciate the nature of loss and grief in old age, gerontological nurses need to really listen and offer support. Nurses' work must focus on care environments that enhance physical and mental health and wellness, create conditions of hope, and support older adults.

KEY CONCEPTS

- Mental health in later life is difficult to determine, because the accrual of life experiences results in wide variability in the mental health of older adults.
- Mental health is a fluctuating situation for most individuals, with peaks and valleys of happiness and pain.
- The prevalence of mental disorders has increased significantly with the aging of the baby boomers.
- Mental disorders are underreported and underdiagnosed among older adults. Somatic complaints are often the presenting symptoms of mental disorders, making diagnosis difficult.
- The incidence of psychotic disorders with late-life onset is low among older adults, but psychotic manifestations can occur as secondary symptoms in a variety of disorders, the most common of which is Alzheimer's disease.
- Anxiety disorders are common in later life and can be successfully treated.
- Post-traumatic stress disorder is finally being recognized in older adults who have experienced traumatic events.
- Depression is the most common mental disorder of aging and is the most treatable. Unfortunately, it is often neglected or assumed to be a condition of aging that one must "learn to live with." An important nursing intervention is assessment of depression.
- Suicide is a significant problem among older men. Assessment of suicidal intent is important, especially in the light of loss. Many older adults who die of suicide are seen by a health care provider and present with physical complaints shortly before they die.
- Substance use and the misuse of prescription medications are often underrecognized and undertreated in older adults, especially older women. Screening and appropriate assessment and intervention are important in all care settings.
- Problem gambling can have significant consequences for older adults and their families and care partners. Public education and increased awareness are needed for prevention, early identification, and effective treatment.
- Further research is needed to fully understand the cultural and ethnic differences in people's mental health concerns and to appropriately assess and support ethnically and culturally diverse older adults.

ACTIVITIES AND DISCUSSION QUESTIONS

1. List the various stressors you have encountered with the older adults you have cared for and discuss what was done about them.

2. Discuss the three most common mental disorders that older adults are likely to experience and describe appropriate assessment and treatment.

3. Explain what is likely to be different in the appearance of depression in a person who is 70 years old versus that in a person who is 20 years old.

4. Describe the behaviours that are indicative of suicidal intent in an older adult. Discuss the methods of assessment and your reactions to them.

5. Discuss the various situations that may result in an older adult's substance abuse and ways to effectively intervene.

6. Describe the type of teaching on the use of alcohol and medications you would provide to an older adult.

7. Formulate strategies that may be used to promote mental health and wellness in later life.

RESOURCES

Alcohol Use Disorders Identification Test (AUDIT)
https://patient.info/doctor/alcohol-use-disorders-identification-test-audit
Canadian Academy of Geriatric Psychiatry
http://www.cagp.ca
Canadian Coalition for Seniors' Mental Health
https://www.ccsmh.ca
Canadian Mental Health Association
https://www.cmha.ca
Centre for Addiction and Mental Health
https://www.camh.ca
Mental Health Commission of Canada
https://www.mentalhealthcommission.ca
Mood Disorders Society of Canada
https://mdsc.ca/
National Coalition on Mental Health and Aging
http://www.ncmha.org
Network for Aboriginal Mental Health Research. *Mental health programs for Aboriginal peoples in Canada.*
http://www.namhr.ca/mental-health-programs/
Schizophrenia Society of Canada
https://www.schizophrenia.ca

For additional resources, please visit *http://evolve.elsevier.com/Canada/Ebersole/gerontological/*

REFERENCES

Adams, L. Y., Koop, P., Quan, H., et al. (2015). A population-based comparison of the use of acute healthcare services by older adults with and without mental illness diagnoses. *Journal of Psychiatric and Mental Health Nursing, 22*(1), 29–46. doi:10.1111/jpm.12169.

AlAteeq, D., AlDaoud, A., AlHadi, A., et al. (2018). The experience and impact of stigma in Saudi people with a mood disorder. *Annals of General Psychiatry, 17*(1), 51. doi:10.1186/s12991-018-0221-3.

Alexopoulos, G., Young, J., & Shamoian, C. (1988). Cornell scale for depression in Dementia. *Biological Psychiatry, 23,* 271–284. doi:10.1016/0006-3223(88)90038-8.

Alzheimer Society of Canada. (2021). *Delusions and hallucinations.* https://alzheimer.ca/en/help-support/im-caring-person-living-dementia/understanding-symptoms/delusions-hallucinations.

American Psychiatric Association. (2020a). *What is obsessive-compulsive disorder?* https://www.psychiatry.org/patients-families/ocd/what-is-obsessive-compulsive-disorder.

American Psychiatric Association. (2020b). *What is posttraumatic stress disorder?* https://www.psychiatry.org/patients-families/ptsd/what-is-ptsd.

American Psychiatric Association. (2020c). *What is schizophrenia?* https://www.psychiatry.org/patients-families/schizophrenia/what-is-schizophrenia.

American Psychiatric Association. (2020d). *Diagnostic and statistical manual of mental disorders* (5th ed.). Author. https://www.psychiatry.org/psychiatrists/practice/dsm.

Ayers, C., Strickland, K., & Wetherell, J. L. (2015). Evidence-based treatment for late-life generalized anxiety disorder. In P. A. Areán (Ed.), *Treatment of late-life depression, anxiety, trauma, and substance abuse* (pp. 111–139). American Psychological Association.

Battiste, M. (2005). Indigenous knowledge: Foundations for first nations. *WINHEC: International Journal of Indigenous Education Scholarship, 1,* 1–17. https://journals.uvic.ca/index.php/winhec/article/view/19251.

Bohlken, J., Weber, S. A., Siebert, A., et al. (2017). Reminiscence therapy for depression in dementia: An observational study with matched pairs. *GeroPsych: The Journal of Gerontopsychology and Geriatric Psychiatry, 30*(4), 145–151. doi:10.1024/1662-9647/a000175.

Bower, E. S., & Wetherell, J. L. (2015). Late-life anxiety disorders. In P. A. Lichtenberg, B. T. Mast, B. D. Carpenter, et al. (Eds.), *APA handbook of clinical geropsychology, Vol. 2: Assessment, treatment, and issues in later life* (pp. 49–77). American Psychological Association.

Byrd, E. (2005). Nursing assessment and treatment of depressive disorders of late life. In K. Mellilo & S. Houde (Eds.), *Geropsychiatric and mental health nursing* (pp. 147–170). Jones & Bartlett Learning.

Calisgan, E., Cumurcu, H. B., Talu, B., et al. (2020). The effects of physiotherapy methods combined with respiratory and relaxation exercises on patients with major depression. *Medicine, 9*(4), 837–843.

Canadian Coalition for Seniors' Mental Health. (2020). *Opioid use among older adults.* https://ccsmh.ca/wp-content/uploads/2020/09/CCSMH_Opioid_brochure_ENG.pdf.

Canadian Coalition for Seniors' Mental Health. (2021). *Substance use and addiction.* Available from https://ccsmh.ca/substance-use-addiction/opioids/.

Canadian Mental Health Association (CMHA). (2021). *Harm reduction.* https://ontario.cmha.ca/harm-reduction/.

Canadian Coalition for Seniors' Mental Health. (2020). *Opioid use among older adults.* Available from https://ccsmh.ca/wp-content/uploads/2020/09/CCSMH_Opioid_brochure_ENG.pdf.

Canuto, A., Weber, K., Baertschi, M., et al. (2018). Anxiety disorders in old age: Psychiatric comorbidities, quality of life, and prevalence according to age, gender, and country. *American Journal of Geriatric Psychiatry, 26*(2), 174–185. doi:10.1016/j.jagp.2017.08.015.

Ceglowski, J., de Dios, L. V., & Depp, C. A. (2015). Psychosis in older adults. In N. A. Pachana & K. Laidlaw (Eds.), *The Oxford handbook of clinical geropsychology.* Oxford University Press. doi:10.1093/oxfordhb/9780199663170.013.041.

Center for Behavioral Health Statistics and Quality. (2016). *Impact of the DSM-IV to DSM-5 changes on the National Survey on Drug Use and Health.* Substance Abuse and Mental Health Services Administration, US Department of Health and Human Services.

Centre for Addiction and Mental Health (CAMH). (2008). *Improving our response to older adults with substance use, mental health and gambling problems: A guide for supervisors, managers and clinical staff.* Author.

Centre for Addiction and Mental Health (CAMH). (2021). *Addiction.* https://www.camh.ca/en/health-info/mental-illness-and-addiction-index/addiction.

Chen, J., Chen, H., Feng, J., et al. (2018). Association between hyperuricemia and metabolic syndrome in patients suffering from bipolar disorder. *BMC Psychiatry, 18*(1), 390. doi:10.1186/s12888-018-1952-z.

Community Links. (2010). *Seniors and gambling: A hidden problem? A report of the Seniors and Gambling Project.* http://nscommunitylinks.ca/publications/SeniorsandGambling.pdf.

Cook, J. M., & Dinnen, S. (2015). Exposure therapy for late-life trauma. In P. A. Areán (Ed.), *Treatment of late-life depression, anxiety, trauma, and substance abuse* (pp. 133–161). American Psychological Association.

Cuijpers, P., de Wit, L., Kleiboer, A., et al. (2018). Problem-solving therapy for adult depression: An updated meta-analysis. *European Psychiatry, 48*(1), 27–37. doi:10.1016/j.eurpsy.2017.11.006.

Davison, K. M., Lung, Y., Lin, S. L., et al. (2019). Depression in middle and older adulthood: The role of immigration, nutrition, and other determinants of health in the Canadian longitudinal study on aging. *BMC Psychiatry, 19*(1), 329. doi:10.1186/s12888-019-2309-y.

De Pinho, L. G., Pereira, A., & Chaves, C. (2017). Interventions in schizophrenia: The importance of therapeutic relationship. *Nursing & Care Open Access Journal, 3*(6), 00090. doi:10.15406/ncoaj.2017.03.00090.

DiNapoli, E. A., & Scogin, F. R. (2015). Late-life depression. In N. A. Pachana & K. Laidlaw (Eds.), *The Oxford handbook of clinical geropsychology.* Oxford University Press. doi:10.1093/oxfordhb/9780199663170.001.0001.

Dyer, S. M., Harrison, S. L., Laver, K., et al. (2018). An overview of systematic reviews of pharmacological and non-pharmacological interventions for the treatment of behavioral and psychological symptoms of dementia. *International Psychogeriatrics, 30*(3), 295–309. doi:10.1017/S1041610217002344.

Edelstein, B. A., Bamonti, P. M., Gregg, J. J., et al. (2015). Depression in later life. In P. A. Lichtenberg, B. T. Mast, B. D. Carpenter, et al. (Eds.), *APA handbook of clinical geropsychology, Vol. 2: Assessment, treatment, and issues in later life* (pp. 15–59). American Psychological Association.

Erikson, E. H., Erikson, J. M., & Kivnick, H. Q. (1986). *Vital involvement in old age: The experience of old age in our time.* W.W. Norton.

Fiske, A., Smith, M. D., & Price, E. C. (2015). Suicidal behavior in older adults. In P. A. Lichtenberg, B. T. Mast, B. D. Carpenter, et al. (Eds.), *APA handbook of clinical geropsychology, Vol. 2: Assessment, treatment, and issues in later life* (pp. 154–181). American Psychological Association.

Flint, A., Merali, Z., and Vaccarino, F. (Eds.). (2018). *Substance use in Canada: Improving quality of life: Substance use and aging.* Canadian Centre on Substance Use and Addiction.

Franco, C., Amutio, A., Mañas, I., et al. (2017). Reducing anxiety, geriatric depression and worry in a sample of older adults through a mindfulness training program. *Terapia Psicológica, 35*(1), 71–79. doi:10.4067/S0718-48082017000100007.

Gold, S. M., Köhler-Forsberg, O., Moss-Morris, R., et al. (2020). Comorbid depression in medical diseases. *Nature Reviews Disease Primers, 6*(1), 1–22. doi:10.1038/s41572-020-0200-2.

Government of Canada. (2016). *Report on the social isolation of seniors.* https://www.canada.ca/en/national-seniors-council/programs/publications-reports/2014/social-isolation-seniors/page05.html.

Government of Canada. (2017). *About mental illness.* https://www.canada.ca/en/public-health/services/about-mental-illness.html.

Government of Canada. (2018a). *Social isolation of seniors: A focus on new immigrant and refugee seniors in Canada.* https://www.canada.ca/en/employment-social-development/corporate/seniors/forum/social-isolation-immigrant-refugee.html.

Government of Canada. (2018b). *Rights of LGBTI persons.* https://www.canada.ca/en/canadian-heritage/services/rights-lgbti-persons.html.

Government of Canada. (2018c). *Social isolation of seniors: A focus on Indigenous seniors in Canada.* https://www.canada.ca/en/employment-social-development/corporate/seniors/forum/social-isolation-indigenous.html.

Gualano, M. R., Bert, F., Martorana, M., et al. (2017). The long-term effects of bibliotherapy in depression treatment: Systematic review of randomized clinical trials. *Clinical Psychology Review, 58*, 49–58. doi:10.1016/j.cpr.2017.09.006.

Guruge, S., Thomson, M. S., & Seifi, S. G. (2015). Mental health and service issues faced by older immigrants in Canada: A scoping review. *Canadian Journal on Aging, 34*(04), 431–444. doi:10.1017/S0714980815000379.

Han, B. H. (2018). Aging, multimorbidity, and substance use disorders: The growing case for integrating the principles of geriatric care and harm reduction. *International Journal on Drug Policy*, 58(2018), 135–136. doi:10.1016/j.drugpo.2018.06.005.

Han, B. H., & Moore, A. A. (2018). Prevention and screening of unhealthy substance use by older adults. *Clinics in Geriatric Medicine*, 34(1), 117–129.

Havaei, F., Ma, A., Staempfli, S., et al. (2021). Nurses' workplace conditions impacting their mental health during COVID-19: A cross-sectional survey study. *Healthcare*, 9(1), 84. doi:10.3390/healthcare9010084.

Heid, A. R., Christman, Z., Pruchno, R., et al. (2016). Vulnerable, but why? Post-traumatic stress symptoms in older adults exposed to Hurricane Sandy. *Disaster Medicine and Public Health Preparedness*, 10(03), 362–370. doi:10.1017/dmp.2016.15.

Heisel, M. J., & Flett, G. L. (2016). Investigating the psychometric properties of the Geriatric Suicide Ideation Scale (GSIS) among community-residing older adults. *Aging & Mental Health*, 20(2), 208–221. doi:10.1080/13607863.2015.1072798.

Hill, G. (2021). *Indigenous healing: Voices of elders and healers.* J. Charlton Publishing.

Jenkins, E. K., McAuliffe, C., Hirani, S., et al. (2021). A portrait of the early and differential mental health impacts of the COVID-19 pandemic in Canada: Findings from the first wave of a nationally representative cross-sectional survey. *Preventive Medicine*, 145, 106333. doi:10.1016/j.ypmed.2020.106333.

Katzman, M. A., Bleau, P., Blier, P., et al. (2014). Canadian clinical practice guidelines for the management of anxiety, posttraumatic stress and obsessive-compulsive disorders. *BMC Psychiatry*, 14(1), S1. doi:10.1186/1471-244X-14-S1-S1.

Kim, W., Kang, S. Y., & Kim, I. (2015). Depression among Korean immigrant elders living in Canada and the United States: A comparative study. *Journal of Gerontological Social Work*, 58(1), 86–103. doi:10.10 80/01634372.2014.919977.

King, T., Cardinal, T., & Highway, T. (2005). *Our story: Aboriginal voices on Canada's past.* Anchor Publishing.

Kitson, A., & Berglund, L. (2020). Preserving the painful: Lessons on agency, preservation, and dialogue in acknowledging Canadian's Indian residential school sites. *Preservation Education & Research*, 12(2020), 24–47. doi:10.5749/preseducrese.12.2020.0024.

Knockwood, I. (1992). *Out of the depths: The experiences of Mi'kmaw children at the Indian residential school at Shubenacadie, Nova Scotia.* Fernwood Publishing.

Kok, R. M., & Reynolds, C. F. (2017). Management of depression in older adults: A review. *Journal of the American Medical Association*, 317(20), 2114–2122. doi:10.1001/jama.2017.5706.

Kredenster, M. S., Martens, P. J., Chochinov, H. M., et al. (2014). Cause and rate of death in people with schizophrenia across the lifespan: A population-based study in Manitoba, Canada. *Journal of Clinical Psychiatry*, 75(2), 154–161. doi:10.1016/j.apnu.2015.11.005.

Lamoureux-Lamarche, C., Vasiliadis, H. M., Préville, M., et al. (2016). Post-traumatic stress syndrome in a large sample of older adults: Determinants and quality of life. *Aging & Mental Health*, 20(4), 401–406. doi:10.1080/13607863.2015.1018864.

Larose, A. T., & Renner, J. (2016). Alcohol and older adults. In M. A. Sullivan & F. R. Levin (Eds.), *Addiction in the older patient* (pp. 69–104). Oxford University Press.

Lenze, E. J., Hickman, S., Hershey, T., et al. (2014). Mindfulness-based stress reduction for older adults with worry symptoms and co-occurring cognitive dysfunction. *International Journal of Geriatric Psychiatry*, 29(10), 991–1000. doi:10.1002/gps.4086.

Lopez, V., Sanchez, K., Killian, M. O., et al. (2018). Depression screening and education: An examination of mental health literacy and stigma in a sample of Hispanic women. *BMC Public Health*, 18(1), 646. doi:10.1186/s12889-018-5516-4.

MacDonald, C., & Steenbeek, A. (2015). The impact of colonization and Western assimilation on health and wellbeing of Canadian Aboriginal people. *International Journal of Regional and Local History*, 10(1), 32–48. doi:10.1179/2051453015Z.00000000023.

Matheson, F. I., Sztainert, T., Lakman, Y., et al. (2018). Prevention and treatment of problem gambling among older adults: A scoping review. *Journal of Gambling Issues*, 39. doi:10.4309/jgi.2018.39.2.

Mausbach, B. T., & Ho, J. (2015). Schizophrenia in late life. In P. A. Lichtenberg, B. T. Mast, B. D. Carpenter, et al. (Eds.), *APA handbook of clinical geropsychology, Vol. 2: Assessment, treatment, and issues in later life* (pp. 105–129). American Psychological Association.

McKenzie, G. L., & Harvath, T. A. (2016). Late-life depression. In M. Boltz, L. Capezuti, T. T. Fulmer, et al. (Eds.), *Evidence-based geriatric nursing protocols for best practice* (5th ed., pp. 211–232). Springer.

McQuaid, R. J., Bombay, A., McInnis, O. A., et al. (2017). Suicide ideation and attempts among First Nations peoples living on-reserve in Canada: The intergenerational and cumulative effects of Indian residential schools. *Canadian Journal of Psychiatry*, 62(6), 422–430. doi:10.1177/0706743717702075.

Mental Health Commission of Canada (MHCC). (2009). *Towards recovery and well-being: A framework for a mental health strategy for Canada.* Author. https://www.mentalhealthcommission. ca/wp-content/uploads/drupal/FNIM_Toward_Recovery_and_ Well_Being_ENG_0_1.pdf.

Mental Health Commission of Canada (MHCC). (2012). *Changing directions, changing lives: The mental health strategy for Canada.* https://www.mentalhealthcommission.ca/wp-content/uploads/ drupal/MHStrategy_Strategy_ENG.pdf.

Merkouris, S. S., Thomas, S. A., Browning, C. J., et al. (2016). Predictors of outcomes of psychological treatments for disordered gambling: A systematic review. *Clinical Psychology Review*, 48, 7–31. doi:10.1016/j.cpr.2016.06.004.

Moyser, M. (2020). *StatCan COVID-19: Data to insights for a better Canada. Gender differences in mental health during the COVID-19 pandemic.* https://www150.statcan.gc.ca/n1/pub/45-28-0001/2020001/article/00047-eng.htm.

Munir, S., & Takov, V. (2020). *Generalized anxiety disorder.* StatPearls. https://www.ncbi.nlm.nih.gov/books/NBK441870/.

Naegle, M. A., & McCabe, D. (2016). Substance misuse and alcohol use disorders. In M. Boltz, L. Capezuti, T. T. Fulmer, et al. (Eds.), *Evidence-based geriatric nursing protocols for best practice* (5th ed., pp. 457–477). Springer.

Ngo, V. T. H., Camacho, H., & Singh, J. (2019). "You are the one who was beating me": A case report of a patient with postictal psychosis secondary to bilateral temporal lobe epilepsy. *Cureus*, 11(11), e6069. doi:10.7759/cureus.6069.

Pachana, N. A., Byrne, G. J., Siddle, H., et al. (2007). Development and validation of the Geriatric Anxiety Inventory. *International Psychogeriatrics*, 19(1), 103–114. doi:10.1017/S104161020 6003504.

Park, N. S., Jang, Y., & Chiriboga, D. A. (2018). Willingness to use mental health counseling and antidepressants in older Korean Americans: The role of beliefs and stigma about depression. *Ethnicity & Health*, *23*(1), 97–110. doi:10.1080/13557858.2016.1246429.

Parker, G., Lie, D., Siskind, D. J., et al. (2016). Mental health implications for older adults after natural disasters—A systematic review and meta-analysis. *International Psychogeriatrics*, *28*(1), 11–20. doi:10.1017/S1041610215001210.

Pary, R., Sarai, S. K., Micchelli, A., et al. (2019). Anxiety disorders in older patients. *Primary Care Companion to CNS Disorders*, *21*(1), 18nr02335. doi:10.4088/PCC.18nr02335.

Region of Waterloo. (2021). *Consumption and treatment services*. https://www.regionofwaterloo.ca/en/health-and-wellness/consumption-and-treatment-services.aspx.

Registered Nurses' Association of Ontario (RNAO). (2009). *Assessment and care of adults at risk for suicidal ideation and behaviour*. Author. https://rnao.ca/bpg/guidelines/assessment-and-care-adults-risk-suicidal-ideation-and-behaviour.

Registered Nurses' Association of Ontario (RNAO). (2016). *Delirium, dementia, and depression in older adults: Assessment and care* (2nd ed.). Author. https://rnao.ca/bpg/guidelines/assessment-and-care-older-adults-delirium-dementia-and-depression.

Rej, S., Schuurmans, J., Elie, D., et al. (2016). Attitudes towards pharmacotherapy in late-life bipolar disorder. *International Psychogeriatrics*, *28*(6), 945–950. doi:10.1017/S1041610215002380.

Rönnqvst, I., Nilsson, F. K., & Nordenskjöld, A. (2021). Electroconvulsive therapy and the risk of suicide in hospitalized patients with major depressive disorder. *JAMA Network Open*, *4*(7), e2116589. doi:10.1001/jamanetworkopen.2021.16589.

Sachdev, P. S., Mohan, A., Taylor, L., et al. (2016). DSM-5 and mental disorders in older individuals: An overview. *Harvard Review of Psychiatry*, *23*(5), 320–328. doi:10.1097/HRP.0000000000000090.

Sadek, J. (2019). *A clinician's guide to suicide risk assessment and management*. Springer. doi:10.1007/978-3-319-77773-3.

Satre, D. D., & Wolf, J. P. (2015). Alcohol abuse and substance misuse in later life. In P. A. Lichtenberg, B. T. Mast, B. D. Carpenter, et al. (Eds.), *APA handbook of clinical geropsychology, Vol. 2: Assessment, treatment, and issues of later life* (pp. 130–153). American Psychological Association.

Segal, D. L., June, A., Payne, M., et al. (2010). Development and initial validation of a self-report assessment tool for anxiety among older adults: The Geriatric Anxiety Scale. *Journal of Anxiety Disorders*, *24*(7), 709–714. doi:10.1016/j.janxdis.2010.05.002.

Siskind, D. J., Sawyer, E., Lee, I., et al. (2016). The mental health of older persons after human-induced disasters: A systematic review and meta-analysis of epidemiological data. *American Journal of Geriatric Psychiatry*, *24*(5), 379–388. doi:10.1016/j.jagp.2015.12.010.

Statistics Canada. (2016). *Rates of depression, 12 month, by age and sex, Canada, household population 15 and older, 2012*. http://www.statcan.gc.ca/pub/82-624-x/2013001/article/c-g/11855-c-g-01-eng.htm.

Statistics Canada. (2021). *Suicides and suicide rate, by sex and by age group (both sexes rate)*. http://www.statcan.gc.ca/tables-tableaux/sum-som/l01/cst01/hlth66d-eng.htm.

Stinchcombe, A., Wilson, K., Kortes-Miller, K., et al. (2018). Physical and mental health inequalities among aging lesbian, gay, and bisexual Canadians: Cross-sectional results from the Canadian Longitudinal Study on Aging (CLSA). *Canadian Journal of Public Health*, *109*(5–6), 833–844. doi:10.17269/s41997-018-0100-3.

Tamminga, C. (2020). *Schizophrenia*. Merck Manuals. https://www.merckmanuals.com/en-ca/home/mental-health-disorders/schizophrenia-and-related-disorders/schizophrenia.

Tira, C., Jackson, A. C., & Tomnay, J. E. (2014). Pathways to late-life problematic gambling in seniors: A grounded theory approach. *Gerontologist*, *54*(6), 1035–1048. doi:10.1093/geront/gnt107.

US National Institute on Alcohol Abuse and Alcoholism. (2021). *Older adults*. https://www.niaaa.nih.gov/alcohols-effects-health/special-populations-co-occurring-disorders/older-adults.

Valiengo, L. C. L., Stella, F., & Forlenza, O.V. (2016). Mood disorders in the elderly: Prevalence, functional impact and management challenges. *Neuropsychiatric Disease and Treatment*, *12*, 2105–2114. doi:10.2147/NDT.S94643.

van der Mass, M., Mann, R. E., Turner, N. E., et al. (2018). The prevalence of problem gambling and gambling-related behaviours among older adults in Ontario. *Journal of Gambling Issues*, *39*. doi:10.4309/jgi.2018.39.3.

Vasiliadis, H. M., Lamoureux-Lamarche, C., & Guerra, S. G. (2017). Gender and age group differences in suicide risk associated with co-morbid physical and psychiatric disorders in older adults. *International Psychogeriatrics*, *29*(2), 249–257. doi:10.1017/S1041610216001290.

Weiss, D. S., & Marmar, C. R. (1997). The impact of event scale-revised. In J. P. Wilson & T. M. Keane (Eds.), *Assessing psychological trauma and PTSD: A practitioner's handbook* (pp. 399–411). Guilford Press.

Williams, R. J., Leonard, C. A., Belanger, Y. D., et al. (2020). Gambling and problem gambling in Canada in 2018: Prevalence and changes since 2002. *Canadian Journal of Psychiatry*, *66*(5), 485–494. doi:10.1177/0706743720980080.

Wilson, K., & Stinchcombe, A. (2019). *Policy brief: Policy legacies and forgotten histories: Health impacts on LCGTQ2 older adults*. https://www.ourcommons.ca/Content/Committee/421/HESA/Brief/BR10449325/br-external/WilsonKimberley-e.pdf.

Wilson, K., Stinchcombe, A., Kortes-Miller, K., et al. (2016). Support needs of lesbian, gay, bisexual, and transgender older adults in the health and social environment. *Counselling and Spirituality*, *35*(1), 13–29. doi:10.2143/CS.35.1.3189089.

Wisocki, P. A., Handen, B., & Morse, C. (1986). The Worry Scale as a measure of anxiety among homebound and community active elderly. *Behavior Therapist*, *5*, 91–95.

World Health Organization (WHO). (2018, March 30). *Mental health: Strengthening our response*. https://www.who.int/news-room/fact-sheets/detail/mental-health-strengthening-our-response.

World Health Organization (WHO). (2019, November 28). *Mental disorders*. https://www.who.int/news-room/fact-sheets/detail/mental-disorders.

Zimmerman, M., Morgan, T. A., & Stanton, K. (2018). The severity of psychiatric disorders. *World Psychiatry*, *17*, 258–275. doi:10.1002/wps.20569.

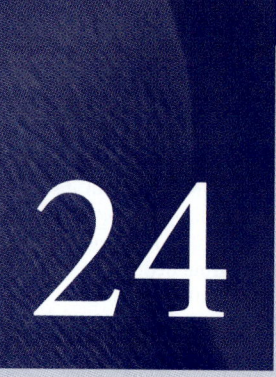

24

ECONOMIC AND LEGAL ISSUES

GLOSSARY

Gross domestic product   The main measure of economic activity, defined as "the total market value of all final goods and services produced within a country in a given period of time (usually a calendar year)" (Black et al., 2009, para. 1).

Intersectoral collaboration   Health care providers working with experts in fields outside the health sector (e.g., housing, employment, justice).

Net income   Income after deductions for certain payments and deductions specified by the Canada Revenue Agency (pensions, union dues, child care expenses, disability support, moving expenses, support payments, employment expenses, and clergy residence costs).

THE LIVED EXPERIENCE

"First of all, if she had a normal income, she would eat fruit. Lots of fruit, lots of vegetables. Because right now she cannot afford it. And then she can save and go to Hajj. Very important, first of all. And then after that, maybe she can go somewhere, see places and have fun. Now with this money we're just staying here, and not properly eating, not properly enjoying, and just living."
Interpreter for participant No. 22, an older adult

Salma, J., & Salamai, B. (2020). "We are like any other people, but we don't cry much because nobody listens": The need to strengthen aging policies and service provision for minorities in Canada. *The Gerontologist, 60*(2), 279–290. doi:10.1093/geront/gnz184.

Canadians represent all levels of education, experience, and income. However, what everyone has in common is the potential need for health care. It is rare to meet an older adult who does not have some experience with both the past and the present Canadian health care systems. The Canadian health care system is in a constant state of flux. Health care financing is a political issue and a topic of debate across Canada. For nurses, it is important to have a basic understanding of how the health care system is financed and what the implications are for our aging society. Contrary to some claims, financial sustainability is possible, even with a growing number of older Canadians.

The Canadian Gerontological Nursing Competencies and Standards of Practice (Canadian Gerontological Nursing Association, 2020) specify that gerontological nurses are expected not only to advocate for the older adult and the health care system but also to identify gaps, barriers, and fragmentation in the health care system and to work to overcome them. This chapter provides an overview of the Canadian health care system, including financing and services for veterans. Social security programs for older Canadians are described, and legal issues of capacity and guardianship are discussed. The final section of the chapter discusses abuse of older adults, which is, sadly, a growing problem in Canada.

THE CANADIAN HEALTH CARE SYSTEM

The Canadian health care system has been evolving for many years. Older adults who grew up in Canada have experienced dramatic changes in the way health care is funded. Before 1947, health care in Canada was privately delivered and funded. People paid for health care out of pocket or through private insurance; people who could not pay relied on charity. In 1947, the government of Saskatchewan introduced a provincial hospital insurance plan, and in 1957, the federal government passed legislation for sharing the costs of hospital services with the provinces and territories. This legislation was extended to physicians' services in 1962, and all provinces and territories had physician insurance plans by 1968.

The *Canada Health Act*

The *Canada Health Act* of 1984 is an amalgamation of previous federal legislation. It sets out the national health insurance plan as well as federal, provincial, and territorial roles in the health care system. Health care is administered and delivered by the provinces and territories; the Canadian "system" consists of 13 interlinked provincial and territorial systems. The responsibilities of the federal government include the following:

- Setting and administering national principles for the health care system through the *Canada Health Act*
- Collaborating with provinces and territories on national health policies, and
- Contributing to the funding of health care services through transfer payments to the provinces and territories.

The transfer of funds for health care from the federal government to provincial governments is contingent on adherence to the principles of the *Canada Health Act* (Box 24.1). The federal government's responsibilities for the provision of health care services are restricted to specific groups (e.g., Indigenous peoples and veterans). Aside from this limitation, the provinces and territories—each of which has its own

---

BOX 24.1
PRINCIPLES OF THE *CANADA HEALTH ACT*

Public administration	The provincial and territorial plans must be administered and operated on a nonprofit basis by a public authority.
Comprehensiveness	The provincial and territorial plans must insure all medically necessary services provided by hospitals, medical practitioners, and dentists working within a hospital setting. If a service is considered medically necessary, the full cost must be covered by the public health care insurance plan.
Universality	The provincial and territorial plans must cover all residents.
Portability	The provincial and territorial plans must cover all insured persons when they move to another province or territory within Canada and when they travel abroad. If a resident moves to another province, they can continue to use their original health care insurance card for up to 3 months. This ensures enough time to register for the new plan and receive their new health insurance card.
Accessibility	The provincial and territorial plans must provide all insured persons reasonable access to medically necessary hospital and physician services without financial or other barriers.

Source: Health Canada. (2016). *Canada's health care system.* https://www.canada.ca/en/health-canada/services/canada-health-care-system.html.

health care insurance plan—are responsible for the management, financing, and delivery of publicly insured health services. Under the *Canada Health Act*, "medically necessary" services are publicly insured, including primary health care, care in hospitals, and dental surgery in hospitals. However, the term "medically necessary" is not explicitly defined and is thus somewhat open to interpretation. Hence, there is variability across the country in the provision of some services such as home care, long-term care (LTC), medications outside of those administered in hospital, physiotherapy, optometry services, and others. The level of funding provided for these services varies across the country. For example, provincial variations in LTC mean that there are differences in the amount that residents pay, the hours of care provided per day (see Chapter 28), and the requirements for length of residency in the province to determine eligibility for government-funded LTC. In some provinces, the cost of LTC for those who need it can at times have a significant impact on the person's family and their plans.

Health Care Financing

According to a report from the Canadian Institute for Health Information (Canadian Institute for Health Information [CIHI], 2020), total health care spending in Canada in 2019 was about $265.5 billion. Government spending consistently accounts for about 70% of total health care spending, while private-sector spending (i.e., private insurance and out-of-pocket expenses) accounts for 30% of spending. Per capita spending varies by province; the highest per-person expenditure ($19,367) is in Nunavut, and the lowest ($6,583) is in British Columbia. At 26.4%, government spending on hospitals accounts for the largest proportion of health expenditures, followed by expenditures on physician services (14.9%) and medications (15.2%).

According to the Canadian Institute for Health Information, health care spending for older adults aged 65 years or older was $11,599 per capita, the second-highest age group after infants younger than a year old ($12,678) (CIHI, 2020). The proportion of government health care expenditures for older adults has been about 45% (CIHI, 2019). In 2016, per capita expenditures for older adults were higher than those for younger adults—$6,481 for people aged 65 to 69 years, and $20,397 for people older than 80 years. Health care

funding has not increased in proportion to inflation or the growth of the Canadian population. With the population continuing to age, CIHI (2019) believes that health care decision makers will need to determine the level of care (hospital, home care, LTC) for older adults to balance access to and quality of care with the cost of care.

Government health care spending as a proportion of **gross domestic product** is not significantly affected by expenditures on older Canadians. Over the years, the biggest cost increase in the health care system has been spending on prescription medications. However, most of this expense is paid out of pocket and by private insurance. The extent to which provincial governments pay for prescription medications for older adults varies considerably from province to province. For example, Albertans aged 65 years and older pay 30% of each prescription, to a maximum of $25 per prescription (Alberta Health, 2017). In Ontario, those aged 65 years and older pay the first $100 of prescription costs and then up to $6.11 for each prescription filled or renewed (Government of Ontario, 2017). The rising costs of prescription medications will have an effect on both government expenditures and individual Canadians. The way in which health services are provided to older Canadians will continue to be monitored, and there will be growing pressure to use research evidence about the best models of health care and health promotion.

SOCIAL SECURITY RETIREMENT INCOME PROGRAMS

Social security retirement income programs are designed to minimize the chances that retirees and older adults will live in poverty. The first publicly funded income support program for older Canadians came with the establishment of the Old Age Security (OAS) program in 1952, which occurred at about the same time as the establishment of the first publicly funded health insurance programs. The Canada Pension Plan (CPP) and the parallel Quebec Pension Plan (QPP) were established in 1966.

Old Age Security Program

The OAS program is an income support program for older Canadians. It includes the OAS pension, the Guaranteed Income Supplement (GIS), the Allowance, and the Allowance for the Survivor. It is federally financed through general tax revenues.

Old Age Security Pension

The OAS pension is a monthly payment available to Canadian citizens and legal residents aged 65 years and older who have lived in Canada for at least 10 years after the age of 18 years. Citizens and legal residents who do not reside in Canada may receive the OAS pension if they have lived in Canada for at least 20 years after the age of 18 years. Older adults must apply to receive the OAS, and they can apply 6 months before they turn 65 years of age. Whether the older adult receives a full or partial OAS pension depends on their length of residency in Canada after the age of 18 years. The full OAS pension is provided to (1) people who have lived in Canada for at least 40 years after turning 18 years of age, and (2) people who have lived in Canada for 10 years immediately before approval of their OAS application and who meet additional residency or immigration status requirements. This means that some people who immigrated to Canada as older adults are not eligible for the OAS for the first 10 years of residence. In 2021, the maximum monthly OAS pension benefit was $615.37. The amount is "indexed" to the cost of living; every four months the amount is adjusted if the cost of living increases. The OAS is taxable income. Persons with an annual **net income** over $129,075 do not receive the OAS. Updated rates for all benefits are available at the Service Canada website (https://www.canada.ca/en/services/benefits/publicpensions/cpp/old-age-security/payments.html#tbl1).

Guaranteed Income Supplement

The GIS, sometimes referred to as "the supplement," is a monthly benefit for OAS recipients who have little or no other income. Recipients apply at the same time they apply for the OAS and must reapply annually. Sponsored immigrants are not eligible for the GIS or the Allowance during the period of their sponsorship (up to 10 years) except under limited conditions. The amount of the benefit depends on the amount of other income, marital status, and whether or not the spouse is receiving the OAS or the GIS; the rate for single persons is higher than that for people who are married or living as common-law partners. In 2021, the maximum monthly benefit was $919.12 for a single person

and $553.28 for the spouse of someone who receives OAS. Like the OAS, the GIS is indexed to the cost of living. Up-to-date information is available at https://www.canada.ca/en/services/benefits/publicpensions/cpp/old-age-security/guaranteed-income-supplement/benefit-amount.html.

Allowance and Allowance for the Survivor

The Allowance is paid to the spouse or common-law partner of an OAS pensioner. The Allowance for the Survivor is paid to the survivor (widow or widower) of an OAS pensioner. It is an income-tested benefit based on the combined yearly income of a couple or the survivor. Persons between the ages of 60 and 64 years who meet Canadian citizenship and residency requirements are eligible to apply and must reapply annually. The benefits are not taxable income and stop at age 65 years, when the person becomes eligible for the OAS. The maximum monthly benefit for the Allowance was $1,168.65 in 2021, and the maximum monthly benefit for the Allowance for the Survivor was $1,393.08. The Allowance and the Allowance for the Survivor are indexed to the cost of living.

Canada Pension Plan and Quebec Pension Plan

The CPP and the QPP provide retirement pensions and disability benefits for persons who have made contributions to the plans. When a contributor to the plan dies, the CPP and QPP also provide survivor benefits for eligible spouses, common-law partners (including same-sex partners), and dependent children. The CPP and the QPP were established after years of provincial–federal negotiations. Provinces may opt out of the CPP (the federal pension plan). Quebec is the only province with its own plan, the QPP. The CPP and the QPP are similar; neither is funded from tax revenues but rather from mandatory contributions from all employers, employees, and self-employed persons.

Older adults are eligible to receive the CPP or the QPP retirement pension (1) if they have contributed to one of the plans and they are either 65 years old or more or (2) if they are between 60 and 64 years of age and meet additional requirements. To receive the CPP or QPP between 60 and 64 years of age, the person either must stop working and have no earnings for 1 month before the pension begins or must earn less than the current monthly CPP retirement pension amount. A person must apply to receive the CPP or QPP retirement pension. The amount received depends on how much and how long the person contributed to the CPP or QPP and on their age when they start receiving the pension. The maximum monthly benefit was $1,203.75 in 2021; this amount is indexed to the cost of living and is adjusted annually. The maximum amount is less for persons who start receiving the pension before age 65. The average monthly CPP benefit for new beneficiaries in 2020 was $61.21 (Service Canada, 2021).

Survivor benefits include the CPP death benefit, the CPP survivor's pension, and the CPP children's benefit. The CPP death benefit is a maximum $2,500 payment to the deceased contributor's estate. The CPP survivor's pension is a monthly payment to the spouse or common-law partner of a person who received or was eligible to receive the CPP. The amount of the survivor pension benefit depends on contributions the spouse made to the CPP and on the surviving spouse's age and income. If the surviving spouse is 65 years or older and is not receiving other CPP benefits, then they receive 60% of the contributor's CPP pension. The benefit amount for surviving spouses who are aged 64 years or less depends on a number of other conditions.

Workers between the ages of 65 and 70 years can continue to contribute to CPP and QPP funds. It may be possible for people who made contributions to a social security system in a country with which Canada has a social security agreement to use those contributions to meet minimum qualifying conditions. For further information about the QPP, see http://www.retraitequebec.gouv.qc.ca. For information about the CPP, see https://www.canada.ca/en/services.html.

Financing OAS, CPP, and QPP

The OAS program is financed through federal tax revenues. The CPP and QPP programs are financed through mandatory contributions from employers, employees, and self-employed workers and from revenue from investments of funds in the CPP and QPP. Funds in the CPP and QPP are independently managed by the Canada Pension Plan Investment Board and by la Caisse de dépôt et placement du Québec (referred to as the "Caisse"), respectively. Both fund-management bodies operate at arm's length from the

government, are accountable to the public, and are responsible for maximizing returns on investment without undue risk.

The amount that employers, employees, and self-employed workers contribute to the CPP and QPP is set to ensure the long-term viability of the pension programs. Employee and employer contribution rate for CPP in 2021 was 5.45% with maximum contributory earnings of up to $58,100 (Government of Canada, 2020). For QPP in 2021, the maximum contribution rate was 5.90% with maximum contributory earnings of $58,100 (Revenu Québec, 2021). Self-employed workers contribute the full amount. In the case of employees, the employee and the employer each contribute half of the maximum amount. Pensions to current pensioners are paid from contributions of current workers and employers; the surplus is added to the CPP and QPP fund and invested.

Public opinion surveys indicate that Canadians are not well informed about the CPP and have doubts about the future viability of the CPP (Press, 2017). However, since reforms to the contribution system were made in 1996, actuarial reports and audits of the fund have consistently shown that the CPP and QPP are financially sound. As of 2019, the CPP fund was $392 billion (Canada Pension Plan [CPP] Investments, 2021). It is projected that additional contributions to the CPP fund will be higher than additional payouts and costs to run the fund until 2058. By that time, the fund will have grown considerably, producing more investment income to continue to finance pensions (Office of the Chief Actuary, 2016; CPP Investment Board, 2016). The Chief Actuary of Canada asserts that the CPP is sustainable over a very long term (Office of the Chief Actuary, 2016). As with Medicare, the growing number of older Canadians will not "bankrupt" the current CPP and QPP pensions.

IMPLICATIONS FOR GERONTOLOGICAL NURSING AND HEALTHY AGING

Medicare and the social security income programs that are part of the social safety net in Canada directly affect the health of older Canadians. Medicare is designed to ensure that Canadians receive necessary health care regardless of their financial means. The OAS programs and the CPP and QPP are designed to ensure that older Canadians do not live in poverty.

Gerontological nurses will nonetheless find that, despite the principles of universality and accessibility enshrined in the *Canada Health Act*, the health care services that older adults need are not always equally available across the country. Many services that support older adults' health are not deemed "medically necessary" as defined by the *Canada Health Act* and may fall outside provincial/territorial health plans. This does not mean that these services are unavailable; rather, access may depend on the older adult's income or on where they live. For example, the amount that residents pay for accommodation in LTC homes varies across provinces and territories (see Chapter 28); access to respite services is limited in rural and remote areas (see Chapter 25); access to end-of-life care is uneven, especially for those living in rural and remote areas (see Chapter 27); and culturally and ethnically specific services for older adults are limited (see Chapter 25). Gerontological nurses have a role in individually and collectively advocating for policies that improve access to health care services for older Canadians.

The OAS program and the CPP and QPP are two "pillars" of financial security in retirement. The third pillar of financial security is private savings, including Registered Retirement Savings Plans (RRSPs). Not everyone has adequate retirement savings; many older women are not eligible for CPP or QPP, and some immigrants may not be eligible for the OAS or for CPP or QPP. Consequently, 14.5% of Canadians aged 65 years and older live under low-income circumstances (Statistics Canada, 2017).

The two commonly used measures of poverty in Canada are the low income cut-off (LICO) and the low income measure (LIM). (The latter is now favoured by Statistics Canada.) The LICO is the point at which a family is spending 70% or more of their income on necessities (i.e., food, clothing, and shelter). The LICO depends on family size and community size. In 2019, the LICO after-tax for one person living alone ranged from $14,325 for a person living in a rural area to $21,899 for a person living in an area with a population of 500,000. For two-person families, the corresponding LICOs were $17,436 to $26,653 (Statistics Canada, 2021).

The poverty rate for older adults aged 65 years or older was 3.5% in 2018 (Hillel, 2020). Compared to single households, couples have a lower incidence of poverty (El-Attar & Fonseca, 2020). Fair to poor health also contributes to a higher incidence of poverty (El-Attar & Fonesca, 2020).

The process of applying for the GIS, the Allowance, and the Allowance for the Survivor can be challenging. A significant number of older Canadians miss out on benefits they are entitled to and need because of late applications or missed renewal application deadlines. Nurses' assessments should include information about total income, all sources of income, and the person's knowledge about the process of applying for OAS and CPP or QPP benefits. Because some older adults may be reluctant to reveal the extent of their financial need, assessment in the context of the therapeutic relationship is important. Nurses can provide the person with information about income supports and the process of applying. Detailed information is available on the Service Canada website (https://www.canada.ca/en.html).

Receiving the GIS may entitle the recipient to additional benefits from their province or territory. Gerontological nurses should be aware of additional benefits that older adults with low income can apply for in their province or territory and be familiar with the process of applying for these benefits. Recipients must reapply for the GIS and the Allowance every spring. They can reapply by completing an income tax return. If a tax return is not filed by April 30, a renewal form is mailed to the recipient. Completing a tax return may also be tied to other entitlements, such as provincial tax rebates. In many communities, nurses can provide older adults with information about charitable organizations that help people with a low income complete and file tax returns.

Gerontological nurses can promote age-friendly attitudes and combat ageism by being knowledgeable about the financing of both the health care system and the pension system. Statements that older adults will overwhelm either system are unfounded.

HEALTH CARE AND SERVICES FOR VETERANS

The Canadian health care system includes services for veterans that are provided or funded directly by the federal government. A "veteran" is a person who served in the Canadian Forces.

"Traditional" veterans are those who served in the First World War (of which there are no living survivors), the Second World War, and the Korean War. The average age of the 26,300 WWII veterans is 95 years; the average age of the 5,900 Korean War veterans is 88 years (Veterans Affairs Canada, 2020). "Nontraditional" veterans are those who served in the Regular Forces or Primary Reserves after 1947 (except those who served in the Korean War). The average age of the 597,200 Canadian Forces Veterans (Regular Forces and Primary Reserves) is 59 years (Veterans Affairs Canada, 2020).

The federal government, through Veterans Affairs Canada, provides treatment and other health-related benefits and services to veterans and to civilians who served in wartime. It also provides services to retired members of the Royal Canadian Mounted Police. Services and benefits include disability pensions; War Veterans Allowance (WVA); home care services; financial support for LTC homes; counselling; personalized case planning; medical needs assessment, advice, information, and referral; legal help with pension or allowance matters; and help with the cost of funerals and burials. Health care services are provided directly or through community or contract facilities. There are some differences in eligibility for and types of services provided for traditional and nontraditional veterans.

War Veterans Allowance and Disability Pension

The WVA is a tax-free monthly payment designed to meet basic financial needs, in recognition of the war service of veterans and qualified civilians. Veterans and civilians who meet one of the following war service requirements are eligible to receive the WVA:

1. Canadian Armed Forces veterans and Merchant Navy veterans who served in the First or Second World War or in the Korean War
2. Veterans of allied countries who served in the First or Second World War or in the Korean War and lived in Canada either before or after the war, or
3. Civilians who served in close support of the Canadian Armed Forces during wartime.

Eligibility is based on age or health, income, and residency in Canada at the time of application. The WVA is an income-tested benefit that supplements income up to a maximum ceiling. Surviving spouses, common-law partners, and orphans may also qualify.

Disability pensions are provided to eligible veterans who have a medical disability related to their service. Eligibility for the disability pension and eligibility for the WVA are based on the same three criteria. Disability pensions are monthly payments; additional payments to disability pensioners, depending on the pensioner's eligibility, may include the exceptional incapacity allowance, the attendance allowance, and the clothing allowance. Veterans who served after 1947 and were disabled as a result of their service are eligible for a lump-sum disability payment rather than a monthly disability pension.

Veterans Health Care Program

Persons who receive the WVA and some recipients of disability pensions are also eligible for other programs and benefits, including health care benefits. The Veterans Health Care Program promotes independence and assists veterans to stay at home and in their communities. This program includes the Veterans Independence Program, treatment benefits, and LTC.

Veterans Independence Program. The Veterans Independence Program complements other federal, provincial, and municipal programs that help veterans to remain in their homes and communities. Services depend on the individual's circumstances and health needs and may include the following: grounds maintenance; housekeeping; personal care services; nutrition services (such as Meals on Wheels); health and support services; outpatient health care, including the provision of adult day programs; payment of transportation costs for adult day programs, social activities, and activities of daily living; and home adaptation. Disabled and low-income survivors of certain categories of veterans are eligible for the housekeeping and grounds maintenance services.

Health Care Benefits. Recipients of the WVA or the disability pension are eligible for treatment benefits. For disability pensioners, eligibility is limited to services that are directly related to the condition for which the disability pension was granted. Treatment benefit programs are listed in Box 24.2.

Long-Term Care. For eligible veterans, Veterans Affairs Canada shares with provincial and territorial LTC programs the cost of care at an LTC home. Veterans pay the cost of accommodations and meals (see Chapter 28). The cost of LTC is subsidized according to the person's military service, the person's income, and whether the person's admission to an LTC home is due to the condition for which they are receiving the disability pension. Veterans Affairs Canada works with veterans, their families, LTC homes, and provincial and municipal governments to ensure that veterans' needs are met. An outreach and visitation program operated by the Royal Canadian Legion provides volunteer visitors to veterans who receive financial assistance and live in LTC homes. For more information, visit https://www.veterans.gc.ca/eng/housing-and-home-life/long-term-care.

IMPLICATIONS FOR GERONTOLOGICAL NURSING AND HEALTHY AGING

Gerontological nurses need to be aware of the services and support that are available for veterans. Currently, people are provided with information about programs and eligibility when they retire. However, this was not the case at the end of the Second World War or the Korean War, and nurses may encounter veterans and family caregivers who may not be aware of the benefits and assistance to which they are entitled. Assessments should include questions about military service or civilian service during wartime. Those people who may be eligible for veterans' benefits can be assisted in obtaining additional information. Veterans and civilians who served during wartime can get information about programs and services by contacting Veterans Affairs Canada. Details regarding eligibility and application procedures for each program are available on the Veterans Affairs Canada website at https://www.veterans.gc.ca/eng.

LEGAL ISSUES IN GERONTOLOGICAL NURSING

Knowledge of the most common legal issues that may arise when working with older adults is as important as knowledge of the financial issues just discussed. The lack of knowledge about health care laws and the misapplication of laws have been cited as a cause of ageist practices (Law Commission of Ontario, 2020a). Legal concerns are most often related to an individual's ability to make financial, personal, or health care decisions and their ability to consent to treatment.

Informed Consent

The health care team must obtain a person's informed consent prior to any examination, assessment, treatment or procedure (College of Physicians and Surgeons of Alberta, 2016). Informed consent means that the person has received information about the benefits and risks of a procedure or treatment. The nurse or other health care provider should be providing this information using clear terminology that is easily understandable (Canadian Nurses Protective Society, 2021). There are times when someone's mental capacity may make it more difficult for them to be fully informed. More information on mental capacity is described in the next section.

Mental Capacity

Mental capacity is the ability to make decisions. It is a legal construct, not a clinical condition. The exact legal definition of capacity varies from province to province and from country to country. In general, to be deemed capable of making a decision, a person must understand information that is relevant to making a decision, evaluate the data, and appreciate the consequences of the decision (or the consequences of not making a decision) (Law Commission of Ontario, 2020b). People are presumed to have capacity unless there is clear evidence to the contrary and the person has been legally deemed incapable.

The concept of capacity applies to different kinds of decisions, including financial decisions; decisions about daily activities, housing, and personal care; and medical and health-related decisions, including consent to treatments and procedures.

Capacity exists on a continuum and is issue or task specific; there is no such thing as global incapacity. A person may have capacity for a particular decision or kind of decision but not for another decision or kind of decision. For example, a person may not be able to adequately take care of day-to-day personal business such as paying bills but may still be able to make personal health care decisions. Capacity can improve, decrease, or fluctuate.

Mental capacity is assessed by different caregivers, depending on the kind of decision being made (e.g., health care consent, admission to an LTC home, or a financial contract) and relevant provincial laws, including health care consent laws, guardianship laws, substitute decision-maker and personal directives laws, privacy and personal information laws, and mental health laws. For example, capacity to provide health care consent is assessed by the nurse or another health care provider offering the health care. Under mental health laws, whenever a person is admitted to a psychiatric facility, a physician assesses the person's capacity to provide health care consent and capacity (sometimes referred to as *competency*) to manage their property. The mechanisms by which a person can dispute a finding of incapacity vary from province to province and within provinces according to the type of decision.

For persons who are unable to speak for themselves or are not able to understand the consequences of their decisions, legal protection may be needed. However, every attempt should be made to match the level of protection to the person's need, taking actions that provide the needed protection with the minimum restriction of personal autonomy.

Legal protection of the person with impaired capacity ranges includes power of attorney (POA) for finances, power of attorney for personal care, and guardianship (a mechanism by which the person becomes a "ward" under the protection of a guardian).

Power of Attorney

A POA is a legal document in which one person designates another person (e.g., a family member or a friend) to act on their behalf. The appointed person is called the *attorney* and may or may not be a lawyer. The two types of POA for financial affairs are *continuing* or *enduring* POA and *noncontinuing* POA (appointed for a limited time, such as when the person is out of the country). An attorney for financial affairs does not have the authority to make decisions about the person's health or personal care. (Information about relevant provincial and territorial laws are available on the websites of the respective Public Guardians and Trustees.)

An individual may appoint an attorney with a POA for personal care (who is also referred to as the personal guardian, agent, or delegate for personal care). The attorney has the authority to make health-related decisions for the individual when that individual is unable to do so themselves. The attorney with POA is expected to use "substituted judgement" in making decisions; that is, the decision is expected to be the decision the person would make were the person able to do so and not the decision the attorney would make for themselves in the same situation. Therefore, it is always advisable that the person selected as attorney be someone who knows and is willing to uphold the wishes and preferences of the individual.

A POA for finances comes into effect as soon as it is signed, unless the document clearly indicates that it takes effect only after the individual becomes mentally incapable of managing finances. A POA for personal care comes into effect when the individual becomes mentally incapable of making decisions about personal care. An important aspect of POA is that the person who is given decision-making rights is chosen by the older individual rather than by a court. This type of advance planning is generally recommended because it is the least restrictive and is most likely to ensure that the wishes of the older adult are followed. It does not, however, ensure that the POA will not be misused.

Guardians

When a person becomes mentally incapable of managing personal or financial affairs and does not have a

POA in place, a guardian may be appointed. Guardians may have responsibility for finances and property, personal care, or both. The appointment is made at a court hearing in which someone provides evidence of the incapacity of the person, who often is not present. Such a person is declared *incapacitated* (sometimes called *incompetent*) in a process that differs by province and territory. The guardian continues in the role until the court rescinds the order. When there is no suitable person to be appointed guardian, a provincial (or territorial) public guardian or trustee may be appointed.

IMPLICATIONS FOR GERONTOLOGICAL NURSING AND HEALTHY AGING

Nurses are responsible for assessing the person's capacity to consent to health care and for obtaining consent from the appropriate legal designate when a person is not capable of providing consent. There is no specific test for capacity, such as a score on an assessment of cognitive functioning. Nurses must be fully informed about the laws in their province or territory that are related to consent, capacity, and substitute consent, and they must also be aware that the laws are changing.

Nurses who are consulted by older adults and their families about legal issues should not attempt to provide legal advice. Instead, nurses should refer them to legal resources, legal clinics, or specialized lawyers. The provincial or territorial bar association is a resource for nurses and for older adults and their advocates (https://www.cba.org). A number of organizations dedicated to legal issues and advocacy for older adults are listed in the Resources section at the end of this chapter.

ABUSE, MISTREATMENT, AND NEGLECT OF OLDER ADULTS

Elder abuse is "any action by someone in a relationship of trust that results in harm or distress to an older adult. Neglect is a lack of action by that person in a relationship of trust with the same result" (Government of Canada, 2016, para. 2). Abuses of older adults include physical abuse, sexual abuse and exploitation, neglect, psychological or emotional abuse, economic or financial abuse, and spiritual abuse (Table 24.1). A person may experience more than one form of abuse. The abuse may occur in private homes, in places where the older adult lives alone or with other persons, or in care homes and health care facilities. The abuse of persons living in LTC homes or retirement care facilities is called *institutional abuse*. It "involves inadequate care and nutrition, low standards of nursing care, inappropriate and aggressive staff–client interactions, or substandard, overcrowded or unsanitary living environments" (Department of Justice Canada, 2015).

The most common form of abuse of older adults is financial abuse (Elder Abuse Prevention Ontario, 2021). Financial abuse is defined as "any improper conduct, done with or without the informed consent of the senior that results in a monetary or personal gain to the abuser and/or monetary or personal loss for the older adult" (Elder Abuse Prevention Ontario, 2021, para. 1). Most often, financial abuse happens between family members.

Accurate prevalence of elder abuse is difficult to ascertain because of underreporting and differences in the ways this abuse is defined and measured. Some studies have shown that up to 10% of older Canadians are abused (Canadian Association of Retired Persons [C.A.R.P.], 2016; Conroy, 2017); only 20% of these cases are reported to someone who is able to assist (C.A.R.P., 2016; Conroy, 2017). A 2015 national survey found that 8.2% of community-dwelling older Canadians had experienced abuse or neglect in the previous year (National Initiative for Care of the Elderly [NICE], 2015). The rate of family violence was lower for persons aged 75 years and older than for those between 65 and 74 years of age. Persons who have cognitive impairment are more likely than those who are not cognitively impaired to experience abuse (Han et al., 2019). Experts on elder abuse caution that prevalence estimates are probably low because older adults are reluctant to report and disclose abuse and because people who are more vulnerable are less likely to participate in surveys of the abuse of older adults (Han et al., 2019).

The abuse of older adults is a complex problem. Psychological, social, and economic factors, along with the mental and physical conditions of the victim and the perpetrator, contribute to the occurrence of the abuse of the older adult (Registered Nurses' Association of Ontario [RNAO], 2014). Most abuse of older adults is committed by family members (Elder Abuse Prevention Ontario, 2021). Older women are most

TABLE 24.1
Types of Abuse of Older Adults

Definition	Examples	Indicators
Emotional (Psychological) Abuse Using words or actions to control, frighten, isolate, or erode a person's self-respect.	■ Threatening ■ Blaming, insulting, lying ■ Deciding what the person can or cannot do ■ Not keeping promises ■ Humiliating the person ■ Alienating others from the older adult ■ Making fun of the person's heritage, traditions, or religious or spiritual beliefs ■ Constant yelling	■ Fear, anxiety, withdrawal ■ Depression ■ Cowering ■ Reluctance to talk openly ■ Fearful interaction with caregiver ■ Family or caregiver talking on behalf of the person and not allowing privacy
Financial Abuse Acting without the older adult's consent in a way that benefits the abuser at the expense of the older adult through threats, intimidation, or deceit. Most forms of financial abuse are crimes.	■ Misuse of power of attorney ■ Theft ■ Misusing control over a person's funds by not providing them for the person's benefit ■ Pressuring the person to provide financial support ■ Making the person sign a legal document ■ Overcharging for services ■ Failing to repay loans ■ Pressuring the person to sign over house or property	■ Standard of living inconsistent with income or assets ■ Theft or missing property noted ■ Unusual or inappropriate activity in bank accounts ■ Forged signatures on cheques ■ Overdue bills ■ Missing mail
Physical Abuse Using physical force against a person without the person's consent. It can cause pain, injury, or impairment.	■ Hitting, punching, slapping, pushing, biting, or throwing the older adult ■ Burning the person ■ Confining the older adult, including unnecessary use of restraints ■ Throwing objects at the older adult	■ Unexplained injuries (bruises, burns, bites, fractures) ■ Untreated medical problems ■ History of "accidents" ■ Signs of overuse or underuse of medication ■ Wasting ■ Dehydration
Neglect Failing to adequately provide necessities or care for a dependent older adult.	■ Failing to provide adequate nutrition, personal care, or a clean, warm, safe environment ■ Withholding medical services or treatments ■ Failing to provide proper needed supervision ■ Failing to prevent physical harm	■ Unkempt appearance ■ Inappropriate or dirty clothing ■ Signs of infrequent bathing ■ Unhealthy living conditions ■ Dangers or disrepair in home environment ■ Hoarding ■ Lack of social contact ■ No regular health care appointments

Sources: Adapted from Department of Justice Canada. (2015). *Elder abuse is wrong.* http://www.justice.gc.ca/eng/rp-pr/cj-jp/fv-vf/eaw-mai/index.html; National Initiative for Care of the Elderly. (n.d.). *Elder abuse: Assessment and intervention reference guide.* https://www.nicenet.ca/product-page/elder-abuse-assessment-and-intervention-reference-guide.

likely to be abused by their spouse or adult children (HealthLink BC, 2018). Intimate partner violence in older age is most likely to be a continuation of domestic violence that began earlier in the relationship (HealthLink BC, 2018).

Older women are more likely than older men to experience abuse (HealthLink BC, 2018). (Other risk factors for the abuse and neglect of older adults are listed in Box 24.3.) Some risk factors may be more relevant to a particular type of abuse or neglect. A recent national survey of more than 8,000 older Canadians indicated that the following factors are independently associated with abuse: being depressed, having been abused at another age (i.e., childhood, youth, or middle age), feeling unsafe with the people who are closest, having unmet needs in regard to activities of daily living and instrumental

BOX 24.3

RISK FACTORS FOR ABUSE AND NEGLECT

- Isolation
- Lack of support
- Cognitive impairment (i.e., dementia)
- Responsive behaviours
- Living with a person who has a mental illness
- Living with people who engage in excessive consumption of alcohol or illegal drugs
- Dependency on others to complete activities of daily living (including banking)
- Recent worsening of health
- Arguing frequently with relatives

Source: Extracted from Registered Nurses' Association of Ontario. (2014). *Preventing and addressing abuse and neglect of older adults: Person-centred, collaborative, system-wide approaches* (p. 26, Table 2). Author.

activities of daily living, being unmarried, and being female (NICE, 2015).

Abusers are often dependent on victims for financial assistance or shelter. Personal problems or stressors may increase a person's likelihood of abusing an older adult. Elder abuse may be associated with caregiver stress, but caregiver stress should never be an excuse to abuse (Lumacare, 2021).

Most often, older victims are unwilling or afraid to report the problem because of shame, embarrassment, intimidation, or fear of retaliation. The abuser may be the only caregiver available; reporting or complaining could leave the victim without any care at all. The abuse may be part of a lifelong pattern in which the victim has always felt somewhat at fault; thus, they will remain in the abusive situation.

Institutional Abuse

Older adults who live in LTC homes, hospitals, or retirement homes are vulnerable to abuse because of their isolation and dependence and because of the characteristics of some facilities. There are two types of institutional abuse: *resident-to-resident abuse* and *staff-to-resident abuse.*

Resident-to-resident abuse (also known as resident-to-resident aggression, violence, or mistreatment) differs from the typical abuse of older adults because of its potential harm to both residents and because abuse

is typically defined as occurring in the context of a relationship of trust (which does not apply to resident-to-resident relationships) (McDonald et al., 2015). Resident-to-resident abuse is a relatively new area of research. A recent review indicated that 1% to 41% of residents experienced resident-to-resident abuse (McDonald et al., 2015). According to the review by McDonald and colleagues (2015), resident-to-resident abuse is less frequently reported than staff-to-resident abuse, but it makes up the majority of cases that are reported to the police. Sexual abuse that is reported is more likely to be caused by another resident than a staff member. In a Canadian study by Berry and colleagues (2017), researchers used the Aggressive Behavior Risk Assessment Tool and the Aggressive Behavior Scale to predict aggression among residents of LTC homes in Canada. They found that 8.5% of residents in their sample had at least one aggressive incident (Berry et al., 2017). Most resident-to-resident abuse involves one or more residents with cognitive impairment (Joyce, 2019). In addition, female residents and wandering behaviour are also associated with a higher risk for resident-to-resident abuse. Less is known about perpetrators' characteristics (McDonald et al., 2015). Frequently, residents are unlikely or unable to report abuse.

Surveys confirm that institutional abuse is a problem, but their research methods make it difficult to conclusively quantify the problem. Much of the research asks how many staff members have observed resident abuse (36% to 80% have witnessed resident abuse), not how many incidents of abuse occur (Castle et al., 2015).

Risk factors for institutional abuse include the environment and organizational culture, staff characteristics, and resident characteristics (Hutchison & Kroese, 2015), factors that interact. For example, important organizational-level risk factors (such as how work is organized, inadequate staffing levels, inadequate or ineffective supervision, intimidation, and a low proportion of qualified staff) influence staff-level risk factors, such as staff burnout. Staff characteristics associated with abuse include workplace stress, dissatisfaction with management or the workplace, emotional exhaustion, job pressures, inexperience, lack of knowledge about older adults, negative attitudes such as ageism, personal problems, a personal history of abuse, alcohol or substance misuse, and deficiencies in communication skills or problem-solving ability (RNAO, 2014; Hutchison & Kroese, 2015). Resident characteristics that are associated with higher risk include aggressive, hyperactive, or responsive behaviours (see Chapter 21); dependency on others to complete activities of daily living; a history of previous abuse; social isolation; and impaired communication (RNAO, 2014; Hutchison & Kroese, 2015).

IMPLICATIONS FOR GERONTOLOGICAL NURSING AND HEALTHY AGING

Assessment

The importance of skillful communication (see Chapter 3), the therapeutic relationship, and the establishment and maintenance of trust cannot be understated in the context of preventing the abuse of older adults. Nurses must be vigilant and sensitive to the potential for abuse and neglect, watching for signs and symptoms in all their interactions with older adults (see Table 24.1). In addition to signs of physical abuse, attention should be paid to the more subtle signals. Is there an unusual delay between the beginning of a health problem and when help is sought? Are appointments often missed without reasonable explanations? Are there inconsistencies between the history given by a dependent older adult and by their caregiver?

Certain behaviours may be suggestive of an abusive situation. Does the family member or caregiver do all of the talking in a situation, even though the older adult is capable? Does the family member or caregiver appear angry, frustrated, or indifferent, while the older adult appears hesitant or frightened? Is either the family member or the older adult aggressive toward the other or the nurse? The nurse should pay particular attention to a caregiver who is alone and has no support from others and no opportunities for respite.

The accuracy of screening tools is questionable and controversial. Nurses and other health care providers who use screening tools for elder abuse should be trained in their use. If abuse is suspected, a full assessment should be done, including a determination of the immediate safety of the victim; the desires of the victim, if capable; and supports available to reduce the person's risk of abuse (RNAO, 2014). Assessment will typically involve the interprofessional health care team and possibly police and legal experts. It should include diagnostic tests and referrals and consultations (RNAO, 2014). Privacy in regard to the person's family and care providers should be ensured. It is important to be nonjudgemental and accepting of the person and the suspected abuser (RNAO, 2014). The questions to ask in the assessment depend on the type of suspected abuse. The questions "Are you afraid of anyone?," "Do you live in a household where there is stress or frustration?," "Do you live with anyone who abuses alcohol or drugs?," and "Do you live with anyone who was abused as a child?" can be asked in most types of assessments (Caceres & Fulmer, 2016). Box 24.4 provides some other questions.

BOX 24.4
QUESTIONS TO ASK WHEN ASSESSING SUSPECTED ABUSE

PHYSICAL ABUSE

Has anyone ever tried to hurt you in any way?
Have you had any recent injuries?
Has anyone ever touched you or tried to touch you without permission?
Have you ever been tied down?

EMOTIONAL ABUSE

Has anyone ever yelled at you or threatened you?
Has anyone been insulting you and using degrading language?
Are you cared for by anyone who abuses drugs or alcohol?

FINANCIAL ABUSE

Who pays your bills? Do you ever go to the bank with this person? Does this person have access to your accounts? Does this person have power of attorney?
Have you ever signed documents you did not understand?
Are any of your family members exhibiting a great interest in your assets?
Has anyone ever taken anything that was yours without asking?

NEGLECT

Are you alone a lot?
Has anyone ever failed you when you needed help?
Does anyone care for you or provide regular assistance to you?
Are you cared for by anyone who abuses drugs or alcohol?

Source: Extracted from Caceres, B. A., & Fulmer, T. (2016). Mistreatment detection. In M. Boltz, E. Capezuti, T. T. Fulmer, et al. (Eds.). *Evidence-based geriatric nursing protocols for best practice* (5th ed., p. 184, Table 13.2). Springer.

Intervention

The goals of intervention are to prevent, detect, and stop the mistreatment and neglect of older adults; provide care and treatment for the effects of the abuse; protect the victim and society from inappropriate and illegal acts; hold abusers accountable; rehabilitate the offender; and order restitution of property and payment for expenses incurred as a result of exploitation. Many interventions are done through the justice system and are beyond the nurse's usual scope of practice. Most importantly, nurses must know how to participate in the prevention and early recognition of abuse; how to refer victims and perpetrators to social, health, and legal services in their community; and how to report the abuse of older adults.

Prevention

Prevention of elder abuse is a priority of the World Health Organization and the Canadian government, and there are international, national, provincial, and local initiatives to increase awareness and prevent the abuse of older adults. Two such initiatives are the International Network for the Prevention of Elder Abuse and the Canadian Network for the Prevention of Elder Abuse. Prevention requires **intersectoral collaboration** between the health, social service, and justice (law enforcement and legal) sectors. Canadian prevention networks include representatives from all sectors as well as members of the public, including older adults.

Gerontological nurses need to be alert to situations that entail risk for the mistreatment of vulnerable older adults and take steps to prevent abuse or neglect. In some situations, the abuse may be preventable. Nurses can develop a safety plan with potential victims to ensure that they know how to get help if needed and know what resources are available to them (Box 24.5). Nurses can also provide support, encouragement, and assurance that it is possible to leave the situation. Unfortunately, few shelters will accept a frail older adult. If the abusive behaviour is a learned behaviour or a response to stress, the situation may allow for change.

Addressing Abuse and Preventing Recurrence

Multiple strategies are likely required to effectively address abuse and prevent recurrence. Older adults who are victims of abuse are often unaware of services that are available to them. Nurses should provide information about local services, such as crisis hotlines, victim support

---

BOX 24.5

DEVELOPING A SAFETY PLAN WITH POTENTIAL VICTIMS OF ELDER ABUSE

Encourage the older adult to do the following:

- Tell someone they trust about what is happening to them.
- Ask others for help, and be specific about the type of help needed.
- Think ahead about what to do if someone is hurting them or if they do not feel safe.
- Do the following for their protection if they are facing possible abuse:
  - Have emergency phone numbers written in a safe place.
  - Have a safe place to go, both inside and outside the house.
- Create an emergency kit containing money, copies of important documents, a list of all medications, and a 3-day supply of medications, extra clothing, and assistive devices.
- Dial 911.

Source: Adapted from Ontario Seniors' Secretariat. (n.d.). *Safety planning for older persons.* https://files.ontario.ca/safety_planning_for_older_persons.pdf.

---

groups, and victim volunteer companions, as well as information about how to access them and about the kinds of support they provide. Some communities, through their elder abuse prevention networks, have created intersectoral, interdisciplinary, and interprofessional networks for responding to the abuse of older adults (for example, the BC Association of Community Response Networks; https://www.bccrns.ca).

If the abuse is associated with caregiving, nurses can be proactive and provide support to all involved in order to reduce caregiver stress. This may include finding respite services, changing the situation entirely (e.g., giving the caregiver permission to give up the role), providing referrals to support groups, teaching about the care recipient's illness, teaching how to use crisis hotlines, and teaching anger management strategies.

Culturally and ethnically appropriate services related to the abuse of older adults need to be developed (Haukioja, 2016). Older adults who are members of minority ethnic groups or are immigrants may be more isolated, more dependent on family members, and less aware of their rights and the resources available to them

(Zhang, 2019; Alvi & Zaidi, 2017). Education and support materials for health care providers working with Indigenous persons have been developed by the Vancouver Coastal Health Authority (http://www.vchreact.ca/aboriginal_manual.htm).

Older adults who have experienced abuse often decline to use the offered services. Failure on the part of the nurse to develop a therapeutic relationship with the older adult can contribute to the person's decision to decline services. Some other reasons why older adults decline to use the offered services are that the person thinks that they do not need help; the person does not think that the services offered will help; the financial and emotional costs of accepting services are too high; the person feels under pressure to maintain the family's reputation; the services are culturally and linguistically inappropriate; the person holds culturally based beliefs that are inconsistent with accepting services; and the cost of legal services is too great.

Criminal Code and Reporting

Many police officers and some lawyers have additional training in how to respond to the abuse of older adults. Canada has legislation and legal tools that protect the rights of older adults. There are at least 19 *Criminal Code* offences that may apply to the abuse of older adults (see

http://www.advocacycentreelderly.org/elder_abuse_-_faq.php). However, lack of awareness of legislation and legal tools is a problem among frontline health care providers and law enforcement professionals who encounter the abuse of older adults. Provincial and territorial laws may require that police be notified when there is evidence of abuse of a person who is incapable of seeking assistance. However, a person with mental capacity has the right to make all personal decisions and can refuse assessment and intervention. In most provinces and territories, the reporting of suspected abuse or neglect of residents in LTC homes and assisted-living facilities is mandatory. More information on mandatory reporting for specific provinces and territories can be found in Table 24.2.

Preventing Institutional Abuse

Much of the responsibility for preventing the abuse of older adults in health care settings rests with the organizations and their leadership. Management practices can address risk factors, such as organization of work, staffing levels, staff qualifications, quality of supervision, staff well-being, and job pressures, all of which are thought to be underlying causes of institutional abuse (Hutchison & Kroese, 2015). Approaches to culture change are consistent with recommendations to adopt person-centred approaches (see Chapter 28).

TABLE 24.2

Reporting Elder Abuse: Reporting Structures in Provinces and Territories*

Province or Territory	Legislation
Alberta	■ Under the *Protection for Persons in Care Act*, any person who has reasonable grounds to believe that there is or has been abuse involving an adult receiving care from a hospital or long-term care home must report the abuse. ■ Report to a Complaints Officer, Police, or other Authorized Person. For more information: https://www.qp.alberta.ca/documents/Acts/P29P1.pdf
British Columbia	■ There is no public duty to report abuse. ■ Call the Seniors Abuse and Information Line or VictimLink BC if abuse is suspected. For more information: https://www2.gov.bc.ca/gov/content/family-social-supports/seniors/health-safety/protection-from-elder-abuse-and-neglect/where-to-get-help
Manitoba	■ It is mandatory to report suspected abuse and neglect under the *Protection for Persons in Care Act*. ■ Report to the Protection for Persons in Care Office of Manitoba Health, Seniors and Active Living. For more information: https://www.gov.mb.ca/health/protection/index.html
New Brunswick	■ Call the closest Regional Office if there is suspected abuse, neglect, or self-neglect to make an Adult Protection referral. For more information: https://www2.gnb.ca/content/gnb/en/services/services_renderer.9335.Adult_Protection.html

TABLE 24.2

Reporting Elder Abuse: Reporting Structures in Provinces and Territories—cont'd

Province or Territory	Legislation
Newfoundland	■ Under the *Adult Protection Act*. ■ It is a legal obligation to report suspected abuse or neglect. ■ Call the local police. For more information: https://www.gov.nl.ca/cssd/apa/#neglect
Northwest Territories	■ There is no duty to report abuse and neglect. ■ May need consent from older adult before disclosing personal or health information. ■ Call the Police or Seniors' Information Line. For more information: https://www.hss.gov.nt.ca/en/services/protecting-elders-abuse-and-neglect/getting-help-elder-abuse
Nova Scotia	■ Under the *Adult Protection Act*, one must report cases where they know of or suspect a vulnerable adult is being abused or neglected or experiencing self-neglect. ■ Report to Adult Protection Services. For more information: https://novascotia.ca/seniors/stopabuse/pdf/Toolkit_Sections/Toolkit-Section6.pdf
Nunavut	■ There are no statutory protections for a person who reports abuse. ■ May need consent from older adult before disclosing personal or health information. ■ Call the police. For more information: http://itsnotright.ca/provincial-territorial-initiatives/nunavut
Ontario	■ Mandatory reporting is required according to the *Ontario Long Term Care Homes Act*, 2007. ■ Call the police. For more information: https://www.ontario.ca/laws/regulation/100079#BK127
Prince Edward Island	■ The *Adult Protection Act* (s. 4(1)) states that any person may report to the Minister of Health and Wellness if they have reasonable grounds for believing a person is, or is at risk of being, in need of assistance or protection. ■ Consent or permission must be obtained before disclosing personal or health information. For more information: https://www.princeedwardisland.ca/en/information/family-and-human-services/elder-abuse-awareness
Quebec	■ Must normally need consent from an older adult before disclosing personal or health information. ■ Call the Elder Mistreatment Helpline. For more information: https://www.quebec.ca/en/family-and-support-for-individuals/assistance-and-support/mistreatment-of-older-adults
Saskatchewan	■ There is no general duty to respond to abuse of older adults. ■ May need consent from older adult before disclosing personal or health information. ■ Call the police. For more information: https://agefriendlysk.ca/senior-neglect/
Yukon	■ Under the *Adult Protection and Decision Making Act* (s. 61[1]), any person may make a report to the Seniors' Services/Adult Protection Unit when an older adult is being abused or neglected and is unable to seek support or assistance. ■ May need consent from older adult before disclosing personal or health information. ■ Call the RCMP. For more information: https://yukon.ca/en/legal-and-social-supports/supports-adults-and-seniors/get-help-senior-or-adult-being-abused-or

*Call 911 or emergency line if there is immediate danger.

Source: Some information retrieved from Canadian Centre for Elder Law. (2011). *A practical guide to elder abuse and neglect law in Canada*. https://www.bcli.org/project/practical-guide-elder-abuse-and-neglect-law-canada.

Employers should ensure that all staff are educated about ageism; residents' rights; abuse, neglect, and the factors that contribute to them; and staff members' responsibilities to report abuse (RNAO, 2014). Health care providers within LTC homes should be educated about assessing and responding to abuse; their roles and responsibilities; relevant laws; positive care approaches; managing responsive behaviours; and fostering a safe and healthy work environment. Collaborative teams, including experts from outside the facility, should be in place to work on the prevention of and response to abuse. Policies and procedures for recognizing and responding to abuse should be explicit. A no-blame process for reporting abuse and neglect is important. A combination of approaches is required, as outlined in Box 24.6.

SUMMARY

Nurses are expected to provide safety and security for the persons under their care to the extent possible, regardless of the capacity of the person. This responsibility increases as the limitations of the older adult increase. The nurse is often the one who provides much of the information that older adults and their significant others need in order to make informed decisions; it is essential that this exchange be documented in the health care record (see Chapter 5). The nurse often deals with difficult and problematic legal and ethical issues when providing care to older adults and when interacting with the families of these persons. Nurses must be knowledgeable about the rights of older adults with respect to access to health care and social security programs. Nurses are responsible for acting in accordance with laws pertaining to capacity and consent. There is growing recognition that elder abuse is a problem in our society. Interprofessional and intersectoral collaboration is required to prevent the abuse and neglect of older adults and to effectively intervene in such cases. Providing appropriate care within the context of a person's changing cognitive capacity and judgement is at the core of many ethical and legal dilemmas in gerontological nursing.

KEY CONCEPTS

- The Canadian health care system is made up of 13 interlinked provincial and territorial systems. The extent to which health services other than hospital-based care, primary care, and some dental surgery are part of provincial and territorial health insurance plans varies across the country.
- The Old Age Security program provides eligible persons with a regular income after the age of 65 years. Benefits from the Canada Pension Plan are available only to people who contributed to the plan when they worked; the benefit amount depends on the number of years a person contributed to the plan.
- Through power of attorney and guardians, protective measures are available for persons with limited or absent capacity.
- The nurse has a responsibility to ensure the safety and security of those persons to whom care is provided. This responsibility does not alter with changes in the person's legal status or capacity.
- At least 10% of older Canadians experience abuse or neglect, most often perpetrated by family members.
- Abuse of older adults occurs in all types of health care settings, and some of it is resident-to-resident bullying and abuse.
- In most jurisdictions, the nurse is required to report suspicions of abuse of older adults who live in care homes.

ACTIVITIES AND DISCUSSION QUESTIONS

1. Interview an older adult who receives benefits from the Old Age Security (OAS) program and the Canada Pension Plan or Quebec Pension Plan about what difference these programs make in their daily life. Compare your findings with those of a classmate.

2. Explain the fundamentals of the OAS program sufficiently to assist older adults in applying for benefits.

3. Learn about the laws regarding capacity, consent, and guardianship in your province or territory. Compare these laws to practices you have experienced in clinical settings. Discuss with your classmates.

4. Learn about the laws pertaining to reporting the abuse of older adults in your province or territory.

5. Find legal resources for older adults in your community, and obtain information about the costs of these services to the older adult and how to access them.

6. Interview a member of your local elder abuse prevention network. Find out what motivates them to do this work, what initiatives are in place in your community, what challenges are being faced by the network, and what priorities for future work have been decided upon.

7. Review the instructions for assessing the abuse of older adults. Take turns with classmates in conducting role-play interviews in which you are screening for elder abuse. Discuss what it was like to participate in the role playing.

RESOURCES

Advocacy Centre for the Elderly
http://www.advocacycentreelderly.org
Canadian Association of Retired Persons (C.A.R.P.)
https://www.carp.ca
Canadian Centre for Elder Law
https://www.bcli.org/ccel
Canadian Network for the Prevention of Elder Abuse
https://cnpea.ca/en/
Centre for Public Legal Education Alberta. *Legal resources by province and territory.*
https://www.oaknet.ca/abuse/resources/
Centre for Public Legal Education Alberta. *OakNet: Canadian law for older adults.*
https://www.oaknet.ca/
Employment and Social Development Canada. *Provincial and territorial resources on the abuse of older persons.*
https://www.canada.ca/en/employment-social-development/corporate/seniors/forum.html
Government of Nova Scotia. *Personal directives.*
https://novascotia.ca/just/pda/_docs/PersonalDirective_Booklet.pdf
Public Health Agency of Canada. *Elder abuse: It's time to face the reality.*
https://www.canada.ca/en/public-health/services/health-promotion/stop-family-violence/prevention-resource-centre/prevention-resources-older-adults/elder-abuses-time-face-reality.html

For additional resources, please visit *http://evolve.elsevier.com/Canada/Ebersole/gerontological/*

REFERENCES

Alberta Health. (2017). *Seniors health benefits.* https://www.alberta.ca/seniors-health-benefits.aspx.

Alvi, S., & Zaidi, A. U. (2017). Invisible voices: An intersectional exploration of life for elderly South Asian immigrant women in a Canadian sample. *Journal of Cross-Cultural Gerontology, 32,* 147–170. doi:10.1007/s10823-017-9315-7.

Berry, B., Young, L., Kim, S. C. (2017). Utility of the aggressive behavior risk assessment tool in long-term care homes. *Geriatric Nursing, 38*(5), 417–422. doi:10.1016/j.gerinurse.2017.02.004.

Black, J., Hashimzade, N., & Myles, G. (2009). Gross domestic product. In N. Hashimzade, G. Myles, & J. Black (Eds.), *A dictionary of economics* (5th ed.). Oxford University Press. doi:10.1093/acref/9780198759430.001.0001.

Caceres, B. A., & Fulmer, T. (2016). Mistreatment detection. In M. Boltz, E. Capezuti, T. T. Fulmer, et al. (Eds.), *Evidence-based geriatric nursing protocols for best practice* (5th ed., pp. 179–194). Springer.

Canada Pension Plan (CPP) Investment Board. (2016). *Sustainability of the CPP.* http://www.cppib.com/en/our-performance/cpp-sustainability/.

Canada Pension Plan (CPP) Investments. (2021). *CPP fund totals $392.0 billion at 2019 fiscal year-end.* https://www.cppinvestments.com/public-media/headlines/2019/cpp-fund-totals-3920-billion-2019-fiscal-year-end.

Canadian Association of Retired Persons (C.A.R.P.). (2016). *Elder abuse: How widespread is the problem?* https://www.carp.ca/2016/10/14/elder-abuse-widespread-problem/.

Canadian Gerontological Nursing Association (CGNA). (2020). *Gerontological nursing competencies and standards of practice* (4th ed.). Author.

Canadian Institute for Health Information (CIHI). (2019). *National health expenditures, 1975 to 2018*. Author. https://www.cihi.ca/sites/default/files/document/nhex-trends-narrative-report-2019-en-web.pdf.

Canadian Institute for Health Information (CIHI). (2020). *National health expenditure trends, 2020*. Author. https://www.cihi.ca/en/national-health-expenditure-trends.

Canadian Nurses Protective Society. (2021). *InfoLAW: Consent to treatment: The role of the nurse*. https://cnps.ca/article/consent-to-treatment/.

Castle, N., Ferguson-Rome, J., & Teresi, J. A. (2015). Elder abuse in residential long-term care: An update to the 2003 National Research Council report. *Journal of Applied Gerontology, 34*(4), 407–443. doi:10.1177/0733464813492583.

College of Physicians and Surgeons of Alberta. (2016). *Standards of practice: Informed consent*. https://cpsa.ca/wp-content/uploads/2020/05/Informed-Consent.pdf.

Conroy, S. (2017). *Section 5: Police-reported family violence*. https://www150.statcan.gc.ca/n1/pub/85-002-x/2017001/article/14698/05-eng.htm.

Department of Justice Canada. (2015). *Elder abuse is wrong: Institutional abuse or neglect*. http://www.justice.gc.ca/eng/rp-pr/cj-jp/fv-vf/eaw-mai/p9.html.

El-Attar, M., & Fonseca, R. (2020). *Public pensions and low income dynamics in Canada*. https://creei.ca/wp-content/uploads/2020/02/cahier_20_02_public_pensions_low_income_dynamics_canada.pdf.

Elder Abuse Prevention Ontario. (2021). *Forms of abuse*. http://www.eapon.ca/what-is-elder-abuse/forms-of-abuse/.

Government of Canada. (2016). *Elder abuse: It's time to face the reality*. https://www.canada.ca/en/employment-social-development/campaigns/elder-abuse/reality.html.

Government of Canada. (2020). *CPP contribution rates, maximums and exemptions*. https://www.canada.ca/en/revenue-agency/services/tax/businesses/topics/payroll/payroll-deductions-contributions/canada-pension-plan-cpp/cpp-contribution-rates-maximums-exemptions.html.

Government of Ontario. (2017). *What you pay*. https://www.ontario.ca/page/get-coverage-prescription-drugs#section-6.

Han, S. D., Olsen, B. J., & Mosqueda, L. A. (2019). Elder abuse identification and intervention. In L. D. Ravdin & H. L. Katzen (Eds.), *Handbook on the neuropsychology of aging and dementia* (pp. 197–203). Springer.

Haukioja, H. (2016). Exploring the nature of elder abuse in ethno-cultural minority groups: A community-based participatory research study. *Arbutus Review, 7*(1), 51–67. doi:10.18357/tar71201615681.

HealthLink BC. (2018). *Abuse and neglect of older adults: Understanding gender differences*. https://www.healthlinkbc.ca/healthlinkbc-files/older-adult-abuse-gender.

Hillel, I. (2020). Holes in the social safety net: Poverty, inequality and social assistance in Canada. Centre for the Study of Living Standards. *CSLS Research Report 2020-06*. http://www.csls.ca/reports/csls2020-06.pdf.

Hutchison, A., & Kroese, B. S. (2015). A review of the literature exploring the possible causes of abuse and neglect in adult residential care. *Journal of Adult Protection, 17*(4), 216–233. doi:10.1108/JAP-11-2014-0034.

Joyce, C. M. (2019). Prevalence and nature of resident-to-resident abuse incidents in Australian residential aged care. *Australasian Journal on Ageing, 29*, 269–276. doi:10.1111/ajag.12752.

Law Commission of Ontario. (2020a). *Examples of ageism in law, policy and practice*. https://www.lco-cdo.org/en/our-current-projects/a-framework-for-the-law-as-it-affects-older-adults/older-adults-funded-papers/ageism-and-the-law-emerging-concepts-and-practices-in-housing-and-health/v-examples-of-ageism-in-law-policy-and-practice/.

Law Commission of Ontario. (2020b). *"Legal capacity": Setting the standard*. https://www.lco-cdo.org/en/our-current-projects/legal-capacity-decision-making-and-guardianship/legal-capacity-decision-making-and-guardianship-discussion-paper-2/i-legal-capacity-setting-the-standard/.

Lumacare. (2021). *Elder abuse prevention guide for caregivers*. https://lumacare.ca/wp-content/uploads/2021/03/ONLINE_Elder_Abuse_Guidebook_Caregiver_Edition.pdf.

McDonald, L., Sheppard, C., Hitzig, S. L., et al. (2015). Resident-to-resident abuse: A scoping review. *Canadian Journal on Aging, 34*(2), 215–236. doi:10.1017/S0714980815000094.

National Initiative for Care of the Elderly (NICE). (2015). *Into the light: National survey on the mistreatment of older Canadians*. Author. https://cnpea.ca/images/canada-report-june-7-2016-pre-study-lynnmcdonald.pdf.

Office of the Chief Actuary. (2016). *27th actuarial report on the Canada Pension Plan as at 31 December 2015*. Author. http://www.osfi-bsif.gc.ca/Eng/Docs/cpp27.pdf.

Press, J. (2017, January 25). *Most Canadians have a poor understanding of CPP, reports show*. Toronto Star. https://www.thestar.com/news/canada/2017/01/25/most-canadians-have-a-poor-understanding-of-cpp-reports-reveal.html.

Registered Nurses' Association of Ontario (RNAO). (2014). *Preventing and addressing abuse and neglect of older adults: Person-centred, collaborative, system-wide approaches*. Author. http://rnao.ca/bpg/guidelines/abuse-and-neglect-older-adults.

Revenu Québec. (2021). *Principal changes for 2021*. https://www.revenuquebec.ca/en/businesses/source-deductions-and-employer-contributions/employers-kit/principal-changes-for-2021/.

Service Canada. (2021). *Canada Pension Plan—How much you could receive*. https://www.canada.ca/en/services/benefits/publicpensions/cpp/cpp-benefit/amount.html.

Statistics Canada. (2017). *Income highlight tables, 2016 census*. https://www12.statcan.gc.ca/census-recensement/2016/dp-pd/hlt-fst/inc-rev/Table.cfm?Lang=Eng&T=306&S=126&O=D&RPP=25.

Statistics Canada. (2021). *Low income cut-offs (LICOs) before and after tax by community size and family size, in current dollars*. https://www150.statcan.gc.ca/t1/tbl1/en/tv.action?pid=1110024101.

Veterans Affairs Canada. (2020). *Demographics*. https://www.veterans.gc.ca/eng/about-vac/news-media/facts-figures/ 1-0.

Zhang, W. (2019). Perceptions of elder abuse and neglect by older Chinese immigrants in Canada. *Journal of Elder Abuse & Neglect, 31*(4–5), 340–362. doi:10.1080.08946566.2019.1652718.

25

RELATIONSHIPS AND ROLES

LEARNING OBJECTIVES

Upon completion of this chapter, the reader will be able to:

- Identify the various relationships that people identify as constituting "family."
- Examine family relationships in later life.
- Describe the various roles of grandparents.
- Explain the issues involved in adapting to a major transition such as retirement or widowhood.
- Identify the variety of caregiving situations and associated potential challenges and opportunities.
- Discuss nursing responses to older adults and their family members who are assuming caregiver roles or experiencing transitions.

GLOSSARY

Capacity The ability to understand and appreciate the reasonably foreseeable consequences of decisions or lack of decisions.

Caregiving The act of assisting those who are unable to care entirely for themselves. Caregivers, also referred to as carers or care partners, may be informal (family, friends, and others who volunteer this service) or formal (persons hired to provide the care).

Filial piety Respecting parents and feeling gratitude toward them, placing family needs above individual needs, and caring for parents. Filial piety is a fundamental value in Confucian ethics and is part of other cultures as well.

Familism A "strong identification and solidarity of individuals with their family as well as strong normative feelings of allegiance, dedication, reciprocity, and attachment to their family members, both nuclear and extended" (Sayegh & Knight, 2010, p. 3).

Respite Relief in caregiving, providing benefit to both the caregiver and the care recipient.

THE LIVED EXPERIENCE

"It is so irritating when Madge tries to help me do things. After all, I have lived 85 years and have done very well. I think she wants to put me away somewhere. I wish she would just leave me alone. I'm sure I could manage if she just wouldn't interfere."
John, the father

"I just can't stand watching as my father becomes weaker and is unable to do the things he always did so naturally and well. Yesterday he got lost on his way to the market. He was always my guide and protector. I knew I could count on him no matter what. It makes me feel sort of alone in the world."
Madge, the daughter

RELATIONSHIPS AND ROLES

This chapter focuses on the various relationships and roles that characteristically play a part in later life. Concepts of family structure and function and the transitions of retirement, widowhood, and **caregiving** are examined. Nursing responses to supporting older adults in maintaining fulfilling roles and relationships are discussed.

FAMILIES

The idea of family evokes strong impressions of whatever an individual believes the typical family should be. Because everyone comes from a family, these impressions have powerful symbolic meaning. However, in today's world, the definition of a family is in a state of flux. As recently as 100 years ago, the norm was the extended family, made up of parents, grown children, and the children's children—often living together and sharing resources, strengths, and challenges. As cities grew and adult children moved to them in pursuit of work, parents did not always come along, and the primacy of the nuclear family evolved. The norm in North America became two parents with two children. This pattern has not been as common in many Indigenous families or immigrant families.

Other variations on the idea of family have developed, and today there is no typical Canadian family. Approximately 38% of today's families are couples without children. The high divorce and remarriage rate results in households made up of blended families, with children from both previous and new marriages. Lone-parent families, blended families, and child-free couples are common. Multigenerational families are becoming more common; the number of three-generation households has increased, in part because of a higher proportion of three-generation households among recent Canadian immigrants (Statistics Canada, 2017a). Still other families are composed of couples of the same gender and may or may not include children. Others without biological families (either by choice or by circumstance) have created their own "families" through communal living with siblings, friends, or others.

Family members, however they are defined, form the nucleus of relationships for the majority of older adults and, if they become dependent, their support systems. A longstanding myth in society is that families are alienated from their older members and abandon them to institutions. Nothing could be further from the truth; family relationships remain strong in a family member's old age. Most older adults have frequent contact with their families and possess a large intergenerational web of significant people, including sons, daughters, stepchildren, in-laws, former in-laws, nieces, nephews, grandchildren, and great-grandchildren, as well as partners and former partners of their family members. All of

these people may play an important part in maintaining a person's satisfaction in later life.

As families change, the roles of the family members or their expectations of one another may change as well. Grandparents may assume parental roles for their grandchildren if their children are unable to care for them, or grandparents and older aunts and uncles may assume temporary caregiving roles while the children, nieces, and nephews work. Adult children of any age may provide limited or extensive caregiving to their own parents or aging relatives when needed. A spouse or sometimes a sibling may become a temporary or long-term caregiver when needed. Close-knit families are more aware of the needs of their members, work to resolve problems, and find ways to meet the needs of other family members, even if they are not always successful. Emotionally distant families are less available in times of need and have greater potential for conflict. If the family has never been close and supportive, it will not magically become so when members have unmet needs. Resentments long buried may crop up and produce friction or psychological pain. Long-submerged conflicts and feelings may return if the needs of any one family member exceed those of the others.

In coming to know the older adult, the gerontological nurse comes to know the family as well, learning of their special gifts and life challenges. Knowledge about families and family relationships, the ability to establish and maintain therapeutic relationships with older adults and their family members, and the ability to work collaboratively with older adults and their family members are required to meet the standards of the Canadian Gerontological Nursing Standards of Practice and Competencies (Canadian Gerontological Nursing Association, 2020). The nurse works with the older adult within the culture of the person's family of origin, present family, and support networks, including friends.

Relationship Statuses

Marriage

The marital or partnered relationship is a critical source of support for older adults. In 2020, about 56% of Canadians aged 65 years and older were legally married, the highest statistic among all marital statuses of older adults (Statistics Canada, 2021a). Among those over 65 years of age, about 56% of men and 46% of women were legally married (Statistics Canada, 2021a). Older women are more likely to be widows; about 34% of older women identified as widowed in 2020, compared with 23% of older men (Statistics Canada, 2021a). A man who survives his spouse into old age ordinarily has more than one opportunity to remarry if he wishes; a woman is less likely to have an opportunity for remarriage in later life. Often, older couples live together but do not marry owing to economic and inheritance reasons.

The needs, tasks, and expectations of couples in late life differ from those in their earlier years. Some couples have been married more than 60 years. These years together may have been filled with love and companionship, abuse and resentment, or anything in between. However, in general, being married (or the presence of a long-term partner) is positively related to health, life satisfaction, and well-being. For all couples, the normal physical and sociological circumstances in late life present challenges. Some of the issues that strain many of these relationships are (1) the deteriorating health of one or both partners, (2) limitations in income, (3) conflicts with children or other relatives, (4) incompatible sexual needs, and (5) mismatched needs for activity and social activities.

Divorce

In the past, divorce was considered a stigmatizing event. However, it is so common today that nurses may forget the ostracizing effects of divorce 50 years ago. In 2020, 12% of older adults were legally divorced and 2% were legally separated (Statistics Canada, 2021a). While there are generational and individual differences in people's expectations of marriage, older couples are becoming less likely to stay in unsatisfactory marriages. Nurses need to avoid making assumptions and be alert to the possibility of marital dissatisfaction in old age. Nurses should ask, "How would you describe your marriage?"

Long-term relationships are varied and complex, and many factors keep people together. Marital breakdown may be more devastating in old age because it is often unanticipated and may occur concurrently with other significant losses. Nurses should support people's decisions to divorce and assist them in seeking counselling in the transition. The person should be informed that divorce will bring on a grieving process similar to

that brought on by the death of a spouse, and that a severe disruption in coping **capacity** may occur as the person adjusts to a new life. The grief may be more difficult to cope with because socially sanctioned patterns of grief have not been established, as is the case with widowhood. In addition, tax and fiscal policies favour married couples, and many divorced older women are at a serious economic disadvantage.

LGBTQ2 Relationships

As the variations in families grow, so too do the types of couple relationships. Among the types of couples we see today are those made up of people who identify as lesbian, gay, bisexual, transgender, queer or questioning, and Two-Spirit (LGBTQ2). Although the accurate number of LGBTQ2 people of any age remains difficult to determine, in the 2016 Canadian Census, 0.9% of all couples identified as same-sex couples, and one-third of these same-sex couples were married (Statistics Canada, 2017b). Between 2006 and 2016, the number of same-sex couples increased by 60.7% (Statistics Canada, 2017b).

In the 2014 Canadian Community Health Survey, 3% of adult Canadians between the ages of 18 and 59 years self-identified as gay or lesbian or bisexual (Statistics Canada, 2018). This is likely an underestimate because of the hesitancy of some persons to publicly identify as being LGBTQ2. According to Statistics Canada (2018), there is currently no data regarding the number of Canadians aged 65 years or older who identify as a member of the LGBTQ2 community.

Although these couples are less often seen in the aging population, they are there. They may not be obvious owing to longstanding discrimination and fear. The experiences of younger LGBTQ2 individuals are considerably different from those of older adults. Older LGBTQ2 individuals did not have the benefit of antidiscrimination laws and support for same-sex partners. They were also more likely to keep their sexual orientation, gender identity, and relationships "hidden." A timeline of rights events in the life of a 77-year-old Canadian is presented in Table 25.1.

Many older members of the LGBTQ2 community have been part of a live-in couple at some time during their life. However, they are more likely to live alone in their older years. Some may have social networks consisting of friends, members of their family of origin, and the larger community, but many lack

TABLE 25.1
Timeline of LGBTQ Rights Events for a 77-Year-Old Canadian

Years	LGBTQ Rights Event	Age (Years)
1969	Decriminalization of same-sex acts between consenting adults	29
1973	Homosexuality removed from list of mental illnesses	33
1974	LGBTQ people allowed to immigrate to Canada	34
1977–1998	Provinces and territories prohibit discrimination on basis of sexual orientation	37–58
2003	Ontario legalizes same-sex marriage	63
2005	Ontario opens door to same-sex marriage and immigration	64
2012	Ontario includes protection of gender expression under the *Human Rights Code*	72

LBGTQ, lesbian, gay, bisexual, transgender, and queer.
Source: Extracted from Moore, D. (2017, February). *Older adults: Considerations for care* [PowerPoint presentation]. Brock University, St. Catharines, ON.

social support. In some cases, they may be estranged from their families of origin and come to later life with a network of close friends who make up their self-defined "family." These nonrelatives become a surrogate family and take on the instrumental and affective attributes of a family. Because these family members are not relatives in the traditional sense, they may not be recognized by the health care system, leading to considerable stress for all involved.

Some research indicates the possibility that older lesbian women and gay men may adapt more successfully to old age because of having coped with discrimination and prejudice over a lifetime. However, other research appears to indicate that a lifetime of managing stigma can have significant negative health effects.

Older gay and lesbian adults have described their experience of invisibility in senior organizations, health care, and society (Daley et al., 2017). Experiences of discrimination and prejudice from health care agencies and the resultant realistic fears of disclosing LGBTQ2 identity are barriers to accessing health care

services, including mental health, long-term care and assisted living, palliative care, services for persons infected with human immunodeficiency virus (HIV), and caregiver support (Daley et al., 2017). Gerontological nurses and the health care organizations for which they work can improve accessibility and create a welcoming, safe environment for older person who identify as LGBTQ2 by engaging older LGBTQ2 community members; advocating openness and acceptance; using inclusive language, positive messages, and images of LGBTQ2 older adults in documents and brochures and on websites; enacting inclusive policies; hiring LGBTQ2 staff; and providing education and training for staff and volunteers (Daley et al., 2017).

Older lesbian women and gay men have identified other concerns, such as pension benefits, health insurance, and access to appropriate housing and services. Most research has involved gay and lesbian couples; much less is known about partnerships of bisexual or transgender older adults. More knowledge of cohort, cultural, and generational differences among age groups is needed to understand the recent dramatic changes in family configurations among LGBTQ2 individuals. Few organizations are designed for LGBTQ2 older adults. Aînés et retraités de la communauté, in Montreal, Quebec, is one such group. Some organizations, such as The 519 (an LGBTQ2 agency in Toronto), have programs for older adults.

Older Adults and Their Adult Children

In adulthood, relationships between the generations become increasingly important for most people. Older parents enjoy being told about the various activities and successes of their offspring, and these adult children begin to see aspects of themselves that have developed from their parents. At times, the relationships may become strained because the younger adults are more concerned with their own spouses, partners, and children. The parents are no longer central to the younger adults' lives, although they may be central to their parents' lives. The most difficult situations occur when the older parents are openly critical or judgemental about the lives of their adult children. In the best of situations, adult children shift to the roles of friend, companion, and confidante to the older adult, a concept known as *filial maturity*.

Most older adults see their children on a regular basis. Even children who do not live close to their older parents can maintain their close connections, and "intimacy at a distance" can occur.

Older Adults Who Have Never Married

Approximately 5% of older adults today have never married (Statistics Canada, 2016). Older adults who have lived alone most of their lives often develop supportive networks with siblings, friends, and neighbours. As a result of their independence, older adults who have never married may be resilient to the challenges of aging and may not feel lonely or isolated. Furthermore, they may have longer lifetime employment and enjoy greater financial security as they age.

Hamedanchi and colleagues (2020) conducted a review of studies identifying the characteristics of older adults who have never been married. Some findings were contradictory. For example, some studies found that older adults who have never been married had larger social networks, closer connections with family and friends, were satisfied with life, and had better mental health (Hamedanchi et al., 2020). Other studies found higher depression rates, less happiness and life satisfaction, and greater risk of frailty among those who were not married (Hamedanchi et al., 2020). It is important to look at each person and their situation.

Grandparenting

Grandparenthood and, increasingly, great-grandparenthood are experienced by most older adults. There are over 7.5 million grandparents in Canada (Statistics Canada, 2019a). The average age at which Canadians become grandparents is increasing because of the older ages at which people have had children over the past several decades. The share of grandparents aged 85 years and older has nearly tripled since 1995, from 3% to 8% (Statistics Canada, 2019a).

In 2016, about 9% of children 14 years old or under lived with grandparents. Approximately 6% lived with both parents and grandparents, about 3% lived with one parent and grandparents, and less than 1% lived with grandparents only (Statistics Canada, 2017c).

As the term implies, "grands" are a step ahead of parents in their concerns, exposure, and responsibility. Most grandparents derive great emotional satisfaction from their grandchildren. Historically, the emphasis has been on the aging of the grandparent as it affects the relationship with the grandchild, but little has been said about the effects of the growth and maturation of the grandchild in the relationship. Many young adults who have had close contact with their grandparents report that this relationship has been very meaningful in their lives. Growing numbers of adult grandchildren are assisting in caregiving for frail grandparents.

The age, vitality, and proximity of both the child and grandparent produce a kaleidoscope of possible activities and interactions as both progress through the aging process. Approximately 80% of grandparents see a grandchild at least monthly, and nearly 50% do so weekly. Geographic distance does not significantly affect the quality of the relationships between grandparents and their grandchildren. The Internet is increasingly being used by distant grandparents as a way of staying involved in their grandchildren's lives and forging close bonds.

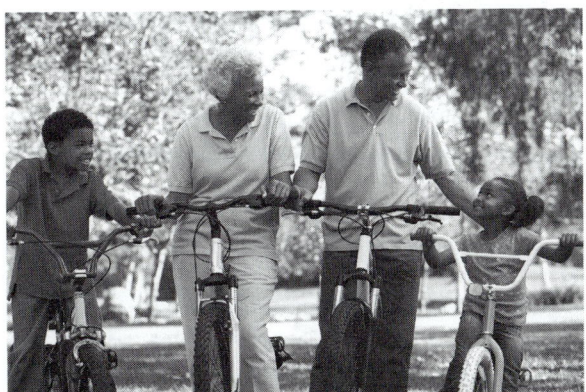

Many grandparents develop close, engaged relationships with their grandchildren—staying in touch in person or virtually. © CanStock Photo Inc. / monkeybusiness.

Younger grandparents and grandparents who live near their grandchildren are more likely to be involved in child care and recreational activities (Margolis & Wright, 2016). About 75% of grandparents provide financial assistance to their adult children or grandchildren (Margolis & Wright, 2016). As of the 2016 Census of Canada, approximately 17.6% of Indigenous children aged 0 to 4 years of age lived in a household with at least one grandparent, and 10.5% of children who identify as Métis lived with at least one grandparent (Statistics Canada, 2019b). Living with grandchildren is more common among the Inuit (22.8%) and First Nations (21.2%) communities (Statistics Canada, 2019b).

Siblings

Sibling relationships in late life are poorly understood and have been neglected by researchers. As individuals age, they often have more contact with siblings than they did in the years when family and work demands were more pressing. About 80% of older adults have at least one sibling, and siblings are often strong sources of support in the lives of never-married older adults, widowed persons, and those without children. For many older adults, these relationships become increasingly important because siblings have a long history of memories, are of the same generation, and have similar backgrounds. Sibling relationships become particularly important when siblings are part of the support system, especially for single or widowed older women living alone. The strongest sibling bond is thought to be the relationship between sisters. Sibling relationships remain important into late old age. Nurses should ask about sibling relationships of past and present significance.

The death of a sibling has a profound effect on a person's awareness of their own mortality, particularly when the sibling is of the same gender. When an older adult reaches the age of the sibling who died, the reaction can be quite disruptive. Grieving is activated, and a rehearsal of the person's own death may occur. In some cases, when an older sibling survives younger ones, there may be not only deep grief but also pangs of guilt—"Why them and not me?" (see Chapter 27).

Other Kin

Interaction with collateral kin (cousins, aunts, uncles, nieces, and nephews) generally depends on proximity, preference, and the availability of primary kin. The quality of relationships varies but is still a potential source of joy, support, assistance, or conflict. These relatives may provide a reservoir of kin from which to find replacements for missing or lost intimate relationships for single or childless people as they grow older.

LATE-LIFE TRANSITIONS

Transition is "a process of convoluted passage during which people redefine their sense of self and develop self-agency in response to disruptive life events" (Kralik et al., 2006, p. 321). Transitions are classified as developmental (e.g., retirement, grandparenthood), situational (e.g., widowhood, becoming a caregiver, moving to

seniors' housing, moving to receive care), or health–illness (e.g., experiencing persistent illness, transition between hospital and home, transition from home to long-term care) (Schumacher & Meleis, 1994). Often, transitions are not discrete; people experience one or more related transitions at the same time.

Transitions may occur predictably or may be imposed by unanticipated events. Retirement is a predictable event that can and should be planned long in advance; for some persons, however, it can occur unexpectedly as a result of illness, disability, or being terminated from a job. To the degree that an event is perceived as expected and occurring at the "right" time, a transition may be comfortable and even welcomed. Persons who must retire "too early" or are widowed "too soon" will have more difficulty adapting than those who are at an age when these events are expected.

The speed and intensity of a major change may make the difference between a transitional crisis and a gradual, comfortable adaptation. The most difficult transitions are those that incorporate losses rather than gains in status, influence, and opportunity. The move from independence to dependence and becoming a care recipient is particularly difficult.

Conditions that influence the process and outcome of transitions include personal meanings, expectations, knowledge, planning, socioeconomic status, and emotional and physical reserves, as well as community and societal conditions. Cohort, cultural, and gender differences are inherent in all of life's major transitions. Transitions that make use of past skills and adaptations may be less stressful. The ideal outcome occurs when gains in satisfaction and new roles offset losses.

Retirement

Historically, retirement was compulsory at the age of 65 years. However, Canada does not have a mandatory retirement age. "Retirement" no longer simply means a few years of rest from the rigours of work before death. It is a developmental stage that may occupy 30 or more years of a person's life and may involve many stages. The transitions are blurring, and the numerous patterns and styles of retiring have produced more varied experiences of retirement. Over the past decade, there has been a trend for people to retire at a later age; in 2015, about 20% of Canadians aged 65 years and older worked during the year (Statistics Canada, 2017d).

Many retirees work for pay at some point after retirement. Some do so because of economic need, whereas others want to remain involved and productive.

Obviously, health and financial status affect people's abilities and decisions to work or to engage in new work opportunities. The "baby boomers" increasingly face the prospect of working longer, and many are concerned about the possibility of outliving their retirement savings. The Canadian government estimates that 24% of persons approaching retirement will not have sufficient income to maintain their standard of living (Department of Finance Canada, 2016).

Older adults who did not expect to retire when they did may experience detrimental effects and need counselling or assistance. Some may experience job separation as a crisis and a traumatic role transition triggered by an unplanned job termination—for example, as a result of illness or company downsizing. Others, given the opportunity to work past retirement age, must weigh the benefits of doing so. Part-time work during retirement may be an option. Employers value older workers because they are experienced and dependable. Canadians older than 65 years can earn any amount without endangering their Canada Pension Plan (CPP) benefits. A portion of Old Age Security (OAS) benefits is repaid if income is over $77,580.

Retirement Planning

Current research indicates that retirement may have positive effects on life satisfaction and health, although this may vary depending on the individual's circumstances. Decisions to retire are often based on financial resources, age, health, attitude toward work, and self-perceptions of the ability to adjust to retirement. Retirement planning is advisable during early adulthood and is essential in middle age. However, people differ in their focus on the past, present, and future and in their realistic ability to "put away something" for future needs.

Retirement preparation programs are usually aimed at employees with high levels of education and occupational status, those with private pension coverage, and government employees. Thus, the people with the fewest resources for retirement—those who are most in need of planning assistance—may be least likely to have access to such assistance. People who are retiring in poor health, people who live at lower socioeconomic levels, and ethnoculturally diverse persons may have greater financial concerns in retirement and may need specialized counselling. These groups are often neglected in retirement planning programs.

Working couples must plan together for retirement. Decisions will depend on their career goals, their shared future interests, and the quality of their interpersonal relationship. The following are some questions a person must weigh when deciding to retire or continue working:

- What do I want to do?
- Who needs me, and what are my best opportunities?
- What am I best able to do?
- What is the meaning of my life?
- What should my life accomplish or contribute?
- Will I be financially secure for the rest of my life if I live 30 or more years?
- Can I afford to completely retire from paid work?

Information about retirement planning is supplied through group lectures, individual counselling, booklets, and online resources. However, in light of the current economy and the many financial hazards people will experience before retirement, planning for retirement is often insufficient. Many individuals have very high expectations for the final third of their lives. Federal tax laws encourage contributions to private savings plans such as Registered Retirement Savings Plans (RRSPs); in any given year, however, less than 25% of Canadians who file a tax return make RRSP contributions (Statistics Canada, 2021b). When considering retirement, people need to consider the adequacy of (1) employer-provided retirement benefits, (2) government pension benefits, (3) employer-provided postretirement health care, and (4) personal savings.

The adequacy of retirement income depends not only on a person's work history but also on marital history and marital status. The poverty rates of women are excessively high. Couples who had previous marriages and divorces may have significantly fewer economic resources available than couples in first marriages. Child support, divorce settlements, and pension apportionment to former spouses may result in diminished retirement income. This problem is an ever-increasing impediment to retirement, as less than half of couples presently approaching retirement age are in a first marriage. Policies based on the traditional lifelong marriage are no longer appropriate.

Special Considerations in Retirement

Retirement security depends on the following "three pillars" or "three-legged stool" of income protection: (1) the federal OAS and Guaranteed Income Supplement (GIS) programs; (2) income from the CPP or Quebec Pension Plan (QPP); and (3) income from private retirement savings, including investments and savings, RRSPs, and Tax-Free Savings Accounts (TFSAs) (Government of Canada, 2018).

People with higher incomes are most likely to participate in retirement savings plans. Canadians are eligible to receive CPP or QPP payments if they have worked and made contributions to the plan and are at least 60 years old. The amount received depends on the amount contributed, how long the person has been making contributions, and the person's age at retirement. The OAS pension, the GIS, and the Allowance are provided to Canadian citizens or legal residents who have lived in Canada for at least 10 years. Eligibility does not depend on work history. Persons with very low income or no sources of income are eligible for an income supplement benefit (see Chapter 24).

Older adults with disabilities, persons who lacked access to education or held low-paying jobs that provided no benefits, and persons who are not eligible for CPP or QPP benefits are at economic risk during their retirement years. In addition, older adults who are members of an ethnocultural minority group, women (especially widows and divorced or never-married women), immigrants, and LGBTQ2 persons often face greater difficulties in obtaining adequate income and benefits in retirement than others.

Inadequate coverage for women in retirement is common because their work histories are sporadic and diverse. Women often retire earlier than anticipated because of family needs. Whereas most men have always worked outside the home, only within the past 30 years has this been expected of women. When today's retired women were working, they earned significantly less than men; therefore, large cohort differences exist. Traditionally, the variability of women's work histories, interrupted careers, the residuals of sexist pension policies, pension inequities, and low-paying jobs created hazards for adequate income in retirement. Older women are likely to have several years of no earnings included in the averages that determine the amount of their CPP or QPP benefits.

Barriers to equal treatment for LGBTQ2 couples include job discrimination and historically unequal treatment under government pension plans. To help rectify this situation, Canadian legislation introduced in 2000 extended benefits to persons in same-sex common-law relationships, giving them access to CPP and OAS survivor benefits (McLaren & Manery, 2001).

IMPLICATIONS FOR GERONTOLOGICAL NURSING AND HEALTHY AGING

Successful retirement adjustment depends on socialization needs, energy levels, health, adequate income, a variety of interests, the amount of self-esteem derived from work, the presence of intimate relationships, social support, and general adaptability. Nurses may have the opportunity to work with older adults in different phases of retirement or participate in retirement education and counselling programs. Talking with people older than 50 years of age about retirement plans, providing proactive guidance in the transition to retirement, identifying those who may be at risk for lowered income and health concerns, and referring individuals to appropriate resources for retirement planning and support are important nursing interventions.

It is important to build on the strengths of older adults' life experiences and coping skills and to provide appropriate counselling and support to help older adults continue to grow and develop in meaningful ways during the various transitions. In ideal situations, retirement offers older adults the opportunity to pursue interests that may have been neglected while fulfilling other obligations. However, for too many older adults, retirement presents challenges that affect both health and well-being, and nurses must be advocates for policies and conditions that allow all older adults to maintain their quality of life in retirement.

Widows and Widowers

Widowhood is common; 34% of all women and 11% of all men aged 65 years and older are widowed (Statistics Canada, 2021a). The rate is lower for men because men are more likely to remarry after a spouse dies. Losing a partner after a long, close, and satisfying relationship is one of the most difficult transitions a person can face. The transition involves grief—the psychological and physical reactions to the loss—as well as the process of grieving—coping with the loss and reconstructing meaning. Over time, most people come to terms with bereavement. However, even widows and widowers who reorganize their lives and invest in family, friends, and activities often find that many years later they still profoundly miss their "other half."

The core features of grief are depression, anxiety, and loneliness. Table 25.2 presents four dimensions—affective, cognitive, behavioural, and physiological–somatic—of the many symptoms of normal, uncomplicated grief. Note that not every grieving person experiences all of these reactions. Furthermore, the intensity, duration, and impact of these reactions vary from person to person and across cultures.

The bereaved partner experiences stress from the loss of the loved person and their companionship, as well as stress, a secondary consequence of the loss (Stroebe & Schut, 2010). Thus, grieving involves two kinds of coping: (1) dealing with the loss of the partner and (2) adjusting to secondary losses, such as changes in living arrangements; loss of income; no longer having a partner who does certain tasks (e.g., cooking, doing chores, or managing finances); and changes in identity, from being a spouse or partner to being a widow or widower and from being part of a couple to being single. Grieving involves moving back and forth between these two kinds of coping; the person copes with loss, adjusts to secondary losses, and establishes new activities and relationships.

A person's bereavement is influenced by the circumstances of the spouse's death, by other stressors (such as financial stress or social isolation), and by the supports that are available to the person. There are gender differences in regard to bereavement. Bereaved husbands may be more socially and emotionally vulnerable. Suicide risk is highest among men over 80 years of age who have experienced the death of a spouse. Widowers adapt more slowly than widows to the loss of a spouse and often remarry quickly. Loneliness and the need to be cared for are factors influencing widowers to seek out new partners. Associating with family and friends, being members of a faith community, and continuing to work or engage in activities can all be helpful for men in the adjustment period following the death of a spouse. Widows are more likely to experience financial hardship and poverty. Adjusting to social life as a single person is difficult for both men and women.

IMPLICATIONS FOR GERONTOLOGICAL NURSING AND HEALTHY AGING

Assessment

Nurses interact with bereaved older adults in many settings. When working with widows and widowers, nurses need to understand the complexity and variability of

TABLE 25.2	
Four Dimensions of Grief Reactions	
Reaction	**Symptoms**
Affective	Depression, despair, dejection, distress Anxiety, fear, dread Guilt, self-blame, self-accusation Anger, hostility, irritability Anhedonia (loss of pleasure) Loneliness Yearning, longing, pining Shock, numbness
Cognitive	Preoccupation with thoughts of the deceased, intrusive ruminations Sense of presence of the deceased Suppression, denial Lowered self-esteem Self-reproach Helplessness, hopelessness Sense of unreality Memory, concentration problems
Behavioural	Agitation, tenseness, restlessness Fatigue Overactivity Searching Weeping, sobbing, crying Social withdrawal
Physiological–somatic	Loss of appetite Sleep disturbances Energy loss, exhaustion Somatic complaints Physical complaints similar to those of the deceased Immunological and endocrine changes Susceptibility to illness, disease

Source: Extracted from Hansson, R. O., & Stroebe, M. S. (2007). *Bereavement in late life: Coping, adaptation, and developmental influences* (p. 14). American Psychological Association.

normal grief reactions, as well as the resilience of older adults. It is important to avoid judging people's coping behaviours as being adaptive or maladaptive. Rather, the nurse should focus on understanding the meaning of the loss, the resources available to the person, and the strategies the person is using to cope.

Assessment should include the person's grief and response to the loss of the spouse, as well as how the person is adjusting to secondary losses and role changes. Grief reactions must be accepted as personally valid and useful evidence of healing. Intense emotions in the weeks after the death of the spouse are common. Emotions commonly experienced over a longer period include loneliness, shock, pain, sadness, anger, and regret. Sleep difficulties are common and may persist for up to 2 years. Loss of appetite and weight loss are also common, especially in the first few months of bereavement (O'Connor, 2020). Many widows and widowers are comforted by ongoing bonds and connections with their departed spouse (e.g., dreaming of them, conversing with them, taking up an activity their spouse engaged in, or keeping objects that belonged to their spouse) long after the spouse's death. Grief is not a linear process; each person has a unique grief and adjustment experience. However, there are patterns of adjustment and reintegration that can usually be expected in 2 to 4 years.

Interventions

People respond to losses in ways that reflect the nature and meaning of the lost relationships, as well as the unique characteristics of the bereaved. To support grieving persons, nurses need to extend themselves with warmth and caring in order to connect with the person.

With the support of friends and family, most people cope and grieve without complication and without professional help. Some may find that grief counselling or bereavement support groups facilitate normal, uncomplicated grieving. Information in Box 25.1 can be used to plan interventions to support widows and widowers.

People with little family or social support may need professional help to get through the early months of grief. Widows and widowers may need more support with the secondary stressors of grief—finding new ways to manage at home, seeking social support, or managing financial hardship. (See Chapter 27 for additional information about dying, death, and grief.)

BOX 25.1
PATTERNS OF ADJUSTMENT TO WIDOWHOOD

STAGE ONE: REACTIONARY (FIRST FEW WEEKS)

Disbelief, anger, indecision, detachment, and inability to communicate in a logical, sustained manner are common. Searching for the partner, visions, hallucinations, and depersonalization may be experienced.

Interventions: Support, validate, be available, listen to talk about the partner, and reduce the person's expectations.

STAGE TWO: WITHDRAWAL (FIRST FEW MONTHS)

Depression, apathy, physiological vulnerability occur; movement and cognition are slowed; insomnia, unpredictable waves of grief, sighing, and anorexia occur.

Interventions: Protect against suicide, and involve the person in support groups.

STAGE THREE: RECUPERATION (SECOND 6 MONTHS)

Periods of depression are interspersed with characteristic capability. Feelings of personal control begin to return.

Intervention: Support accustomed lifestyle patterns that sustain and assist the person in exploring new possibilities.

STAGE FOUR: EXPLORATION (SECOND YEAR)

The person begins new ventures, testing the suitability of new roles. Wedding anniversary, holidays, birthdays, and the anniversary of the death may be especially difficult.

Intervention: Prepare the individual for unexpected reactions during anniversaries. Encourage and support new trial roles.

STAGE FIVE: INTEGRATION (FIFTH YEAR)

The person will feel fully integrated into new and satisfying roles if grief has been resolved in a healthy manner.

Intervention: Help the person recognize and share their own pattern of growth through the trauma of loss.

CAREGIVING

Former First Lady Rosalynn Carter said, "There are only four kinds of people in the world: those who have been caregivers, those who currently are caregivers, those who will be caregivers, and those who will need caregivers" (Alzheimer Society, 2017, para. 1).

Family caregiving has become a normative experience (similar to marriage, work, or retirement) for many families and cuts across racial, ethnic, and social class distinctions. Gerontological nurses are most likely to encounter older adults and their family and friends in situations related to caregiving of some kind. In 2018, 7.8 million Canadians provided care to someone with a health condition, someone with a physical or mental disability, or an older adult (Statistics Canada, 2020). Most of these caregivers provide care for at least a year; periods longer than 4 years are common. Informal caregivers include friends, unpaid workers, and volunteers in the home.

Family caregiving activities vary. They can include assistance with activities of daily living and instrumental activities of daily living; illness-related care such as carrying out treatments, managing symptoms, and managing equipment; and case management, including care coordination, communication with health care providers, and advocacy. Most caregivers (64%) spend less than 10 hours a week doing caregiving, while 15% spend 10 to 19 hours, and 21% spend 20 hours or more (Statistics Canada, 2020). Our health care system relies heavily on family caregiving. The value of caregiving is estimated to be at least $25 billion per year (National Seniors Strategy, 2015). The cost of replacing family caregiving with formal care within the health care system would be devastating for society.

Just over half (54%) of family caregivers are women (Arriagada, 2020). Women are more likely than men to spend 20 or more hours per week giving care (Arriagada, 2020). They are also more likely to provide personal care, assist with medical treatments, and complete household tasks. In addition to these responsibilities, caregiving can also be a financial burden, and women who are family caregivers are more likely to live in poverty than those who are not caregivers. Even though caregiving is generally considered a women's issue, more and more men, including those who are not spouses (e.g., brothers, nephews, and sons), are assuming the full range of caregiving roles. Forty-six percent of caregivers are men, and more research is needed to identify their particular needs and challenges.

Caregiving is considered a major public health issue, and the physical and mental health of caregivers is receiving increased attention. The aging of the population, medical advances, shorter hospital stays, and the expansion of home care technology will increase the demand for family caregivers. At the same time, however, the number of family members who are available to provide care will decrease.

Impact of Caregiving

Although caregiving is a way to "give back" to a loved one and joy can be found in the giving, it is also stressful and can be physically and emotionally demanding, leading to greater risks for illness and mortality. There is said to be a "hidden health crisis" amongst the family caregiving population (Sterling & Baumblatt, 2019). Family caregiving is associated with increased depression and anxiety (Sterling & Baumblatt, 2019). Often, family caregivers neglect their own health and prioritize their caregiving responsibilities:

Caregiving is a very complex issue, and assuming a caregiving role is a time of transition that requires a restructuring of one's goals, behaviors, and responsibilities. It requires taking on something new but it is also about loss—of what was and what could have been. (Lund, 2005, p. 152)

The financial consequences of caregiving can be significant. A systematic review by Stewart (2020) found several studies describing how 20% of caregivers, and specifically spousal caregivers, reported financial hardships. This affected women most often, as 42% of women who were spousal caregivers found it difficult to meet their financial basic needs. Stewart (2020) also described studies indicating that those who felt financially secure reported better mental health.

Most caregivers report that they can cope with the demands of caregiving—caregiving does not necessarily result in negative outcomes. However, the circumstances that are more likely to cause problems with caregiving include competing role responsibilities (e.g., work, home, parenting), advanced age of the caregiver, high-intensity caregiving needs, insufficient resources, a care recipient with dementia, and prior relational conflicts between the caregiver and care recipient. Caregivers of persons with dementia may experience even greater emotional and physical stress than other caregivers experience. Suggestions for reducing caregiver stress are presented in Box 25.2.

Some research indicates that caregiving intensity or time spent caregiving may be higher in racial/ethnic minority groups such as African American and Latino caregivers (Rote et al., 2019). **Filial piety** and **familism**—prevalent values in Asian, Indigenous, and other minority ethnic cultures in Canada—play an important role

BOX 25.2

10 STRATEGIES TO REDUCE CAREGIVER STRESS

1. If your loved one has a disease, learn about the disease. This will prepare you, as their caregiver, to understand how the disease will affect your loved one and yourself.
2. Be realistic about the disease and how it will affect your loved one over time. This will allow you to adjust any expectations.
3. Be realistic about yourself and how much you can do as a caregiver.
4. Accept your feelings. Having mixed feelings may be confusing, but they are normal. Recognize that you are doing the best you can.
5. Share information and feelings with family and friends so that they can better understand how to help and support your needs. Find someone with whom you feel comfortable talking about your feelings. This may be a close friend, family member, someone from a support group, member of a religious community, or health care provider.
6. Be positive and try to look at the positive side of things. Focus on what your loved one can do as opposed to the abilities they have lost. Try and make the day count.
7. Look for humour. Find situations that have a bright side to them. Maintaining a sense of humour can be a good coping strategy.
8. Take care of yourself. Your health is important. Do not ignore it. Eat properly, exercise regularly, and find ways to relax and get the rest you need. Make regular appointments with a health care provider for checkups.
9. Get help. This may mean someone whom you can share thoughts and feelings with (individual, health care provider, support group). This may also mean practical help from family or friends, or programs in the community.
10. Plan for the future. Choices relating to health and personal care decisions should be considered and recorded. Legal planning should also be discussed. As well, think about an alternate caregiving plan in the event that you are unable to provide care in the future.

Source: From Alzheimer Society of Canada. (2021). The importance of reducing stress. https://alzheimer.ca/en/help-support/im-caring-person-living-dementia/looking-after-yourself/reducing-caregiver-stress#10_tips_to_reduce_stress.

in family caregiving (Liu & McDaniel, 2015). Further research into ethnicity, culture, and caregiving is needed in light of the increasing ethnocultural diversity of older Canadians.

Some of the benefits of caregiving are enhanced self-esteem, well-being, and ability to empathize with others; personal growth, satisfaction, and pride in caregiving; finding meaning or making meaning through caregiving; and the development of an interest in activism (Pristavec, 2019). Further research is needed to understand the factors that influence how family caregivers perceive the experience. Most attention in caregiving research has focused on the caregiver. Less attention has been given to the care recipient or to the relationship between caregiver and care recipient.

Several researchers have studied caregiving as a role, examining how the relationships between the family caregiver and care recipient and the preparation of the family caregiver influence reactions to caregiving. Family caregivers who have a positive relationship with the care recipient experience less stress and find caregiving more meaningful. Nursing interventions to assist in preparing a person for the caregiving role, particularly at the time of the patient's discharge from hospital, also seem to prevent or reduce role strain. Further research is needed to understand the complexities of these roles.

Spousal Caregiving

Of family caregivers over 60 years of age, spouses provide the most care, and 80% of persons who live with spouses with disabilities provide care for them. Many have health problems that are neglected in deference to the needs of the spouse. Although spousal caregivers provide more intensive, time-consuming care than other family caregivers, the spouse may need care that is beyond the capabilities of their partner.

A comparison of the needs of spouses and adult children who were primary caregivers for persons living with dementia found that for both groups of caregivers, the burden of caregiving was associated with needing more support from family, feeling lonely, and feeling underappreciated. For spouses, having a poor relationship with the person before the person became ill was associated with a greater burden, as was caring for a person experiencing agitation or sleep problems (Chappell et al., 2014).

Older family caregivers are at greater risk for negative consequences. The nurse should be alert for situations in which health care providers may be able to provide supports and resources that make it possible for a family caregiver to assume new responsibilities without being totally overwhelmed. When a spouse is ill and the partner needs to take over functions for both of them, someone must be available to provide reinforcement, encouragement, and relief. An adult day program, **respite** care services, routine visits from a community health nurse, or periodic assistance from a home health aide or a housekeeper may make it possible for the couple to continue to live together. It is important to pay attention to the physical and mental health needs of the caregiver as well as those of the care recipient. Several assessment tools exist to assess the level of caregiver needs—these are discussed later in this chapter.

Aging Parents Caring for Adult Children

Although we tend to think of caregivers as middle-aged adults caring for older adults, an unknown number of older adults are caring for their middle-aged children who are physically or mentally disabled. Earlier in the last century, children with chronic illnesses or developmental disabilities usually died before reaching adulthood. Now, with improved care, they are surviving.

With increased survival, adults with developmental disabilities are also at risk for developing chronic illness, and thus they are in greater need of care and services. For example, people with Down syndrome are much more likely to develop dementia, and they develop it at a younger age. Often, the responsibility for managing or providing care is carried by parents for their entire adult life, ending only with the death of the parent or the adult child. The most stressful issues for parents are long-term planning for care of the adult child after the parent dies, planning for emotional and social support, handling financial concerns, and creating opportunities for their child to socialize. Families also report lack of access to sufficient respite care (Smith et al., 2017). The phenomenon of an aging parent caring for an aging child is beginning to receive more attention both from organizations for aging and from advocacy organizations.

Grandparents Raising Grandchildren

In recent years, more grandparents have become primary caregivers for their grandchildren when the parents are unable to provide needed care. The reasons include child abuse, teen pregnancy, imprisonment, joblessness, military deployment, drug and alcohol addictions, illness, death, and other social problems. In Canada in 2016, 32,520 children aged 0 to 14 years lived solely with their grandparents (Statistics Canada, 2017c).

Caregiving by grandparents is a common role among Indigenous peoples. This is partly a reflection of Indigenous cultures in which grandmothers are traditionally involved in child rearing, yet it is also a result of historical and current government policies (see Chapter 4). One scoping review by Hsieh and colleagues (2017) found that Indigenous grandparents highly valued their role as caregivers to their grandchildren because they see it as a way to pass on traditional wisdom and values. Box 25.3 describes a research study exploring the experiences of Yup'ik grandparents raising their grandchildren.

For many grandparents, the economic, health, and social challenges associated with caregiving include limited income and financial support through the welfare system, lack of informal support systems, loss of leisure and social activities in retirement, and shame or guilt related to their children's inability to parent. Research on the physical and mental health consequences of grandparents' raising grandchildren is limited, but some of the research suggests that custodial grandparents are at risk for psychological distress and depression, especially in a context of poverty (Taylor et al., 2017). Many custodial grandparents are happy and satisfied with their roles (Hsieh et al., 2017), but they also experience caregiver stress, particularly when resources are inadequate, there is conflict with the child's parents, or the grandchild has emotional or health problems (Hsieh et al., 2017). Too often, both the children and their grandparents need help. Children in the care of a custodial grandparent are more likely to have emotional or behavioural problems than are children in two-parent families.

Routine screening for psychological distress in custodial grandparents is important, as is offering support and referrals to reduce stressors. Box 25.4 provides guidelines for older adults who are providing primary care to their grandchildren. Nurses can be instrumental in collaborating with community organizations to provide needed support. Resources and online information

BOX 25.3

RESEARCH FOR EVIDENCE-INFORMED PRACTICE: "WE RAISE OUR GRANDCHILDREN AS OUR OWN:" ALASKA NATIVE GRANDPARENTS RAISING GRANDCHILDREN IN SOUTHWEST ALASKA

Problem: Families in which grandparents are caring for their grandchildren experience unique challenges. Furthermore, grandparents raising grandchildren is high among ethnic minority groups, such as Indigenous families. However, very little is known about the experiences of Indigenous coastal grandparents raising grandchildren.

Methods: Researchers completed a qualitative study consisting of 20 semi-structured interviews with Yup'ik grandparents, a Native community in the Bristol Bay region of southwest Alaska. Participant ages ranged from 46 to 95 years. Fourteen women and six men participated. Participants were the primary caregivers of their grandchildren. Researchers wanted to answer the following questions: (1) What are Yup'ik grandparents' understandings of their role in raising grandchildren? (2) What has influenced the Yup'ik grandparents' understandings of this role?

Findings: The overall role of grandparents was best understood through the theme "as our own." This meant that grandparents did not make a distinction between their own children and their grandchildren. Grandparents took care of their grandchildren as if they were their own children. The roles of grandparents included being a family provider (buying food and necessities), teacher of appropriate behaviour, and a role model for others. Grandparents also described themselves as being a wisdom bearer, instilling the values of traditional Yup'ik life in their grandchildren. Education and nontraditional activities such as school were important to grandparents, but at times meant they had less time together and fewer opportunities to instill traditional activities. Having to work outside of the home to support children and grandchildren was important to grandparents, but was also sometimes seen as a challenge.

Implications for Nursing Practice: It is important to understand how the roles of grandparents are influenced by ethnicity and culture. Understanding grandparents' unique experiences opens the doors to providing individualistic and person-centred nursing care.

Source: Lewis, J. P., Boyd, K., Allen, J., et al. (2018). "We raise our grandchildren as our own:" Alaska Native grandparents raising grandchildren in Southwest Alaska. *Journal of Cross-Cultural Gerontology, 33,* 265–286. doi:10.1007/s10823-018-9350-z.

BOX 25.4
GUIDELINES FOR GRANDPARENT CAREGIVERS

1. Acknowledge your feelings, both positive and negative.
2. Take care of yourself and get the support you need for your own mental and physical health.
3. Grandchildren will have mixed feelings too, and it is important to understand that grandchildren also need time to adjust.
4. Focus on creating a stable environment by establishing a routine, setting clear house rules, and making sure each grandchild has a private space.
5. Encourage open and honest communication by planning regular times to sit and talk with grandchildren; encourage them to share their feelings and identify their emotions.
6. Encourage contact with parents if possible. Make visits part of your grandchildren's routines and be sensitive to your grandchildren's feelings.

Source: Smith, M., & Segal, J. (2020). *Grandparents raising grandchildren.* https://www.helpguide.org/articles/parenting-family/grandparents-raising-grandchildren.htm.

are available for custodial grandparents (see the Resources section at the end of this chapter).

Long-Distance Caregiving

Because of the increasing mobility of today's society, more children move away from home for education or employment. Help for a parent must therefore be provided "long distance." Caregivers at a distance provide similar types of assistance and care, although they do so less frequently than those living closer to the older adult. Distance caregivers incur more expenses for caregiving and have higher incomes. This is perhaps one of the most difficult situations, and it presents unique challenges. See Chapter 28 for a discussion of care options for older adults, including moving in with an adult child.

A caregiving industry is emerging to assist the geographically distant family member to ensure that an older relative will be cared for; this industry is made up of geriatric care managers, some of whom are nurses or social workers. The services are provided on a fee-for-service basis.

IMPLICATIONS FOR GERONTOLOGICAL NURSING AND HEALTHY AGING

Nurses are often care providers and case managers for older adults and their families, both in the home and in retirement homes, assisted living, and long-term care. Support for families in the caregiving role is an important nursing intervention.

Assessment

Family Assessment

A comprehensive assessment of the older adult includes an assessment of the family—its members; family history; usual roles; family members' strengths and contributions; and deterrents to the functioning of the family unit. In order to know the family and design responses that may strengthen the family unit, the nurse must assess the family's needs and strengths and the meaning family members assign to caregiving, as well as their sources of stress, particular methods of coping, cultural values, support system, and family dynamics.

Often, nurses see families in times of crisis, when an older family member needs care. It is important that nurses encourage the expression of feelings from all involved family members as well as from the older adult and that they maintain a nonjudgemental attitude. The nurse must also be aware of their vision of what a family should be and do. The nurse's values should not enter into assessment and intervention, and nurses should not label families as "dysfunctional." As Meiner (2011, p. 113) stated, "It is necessary to identify the strengths within each family and to build on those strengths while recognizing the family's limitations in providing support and caregiving." Thus, the nurse's role is to teach, monitor, and strengthen the family system so as to maintain the health and wellness of the entire family.

Caregiver Assessment

The stresses, expectations of future needs and problems, and positive aspects of the caregiving situation should be explored with family caregivers. Assessing a caregiver includes determining how the caregiver can help the care recipient and how the health care team can help the caregiver. In light of the physical and emotional stressors often associated with the caregiving role, nurses need to monitor the physical and emotional health of both the caregiver and the care recipient and provide support as necessary. A partnership model "blending the nurse's knowledge and expertise in health care with the caregiver's knowledge of the family members and the caregiving situation" is necessary (Messecar, 2016, p. 152).

The assessment focuses on identifying the caregiver's priorities and includes (1) the caregiving context (i.e., relationship of caregiver to care recipient, roles and responsibilities, home and physical environments, financial status, potential caregiving resources, and cultural background); (2) the caregiver's perception of the health and functional status of the care recipient; (3) the caregiver's preparedness for caregiving; (4) the quality of family relationships; (5) indications of challenges with quality of care; (6) the caregiver's physical and mental health; and (7) the caregiver's strengths (Messecar, 2016). Several validated caregiver assessment instruments are available in the "Try This: Series" section of the *Consult-Geri* website, which includes the Modified Caregiver Strain Index, Let's PREPARE, and the Elder Assessment Instrument (https://hign.org/consultgeri-resources/try-this-series). Box 25.5 presents a research-based model to guide nursing interventions with caregivers.

Interventions

Caregiver interventions have the goal of either reducing the amount of caregiving provided by a caregiver or improving the caregiver's well-being and coping. Some interventions aim to achieve both outcomes. The six types of caregiver interventions are psychoeducational interventions, supportive interventions, respite interventions, psychotherapy interventions, interventions to improve care receiver competence, and multicomponent interventions. These interventions have all been tested for their effects in regard to caregiver burden, depression, and well-being; the care provider's satisfaction with caregiving; the caregiver's knowledge and caregiving ability; and the care receiver's functioning. Caregiver interventions are not equally effective, with their effectiveness varying according to the characteristics of the caregiver and the care recipient (Messecar, 2016).

In general, caregiver interventions have a bigger effect on caregiver knowledge than on other outcomes. Group interventions are less effective than individual interventions. Psychoeducation, counselling, and interventions with multiple components show the strongest evidence

BOX 25.5

NURSING ACTIONS TO CREATE AND SUSTAIN A PARTNERSHIP WITH CAREGIVERS

1. Reflect with the family on expectations of the conversation, and jointly set the goals of the conversation.
2. Get to know each other, who is present, and who is absent.
3. Explore the family structure and find out who is part of the family.
4. Explore the relationships within the family and relationships between the family and others.
5. Invite each family member to share their story and narrate expectations, needs, and emotions.
6. Formulate shared questions or problems.
7. Acknowledge painful experiences and events related to emotions.
8. Provide recommendations about family strengths, competencies, and resources.
9. Stimulate open communication between family members, even about difficult topics.
10. Discuss family members' beliefs related to the care situation.
11. Summarize central issues that have been raised.
12. Set goals and agreements.

Sources: Broekema, S., Paans, W., Roodbol, P.F., et al. (2019). Nurses' application of the components of family nursing conversations in home health care: A qualitative content analysis. *Scandinavian Journal of Caring Sciences*, 34(2), 322–331. doi:10.1111/scs.12731; Östlund, U., Bäckström, B., Lindh, V., et al. (2015). Nurses' fidelity to theory-based core components when implementing family health conversations—A qualitative inquiry. *Scandinavian Journal of Caring Sciences*, 29(3), 582–90. soi: 10.1111/scs.12178.

restore the balance of the system to the greatest extent possible and to support caregivers in their caring. The family can be visualized as a mobile with many parts; when the mobile is touched, each part shifts to regain the balance. The intrusion of health care providers into a family system will temporarily unbalance the system but may provide an opportunity to restore the balance in a healthier manner, sometimes by adding an element or by increasing the weight of one and decreasing the weight of another.

When the nurse works with a family whose culture is different from their own—for instance, a culture whose rituals and routines are unfamiliar to the nurse—the nurse must be particularly careful to respect the differences. The nurse can work with the family to make the best use of their strengths; each family member can be valued for what they bring to the situation.

KEY CONCEPTS

- The ability to successfully negotiate transitions and develop new and gratifying roles depends on personal and environmental supports, timing, clarity of expectations, personality, and the degree of change required.
- Older adults and their family members carry a long history. Current family dynamics must be understood within the context of family history.
- Sibling relationships may increase in importance during old age as individuals cope with various losses.
- Grandparenting is a significant role among older adults. In an increasing number of families, grandparents are the primary providers for young children and function as parents.
- Caregiving is one of the major social issues of our times. Most spouses or partners will spend some time caring for one another, and most adult children will spend some time caring for aged parents.

of effectiveness. The effectiveness is less when care receivers have dementia or other illness conditions that worsen over time (Messecar, 2016).

Interventions with caregivers must always be made with consideration of the great variability in family structures, resources, traditions, and history. The range of adaptations is enormous, and the goal is always to

ACTIVITIES AND DISCUSSION QUESTIONS

1. Discuss your position in the family and how that has affected your relationship with siblings and parents.

2. What do you suppose your role will be when your parent or parents need help?

3. What would you find most difficult in regard to assisting your older parent?

4. What resources are available for older LGBTQ2 persons in your community?

RESOURCES

Grandparents raising grandchildren
https://www.helpguide.org/articles/grandparenting/grandparents-as-parents.htm
Parent Support Services Society of BC. *Resources for grandparents raising grandchildren.*
http://www.parentsupportbc.ca/for-grandparents/
Rainbow Health Ontario. *LGBT2SQ health education, training, research, and policy.*
http://www.rainbowhealthontario.ca/
SAGE—Advocacy & Services for LGBT Elders. *Resources for LGBT older people and those interested in LGBT aging issues.*
http://www.sageusa.org/index.cfm
Senior Pride Network of Toronto
https://www.seniorpridenetwork.ca/

For additional resources, please visit *http://evolve.elsevier.com/Canada/Ebersole/gerontological/*

REFERENCES

Alzheimer Society. (2017). *You are not alone!* http://alzheimersocietyblog.ca/you-are-not-alone/.

Arriagada, P. (2020). *The experiences and needs of older caregivers in Canada.* https://www150.statcan.gc.ca/n1/pub/75-006-x/2020001/article/00007-eng.htm.

Canadian Gerontological Nursing Association. (2020). *Gerontological nursing standards of practice and competencies* (4th ed.). https://cgna.net/standards.

Chappell, N. L., Dujela, C., & Smith, A. (2014). Spouse and adult child differences in caregiver burden. *Canadian Journal on Aging, 33*(4), 462–472. doi:10.1017/S0714980814000336.

Daley, A., MacDonnell, J. A., Brotman, S., et al. (2017). Providing health and social services to older LGBT adults. *Annual Review of Gerontology & Geriatrics, 37*(1), 143–160. doi:10.1891/0198-8794.37.143.

Department of Finance Canada. (2016). *Backgrounder: Canada Pension Plan (CPP) enhancement.* https://www.canada.ca/en/department-finance/news/2016/09/backgrounder-canada-pension-plan-cpp-enhancement.html.

Government of Canada. (2018). *Enhancing retirement security for Canadians: Consultation document.* https://www.ic.gc.ca/eic/site/116.nsf/eng/00001.html.

Hamedanchi, A., Khankeh, H. R., Momtaz, Y. A., et al. (2020). The gray never married: An integrative review. *Journal of Clinical and Diagnostic Research, 14*(10), LE01–LE08. doi:10.7860/JCDR/2020/45141.14119.

Hsieh, J. Y., Mercer, K. J., & Costa, S. A. (2017). Parenting a second time around: The strengths and challenges of Indigenous grandparent caregivers. *GrandFamilies: The Contemporary Journal of Research, Practice and Policy, 4*(1), 76–114. http://scholarworks.wmich.edu/grandfamilies/.

Kralik, D., Visentin, K., & van Loon, A. (2006). Transition: A literature review. *Journal of Advanced Nursing, 55*(3), 320–329.

Liu, L. W., & McDaniel, S. A. (2015). Family caregivers for immigrant seniors living with heart disease and stroke: Chinese Canadian perspective. *Health Care for Women International, 36*(12), 1327–1345. doi:10.1080/07399332.2015.1038346.

Lund, M. (2005). Caregiver, take care. *Geriatric Nursing, 26*(3), 152–153. doi:10.1016/j.gerinurse.2005.03.009.

Margolis, R., & Wright, L. (2016). Older adults with three generations of kin: Prevalence, correlates, and transfers. *Journals of Gerontology. Series B, Psychological Sciences and Social Sciences, 72*(6), 1067–1072. doi:10.1093/geronb/gbv158.

McLaren, A. T., & Manery, M. M. (2001). *Factors affecting the economic status of older women in Canada: Implications for mandatory retirement.* British Columbia Human Rights Commission. https://books.google.ca/books/about/Factors_Affecting_the_Economic_Status_of.html?id=evqDvgAACAAJ&redir_esc=y.

Meiner, S. E. (2011). *Gerontological nursing* (4th ed.). Mosby.

Messecar, D. C. (2016). Family caregiving. In M. Boltz, E. Capezuti, T. T. Fulmer, et al. (Eds.), *Evidence-based geriatric nursing protocols for best practice* (5th ed., pp. 137–163). Springer Publishing Company.

National Seniors Strategy. (2015). National Seniors Strategy evidence informed policy brief: Ensuring caregivers are not unnecessarily financially penalized for taking on caregiving roles. http://www.nationalseniorsstrategy.ca/wp-content/uploads/2015/02/NSS-SupportforCaregivers.pdf.

O'Connor, M. F. (2020). Bereavement. In K. Seeeny, M. L. Robbins, & L. M. Cohen (Eds.), *The Wiley encyclopedia of health psychology* (pp. 43–46). Willey Online Library.

Pristavec, T. (2019). The burden and benefits of caregiving: A latent class analysis. *Gerontologist, 59*(6), 1078–1091.

Rote, S. M., Angel, J. L., Moon, H., et al. (2019). Caregiving across diverse populations: New evidence from the National Study of Caregiving and Hispanic EPESE. *Innovation in Aging, 3*(2), 1–11. doi:10.1093/geroni/igz033.

Sayegh, P., & Knight, B. G. (2010). The effects of familism and cultural justification on the mental and physical health of family caregivers. *Journals of Gerontology. Series B, Psychological Science and Social Sciences, 66B*(1), 3–14. doi:10.1093/geronb/gbq061.

Schumacher, K. L., & Meleis, A. I. (1994). Transitions: A central concept in nursing. *IMAGE-The Journal of Nursing Scholarship, 26*(2), 119–127. doi:10.1111/j.1547-5069.1994.tb00929.x/pdf.

Smith, C. H., Graham, C. A., & Herbert, A. R. (2017). Respite needs of families receiving palliative care. *Journal of Paediatrics and Child Health, 53*(2), 173–179.

Statistics Canada. (2016). *Marital status (13), age (16), and sex (3) for the population 15 years and over of Canada, provinces and territories and census metropolitan areas, 1996 to 2016 censuses—100% data.* https://www150.statcan.gc.ca/n1/en/catalogue/98-400-X2016031.

Statistics Canada. (2017a). *Children with an immigrant background: Bridging cultures.* https://www12.statcan.gc.ca/census-recensement/2016/as-sa/98-200-x/2016015/98-200-x2016015-eng.cfm.

Statistics Canada. (2017b). *Same-sex couples in Canada in 2016.* https://www12.statcan.gc.ca/census-recensement/2016/as-sa/98-200-x/2016007/98-200-x2016007-eng.cfm.

Statistics Canada. (2017c). *Families, households and marital status highlight tables.* https://www12.statcan.gc.ca/census-recensement/2016/dp-pd/hlt-fst/fam/Table.cfm?Lang=E&T=42&Geo=00.

Statistics Canada. (2017d). *Working seniors in Canada.* https://www12.statcan.gc.ca/census-recensement/2016/as-sa/98-200-x/2016027/98-200-x2016027-eng.cfm.

Statistics Canada. (2018). *Social isolation of seniors: A focus on LGBTQ seniors in Canada.* https://www.canada.ca/en/employment-social-development/corporate/seniors/forum/social-isolation-lgbtq.html.

Statistics Canada. (2019a). *Family matters: Grandparents in Canada.* https://www150.statcan.gc.ca/n1/daily-quotidien/190207/dq190207a-eng.htm.

Statistics Canada. (2019b). *Diverse family characteristics of Aboriginal children aged 0 to 4.* https://www12.statcan.gc.ca/census-recensement/2016/as-sa/98-200-x/2016020/98-200-x2016020-eng.cfm.

Statistics Canada. (2020). *Caregivers in Canada, 2018.* https://www150.statcan.gc.ca/n1/daily-quotidien/200108/dq200108a-eng.htm.

Statistics Canada. (2021a). *Table 17-10*-0060-01: Estimates of population as of July 1st, by marital status or legal marital status, age and sex. doi:10.25318/1710006001-eng.

Statistics Canada. (2021b). *Table* 111-0039: Registered Retirement Savings Plan (RRSP) contributions, by contributor characteristics. doi:10.25318/1110004401-eng.

Sterling, M., & Baumblatt, G. L. (2019). The hidden health crisis: What family caregivers want you to know. *Caregiver's Perspective, 20*(2), 17–18. doi:10.1016/j.carage.2019.02.011.

Stewart, S. (2020). Spousal caregiving in community settings in Canada: Implications for nursing professionals. *Gerontology & Geriatric Medicine, 6,* 1–8. doi:10.1177/2333721420914476.

Stroebe, M., & Schut, H. (2010). The dual process model of coping with bereavement: A decade on. *Omega, 61*(4), 273–289. doi:10.2190/OM.61.4.b.

Taylor, M. F., Marquis, R., Coall, D. A., et al. (2017). The physical health dilemmas facing custodial grandparent caregivers: Policy considerations. *Cogent Medicine, 4*(1), 1292594.

26

SEXUAL HEALTH AND WELL-BEING

LEARNING OBJECTIVES

Upon completion of this chapter, the reader will be able to:

- Discuss intimacy and sexuality in later life and provide the appropriate nursing responses.
- Describe the biological changes that come with age that affect sexual health and well-being.
- Explain factors that impact sexual health in later life.
- Describe cohort and cultural influences on sexual health for older adults.
- Examine intimacy and sexuality for those living in long-term care homes.

GLOSSARY

Gender A social construct of characteristics, behaviours, and roles associated with being a woman or a man.

Intimacy Emotional closeness; close familiarity to someone.

Sex Identity based on reproductive functions (male, female, or intersex). This term can also be used to reference sexual activity.

Sexual intercourse Sexual contact between people. Involves penetration, typically insertion of an erect penis into a vagina.

Sexuality A person's identity in relation to whom they are attracted to.

THE LIVED EXPERIENCE

"He gives me affection, kisses and he is always holding me at home. We always sit on the sofa, and he says to me 'my beautiful face,' 'my love,' it's just that. We've always got on really well."

Ana, 64 years old, care partner to her husband living with dementia

Pinho, S., & Pereira, H. (2019). Sexuality and intimacy behaviors in the elderly with dementia: The perspective of healthcare professionals and caregivers. *Sexuality and Disability, 37,* 489–509. doi: 10.1007/s11195-019-09589-0.

SEXUALITY AND WELL-BEING

This chapter focuses on sexual health and well-being in later life. The factors influencing the sexual health of older adults are explored. This chapter also examines sexuality for residents living with dementia in long-term care (LTC) homes. Lastly, this chapter discusses nursing responses that support older adults to maintain their sexual health.

Sex and the Constructs of Gender

It is important for nurses to understand the difference between **sex** and **gender**. Sex and gender are separate personal characteristics (Government of Canada, 2019). Biological characteristics determine the sex of a person. Sex can be male, female, or intersex. By contrast, gender is a social construct that refers to one's social identity. Gender identities include man, woman, nonbinary, or Two-Spirit (Government of Canada, 2019). People who identify as nonbinary may feel like they do not fit into the category of "man" or "woman." Instead, they may feel a blend of being male and female, or a gender other than male and female (National Center for Transgender Equality, 2018). Indigenous peoples who identify as Two-Spirit possess both masculine and feminine spirits. They use this term to describe their gender, sexual, or spiritual identity (University of Toronto and Centre for Addiction and Mental Health, 2021).

Transgender Older Adults

Transgender is a broad term that can be used to describe people whose gender identity is different from the sex they were assigned at birth (Government of Alberta, 2020). In 2018, 0.24% of Canadians aged 15 and older identified as transgender (Statistics Canada, 2020). Transgender people in Canada are more likely to experience violence, mental illness, health disparities, and barriers to adequate health care (Government of Alberta, 2020).

Nurses' Role

Nurses must be respectful of older adults, the gender they identify with, and the pronouns they prefer to use. It is important to support transgender older adults by caring for them according to their gender identity and not according to their sex at birth (National Center for Transgender Equality, 2018). The Government of Alberta (2020) has outlined some strategies for inclusion of older adults who identify as lesbian, gay, bisexual, transgender, queer, and Two-Spirit (LGBTQ2). Nurses should remain person-centred and support older adults by building on their strengths and resilience. Nurses should also understand that transgender older adults may have had traumatic health care experiences in the past. It is very important to remain sensitive to and respectful of their needs.

INTIMACY AND SEXUALITY

Intimacy

The term **intimacy** stems from the Latin word "intimare," which means to "impress" or "make familiar." Intimacy is a close, family-like connection and a warm, meaningful feeling of joy. Intimacy involves the need for close friendships along with relationships with family, friends, and formal caregivers. Intimacy is expressed through open communication, active listening, and nonjudgmental support (Princeton University, 2021).

Older adults may be concerned about changes in sexual intimacy, but social relationships with the people who are important in their lives, the ability to interact intellectually with people who share similar interests, the supportive love that grows between human beings (whether romantic or platonic), and physical nonsexual intimacy are equally—and in many instances more—important than the physical intimacy of direct sexual relations. Intimacy needs with others change over time, but intimacy and satisfying social relationships are important components of successful aging.

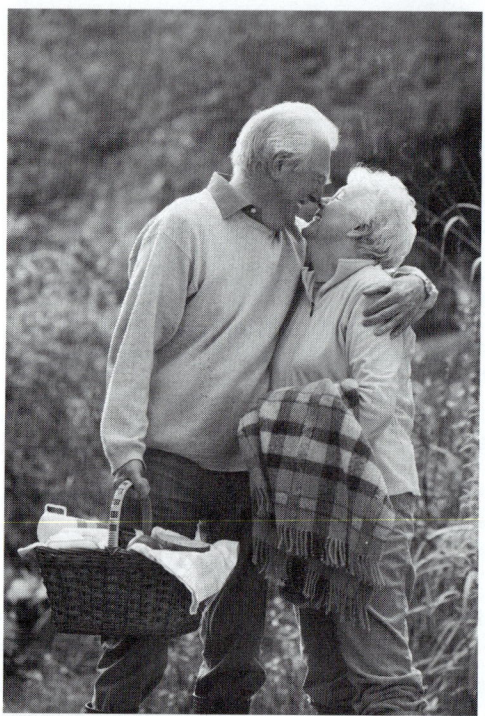

Love and affection are important to older adults. From Sorrentino, S. A., & Wilk, M. (2022). *Sorrentino's Canadian textbook for the support worker* (5th ed.). Elsevier Inc.

Sexuality

Sexuality is a central aspect of being human throughout life and encompasses sex, gender identities and roles, sexual orientation, eroticism, pleasure, intimacy, and reproduction (World Health Organization [WHO], 2021). As a major aspect of intimacy, sexuality includes the physical act of intercourse, as well as many other intimate activities. Sexuality provides the opportunity to express passion, affection, admiration, and loyalty; it can also enhance personal growth and communication. Sexuality also allows a general affirmation of life and a continuing opportunity to search for new growth and experiences.

Sexuality, like food and water, is a basic human need, yet it goes beyond the biological realm and has psychological, social, and moral dimensions. The constant interactions among these spheres of sexuality produce harmony. The linkage of the four dimensions makes up the holistic quality of an individual's sexuality.

The social dimension of sexuality is the sum of cultural factors that influence the individual's thoughts and actions with respect to interpersonal relationships and the individual's ideas and learned behaviour related to sexuality. Social media, television, art, literature, and the more traditional sources of family, school, peer group, and religious teachings combine to influence social sexuality. A person's beliefs about what constitutes masculinity and femininity is deeply rooted in cultural factors.

The psychological domain of sexuality reflects a person's attitudes, feelings toward self and others, and learning from experiences. From birth, people are bombarded with cues and signals instructing them how a person should act and think about the use of "dirty words" or body parts. Conversation is self-censored in the presence of or in discussion with certain people. The moral aspect of sexuality (the "I should" or "I shouldn't") is based in religious beliefs or in a pragmatic or humanistic outlook.

The final dimension, biological sexuality, is reflected in physiological responses to sexual stimulation, reproduction, puberty, and growth and development.

Because of their interrelatedness, these dimensions affect each other directly or indirectly whenever an aspect of sexuality is out of harmony. Sexuality is a vital aspect to consider in the care of the older adult, regardless of the setting. Sexuality exists throughout life in one form or another in everyone. All older adults have a need to express sexual feelings, whether the individuals are healthy and active or frail. Sexuality in the older adult shifts from a focus on procreation to a focus on companionship, physical nearness, intimate communication, and a pleasure-seeking physical relationship.

Sexual Health

The World Health Organization defines sexual health as a state of physical, emotional, mental, and social well-being related to sexuality (WHO, 2021). This definition illustrates the multifaceted nature of the biological, psychosocial, cultural, and spiritual components of sexuality and implies that sexual behaviour has the capacity to enhance the self and others. Sexual health is individually defined and wholesome if it leads to intimacy (not necessarily coitus) and enriches the involved parties.

Factors Influencing Sexual Health

Expectations. A large number of cultural, biological, psychosocial, and environmental factors influence older adults' sexual expression and sexual behaviour. Factors affecting a person's attitudes toward intimacy and sexuality include family dynamics and upbringing and cultural and religious beliefs. Older adults often internalize the broad cultural proscriptions of sexual behaviour in late life that hinder the continuation of sexual expression. Much sexual behaviour stems from the incorporation of other people's reactions. Older adults may be influenced to feel asexual when encountering others who consider them to be old and thus asexual.

Normal sexual interest and activity in the older population are sometimes regarded as deviant behaviour. By comparison, the same activity engaged in by a younger person is viewed as appropriate. The following often-quoted statement by Alex Comfort (1974) sums it up nicely: "In our experiences, old folks stop having sex for the same reasons they stop riding a bicycle—general infirmity, thinking it looks ridiculous, so no bicycle." Box 26.1 presents some of the myths about sexuality in older adults that may be held by older adults themselves and by society in general.

Activity Levels. While sexual desire may change as people age, older adults remain sexually active and interested and find their sexual lives satisfying. A Dutch study involving older participants aged 65 or older found that about half of those who were in a partnered relationship had engaged in sexual activity within the past 6 months (Freak-Poli et al., 2017; Freak-Poli, 2020). Only 1% of unpartnered women had engaged in sexual activity within the past 6 months (Freak-Poli et al., 2017; Freak-Poli, 2020). Sexual activity was found to decrease slightly with increasing age (Freak-Poli et al., 2017; Freak-Poli, 2020). A US-based study found that those who engaged in sexual activity within the

BOX 26.1
SEXUALITY AND AGING: COMMON MYTHS AND REALITIES

Myth: Older adults do not have sex.
Reality: Many older adults have intimate connections and sexual relationships.

Myth: The desire for sex decreases with age.
Reality: Sex is no less pleasurable with age.

Myth: Older adults do not need to worry about sexually transmitted infections.
Reality: Sexuality transmitted infections do not discriminate based on age. Sexually transmitted infections among older adults exist and condoms should be used.

Myth: Erectile dysfunction is uncommon.
Reality: A man's testosterone decreases every year beginning at age 25. As a result, erectile dysfunction is common among older men.

Myth: Older adults do not masturbate.
Reality: Masturbation is a natural, healthy behaviour that people often condemn in long-term care.

Source: Adapted from Seasons Retirement Communities. (2018, August 21). *7 myths about seniors and sex.* https://www.seasonsretirement.com/tips/7-myths-about-seniors-and-sex/.

past year had significantly higher life satisfaction compared with those who were not sexually active (Smith et al., 2019). Concerns about sex life and sexual health were found to be strongly associated with lower levels of life satisfaction, especially among men (Smith et al., 2019). **Sexual intercourse,** kissing, petting, and fondling were associated with greater life satisfaction among men, whereas kissing, petting, and fondling were associated with greater life satisfaction among women (Smith et al., 2019).

Cohort and Cultural Influences. The era in which a person was born also influences their attitudes about sexuality. Women who are in their eighties today may have been influenced by the conservative atmosphere of their youth, when sexuality was not openly discussed. The next generation of older adults (the "baby boomers") experienced the women's movement, increasing numbers of gay and lesbian couples,

more divorced adults, more liberal attitudes toward sexuality, and the human immunodeficiency virus (HIV) epidemic, all of which have affected their views and attitudes as they have aged. Boomers and future generations, as they find themselves experiencing sexuality, may alter society's perceptions of aging and sexuality.

Most of what is known about sexuality and aging has been gained through research with well-educated, healthy, White older adults. More research needs to be done on culturally, socially, and ethnically diverse older adults; those with persistent illness; and LGBTQ2 persons. It is important to know and understand older adults within their social and cultural backgrounds and not to make judgements based on one's own belief system.

Older LGBTQ2 Adults. Older LGBTQ2 persons are as diverse as the heterosexual older population. Most age successfully, are healthy and active, and have satisfying lives. Some people live as couples, have children, and are open about their sexual orientation. Some of these individuals have only recently "come out"; others have been "out" most of their lives; and some find themselves isolated in the larger society. Older gay persons and lesbians are more likely to have kept their relationships hidden than those who grew up in the modern-day gay liberation movement (Daley et al., 2017).

One study by Fleishman and colleagues (2019) explored sexual satisfaction, resilience, and internalized homophobia in older adults who were in gay and lesbian relationships. The authors found that relationship satisfaction was positively associated with sexual satisfaction. They also found that the sample of older adults had low levels of internalized homophobia and high levels of resilience and relationship satisfaction (Fleishman et al., 2019).

Another study looked at sexual satisfaction in lesbian, gay, and bisexual men and women and found that relationship commitment was more likely to predict sexual satisfaction for women than for men (Shepler et al., 2018). A second influence that was predictive of sexual satisfaction was identity pride and feeling comfortable with one's sexual identity (Shepler et al., 2018).

Older LGBTQ2 adults are less likely to access needed health and social services or to identify themselves as gay, lesbian, bisexual, transgender, or queer to health care providers (Casey, 2019). Health care providers may assume that their LGBTQ2 patients or clients are heterosexual and thus neglect to obtain a sexual history, discuss sexuality, or develop awareness of their particular sexual health needs.

Health care providers receive little education and training on the needs of this population and may lack sensitivity when caring for older LGBTQ2 individuals. Sensitivity is of utmost importance when obtaining a health history. Asking open-ended questions such as "Who is most important to you?" or "Do you have a significant other?" is much better than asking "Are you married?" This form of questioning allows a nurse to be open to diverse responses. Euphemisms (e.g., roommate or close friend) are frequently used to describe a life partner. Asking individuals if they consider themselves to be primarily heterosexual, bisexual, or gay (or lesbian) conveys the questioner's recognition and acceptance of sexual variety. An older lesbian woman in a health care situation may refer to herself indirectly by saying "people like us." Nurses must be aware of these nuances and try to understand the fear of discovery that is felt by older LGBTQ2 individuals, many of whom may still be "closeted" because of the homophobic experiences they had in their younger years.

Better support and care services for older LGBTQ2 adults by care providers should include the care providers working through any personal homophobic attitudes and discomfort when discussing sexuality, learning about special challenges facing older gay men and lesbians, and becoming aware of resources for LGBTQ2 persons in the community. Programs to increase awareness of the needs of LGBTQ2 older adults and to reduce discrimination are necessary. One Toronto-based community organization, The 519, promotes inclusion, understanding, and respect toward older LGBTQ2 adults, including by providing tips for care providers on how to support them. More information can be found at https://www.the519.org/programs/senior-pride-network. The Government of Alberta (2020) has also published a resource for improving services to older LGBTQ2 adults—*Aging With Pride: A Guide to Creating Inclusive Services for LGBTQ2S+ Older Adults.*

Biological Changes With Age. Acknowledgement and understanding of the age-related changes that influence a person's sexuality may partially explain alterations in

sexual behaviour that accommodate these changes and facilitate the continuation of pleasurable sex (see Chapter 6). Characteristic physiological changes during the sexual response cycle do occur with aging, but these changes vary from person to person, depending on general health factors. The more sexually active a person is, the fewer changes they are likely to experience in their patterns of sexual response. Illness and medication also affect sexual response. In a study by de Mello and colleagues (2020), older women reported that caring aesthetically for their body, face, and hair provided self-esteem and satisfaction. Feeling attractive provided further motivation to deal with life challenges. This could be linked to thoughts, feelings, and perceptions from experiences and sociocultural influences (de Mello et al., 2020).

Older adults who do not understand the physical changes that affect sexual activity become concerned that their sex life is approaching its natural conclusion. Some women make this assumption with the onset of menopause. Men may assume so when they discover a reduced firmness of their erection, less need for ejaculation with each orgasm, or a lengthier refractory period between episodes of intercourse. A major nursing role is to provide information about these changes, as well as appropriate assessment and counselling in the context of the individual's needs.

Sexual Dysfunction

"Sexual dysfunction," defined as the impairment of normal sexual functioning, can have both physical and psychological causes. Sexual disorders have not been well studied among older adults, but the following four groupings are generally described: hypoactive sexual desire disorder, sexual arousal disorder, orgasmic disorder, and sexual pain disorders.

Male Sexual Dysfunction. Erectile dysfunction is the inability to achieve and sustain an erection sufficient for satisfactory sexual intercourse in at least 50% of attempts. It is the most prevalent sexual problem in men. Erectile dysfunction (ED) occurs transiently to men of all ages at some point in their life. However, the prevalence of ED increases with age, affecting as many as 76.5% of men (Kessler et al., 2019).

For most older men, ED is caused by an underlying medical condition. The interaction among the hormonal, vascular, and nervous systems governs an erection; a problem in any of these systems can cause ED. In nearly one-third of cases, ED is a complication of diabetes. Alcoholism, depression, medications, and prostate disease and treatment are also causes of ED in older men. Various medications that affect the sympathetic and parasympathetic nervous systems interfere with the capacity to have an erection or to ejaculate. Erectile dysfunction is associated with the prescription of vasodilators, selective serotonin reuptake inhibitor (SSRI) antidepressants, and cardiac, antihypertensive, and antihyperglycemic medications (Razdan et al., 2018).

Because of health care providers' discomfort with discussing sexuality or because of a lack of knowledge about the sexuality of older adults, medications are often prescribed to older adults without consideration of sexual side effects. If medications that affect sexual function are necessary, then the adjustment of doses, the use of alternative drugs, and the prescription of antidotes to reverse sexual side effects are important.

The use of phosphodiesterase type 5 inhibitors such as sildenafil (Viagra), vardenafil (Levitra), and tadalafil (Cialis) has revolutionized the treatment of ED regardless of cause. Contraindications to the use of these medications include nitrate therapy, heart failure with low blood pressure, certain antihypertensive regimens, and other medications and cardiovascular conditions. (See Chapter 14 for a discussion of contraindications and side effects.) Penile implants of the semi-rigid, adjustable–malleable, or hinged and inflatable types are available when impotence does not respond to other treatments or is irreversible.

Female Dysfunction. Female dysfunction may include painful intercourse, painful contractions (spasm) of vaginal muscles, and problems with sexual desire and orgasm (National Health Service, 2019). Female sexual function can be influenced by culture, ethnicity, emotional state, age, and previous sexual experiences, as well as by changes in sexual response with normal aging. For women, the frequency of intercourse depends more on the age, health, and sexual function of the partner or on the availability of a partner than it does on their own sexual capacity.

Pain resulting from vaginal atrophy and dryness can result in painful intercourse (dyspareunia) and the avoidance of sexual activity. The use of water-soluble lubricants such as K-Y Jelly, Astroglide, and HR lubricating jellies can help with vaginal dryness. Topical low-dose estrogen creams, rings, or pills that are introduced into the vagina may also help to plump tissues and restore lubrication, with less absorption than with oral hormones (Robb-Nicholson, 2021).

Women can experience arousal disorders that result from the use of medications such as anticholinergics, antidepressants, and chemotherapeutic agents and from a lack of lubrication resulting from radiation, surgery, or stress. Orgasmic disorders also may result from medications used to treat depression. Prolapse of the uterus, rectoceles, and cystoceles can be surgically repaired to facilitate continued sexual activity. Urinary incontinence (UI) is another condition that may affect sexual activity for both men and women. Appropriate assessment and treatment are important because many causes of UI are treatable (see Chapter 9).

Intimacy and Persistent Illness

Persistent chronic illnesses and their related treatments may bring many challenges to intimacy and sexual activity. Some research has been done on the effects of myocardial infarction on sexual function. Often, older adults and their partners are given little or no information about the effect of illnesses on sexual activity or about strategies for continuing sexual activity within functional limitations. The timing of intercourse (e.g., mornings or when energy level is highest); oral or anal sex; masturbation; appropriate pain relief; different sexual positions; and the use of sex toys may all help individuals continue sexual activity. If pain due to arthritis is a concern, taking pain medications or a warm bath prior to lovemaking may be helpful. Alternate sexual positions such as side-by-side, straddling the male partner if he is the one with arthritic issues, or propping bent knees up with pillows for the woman with arthritis require less flexion of the hip and knee (Conrad Stöppler, 2016). Male partners who have had a stroke may prefer side-by-side positions, having both partners facing one another with legs interlaced, or having the affected male partner on top (Conrad Stöppler, 2016). Table 26.1 presents other suggestions for individuals with chronic illness.

Intimacy and Sexuality in Long-Term Care Homes

Surveys indicate that a significant number of older adults residing in long-term care homes might choose to express themselves sexually and, if they had privacy

TABLE 26.1
Chronic Illness and Sexual Function: Effects and Interventions

Illness	Effects and Problems	Interventions
Arthritis	Pain, fatigue, limited motion. Steroid therapy may decrease sexual interest or desire.	Advise the person to perform sexual activity at a time of day when they are less fatigued and most relaxed. Suggest use of analgesics and other pain-relief methods before sexual activity. Encourage use of relaxation techniques before sexual activity, such as a warm bath or shower or the application of hot packs to affected joints. Advise the person to maintain optimum health through a balance of good nutrition, proper rest, and activity. Suggest that the person experiment with different positions or use pillows for comfort and support. Recommend use of a vibrator if massage ability is limited. Suggest the use of water-soluble jelly for vaginal lubrication.
Cancer Breast cancer	No direct physical effect. Psychological effects: ■ Loss of sexual desire ■ Body-image change ■ Depression ■ Reaction of partner	Encourage individual or group counselling.
Most other cancers	Temporary loss of sexual desire. In men, potential erectile dysfunction; dry ejaculation; retrograde ejaculation. In women, potential vaginal dryness or dyspareunia. Anxiety, depression, pain, or nausea from chemotherapy, radiation, pelvic surgery, or hormone therapy, or nerve damage from pelvic surgery.	
Cardiovascular disease	Most men have no change in physical effects on sexual function. One-fourth may not return to pre–heart attack function; one-fourth may not resume sexual activity. Women do not experience sexual dysfunction after a heart attack. Fear of another heart attack (or death) during sex. Shortness of breath.	Encourage counselling about realistic restrictions that may be necessary. Teach the person alternative positions that avoid strain. Suggest that the person avoid large meals for several hours before sex. Advise the person to relax. Plan medications for effectiveness during sex.
Cerebrovascular accident (stroke)	Depression. May or may not have changes in sexual activity. Often, erectile disorders; decrease in frequency of intercourse and sexual relations. Change in role and function of partners. Fatigue, decreased physical endurance. Mobility and sensory deficits. Perceptual and visual deficits. Communication deficit. Cognitive and behavioural deficits. Fear of relapse or sudden death.	Encourage counselling. Instruct the person to use alternative positions. Suggest the use of a vibrator if massage ability is limited. Suggest the use of pillows for positioning and support. Suggest the use of water-soluble jelly for lubrication. Instruct the person to use alternative forms of sexual expression.

Continued

TABLE 26.1
Chronic Illness and Sexual Function: Effects and Interventions—cont'd

Illness	Effects and Problems	Interventions
Chronic obstructive pulmonary disease	No direct impairment of sexual activity, although coughing, exertional dyspnea, positions, and activity intolerance can have an effect. Medications may lead to erectile difficulties.	Encourage the person to plan sexual activity when energy is highest. Instruct the person to use alternative positions. Advise the person to plan sexual activity at a time when medications are most effective. Suggest that the person use oxygen before, during, or after sex, depending on when it provides the most benefit.
Diabetes	Sexual desire and interest unaffected. Erectile function interference from neuropathy, vascular damage, or both. (About 50% to 75% of men have erectile disorders; a small portion have retrograde ejaculation. Some men regain function if diagnosis of diabetes is well accepted, if diabetes is well controlled, or both. Women have less sexual desire and vaginal lubrication.) Potential decrease in orgasms, or absence of orgasm. Less frequent sexual activity. Local genital infections.	Recommend possible candidates for penile prosthesis. Instruct the person to use alternative forms of sexual expression. Recommend immediate treatment of genital infections.

and an available partner, would be sexually active (Aguilar, 2017). Intimacy and sexuality among residents encompasses not only coitus but also other forms of intimate expressions, such as hugging, kissing, handholding, and masturbation. Wallace (2003) commented that the sexual needs of older adults in LTC homes should have the same priority as nutrition, hydration, and other well-accepted needs. A person who lives in an LTC or assisted-living home has the same right to engage in or abstain from sexual activity as a person living in the community.

Depending on the province or territory, LTC homes may be required by law to offer a shared room to residents who are married or in a relationship. Residents also have the right to meet privately with their spouse or partner. Participants of studies on older gays and lesbians and their families have reported being terrified of going into care homes and having to hide their relationships or losing their partners and friends. A study by Sussman and colleagues (2018) discussed the importance of LGBT inclusivity in all congregate living environments, particularly LTC. One participant in their study described how relocations to LTC is based on bed availability and not choice, and how this would mean being separated from their partner (Sussman et al., 2018).

Lack of privacy is a major issue in LTC and assisted-living homes, as it can prevent the fulfillment of intimacy and sexual needs. Suggested actions for providing privacy and an atmosphere accepting of sexual activity include making a private room available, not interrupting when doors are closed or sexual activity is taking place, not interfering when residents have sexually explicit materials in their rooms, and providing adaptive equipment such as side rails and double beds when needed.

Attitudes about intimacy and sexuality among LTC home staff and, often, family members may reflect general societal attitudes that older adults do not have sexual needs or that their engagement in sexual activity is inappropriate. Family members may have difficulty understanding that their older relative may want to have a new relationship. Health care providers often view residents' sexual acts as problems rather than expressions of the need for love and intimacy. Reactions may include disapproval, discomfort, and embarrassment, and health care providers may explicitly or implicitly discourage or deny intimacy needs.

It is important that LTC staff and resident programs promote awareness, provide education on sexuality and intimacy in late life, involve residents and their families in discussions of sexuality, and discuss interventions that respond to residents' needs. Staff education should also include the opportunity to discuss personal feelings about sexuality, normal changes of aging, and the impact of diseases and medications on sexual function, as well as skill training in sexual assessment and intervention.

Intimacy, Sexuality, and Dementia

Intimacy and sexuality remain important in the lives of persons living with dementia and their partners throughout the illness. Intimacy and sexuality may serve as a nonverbal form of communication when other cognitive skills and functions have declined. As dementia progresses, particularly in persons living in LTC homes, intimacy and sexuality issues may present challenges, especially in regard to the person's ability to consent to sexual activity; consent requires accurate assessment and documentation. Issues of intimacy and sexuality of persons with dementia in LTC homes are complex. Practice standards and applicable legislation must guide nursing practice (Bauer et al., 2018; Brassolotto et al., 2020).

Determination of a cognitively impaired person's ability to consent to participation in a sexual activity involves consideration of (1) the person's mental capacity, (2) the risks and benefits of such activity for the person, and (3) what constitutes voluntary participation. Assessing the person's capacity to consent to sexual activity involves assessing the resident's awareness of the relationship, ability to avoid exploitation, and awareness of potential risks (Rector et al., 2020). If the person does not have the capacity to consent to sexual activity, the LTC home has a duty to protect that person from abuse and harm (Rector et al., 2020). An interprofessional working group in Hamilton, Ontario, has created a toolkit for developing policies about intimacy, sexuality, and sexual behaviour in older adults with dementia in LTC homes (http://www.rgpc.ca/resources/#resource-535).

Persons living with dementia in LTC homes may express their sexuality by holding hands, cuddling, having sexual intercourse, and using sexual language, as well as by engaging in behaviour that may be labelled inappropriate (e.g., exposing themselves, masturbating in public, or making inappropriate sexual advances or comments). These behaviours can be distressing to staff, residents, and families. The extent to which sexual expression and the sexual behaviour of residents who live with dementia are accepted varies between settings (Makimoto et al., 2015). When sexually inappropriate behaviour occurs, it should be assessed (as is any other behaviour) for cause, precipitating factors, and response to interventions. Encouraging family and friends to touch, hug, kiss, and hold hands when visiting may help to meet touch and intimacy needs and reduce inappropriate sexual behaviour. Also, allowing the person with dementia to stroke a pet or hold a stuffed animal may be helpful. Providing an environment that allows for the expression of sexuality in private may also be a solution (Rector et al., 2020). It is important to provide staff with opportunities for discussion, assistance with interventions, and education about written policies on sexuality and capacity assessment (Rector et al., 2020).

SEXUALLY TRANSMITTED INFECTIONS

The prevalence of sexually transmitted infections (STIs) such as chlamydia, gonorrhea, syphilis, human immunodeficiency virus (HIV), and genital herpes is increasing in Canada. Although younger Canadians have the highest incidence of STIs, older Canadians are also at risk. Among Canadians aged 60 years and older, the rates for chlamydia are 12.5 and 3.8 per 100,000 for men and women, respectively; for gonorrhea, the rate is 10.3 and 1.1 per 100,000 for men and women, respectively; and for syphilis, the rate is 5.1 and 0.1 per 100,000 for men and women, respectively (Government of Canada, 2020).

In the context of reporting HIV infection statistics, the Public Health Agency of Canada, along with other international reporting bodies, considers an older adult to be a person older than 50 years. In 2018, persons aged 50 years and older accounted for 22.5% of HIV cases in Canada, a statistic that remained stable over the previous 5 years (Haddad et al., 2019). The proportion of HIV cases in men and women were similar (Haddad et al., 2019).

The compromised immune system of older adults, which is associated with normal age-related changes, makes them more susceptible than younger adults to HIV or acquired immunodeficiency syndrome (AIDS). AIDS is not exclusively a young person's disease, but it is frequently underreported in the older population because the symptoms of fatigue, weakness, weight loss, and anorexia are common to other disease conditions or may be falsely attributed to "normal aging." Older adults are often diagnosed in the later stages of HIV infection (Haddad et al., 2019), which may result in an AIDS diagnosis. Lack of knowledge about HIV and AIDS and a belief that it "just does not happen in my generation" contribute to underreporting and late diagnosis. In addition, the idea that older adults are not sexually active limits health care providers' objectivity and thus their ability to recognize HIV infection and AIDS as possible diagnoses.

Older adults who are sexually active are at risk for HIV infection and AIDS and other sexually transmitted infections. For older men, gay or bisexual encounters were the most common mode of HIV transmission (48%), followed by heterosexual contact (32%) and drug use (14%) (Haddad et al., 2019). For women, heterosexual contact (75%) was the most common mode of HIV transmission, followed by drug use (29%) (Haddad et al., 2019). Older women who are sexually active are at high risk for HIV infection and for AIDS and other STIs from an infected partner, resulting in part from the normal age-related changes of the vaginal tissue (such as a thinner, drier, and more friable vaginal lining). They are also less likely than younger women to use condoms.

Testing for HIV is less common among older adults. However, assessment and screening for other STIs should be part of primary care for sexually active older adults. If symptoms of another STI arise, HIV testing should be done as well.

Nurses and other health care providers must become comfortable with taking a complete sexual history, talking about sex and STIs with older adults, and providing education about condom use and safer sex practices. (Websites with specific information about HIV, AIDS, and older adults for prevention and education are listed in the Resources section at the end of this chapter.)

IMPLICATIONS FOR GERONTOLOGICAL NURSING AND HEALTHY AGING

Nurses have many roles in the area of sexuality and older adults. The nurse is a facilitator of a milieu that is conducive to the older adult asking questions and expressing sexuality. The nurse has the responsibility to help maintain the sexuality of older adults by offering an opportunity for discussion. Some older adults remain or want to remain sexually active, whereas others do not see this as an important part of their lives. Nurses should open the door to discussions of sexual concerns in a nonjudgemental manner, relieving any anxiety or discomfort of having discussions about sexual health (Bauer et al., 2016). Nurses should promote open sharing of information (Bauer et al., 2016), supporting those who want to continue to be sexually active and making it clear to others that stopping sex is an acceptable option. The nurse should be an educator, providing information and guidance to older adults who need it.

Assessment

To assist and support older adults' sexual needs, nurses should be aware of their own feelings about sexuality and their attitudes toward intimacy and sexuality in older adults, whether those persons are single, married, or LGBTQ2. Only after nurses confront their own attitudes, values, and beliefs can they provide support without being judgemental. Sexual histories are rarely elicited from older adults, and physical examinations often do not include the reproductive system unless it is directly involved in a current illness. However, when questions about sexual issues are asked or when an older adult is assessed, the nurse needs to be particularly cognizant of the era the person has lived through and the person's culture in order to understand the factors affecting the person's conduct.

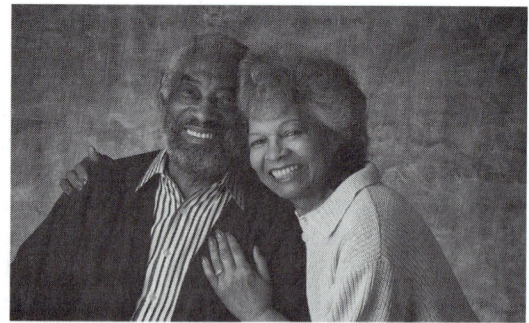

Sexuality is an important need in late life—it affects pleasure, adaptation, and a person's general feeling of well-being. © Getty Images.

Older adults should be asked about their sexual satisfaction because they may not mention it voluntarily. Anticipating problems in older adults' sexual experiences can ward off anxiety, misconceptions, and an arbitrary cessation of pleasurable sexual activity. The normalcy of sexual activity may need validation. Also needed may be a discussion of the physiological changes that occur with age or of the effects of illness and treatment that may interfere with sexual activity by altering its routine or interfering with physical performance. Counselling may also be needed for the older adult to adapt to natural physiological changes and image-altering surgical procedures. Assessment of any medical conditions or medications that are associated with poor sexual health and functioning, screening for HIV infection and for AIDS and other STIs, and education about safer sex are also important.

Discussion of sexuality and sexual dysfunction may be uncomfortable for the nurse or the older adult. Nonetheless, it is important that the nurse learn the significance that sexual function has for the older adult and the person's perception of sexual function without bringing the nurse's own biases into the interaction.

The PLISSIT model (Annon, 1976) and *Sexuality Assessment for Older Adults* (Smyth, 2018) (see Box 26.2) are two useful resources for the discussion of sexuality.

Interventions

Interventions will vary depending on the needs identified by the assessment. Following a comprehensive assessment, interventions may centre on the following categories: (1) education regarding age-associated changes in sexual function, (2) ways of compensating for normal age-related changes, (3) effective management of the effects of acute and chronic illness on sexual function, (4) removal of barriers associated with difficulty in fulfilling sexual needs, and (5) special interventions to promote sexual health in cognitively impaired older adults (Steinke, 2016).

Education about the prevention of HIV infection and STIs is also important for sexually active older adults.

BOX 26.2
THE PLISSIT MODEL

P	Having **P**ermission from the person to initiate sexual discussion.
LI	Providing the **L**imited **I**nformation needed to function sexually.
SS	Giving **S**pecific **S**uggestions to the individual for proceeding with sexual relations.
IT	Providing **I**ntensive **T**herapy around the issues of sexuality for the person. (This may mean referral to specialist.)

Sources: Adapted from Annon, J. (1976). The PLISSIT model: A proposed conceptual theme for behavioral treatment of sexual problems. *Journal of Sexual Education & Therapy, 2*(2), 1–15; Smyth, C. (2018). *Sexuality assessment for older adults.* Try This Series (Issue 10). https://hign.org/sites/default/files/2020-06/Try_This_General_Assessment_10.pdf.

KEY CONCEPTS

- Sexuality comprises love, sharing, trust, and warmth, as well as physical acts. Sexuality provides a person with self-identity and affirms life.
- Sexuality continues in late life, although older adults need support to adapt to age-related changes and the effects of chronic illness.
- Further research is needed to promote knowledge and understanding of the sexual health of older LGBTQ2 adults.
- Awareness of HIV and AIDS and the practice of safer sex among older adults are still lacking. Older adults and health care providers may not consider the risk for HIV infection and AIDS, even though the incidence of both in the older population is increasing.
- To optimize the sexuality of older adults in the community or in an LTC home, the nurse provides education and counselling about sexual function, adaptations for age-related changes and chronic conditions, the prevention of HIV infection and AIDS and other STIs in sexually active older adults, and the maintenance of intimacy and sexuality for the older adult who desires them.

ACTIVITIES AND DISCUSSION QUESTIONS

1. With a classmate, role play how you would conduct a review of systems in the area of sexual health with an older adult. What would be the most important factors to consider when teaching about sexuality and sexual health?

2. Discuss how you would approach a conversation about intimacy and sexuality with an older adult with a chronic illness in your care.

3. What is your role as a nurse in informing an older adult in your care about biological changes that affect sexual health and well-being?

4. What would you find most difficult about discussing cultural influences on sexual health with an older adult?

5. What sexual health resources are available for older LGBTQ adults in your community?

RESOURCES

BC Centre for Disease Control. Sexually transmitted infections.
http://www.bccdc.ca/health-info/disease-types/sexually-transmitted-infections

Centre for Sexuality—Seniors A GOGO (Growing Older, Getting It On) theatre project.
https://www.calgarysexualhealth.ca/programs-workshops/older-adults-seniors/

Hartford Institute for Geriatric Nursing. Sexuality assessment for older adults (streaming video).
https://hign.org/consultgeri/try-this-series/sexuality-assessment-older-adults

Health Canada. Seniors and aging—Sexual activity.
http://publications.gc.ca/collections/collection_2007/hc-sc/H13-7-15-2006E.pdf

Helpguide.org.

Rainbow Health Ontario. Improving health care service to LGBT2SQ communities.
http://www.rainbowhealthontario.ca/

Realize: Fostering positive change for people living with HIV and other episodic disabilities—HIV and aging.
https://www.realizecanada.org/en/our-work/hiv-and-aging/

Senior Pride Network. Volunteer-run organization for LGBTQ2 people in Toronto.
http://www.seniorpridenetwork.com/home.htm

SAGE—Advocacy and Services for LGBT Elders. Resources for LGBT older people and those interested in LGBT aging issues.
http://www.sageusa.org/index.cfm

For additional resources, please visit *http://evolve.elsevier.com/Canada/Ebersole/gerontological/*

REFERENCES

Aguilar, R. A. (2017). Sexual expression of nursing home residents: Systematic review of the literature. *Journal of Nursing Scholarship*, 49(5), 470–477.

Annon, J. (1976). The PLISSIT model: A proposed conceptual theme for behavioral treatment of sexual problems. *Journal of Sexual Education and Therapy*, 2(2), 1–15. doi:10.1016/B978-0-08-020373-7.50019-X.

Bauer, M., Haesler, E., & Fetherstonhaugh, D. (2016). Let's talk about sex: Older people's views on the recognition of sexuality and sexual health in the health-care setting. *Health Expectations*, 19(6), 1237–1250. doi:10.1111/hex.12418.

Bauer, M., Haesler, E., & Fetherstonhaugh, D. (2018). Organizational enablers and barriers to the recognition of sexuality in aged care: A systematic review. *Journal of Nursing Management*, 27(4), 858–868. doi:10.1111/jonm.12743.

Brassolotto, J., Howard, L., & Manduca-Barone, A. (2020). Sexual expression in Alberta's continuing care homes: Capacity, consent and decision-making. *Canadian Journal on Aging*, 40(1), 156–165. doi:10.1017/S0714980819000813.

Casey, B. (2019). *The health of LGBTQIA2 communities in Canada: Report of the Standing Committee on Health.* https://www.ourcommons.ca/Content/Committee/421/HESA/Reports/RP10574595/hesarp28/hesarp28-e.pdf.

Comfort, A. (1974). Sexuality in old age. *Journal of the American Geriatrics Society*, 22(10), 440–442. doi:10.1111/j.1532-5415.1974.tb04811.x.

Conrad Stöppler, M. (2016). *Better sex after 50.* https://www.onhealth.com/content/1/sex_after_50.

Daley, A., MacDonnell, J. A., Brotman, S., et al. (2017). Providing health and social services to older LGBT adults. *Annual Review of Gerontology & Geriatrics*, 37(1), 143–160. doi:10.1891/0198-8794.37.143.

Fleishman, J. M., Crane, B., & Barthalow Koch, B. (2019). Correlates and predictors of sexual satisfaction for older adults in same-sex relationships. *Journal of Homosexuality*, doi:10.1080/00918369.2019.1618647.

Freak-Poli, R. (2020). It's not age that prevents sexual activity later in life. *Australasian Journal on Ageing*, 39(1), 22–29. doi:10.1111/ajag.12774.

Freak-Poli, R., Kirkman, D., De Castro, L. G., et al. (2017). Sexual activity and physical tenderness in older adults: Cross-sectional prevalence and associated characteristics. *Journal of Sexual Medicine*, 14(7), 918–927. doi:10.1016/j.jsxm.2017.05.010.

Government of Alberta. (2020). *Aging with pride: A guide to creating inclusive services for LGBTQ2S+ older adults.* https://open.alberta.ca/dataset/e99b2db8-c11c-41d4-ae26-50908e1315b6/resource/999e894a-c6aa-467e-b5f4-37a83831b61f/download/sh-aging-with-pride-guide-2020.pdf.

Government of Canada. (2019). *Modernizing the Government of Canada's sex and gender information practices: Summary report.*

https://www.canada.ca/en/treasury-board-secretariat/corporate/reports/summary-modernizing-info-sex-gender.html.

Government of Canada. (2020). *Report on sexually transmitted infections in Canada, 2017.* https://www.canada.ca/en/public-health/services/publications/diseases-conditions/report-sexually-transmitted-infections-canada-2017.html.

Haddad, N., Robert, A., & Weeks, A., et al. (2019). *HIV in Canada—Surveillance report, 2018. Canadian Communicable Disease Disease Report, 45*(12), 304–312. doi:10.14745/ccdr.v45i12a01.

Kessler, A., Sollie, S., Challacombe, B., et al. (2019). The global prevalence of erectile dysfunction: A review. *BJU International, 124,* 587–599. doi:10.1111/bjui.org.

Makimoto, K., Kang, H. S., Yamakawa, M., et al. (2015). An integrated literature review on sexuality of elderly nursing home residents with dementia. *International Journal of Nursing Practice, 21*(52), 80–90. doi:10.1111/ijn.12317.

de Mello, M., de Moura Scortegagna, H., & Pichler, N. A. (2020). Care and the impact of aesthetic appearance on the social perception on a group of elderly women. *Revista Brasileira de Geriatria e Gerontolgia, 23*(2), e190271. doi:10.1590/1981-22562020023.190271.

National Center for Transgender Equality. (2018). *Understanding non-binary people: How to be respectful and supportive.* https://transequality.org/issues/resources/understanding-non-binary-people-how-to-be-respectful-and-supportive.

National Health Service. (2019). *Female sexual problems.* https://www.nhs.uk/live-well/sexual-health/female-sexual-problems/.

Princeton University. (2021). Intimacy. https://umatter.princeton.edu/respect/relationships/intimacy.

Razdan, S., Greer, A. B., Patel, A., et al. (2018). Effect of prescription medications on erectile dysfunction. *Postgraduate Medical Journal, 94*(1109), 171–178.

Rector, S., Stiritz, S., & Morley, J. E. (2020). Sexuality, aging, and dementia. *Journal of Nutrition, Health & Aging, 24,* 366–370. doi:10.1007/s12603-020-1345-0.

Robb-Nicholson, C. (2021, August 17). *By the way, doctor: Is vaginal estrogen safe?* https://www.health.harvard.edu/womens-health/by_the_way_doctor_is_vaginal_estrogen_safe.

Shepler, D. K., Smendik, J. M., Cusick, K. M., et al. (2018). Predictors of sexual satisfaction for partnered lesbian, gay, and bisexual adults. *Psychology of Sexual Orientation and Gender Diversity, 5*(1), 25–35. doi:10.1037/sgd0000252.

Smith, L., Yang, L., Veronese, N., et al. (2019). Sexual activity is associated with greater enjoyment of life in older adults. *Sexual Medicine, 7*(1), 11–18. doi:10.1016/j.esxm.2018.11.001.

Smyth, C. (2018). *Sexuality assessment for older adults.* Try This Series (Issue 10). https://hign.org/sites/default/files/2020-06/Try_This_General_Assessment_10.pdf.

Statistics Canada. (2020). *Sexual minority people almost three times more likely to experience violent victimization than heterosexual people.* https://www150.statcan.gc.ca/n1/daily-quotidien/200909/dq200909a-eng.htm.

Steinke, E. (2016). Issues regarding sexuality. In M. Boltz, E. Capezuti, T. T. Fulmer, & D. Zwicker (Eds.), *Evidence-based geriatric nursing protocols for best practice* (5th ed., pp. 165–188). Springer Publishing Company.

Sussman, T., Brotman, S., MacIntosh, H., et al. (2018). Supporting lesbian, gay, bisexual and transgender inclusivity in long-term care homes: A Canadian perspective. *Canadian Journal on Aging, 37*(2), 121–132. doi:10.1017/S0714980818000077.

University of Toronto and Centre for Addiction and Mental Health. (2021). Re:Searching for LGBTQ2S+ Health. Two-spirit community. https://lgbtqhealth.ca/community/two-spirit.php.

Wallace, M. (2003). Sexuality and aging in long-term care. *Annals of Long-Term Care, 11,* 53–59. http://www.managedhealthcareconnect.com/home/altc.

World Health Organization (WHO). (2021). *Sexual health.* https://www.who.int/health-topics/sexual-health#tab=tab_2.

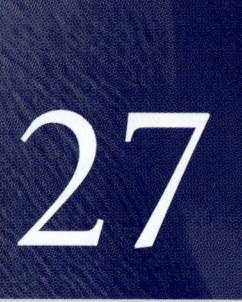

27

COMFORT, PALLIATIVE CARE, DEATH, AND LOSS

LEARNING OBJECTIVES

Upon completion of this chapter, the reader will be able to:

- Differentiate between loss and grief.
- Explain the different types of grief and the dynamics of the grieving process.
- Explain the nursing competencies required to effectively intervene in the older adult's grief and bereavement.
- Describe the principles of hospice palliative care.
- Identify and discuss the needs of people who are in the process of dying, as well as appropriate interventions.
- Explain the role and responsibility of the nurse in advance directives.
- Explain the role of the nurse in medical assistance in dying (MAID).

GLOSSARY

Bereavement overload   Multiple losses occurring in a short period of time.

End-of-life care   Care provided when death is imminent.

Grief   An emotional response to loss.

Hospice palliative care   Care that is directed toward maximizing comfort rather than achieving a cure.

Mourning   The process by which grief is experienced.

THE LIVED EXPERIENCE

"When we were in our sixties, my friends and I met over cards, went on trips, and experienced all of the joys of retirement. We didn't have much time to worry about aches and pains. In our seventies, we had less time to play, because we were busy visiting one another in hospital or in nursing homes. In our eighties, we met frequently again, but it was usually at our friends' funerals, leaving little time for cards or travel. Now that I am in my nineties, hardly any of my friends are still alive; you know, it gets kind of lonely, so you just have to make new younger friends!"
Theresa, 93 years old

Loss, dying, and death are universal, incontestable events of the human experience. Some loss is associated with the normal changes of aging, such as the loss of flexibility in the joints. Loss is also related to normal changes in everyday life and to life transitions such as moving and retirement. Still, other losses are those of loved ones through death. Some deaths, such as those of parents and friends, are considered normative and are expected. Other deaths, such as the deaths of adult children or grandchildren, are non-normative and mostly unexpected.

Regardless of the type of loss, each one has the potential to trigger **grief** and a process called bereavement or **mourning**. "Grief" and "mourning" are usually used synonymously. However, grief is an individual's response to a loss, and mourning is an active and evolving process that includes behaviours through which the experience of loss is incorporated into one's life. Mourning behaviours are strongly influenced by social and cultural norms that prescribe the appropriate or expected ways of both reacting to the loss and coping with it (Thompson et al., 2016; Williams et al., 2015). There is no single way to grieve or respond to loss; each person grieves in their own way. The spiritual search for meaning that confronts individuals when dealing with loss and death is fundamental in many cultures and societies.

Although there are cultural expectations of grief behaviours for loss through death, there are no prescribed guidelines for behaviour when the loss is of another type. For example, an individual who is seriously ill, who moves to a long-term care (LTC) home, or who retires (willingly or unwillingly) may be sad, irritable, and forgetful. The person may be suspected of developing dementia when they are in fact actually grieving. When the losses accumulate in quick succession, **bereavement overload** may result. The griever may become incapacitated and require skilled support and guidance.

Gerontological nurses should be knowledgeable about the grieving process and how to comfort and care for grievers. This includes being able to practise self-care in their own experiences of grief. Knowledge about the dying process is also needed, as are skills related to care of the dying person and the bereaved. This chapter provides the basic information necessary to promote effective grieving, peaceful dying, and good deaths.

THE GRIEVING PROCESS

Researchers have tried for years to understand the grieving process, and their efforts have resulted in a number of proposed models to explain and predict the experience. Most of the models, developed in the 1970s and 1980s, describe how grief is understood by society. Although intended to describe death-related grief, these same models can be applied to other significant and meaningful losses experienced by older adults.

All models recognize similar physical and psychological manifestations of acute grief (i.e., when it is first felt), a middle period when the manifestations of grief (e.g., despair or depression) affect the person's day-to-day functioning, and an ending phase during which the person learns to adjust to life in a new way without that which has been lost. At the same time, it is also recognized that the grieving process is not rigidly structured and that there is not always a predictable pattern of responses.

Worden's Model of Bereavement

The model of bereavement developed by Worden (2008) has been frequently cited and adapted. The model represents the grieving process as a series of evolving tasks that are repeated for all losses or parts of losses. The four tasks are to (1) accept the reality of the loss, (2) work through the physical and emotional pain associated with the loss, (3) adjust to life without the lost person, and (4) find an enduring connection with the deceased person in order to move on with life.

For an example of how to apply this model, consider a hypothetical situation where "Helen" has lost her life partner, "Chris." In this case, the nurse may look for signs that Helen is accepting the reality of Chris's death (e.g., the deceased person is referred to in the past tense rather than the present tense). For example, Helen may speak of Chris as someone who "just loved to garden." Although her working through the pain is an individual process, Helen does have a support network of family, friends, and church members. They encourage her to "tell her story" of not only Chris's life but also their life together, and they gently nudge her to start thinking of her life without Chris. In working through acute grief, the grieving person may try to avoid grief pain by using medications such as anxiolytics (e.g., benzodiazepines). Although these medications may be necessary in some cases to enable the griever to accomplish some needed tasks, they are not recommended for everyday use. These medications interfere with resolution and with dealing with the pain caused by grief and are generally not recommended for older adults (see Chapters 14 and 23).

Adjusting to loss may take a considerable period of time, especially if the relationship with the deceased was a long and close one. Changes in the environment—such as a rearrangement of furniture or a different seating pattern at the dinner table—may be physical, emotional, or spiritual.

As Helen proceeds through the grieving process, her memories of life with Chris will be those of the past, and she will be able to develop new memories of her life without Chris. Although there may be a lot of pain associated with specific days such as birthdays, anniversaries, and holidays without Chris, the pain might lessen with the passing years as the loss is relocated from the present to the past.

Loss Response Model

Jett's Loss Response Model (Jett, 2004) is a modification of a grieving model proposed by Giacquinta for families facing cancer (Giacquinta, 1977). This adapted model incorporates a systems approach that provides a framework for the design of nursing interventions. When loss occurs within a system, such as a family, the experience is one of acute grief. The system's equilibrium is thrown off and undergoes a functional disruption; that is, the system cannot perform its usual activities. Family members are in a state of disequilibrium. The loss seems unreal. The grieving family searches for meaning. Why did this happen? How will they survive the loss? Older adults who are reacting to the loss of a child or a grandchild commonly ask themselves, "Why wasn't it me?"

The family may then become active in informing others. Each time the story is repeated, the loss becomes more real, and the system moves toward a new steady state. The story is also different each time it is told because it is told from a new perspective. Informing others involves engaging emotions that may have been previously withheld or subdued because of the shock of the loss. The expression of emotions can release energy that can be used to reorganize the family structure. As roles change, adaptation and accommodation are necessary. Someone else steps in to perform the roles of the person who is now absent or to complete the tasks of that person. For example, when the older patriarch dies, the eldest child may step up and assume some of the parent's roles and responsibilities.

Finally, if the system is to survive, it needs to redefine itself. One way this is done is through the reframing of memories—that is, families understand that portraits and reunions are still possible, just different from what they were before the loss; or they realize that a person can still be vital, active, and important even after the loss of the ability to drive a car, walk unassisted, or live alone (Fig. 27.1).

Types of Grief

Grieving takes enormous amounts of physical and emotional energy. It is the hardest thing that anyone does and may be especially hard for older adults. Emotions can be intense, and this intensity may manifest as confusion, depression, or a preoccupation with thoughts of the deceased or the loss. This reaction may be mistaken for other conditions, such as dementia. The gerontological nurse will likely work with older adults who are experiencing anticipatory grief, acute grief, or persistent grief.

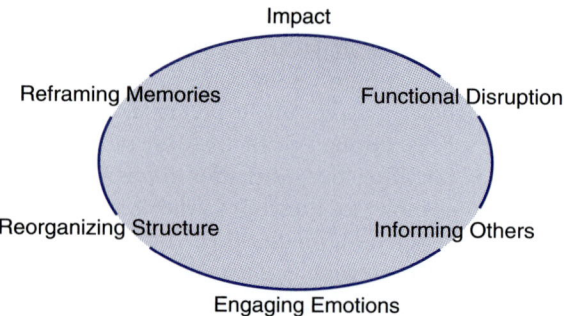

Fig. 27.1 ■ The Loss Response Model. *Source:* Jett, K. F. (2004). *The Loss Response Model* [Unpublished manuscript]. Adapted from Giacquinta, B. (1977). Helping families face the crisis of cancer. *American Journal of Nursing, 77*(10), 1585–1588.

A fourth type, disenfranchised grief, may be hidden but is significant when it does occur.

Anticipatory Grief

Anticipatory grief is the response to a real or perceived loss before that loss occurs. This grief can be in anticipation of a loss, such as loss of belongings (e.g., through the selling of a home), loss of home (e.g., through moving into an LTC home), loss of a body part or function (e.g., through mastectomy or losing the ability to walk), or loss of a spouse or oneself (through dementia or death). The stages of anticipatory grief include (1) experiencing shock about the upcoming loss, (2) denying the reality of the loss, and (3) eventually, for most, acceptance of the loss (Whitley, 2020). Person-centered communication about the loss is associated with anticipatory grief and improved bereavement-related outcomes (Coelho et al., 2018).

When the grieving process occurs in the context of anticipatory grief, it is significantly different in that the loss has not yet occurred. If the loss is certain but no one can say when it will occur, or if it does not occur when or as expected, the person who is awaiting the actual loss or death may become irritable, hostile, or impatient in response to the emotional ups and downs of the waiting.

Anticipatory grief can result in premature detachment from the individual who is dying or from the environment or activity the person will lose. Pattison (1977) called the premature withdrawal of others "sociological death" and the premature withdrawal of the person who is dying "psychological death." In either case, the person who is dying is no longer involved in the day-to-day activities of living and essentially suffers a premature death.

Acute Grief

Acute grief is a crisis. It has a definite syndrome of somatic and psychological symptoms of distress that occur in waves lasting for varying periods of time. These symptoms may occur every time the loss is acknowledged, others are informed, or another person offers condolences. This preoccupation with the loss is similar to daydreaming and is accompanied by a sense of unreality. Depending on the situation, feelings of self-blame or guilt may be present, manifesting as hostility or anger toward friends, depression, or withdrawal.

It is often difficult for people who are acutely grieving to accomplish their usual activities of daily living or to meet other responsibilities (a condition called functional disruption). Even if the tasks are accomplished, the person may complain of feeling distracted, restless, and "at loose ends." Deciding what to wear may seem too complex a task. Often, the signs and symptoms of acute grief eventually diminish. Acute grief is most intense in the months immediately following the loss, especially the first 6 months; the intensity mostly lessens over time (Zisook et al., 2014).

Returning to the previous example, this is how Helen's acute grief manifested: In the first months after Chris died, Helen cried any time he was mentioned. Later on, she was still grieving, but her tears were replaced with a surging sense of loss and sadness. And later still, she experienced more fleeting reactions.

Persistent or Complicated Grief

Although grief may temporarily inhibit some activity, it is considered a normal response to loss. The intermittent pain of grief is often exacerbated on birthdays, holidays, and wedding anniversaries. For the survivors of tragedies such as war, terrorist attacks, natural disasters, or prolonged emotional or physical abuse, the grief may never completely go away. This type of lingering grief has been described as "shadow grief," grief that resurfaces from time to time but does not persist. It produces a temporary grief, usually triggered by a sight, smell, or sound (Fane, 2016).

Some persistent grief is more than shadow grief and evolves into *complicated grief*. Complicated grief is thought to start as an expected grief response, but the evolution toward adjustment and the re-establishment of equilibrium is blocked. The memories resist being reframed. Reactions continue to be very intense and painful, and memories are experienced as recurrent acute grief, over and over again, months and years later. Complicated grief is a chronic and debilitating consequence of bereavement that is associated with clinically significant distress and impairment. The signs of complicated grief include preoccupation with the loss, avoidance of reminders of the loss, the feeling that others are not trustworthy or do not understand the loss, bitterness and anger, numbness or anhedonia, a feeling of shock, and a grief episode that triggers a major depressive episode (Nakajima, 2018). Indigenous peoples, having suffered inequities and multiple traumas, are at higher risk of experiencing complicated grief (Spiwak et al., 2012). Those who have a relative who died from suicide are at greater risk for complicated grief (Andriessen et al., 2020). Complicated grief occurs in up to 7% of bereaved people (Zisook et al., 2014). This type of grief requires the intervention of a professional grief counsellor, a psychiatric nurse practitioner, or a psychologist who is skilled in helping grieving people.

Disenfranchised Grief

Disenfranchised grief is an experience of the person whose loss cannot be openly acknowledged or publicly mourned. The grief is socially disallowed or unsupported and is incongruent with norms of grief in the person's culture (Patlamazoglou et al., 2018; Mughal et al., 2020). The person does not have a socially recognized right to be perceived as a bereaved person or to function as one. The relationship is not recognized, the loss is not sanctioned, or the grieved one is not recognized or cannot be made public. A common theme with disenfranchised grief is that people close to the grieving person do not know about the loss or do not understand the full meaning of the loss to that person.

Situations that are associated with disenfranchised grief include hidden or secret relationships (e.g., some LGBTQ2 relationships and relationships that are part of extramarital affairs) (Patlamazoglou et al., 2018). Disenfranchised grief can also occur when the cause of death is stigmatized (e.g., suicide) or when the loss is not seen as worthy of sympathy (e.g., the death of a pet, retirement). Families grieving the loss of a person who had dementia may also experience disenfranchised grief, particularly when others perceive the death of the person as a blessing and subsequently fail to support the grieving family member, who has struggled for years with losses and anticipatory grief and now must cope with the acute grief of the actual death (Blandin, 2016).

Stages of Grief

In 1969, Elisabeth Kübler-Ross published *On Death and Dying* (Kübler-Ross, 1969). In this book, she describes the five stages of loss. Later, in 2005, Kübler-Ross and David Kessler co-authored *On Grief and Grieving: Finding the Meaning of Grief Through the Five Stages of Loss*, where two additional stages were introduced (Kübler-Ross & Kessler, 1969). The seven stages are (1) shock, (2) denial, (3) anger, (4) bargaining, (5) depression, (6) testing, and (7) acceptance. During the first stage, "shock," the person may be numbed in disbelief and creates an emotional buffer to protect themselves. The second stage, "denial," describes coping with loss through denying the experiences of feelings or denying that the loss has happened. The third stage, "anger," is an important stage of the healing process. Anger can be directed to something or to the person who was lost. Outbursts may occur during this stage. It is important to understand that this is normal and part of the grieving process. The fourth stage, "bargaining," describes the "what ifs" that the person may think about. One example includes "What if this accident never happened?" The person grieving wants life to go back to normal. The fifth stage, "depression," typically occurs after bargaining, where empty feelings come forward and grief moves to a deeper level. In the sixth stage, "testing," people may find solutions for coping with the loss. The seventh stage, "acceptance," describes accepting the new reality. This phase by no means entails that someone is okay with the loss that has happened, but accepts that the loss has actually taken place (Kübler-Ross, 1969, and Kübler-Ross & Kessler, 2005, in Oates and Maani-Fogelman, 2020).

Nurses should understand these stages when caring and supporting older adults who have experienced a loss (Oates & Maani-Fogelman, 2020). Nurses must realize that not everyone experiences every stage of grief nor the order of the stages that Dr. Kübler-Ross presents. Nurses should use their therapeutic communication and educate those in their care on what the person's feelings are, based on the stages of grief (Oates & Maani-Fogelman, 2020).

Death of a Child or Grandchild

Parents and grandparents often believe that a normal life trajectory will allow them to pass away before their younger children and grandchildren. This is not always the case. As a result, older adults are sometimes left grieving the loss of their child or grandchild. Loss of children later in life can result in a conflicting state of emotions – trying to remain strong for the family members who have lost a child, parent, or a sibling, but also mourning the loss of one's own child or grandchild. In one study, older adults who had lost an adult child felt the need to stay strong and put the emotions of other family members first (Lekalakala-Mokgele, 2018). As one participant described:

> "When I cry I am hiding myself from these children, I mean my grandchildren. I had to be strong for them, they have just lost their mother. I'm all by myself, because if you cry and the children cry too, it becomes too chaotic." (Woman, 84 years old; Lekalakala-Mokgele, 2018, p. 153)

When the loss of a grandchild occurs, grandparents can become "neglected mourners," taking on the responsibility of "staying strong" for the child's parents and siblings (Fowler, 2018). Grandparents grieve not only the loss of the grandchild, but also experience grief over their own children's suffering (Fowler, 2018). O'Leary and colleagues (2017) sought to gain insight into the needs of grandparents who had lost a grandchild. They found that grandparents felt isolated and alone and that there was a lack of support to help them with their grief. They felt pressure to not burden their adult child, who was also experiencing a loss (O'Leary et al., 2017). Grandparents felt that there is a lack of information on how to comfort and support their own adult child with loss (O'Leary et al., 2017).

Although with increasing age comes a greater chance of experiencing the loss of a loved one, older adults may not be ready to endure the experiences and grief that come with the loss of younger family members (Lekalakala-Mokgele, 2018). Nurses should understand these situations and consider the difficulty and conflicting emotions that one must cope with when grieving the loss of a child or grandchild. It is important to offer support and empathy and ensure that older adults have a safe space to mourn their loss (Fowler, 2018).

IMPLICATIONS FOR GERONTOLOGICAL NURSING AND HEALTHY AGING

The nursing goal is not to prevent grief but to support those who are grieving. Although the loss will never change, its potential long-term detrimental effects can sometimes be lessened. Working with grieving older adults is part of what gerontological nurses do on a daily basis. Even small actions taken by the nurse can make a large difference in the grieving person's quality of life.

Assessment

In grief assessment, the nurse aims to understand the person's grieving experience so that the person can be appropriately supported. Nurses should assess for signs of grief and loss, and look for those who may not be coping effectively. Building a therapeutic relationship with the person and loved ones is key to ensuring that people feel comfortable discussing their feelings (Oates & Maani-Fogelman, 2020).

A grief assessment is based on knowledge of the grieving process and subsequent mourning. Data are obtained through observation of the person's behaviour, and the assessment is conducted while considering the cultural context (Neimeyer & Holland, 2015). A thorough grief assessment includes questions about recent significant life events, life or religious values, cultural customs and rituals, and the person's relationship to who or what has been lost. It is important to take time to hear the person's account of the death or loss and attend to cues about the meaning of the loss.

Knowing more about the loss and the effect of the loss on the older adult's life enables the nurse to identify those who are at risk for complicated grief and to construct and implement appropriate and caring responses. Box 27.1 provides a pneumonic tool that nurses can use to support older adults and their loved ones in a therapeutic manner.

BOX 27.1
TOOL FOR THERAPEUTIC COMMUNICATION DURING EMOTIONAL CONVERSATIONS: NURSE TECHNIQUE

The American Association of Critical Care Nurses has created the pneumonic *NURSE*. This pneumonic can assist in guiding emotional conversations while maintaining a therapeutic relationship and building rapport. For example, if the person says, "This is overwhelming," the nurse may respond with:

Name: Name what they just said. (*You feel overwhelmed.*)

Understand: Understand their needs. (*There is a lot going on. How can I help you?*)

Respect: Express that you respect them and the situation they are currently experiencing. (*I'm so impressed with how well you are handling everything.*)

Support: Show them that you are there for them. (*I'll be here with you throughout my shift.*)

Explore: Extend the conversation with open-ended questions. (*What is the hardest part?*)

Source: Adapted from Oates, J. R., & Maani-Fogelman, P.A. (2020). Nursing grief and loss. *StatPearls.* https://www.ncbi.nlm.nih.gov/books/NBK518989/.

Interventions

A goal of intervention is to assist the individual, family, and community in attaining a healthy adjustment to the loss experience and in re-establishing equilibrium. Actions that can meet this goal are basic and simple; however, the emotional overlay can make these interventions difficult. For the new nurse who is confronted with a person's grief for the first time, there may be discomfort, fear, and insecurity. The tendency is to be sympathetic rather than empathetic. The following questions may arise in one's mind: What do I say? Should I be cheerful or serious? Should I talk about or even acknowledge the loss?

Nursing interventions, especially when older adults are in crisis, begin with the gentle establishment of rapport. Nurses need to introduce themselves and explain the nature of their roles (e.g., charge nurse, staff nurse) and their availability. If it is the time of impact (e.g., just after a serious diagnosis, at the death of a family member, or upon moving into an LTC home), nurses can provide support and a safe environment and ensure that basic needs are met. The nurse can soften the despair by saying things that foster reasonable hope, such as "You will make it through this, one moment at a time, and I will be here to help."

Nurses need to be observant for *functional disruption* and offer support and direction. They may have to help the person with what has to be done immediately and find ways to support them. The nurse can offer to either complete the task or find a friend or family member who can step in so the disruption does not have any deleterious effects.

As grieving people search for meaning, they may require help to find what they are looking for. Sometimes it is information about a disease, a situation, or a person. Sometimes it is a spiritual search. Sometimes they need help in finding a resource or a place of peace. Often, what is needed most is someone to listen to the "whys" and "hows"—questions that cannot be answered. Healing and addressing grief are often situated within one's cultural values and practices. It is important for nurses to be aware and informed of traditional cultural healing models.

Sometimes nurses offer to contact others on behalf of those who are grieving, assuming that this is something that will help. However, it is far more therapeutic for the grieving person to be the one who informs others, because doing so helps the loss to become real. The nurse can offer to find a phone number, hold the grieving person's hand during the conversation, or just "be there" when the news is being shared. In this way, the nurse can be available to provide support when the grieving person's emotions are difficult.

As the grieving person moves forward in adjusting to the loss (e.g., moving from their home to an LTC home), the nurse can help the person reorganize the structure of their life. For example, the nurse can talk with the person about what was most valued about living at home and what habits were comforting; the nurse can then help the person find ways to incorporate these into the new environment. If, for instance, the older adult always had a cup of tea before bed but now does not have access to a kitchen, addressing this can be a part of the individualized plan of care.

According to the Loss Response Model, memories are reframed as part of the completion of the cycle of grieving. The grandmother who lives in an LTC home who always hosted her granddaughter's birthday party can still host it. The nurse who knows about this important ritual can help the resident reserve a private space, send out invitations, and have the birthday party, just reframed in that it is catered in the grandmother's new "home."

DYING, DEATH, AND COMFORT AND PALLIATIVE CARE

Many people have said that death is not the problem; it is dying that takes the work. This is true for all involved—the person who is dying; the dying person's loved ones; and the professional caregivers, such as nurses and health care aides.

Dying is both a challenging and a very private life experience. How a person deals with dying is a reflection of the person's culture and the way the person has handled earlier losses and stressors. Although not all older adults will feel that they have led fulfilling lives or feel a sense of completion, it is considered normative for older adults to experience transcendence or self-actualization. If the dying process is particularly long or if the death occurs after a painful illness, some people may rationalize the death or view it as a relief, at least in part. Death at a younger age or as the result of trauma or catastrophe is viewed as tragic and sometimes incomprehensible. Death as a result of natural disaster, war, or violence is seldom rationalized; even the deaths of older victims are considered an unacceptable loss of human potential.

Conceptual Models

Just as models have been proposed to explain the grieving process, so too have models been proposed to explain the process of dying. The next section discusses the living–dying interval.

The Living–Dying Interval

Whereas dying physically begins early in life (see Chapter 6), in personal terms, dying begins at a moment called the "crisis knowledge of death" (Pattison, 1977, p. 44) and ends at the moment of physiological death. Pattison (1977) calls the time between these two points the "living–dying interval," a period made up of acute, chronic, and terminal phases. The chronological time of the living–dying interval is accordion-like because of remissions and exacerbations in the terminal illness;

it may last days, weeks, months, or years. The manner in which a person faces dying is an expression of personality, circumstances, illness, and culture.

The "crisis knowledge of death" occurs when someone receives the information that they will not live as long as previously anticipated. It would certainly appear that the greater the discrepancy between the previously assumed length of life and the newly projected length of life, the greater the required adjustment and, perhaps, the greater the intensity of the grief.

The point of crisis is a moment in time that is followed by the acute phase of the living–dying interval. The point of crisis is usually the peak time of stress and anxiety because it is the time when the life and future of the individual and the family are thrown into disequilibrium. Crisis intervention is most effective at this time because the individual, the family, and the caregivers are struggling to come to terms with the knowledge. A significant amount of anticipatory grieving may be observed.

Since no one can withstand a crisis indefinitely, most of the dying time is spent in the chronic phase. During this time, the dying person and those around them are forced to resume some sense of normalcy. Bills still need to be paid, dishes still need to be washed, and life can still be lived. The challenge for people with terminal illnesses and for their families is to work toward living while dying and not toward dying while still living. Entertainment, work, and relationships can be maintained as the individual's condition permits. Life goes on despite the anticipation of its end.

The terminal phase is reached when the speed of the physical dying is accelerated and the person no longer has the energy to maintain the activities of everyday life. The person may withdraw or turn away from the outside world, or the person may engage in coded communication (such as saying "goodbye" instead of the usual "good night," giving away cherished possessions as gifts, or urgently contacting friends and relatives with whom they have not communicated for a long time). The focus then turns to preserving energy and completing life's journey. In some cultures, this period of time is called the "death watch" and is associated with prescribed rituals.

The living–dying interval can reflect an integrated or disintegrated trajectory (Fig. 27.2) (Pattison, 1977). The interval is integrated when each new crisis is dealt with effectively and the quality of life of the person who is dying is preserved. The interval is disintegrated if one crisis tumbles on to the next one without any effective resolution and if the quality of life of the person who is dying is compromised.

IMPLICATIONS FOR GERONTOLOGICAL NURSING AND HEALTHY AGING

Most often, death is not sudden or unexpected. For most people, the dying process lasts from a few weeks to many months. Most people with progressive persistent illnesses experience three distinct illness and death trajectories. Nurses who are aware of these trajectories can anticipate the needs of those who are dying and help them and their families to cope and plan. The first trajectory (typical of cancer) is a short period of decline over weeks, months, and occasionally years. The second trajectory (more typical of conditions such as heart failure and chronic obstructive pulmonary disease) consists of long-term functional limitations and gradual deterioration in health and functioning, with intermittent exacerbations. Death may occur as part of one of these exacerbations, but the timing of death is unpredictable and uncertain. The third trajectory

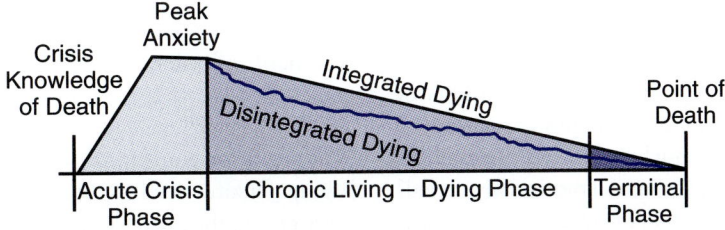

Fig. 27.2 ■ The living–dying interval. **Source:** Pattison, E. M. (1977). *The experience of dying.* Prentice-Hall.

(more typical of dementia or frailty) is called *prolonged dwindling* and lasts for years. Death may occur as a result of an acute condition such as pneumonia, or it may result from a combination of minor physical events that the person does not have the reserve to surmount.

The responsibility of the nurse is to work within the interprofessional team to provide safe conduct as the dying and their families navigate through unknown waters to a good and appropriate death. A good and appropriate death is one that a person would choose (if choosing were possible) and one in which the person's needs are met to the greatest extent possible. There are several ways to approach an understanding of the dying and to meet their needs. The approach discussed here is called the "six Cs approach."

The Six Cs Approach

An older, yet still relevant model is that of Weisman (1984), who identified six needs of those who are dying: care, control, composure, communication, continuity, and closure.

Care

People who are dying should receive the best care possible; this includes expert management of symptoms and support at all times. Care includes the adequate treatment of physical pain (see Chapter 16). Care also addresses the psychological and emotional pain—induced by depression, anxiety, fear, and any other unresolved emotional concern—that can be just as strong and just as real as physical pain. When emotional needs are not met, the total pain experience is intensified. Medications alone cannot relieve pain. Instead, empathic listening and allowing the person to express their thoughts is an important intervention (see Chapter 4). If tears and sadness are present, then gentle touch, closeness, and sitting near the person are helpful when culturally appropriate. As an advocate, the gerontological nurse should make sure that the person receives the care that is needed.

Caring for a dying person also means helping the person conserve energy. Dying calls for great amounts of energy to cope with the emotional and physical assault of illness on the body. How much can the individual do without becoming physically and emotionally taxed? What supports for activities of daily living are most valuable and important for the person to participate in or

receive? How much energy is needed for the person to be able to talk with others or be present without becoming exhausted? Only the person can answer these questions through verbal or nonverbal communication, and the nurse must advocate for the person to have their wishes respected.

Control

As a person proceeds along the living–dying interval, they often feel that their control over their life has been lost. The person is in the process of losing everything they have ever known. The potential loss of identity, independence, and control over bodily functions can lead to a sense of having lost control, dignity, and self-esteem. The person may begin to feel ashamed, humiliated, and like a "burden." There is a strong human need for control—a need to remain in a collaborative role related to one's own living and dying and, where still possible, an active participant in one's own care. The nurse can help the person meet this need by taking every opportunity to return control to the person. Whenever possible, the nurse can have the person decide where, when, and how to receive care, nutrition or hydration, sleep, and so forth. For people living with dementia, it is even more important to protect the person from others who are determining the priorities and activities of the individual. In some cultures, control is given to the eldest son or a family or community member (a priest, Elder, or spiritual or medicine woman) to act as the spokesperson for matters affecting the dying person. Nurses need to be aware of who the liaison is between the family, the health care provider, and the dying person.

Composure

In many cultures, dying is an emotional activity, both for the person who is dying and for those around them. The need for composure is what enables the person to modulate emotional extremes appropriately within cultural norms—not to avoid the sadness, but to have moments of relief.

Communication

The need for communication is broad. It includes the dying person's need to receive information to make decisions and the need to share information. Although the type and content of communication that is acceptable to a person varies by culture, the nurse has a responsibility to make sure that the dying person has an opportunity for the communication they desire (see Chapter 3).

In a study of communication between the dying person, their family, and hospital staff about terminal illness, Glaser and Strauss (1963) identified four types of communication: closed awareness, suspected awareness, mutual pretense, and open awareness. Each type of communication influenced the work on the unit and the care for the dying person.

Closed awareness is described as "keeping the secret." Health care providers, the family, and friends know that the person is dying, but the dying person does not know this or is aware but keeps the secret as well. Generally, caregivers invent a fictitious future for the person to believe in, hoping that this will boost the person's morale. Although this happens less today because of legislation related to patients' rights, it still occurs. In some cultures, it is expected.

In *suspected awareness*, the person suspects they are dying, but because the dying is not discussed, it cannot be confirmed. Inquiries on the part of the person are indirect or are avoided by others. Hints are bandied back and forth, and a contest for control of the information ensues.

Mutual pretense is a situation of "let's pretend." Everyone knows the person has a terminal illness, but no one talks about it; feelings are kept hidden.

Open awareness occurs when the dying person, family, friends, and all health care providers openly acknowledge the eventual death of the person. The person may ask, "Will I die?" and "How and when will I die?" The person is aware of the dying, and the family grieves *with* the person rather than *for* the person. The nurse can encourage open awareness whenever possible, respecting the person's culture at the same time. In some cultures, talking about an anticipated death is deemed helpful. In others, one can be aware of the dying, but talking about it openly may be avoided.

Continuity

Satisfying the need for continuity equates to maintaining as normal a life as possible for the dying person and helping the person transcend the present by leaving a legacy for the future. Sometimes a dying person can feel shut off from the rest of the world at a time when they are still capable of being involved and active in some way. Loneliness is the result of a loss of continuity with one's life. The nurse may ask about the person's life and about those things most valued, and can work with the family and the dying person on a plan to remain engaged in as many activities and past roles as possible. A father who watches a certain ballgame with his son every Sunday can continue to do this, regardless of the need to be in hospital, at home, or in hospice. If the person is at home and bedridden, it may make more sense to have the bed in a central area rather than in a distant room.

One approach people have taken to ensure the continuity of their lives after death is to establish legacies. Legacies can take many different forms. They include the memories that will live on in the minds of others and donations (financial or in-kind) bequeathed to family or loved ones (see Chapter 3). A grandmother who is likely to die before a favourite grandchild's wedding can, by participating in planning the wedding (regardless of the age of the grandchild), leave an enduring and special legacy.

Closure

The need for closure creates an opportunity for reconciliation and transcendence. Closure is not about the end of grief. People often continue to feel grief at least intermittently throughout their lives; there is no absolute closure (Doka, 2016). Reminiscence is one way to move through grief and the reconciliation of loss and to evaluate the pluses and minuses of life. It is a means of resolving conflicts, giving up possessions, and saying final goodbyes. Pain and other symptoms that are not well controlled may interfere with this reconciliation, making the nurse's role of offering appropriate interventions all the more important.

For some, closure means coming to terms with their spiritual selves. If the expressions of the dying person have spiritual overtones, pastoral or spiritual care may be offered but should never be carried out without the person's permission. The nurse can foster transcendence by providing the dying person with the time and privacy for self-reflection as well as an opportunity to talk about whatever they need to talk about, especially the meaning of their life and death.

Care, control, composure, communication, continuity, and closure are necessary to meet the needs of the dying person. Their influence is omnipresent in these needs.

Care and Life Partners, Family, and Loved Ones

Nurses are often present and support the life partners, family, and loved ones at the time of death and in the moments preceding it. Regardless of their ages, the surviving family members, life partners, and loved ones and friends have needs, and nurses have a responsibility to care for them. In one study, newly bereaved people were asked what they had found most helpful (Richter, 1987). Their answers showed that they most appreciated nurses who did the following:

- Kept them informed
- Asked how they were doing and offered support
- Put an arm around them when they cried
- Brought them food
- Knew their name
- Cried with them
- Brought a bed and encouraged them to stay in the room with the dying person
- Told them to hold their dying loved one's hands
- Held their hands
- Got the spiritual or religious leader for them
- Let them take care of their loved one, and
- Stayed with them after the nurse's shift was over.

Although these actions will not provide comfort to all or always be possible, they can be used as starting points. A helpful guide for families, care partners and friends is *When Someone Close to You Is Dying: What You Can Expect and How You Can Help* (available in English, French, and Spanish on the National Initiative for the Care of the Elderly website at https://www.nicenet.ca). The guide was developed to provide information that families and care partners said they needed. It includes information about what the dying person may need, what happens during the last moments of life, pain control, advance care planning (ACP) and substitute health care decision making, and strategies to support the dying person. The guide is also helpful for nursing students and novice nurses who may have limited exposure to the dying process.

End-of-Life Care

Availability of **end-of-life care** across all health care settings and environments is important because, although most deaths occur in hospital (60% in 2019), the proportion of deaths that occur in hospital is decreasing (Statistics Canada, 2021). This decrease is due to more deaths occurring at home, in a hospice, or in an LTC home. One study by Hill and colleagues (2019) found that there has been a corresponding increase in the provision of palliative care with the decreasing rate of deaths in hospital. However, meeting these wishes may be difficult, depending on availability and capacity of those who are able to provide care and support. Family members, care partners, and others often find that there are inadequate resources to support them. Lack of services and funding for palliative care is particularly problematic in rural communities (Pugh et al., 2019).

While most Canadians prefer to die at home, the preferred place of death varies among cultures, and depending on the nature of the illness that a person has, some people may prefer to die in hospital. Nurses working in all health care settings should be knowledgeable about end-of-life care. Box 27.2 describes a study about palliative and end-of-life care in LTC homes.

Hospice Palliative Care

Nurses routinely care for older individuals who have irreversible and progressive conditions such as dementia or Parkinson's disease. Some older adults have exhausted all treatment options or have decided that they want no further treatment for conditions such as cancer or end-stage heart or renal disease. An LTC home resident may elect to remain at the LTC home rather than be transferred to an acute care hospital even if faced with an acute event such as a myocardial infarction or a stroke. These people receive palliative care, care that focuses on comfort rather than cure, on the treatment of symptoms rather than disease, and on quality rather than quantity of life.

Palliative care is "an approach that improves the quality of life of patients and their families facing the problems associated with life-threatening illness, through the prevention and relief of suffering by means of early identification and impeccable assessment and treatment of pain and other problems, physical, psychosocial and spiritual (World Health Organization, 2020).

In 2017, the federal, provincial, and territorial governments agreed to a Common Statement of Principles on Shared Health Priorities (Government of Canada, 2019). This statement included a commitment to improving access to palliative care. The *Framework on Palliative Care*

BOX 27.2
RESEARCH FOR EVIDENCE-INFORMED PRACTICE: DEATH AND DYING IN LONG-TERM CARE HOMES

Problem: The need for palliative care tends to be recognized late for a person living and dying in a long-term care (LTC) home, potentially limiting the preparedness of the family and the comfort of the dying resident. This study investigated how the culture in LTC homes is related to the awareness of impending death and the use of palliative care.

Methods: The study was an ethnographic study of end-of-life practices in three Ontario LTC homes. Residents, family members, and staff were interviewed; documents were reviewed; and a focus group was conducted. The data were analyzed with a constant comparative technique.

Findings: The following four elements of the culture of LTC homes influenced end-of-life care: (1) high care demands and limited resources to meet usual care needs; (2) the belief that LTC homes are for living; (3) the belief that no one should die in pain; and (4) the belief that no one should die alone. Even though 30% of residents died each year, staff members felt it important to counteract fears and negative ideas about LTC homes ("It's an old stigma that this is a place to come to die" [p. 6]) by focusing on the LTC home as a place to live. This focus on LTC homes as a place to live distracted from the acknowledgment of death, dying, and the palliative status of many residents. The findings were seen as being influenced in Canada by a broader cultural force of death denying.

Implications for Nursing Practice: The researchers called for higher staff-to-resident ratios to meet the needs of residents and allow for timely palliative care. The term "palliative care" was narrowly understood to refer to end-of-life care (i.e., care when death is imminent), a view that limited access to palliative care. A palliative approach is consistent with person-centred care that enhances quality of life. However, a reluctance to acknowledge the palliative status of residents may limit the preservation of their quality of life.

Source: Cable-Williams, B., & Wilson, D. M. (2017). Dying and death within the culture of long-term care facilities. *International Journal of Older People Nursing, 12*(1), e1215. doi: 10.1111/opn.12125.

BOX 27.3
GUIDING PRINCIPLES OF THE FRAMEWORK ON PALLIATIVE CARE IN CANADA

1. Palliative care is person- and family-centred care.
2. Death, dying, grief and bereavement are a part of life.
3. Caregivers are both providers and recipients of care.
4. Palliative care is integrated and holistic.
5. Access to palliative care is equitable.
6. Palliative care recognizes and values the diversity of Canada and its peoples.
7. Palliative care services are valued, understood, and adequately resourced.
8. Palliative care is high-quality and evidence-based.
9. Palliative care improves quality of life.
10. Palliative care is a shared responsibility.

Source: Government of Canada. (2019). *Action plan on palliative care.* https://www.canada.ca/en/health-canada/services/health-care-system/reports-publications/palliative-care/action-plan-palliative-care.html.

The federal government is supporting this initiative by funding provincial and territorial governments over 10 years to improve access to palliative care. The federal government has also allocated funding toward improving home and palliative care for Indigenous communities (Government of Canada, 2019).

Hospice palliative care comprises comfort care and may be the heart of caring. The term "hospice" gets its meaning from the medieval concept of hospitality, in which a community assisted a traveller at dangerous points along their journey. The hospice movement has been a vehicle to support the roots of nursing in humane, compassionate care—an ideal that has been the basis of nursing for centuries. People who are dying are indeed travellers—travellers along the continuum of life—and the community consists of friends, family, loved ones, and health care providers, including nurses and others, who are prepared to offer care and services.

Given the complexity of hospice palliative care, it is not surprising that it depends on an interprofessional care team made up of the dying person, care partners, the person's family and loved ones, and professional health care providers. An assessment instrument that

in Canada Act was passed by Parliament in late 2017 (Government of Canada, 2019). The framework was developed by Health Canada through consultations with provincial and territorial governments, the federal government, stakeholders, those living with life-limiting illnesses, their caregivers, and other Canadians. The guiding principles of the framework can be found in Box 27.3.

might be helpful in determining the level of care needed is the Victoria Hospice Palliative Performance Scale (Victoria Hospice, 2001). It consists of an 11-point scale that measures a person's status from 100% (healthy) to 0% (death) on five parameters: ability to do activities, self-care, ambulation, food, and fluid intake and consciousness level (Victoria Hospice, 2021). More information on the Palliative Performance Scale can be found at https://victoriahospice.org/how-we-can-help/clinical-tools/.

Most hospice palliative care is provided at home. The home becomes the primary centre of care and services. Family members, care partners, or friends are supported to provide care for the basic activities of daily living and taught how to administer some of the medication needed to provide comfort for the dying person. Hospice palliative care supports and guides the dying person and the support network. It ensures that the person is not alone and that the network will not be abandoned. Bereavement services for the care partners, family, and loved ones can extend for a period of time on an emergency and regular basis after the death of the person.

Pain control and the opportunity to die at home are the key ideas and activities that people associate with hospice palliative care services. A growing number of inpatient hospice homes exist as well. These care settings have developed from home-based programs that have added small, free-standing inpatient settings for people who have symptoms that cannot be managed at home or for those who have no caregivers or who have limited care capacity. Hospice nurses and others may also care for dying people who are residents in LTC homes, working with staff members to supplement care and provide expertise in symptom management.

Virtual Hospice

Virtual hospice offers people in the process of dying, care partners, family members, and health care providers support and information about palliative and end-of-life care (Virtual Hospice, 2021). The web-based platform of virtual hospice aims to help address gaps in palliative care in Canada. Virtual hospice provides a resource where dying people and family members can ask questions, access resources on symptom management, and access tools for better care (Virtual Hospice, 2021). More information on virtual hospice can be found at https://www.virtualhospice.ca.

The Nurse's Role in Hospice Palliative Care

Nurses provide much of the direct care for a dying person and their family. Additional nursing roles are coordinating the implementation of the interdisciplinary care plan, managing palliative care services, and advocating for the humane care of people who are dying and their families.

The Canadian Nurses Association (CNA) offers certification in hospice palliative care nursing. The Canadian Association of Schools of Nursing entry-to-practice competencies describe the special skills, knowledge, and abilities for palliative and end-of-life care that are expected of graduating nurses. In 2020, the Registered Nurses' Association of Ontario created a best practice guideline entitled *A Palliative Approach to Care in the Last 12 Months of Life* (available at https://rnao.ca/sites/rnao-ca/files/bpg/PALLATIVE_CARE_WEB.pdf). Overarching competencies are presented in Box 27.4. Detailed indicators for each competency are available at https://www.casn.ca/.

DYING AND THE NURSE

Nurses are professional grievers; they invest time and caring. If they are working with older adults, they invest especially in those who are frail and reside in acute and LTC settings. Nurses experience the death of patients and residents over and over again. Some consider the death of a patient, client, or resident a failure because they have "lost" the person they cared for. But good deaths can be viewed as professional successes each time nurses share the special, personal experience of providing care for older dying people and providing gentle care for their survivors. Nurses can use the reminders of their own mortality as motivation to live the best they can with what they have. Nurses can seek support and give support to one another. As grieving people themselves, nurses may need to share their story of caring for the dying person to the health care providers around them, either in formal or in informal support groups. They also must listen to the stories of their colleagues over and over again until the stories become part of the fabric of their colleagues' lives.

Caring for older adults requires knowledge of the grieving and dying processes as well as skills in providing palliative care or relieving symptoms. However, working with grieving or dying people day in and day

> ## BOX 27.4
> ## ENTRY-TO-PRACTICE COMPETENCIES FOR HOSPICE
> ## PALLIATIVE CARE NURSING IN CANADA
>
> 1. Uses requisite relational skills to support decision making and negotiate modes of palliative and end-of-life care on an ongoing basis.
> 2. Demonstrates knowledge of grief and bereavement to support others from a cross-cultural perspective.
> 3. Demonstrates knowledge and skills in holistic, family-centred nursing care of people at end-of-life who are experiencing pain and other symptoms.
> 4. Recognizes and responds to the unique end-of-life needs of various populations, such as elders, children, multicultural populations, those with cognitive impairment, language barriers, those in rural and remote areas, those with chronic diseases, mental illness and addictions, and marginalized populations.
> 5. Applies ethical knowledge skillfully when caring for people at end-of-life and their families while attending to one's own responses such as moral distress and dilemmas, and successes with end-of-life decision making.
> 6. Demonstrates the ability to attend to psychosocial and practical issues such as planning for death at home and after death care relevant to the person and the family members.
> 7. Identifies the full range and continuum of palliative and end-of-life care services, resources and settings in which they are available, such as home care.
> 8. Educates and mentors patients and family members on care needs, identifying the need for respite for family members, and safely and appropriately delegating care to other caregivers and care providers.
> 9. Demonstrates the ability to collaborate effectively to address the patient and family members' priorities within an integrated inter-professional team, including non-professional health care providers, and the patient himself or herself.
>
> *Source:* Extracted from Canadian Association of Schools of Nursing. (2011). *Palliative and end-of-life care: Entry-to-practice competencies and indicators for registered nurses.* Author. http://casn.ca/wp-content/uploads/2014/12/PEOLCCompetenciesandIndicatorsEn1.

out is an art that calls for inner strength and coping skills. The most important coping skills for nurses may be the ability to find meaning and being able to balance seeing the person who is dying as a human being and staying professional throughout the care trajectory (Ingebretsen & Sagbakken, 2016). The effective and caring gerontological nurse has developed a personal philosophy of life and of death; although this outlook can and does change over time, it will help when times are difficult. Emotional maturity enables the nurse to deal with disappointment and the postponement of immediate wants or desires. Maturity also means that the nurse can reach out for help when needed. Finally, in order to provide comfort to grieving people, nurses must be comfortable with their own lives or at least be able to set aside their own sadness and grief while working with the sadness and grief of others.

DECISION MAKING AT THE END OF LIFE

Decision making at the end of life has become a legal, ethical, medical, and personal concern. The lines between living and dying are blurred as a direct result of medical and technological advances; hence, there is ambivalence concerning whether death is to be delayed, fought, or accepted.

The issue of who has the authority to make end-of-life decisions has been the subject of years of research, debate, and legislation. Legal requirements can vary across provinces and territories. Nurses have an obligation to know the legal requirements in their jurisdictions and to work with the older adult and their family to determine how these requirements will fit the family members' cultural patterns and their end-of-life decision making.

The ethical issues of end-of-life care are complex. Nurses observe the CNA *Code of Ethics for Registered Nurses* (Canadian Nurses Association, 2017). The CNA and the Canadian Hospice Palliative Care Association have provided additional resources related to ethics and end-of-life care. (For additional information, see the Resources at the end of this chapter.)

Advance Care Planning

ACP is the process of planning for a time when a person may not have the cognitive capacity to make decisions about health care (Advance Care Planning Canada, 2021) (see Chapter 24). It involves the person's (1) choosing a substitute decision maker and (2) communicating to the substitute decision maker their wishes for future health care, personal care, and living arrangements. Substitute decision makers are required to make decisions based on the person's wishes or, if the person's wishes were not communicated, in the person's best interests. ACP is sometimes referred to as creating a living will or an advance directive; the term "living will" is not a legal term in Canada. The terms used for advance directives and the legal requirements vary across provinces and territories. In some provinces, verbal communication of wishes for future care is sufficient, whereas other provinces require written directives. In all provinces, designating a substitute decision maker requires a written, dated, and signed document. If the person who becomes incapable has not designated a substitute decision maker, a hierarchy of substitute decision makers is mandated by provincial health care consent acts.

For information about advance care planning laws in the provinces and territories, see http://www.virtualhospice.ca/en_US/Main+Site+Navigation/Home/Topics/Topics/Decisions/Advance+Care+Planning+Across+Canada.aspx.

The nurse cannot provide legal information but often serves as a resource person ready to answer many of the questions that people have about end-of-life decision making. The nurse may be called not only to inquire about the presence of an existing advance directive but also to ensure that the directive still reflects the person's wishes and to advocate for those wishes to be followed. The nurse also is responsible for ensuring that existing or newly created advance directives are appropriately located in the health record. Principles of conducting ACP discussions can be found in Box 27.5.

Nurses are often the person others turn to for information on ACP. Yet, a national LTC home study by Heckman and colleagues (2021) indicated that residents, families, administrators, health care providers, and ethicists encountered many challenges navigating differing provincial frameworks for ACP and consent. Consequently, these differences affected planning and care decisions for residents at the end of life. Shared challenges included lacking clarity on the identity of the shared decision maker, lacking clarity on the role of the substitute decision maker, failure to share sufficient

---

BOX 27.5
GENERAL PRINCIPLES OF CONDUCTING ADVANCE CARE PLANNING DISCUSSIONS

1. Ensure that all medical care is based on resident's values, goals, and wishes regarding their care, combined with an understanding of what is realistically achievable for their specific medical situation.
2. Advance care planning (ACP) discussions are best arranged and organized in advance.
3. Before conducting ACP discussions, the nursing home team should meet to ensure that they have a clear and shared understanding of the resident's clinical situation, and of the likely potential trajectories and outcomes that are expected of the resident.
4. The ACP discussion should ideally be inclusive and involve everyone the resident would want to attend, or who has insight into the resident's end-of-life wishes (not just a main shared decision maker).
5. Discussions should be held in a private, quiet, and comfortable location.
6. The shared decision maker(s) should preferably be present in person, though telephone or videoconferencing presence is acceptable.
7. Unless the resident is completely unable to participate, primarily speak with the resident, not the shared decision maker.
8. Use simple language, avoiding jargon or medical abbreviations.
9. If residents or their shared decision maker do not have an adequate understanding of English, have a translator present. This person should be a certified medical translator.
10. Be sensitive to the possible presence of underlying family conflict that may cause the resident to feel coerced into expressing specific care wishes. Carefully observe the resident and family / shared decision maker interactions, watching for language, signs, or body language that suggest that the voice of the resident is being stifled or coerced.

Sources: Adapted from Garland, A., & Heckman, G. (2020). *The BABEL ACP Workbook: Standardized approach to advance care planning in nursing homes*; Heckman, G. A., Boscart, V., Quail, P., et al. (2021). Applying the knowledge-to-action framework to engage stakeholders and solve shared challenges with person-centred advance care planning in long-term care homes. *Canadian Journal on Aging*, 1–11. doi: 10.1017/S0714980820000410.

information to inform care goals formulated by the resident, and failing to communicate decisions during a health crisis. The authors developed several training and knowledge products to foster better conversation and information exchange. All study participants mentioned the importance of ongoing ACP conversations and essential discussions (1) when there is a change in the resident's condition, function or cognition; (2) when there is a deterioration or exacerbation of existing chronic conditions; (3) when the resident requests a discussion; and (4) at regular reviews/intervals for stable residents (Heckman et al., 2021).

Medical Assistance in Dying (MAID)

The recognition of a person's right to refuse life-sustaining medical measures has brought up age-old questions concerning a person's right to make decisions about the continuation of life. Some people, especially those who are suffering unremitting pain from a terminal illness, end their lives. Others ask for assistance in ending life in the most painless way possible.

Medical assistance in dying is legal in Canada, in several other countries, and in several US states. In June 2016, the Government of Canada passed Bill C-14, legalizing medically assisted dying. In Canada, medical assistance in dying occurs when either "a nurse practitioner (NP) or physician provides assistance by administering a medication to a person, at their request, that causes their death (i.e., clinician-assisted medical assistance in dying); or, an NP or physician prescribes or provides a medication to a person, at their request, so that they may self-administer the medication and in doing so cause their own death (i.e., client self-administered medical assistance in dying)" (College of Nurses of Ontario, 2016, p. 2).

The law sets out eligibility criteria and safeguards that must be adhered to. To be eligible for medical assistance in dying, the person must be at least 18 years old; have a grievous and irremediable medical condition; be capable of making their own health-related decisions; request assistance voluntarily; and provide informed consent, having been informed of other options. Medical assistance in dying cannot be requested by a substitute decision maker. The law defines what "grievous and irremediable medical condition" means. Safeguards include requirements for the following: a written request (with limitations on who can witness the request), a second opinion, a waiting period before the request is fulfilled, communication that prescribing physicians and nurse practitioners must have with pharmacists, and format for the completion of a death certificate. In 2021, the Government of Canada modified the eligibility criteria and procedural safeguards in the law governing medical assistance in dying. For example, the law no longer requires a person's natural death to be reasonably foreseeable. More information can be found at https://www.canada.ca/en/health-canada/services/medical-assistance-dying.html.

The nurse's role in medical assistance in dying is to provide nursing care. Nurses are not legally permitted to administer medication in medical assistance in dying; only the person themselves, a nurse practitioner, or a physician may do this. Nurses should refer to their provincial or territorial regulatory body for guidance regarding nurses' roles in medically assisted dying.

Provincial and territorial governments provide information to the public about medical assistance in dying. Information for professional health care providers is available from the provincial and territorial regulatory bodies for nurses, physicians, and pharmacists. (See http://eol.law.dal.ca/?page_id=236 for links to these resources and the law.)

Strong opinions exist about medically assisted dying and about implementing advance directives. Misunderstanding may exist among nurses regarding terminology and the interpretation of the effects the nurse's role may have. Some nurses believe that turning off the ventilator, closing off tube feedings, stopping intravenous fluids, or giving as much pain medication as is needed where death is the outcome—even if directed by the individual themselves—constitute assisted suicide. Another perspective is that withdrawing such devices or treatments allows a natural death to occur, which is very different from actively doing something to cause death. Nurses, individually and collectively, must consider the implication of this issue for themselves and for the profession.

KEY CONCEPTS

- Grief is an emotional and behavioural response to loss. Grief responses are individual; what is appropriate for a person from one ethnocultural group may be considered inappropriate by another person from the same group or from another ethnocultural group.

- Grief is never completely resolved. Instead, the grieving person incorporates the loss into their life.
- Dying is a multifaceted, active process. It affects all involved—the person who is dying; the dying person's care partners, family, friends, and community members; and the professional health care providers.
- The stages or phases of dying and the types of coping are not universal and do not prescribe the way in which a person should die.
- The older dying person has the same needs for good and natural relationships with people as all people have.

- Hospice palliative care is both a concept and a health care approach that focuses on care rather than cure and on the provision of comfort for the dying person and their significant others.
- Advance directives allow a person control over life-and-death decisions through written communication and the appointment of someone (i.e., a proxy) to be the person's advocate when the person is unable to personally communicate their desires.
- The nurse's role in medically assisted dying is to provide care and support for the dying person and their family, care partners, and loved ones.

ACTIVITIES AND DISCUSSION QUESTIONS

1. Explore your response to being given a terminal diagnosis. What coping mechanisms would work for you? With which awareness approach would you be comfortable?

2. Describe how you would work with a dying person and their family when they are very protective of one another.

3. Describe how you would bring up the topic of advance directives.

4. Identify the advance directives that are legally recognized by your province or territory.

5. Describe how you would introduce the topic of dying with a person who is chronically but not terminally ill.

6. Describe how you would provide comprehensive, culturally safe, and sensitive holistic hospice palliative care.

RESOURCES

Association for Death Education and Counselling
https://www.adec.org
Canadian Hospice Palliative Care Association (CHPCA)
http://www.chpca.net
Canadian Hospice Palliative Care Nurses Group
http://www.chpca.net/join-us/nurses.aspx
Canadian Nurses Association. *Code of ethics for registered nurses (2017).*
https://www.cna-aiic.ca/en/on-the-issues/best-nursing/nursing-ethics
Canadian Nurses Association. *Medical assistance in dying.*
https://www.cna-aiic.ca/en/policy-advocacy/palliative-and-end-of-life-care/medical-assistance-in-dying
Canadian Nurses Association. *Palliative and end-of-life care.*
https://www.cna-aiic.ca/en/on-the-issues/better-health/palliative-and-end-of-life-care
Health Canada. *Palliative and end-of-life care resources.*
https://www.canada.ca/en/health-canada/services/health-care-system/palliative-end-life-care/resources.html

Health Law Institute, Dalhousie University. *End-of-life law and policy in Canada.*
http://eol.law.dal.ca/
End of Life Nursing Education Consortium
https://www.aacnnursing.org/ELNEC
Hospice & Palliative Nurses Association
https://advancingexpertcare.org

For additional resources, please visit *http://evolve.elsevier.com/Canada/Ebersole/gerontological/*

REFERENCES

Advance Care Planning Canada. (2021). *Advance care planning in Canada.* https://www.advancecareplanning.ca/?_ga=2.3032240.1660213251.1616005128-175381751.1616005128.

Andriessen, K., Krysinska, K., & Dransart, D. A. C. (2020). Grief after suicide: A health perspective on needs, effective help, and personal growth. *Frontiers in Psychology, 11,* 614405. doi:10.3389/fpsyg.2020.614405.

Blandin, K. (2016). *Dementia grief—Part 1: The unique characteristics.* https://www.dementia.org/dementia-grief-characteristics.

Canadian Nurses Association. (2017). *Code of ethics for registered nurses.* Author. https://hl-prod-ca-oc-download.s3-ca-central-1.amazonaws.com/CNA/2f975e7e-4a40-45ca-863c-5ebf0a138d5e/UploadedImages/documents/Code_of_Ethics_2017_Edition_Secure_Interactive.pdf.

Coelho, A., de Brito, M., & Barbosa, A. (2018). Caregiver anticipatory grief: Phenomenology, assessment and clinical interventions. *Current Opinion in Supportive and Palliative Care, 12*(1), 52–57. doi:10.1097/SPC.0000000000000321.

College of Nurses of Ontario. (2016). *Guidance on nurses' roles in medical assistance in dying.* Author. http://www.cno.org/en/trending-topics/medical-assistance-in-dying/.

Doka, K. J. (2016). *Grief is a journey. Finding your path through loss.* Simon & Schuster.

Fane, B. (2016). *Grief triggers: What are they and what causes them?* https://barbarafane.com/grief-triggers-causes/.

Fowler, K. (2018, January 29). *Coping with the loss of a grandchild.* https://www.aplaceformom.com/caregiver-resources/articles/coping-with-the-loss-of-a-grandchild.

Giacquinta, B. (1977). Helping families face the crisis of cancer. *American Journal of Nursing, 77*(10), 1585–1588.

Glaser, B. G., & Strauss, A. L. (1963). *Awareness of dying.* Aldine.

Government of Canada. (2019). *Action plan on palliative care.* https://www.canada.ca/en/health-canada/services/health-care-system/reports-publications/palliative-care/action-plan-palliative-care.html.

Heckman, G. A., Boscart, V., Quail, P., et al. (2021). Applying the knowledge-to-action framework to engage stakeholders and solve shared challenges with person-centred advance care planning in long-term care homes. *Canadian Journal on Aging,* 1–11. doi:10.1017/S0714980820000410.

Hill, A. D., Stukel, T. A., Fu, L., et al. (2019). Trends in site of death and health care utilization at the end of life: A population-based cohort study. *CMAJ Open, 7*(2), E306–E315. doi:10.9778/cmajo.20180097.

Ingebretsen, L. P., & Sagbakken, M. (2016). Hospice nurses' emotional challenges in their encounters with the dying. *International Journal of Qualitative Studies in Health and Well-being, 11,* 31170. doi:10.3402/qhw.v11.31170.

Jett, K. F. (2004). *The Loss Response Model* [Unpublished manuscript].

Kübler-Ross, E. (1969). *On death and dying.* Macmillan.

Kübler-Ross, E., & Kessler, D. (2005). *On grief and grieving: Finding the meaning of grief through the five stages of loss.* Scribner.

Lekalakala-Mokgele, E. (2018). Death and dying: Elderly persons' experiences of grief over the loss of family members. *South African Family Practice, 60*(5), 151–154. doi:10.1080/20786190.2018.1475882.

Mughal, S., Azhar, Y., & Siddiqui, W. J. (2020). *Grief reaction.* StatsPearls. https://www.ncbi.nlm.nih.gov/books/NBK507832/.

Nakajima, S. (2018). Complicated grief: Recent developments in diagnostic criteria and treatment. *Philosophical Transactions of the Royal Society of London. Series B, Biological Sciences, 373*(1754), 20170273. doi:10.1098/rstb.2017.0273.

Neimeyer, R. A., & Holland, J. M. (2015). Bereavement in later life: Theory, assessment, and intervention. In P. A. Lichtenberg, B. T. Mast, B. D. Carpenter, et al. (Eds.), *APA handbook of clinical geropsychology, Vol. 2: Assessment, treatment, and issues in later life* (pp. 645–666). American Psychological Association. doi:10.1037/14459-025.

Oates, J. R., & Maani-Fogelman, P. A. (2020). *Nursing grief and loss.* StatPearls. https://www.ncbi.nlm.nih.gov/books/NBK518989/.

O'Leary, J. M., Parker, L., & Wimmer, L. J. (2017). Bereaved grandparents—We didn't know our part. *HSOA Journal of Community Medicine & Public Health Care, 4,* 029. doi:10.24966/CMPH-1978-100029.

Patlamazoglou, L., Simmonds, J. G., & Snell, T. L. (2018). Same-sex partner bereavement: Non-HIV-related loss and new research directions. *Omega, 78*(2), 178–196. doi:10.1177/0030222817690160.

Pattison, E. M. (1977). *The experience of dying.* Prentice-Hall.

Pugh, A., Castleden, H., Giesbrecht, M., et al. (2019). Awareness as a dimension of health care access: Exploring the case of rural palliative care provision in Canada. *Journal of Health Services Research & Policy, 24*(2), 108–115. doi:10.1177/1355819619829782.

Richter, J. M. (1987). Support: A resource during crisis of mate loss. *Journal of Gerontological Nursing, 13*(11), 18–22. doi:10.3928/0098-9134-19871101-06.

Spiwak, R., Sareen, J., & Bolton, J. (2012). Complicated grief in Aboriginal populations. *Dialogues in Clinical Neuroscience, 14*(2), 204–209. doi:10.31887/DCNS.2012.14.2/rspiwak.

Statistics Canada. (2021). *Table 13-10-*0715-01: Deaths, by place of death (hospital or non-hospital). doi:10.25318/1310071501-eng.

Thompson, N., Allan, J., Carverhill, P. A., et al. (2016). The case for a sociology of dying, death, and bereavement. *Death Studies, 40*(3), 172–181. doi:10.1080/07481187.2015.1109377.

Victoria Hospice. (2021). *Clinical tools for professionals.* https://victoriahospice.org/how-we-can-help/clinical-tools/.

Virtual Hospice. (2021). *About us.* https://www.virtualhospice.ca/en_US/Main+Site+Navigation/Home+Navigation/About+Us.aspx.

Weisman, A. (1984). *The coping capacity: On the nature of being mortal.* Human Sciences Press.

Whitley, M. (2020). *Anticipatory grief: Learning the signs and how to cope.* https://www.aplaceformom.com/caregiver-resources/articles/anticipatory-grief.

Williams, A. M., Donovan, R., Stajduhar, K., et al. (2015). Cultural influences on palliative family caregiving: Service recommendations specific to the Vietnamese in Canada. *BMC Research Notes, 25*(8), 280. doi:10.1186/s13104-015-1252-3.

Worden, J. W. (2008). *Grief counseling and grief therapy: A handbook for mental health practitioners* (4th ed.). Springer.

World Health Organization. (2020, August 5). *Palliative care.* https://www.who.int/news-room/fact-sheets/detail/palliative-care.

Zisook, S., Iglewicz, A., Avanzino, J., et al. (2014). Bereavement: Course, consequences, and care. *Current Psychiatry Reports, 16*(10), 482. doi:10.1007/s11920-014-0482-8.

CARE ACROSS THE CONTINUUM

LEARNING OBJECTIVES

Upon completion of this chapter, the reader will be able to:

- Compare the major features, advantages, and disadvantages of several living options available to the older adult.
- Assist an older adult or their family or care partners in making an informed choice when planning a move.
- Describe factors influencing the provision of long-term care.
- Discuss the characteristics of long-term care homes and the impact of the culture change movement.
- Name several strategies to ease the transition between care settings for the older adult.

GLOSSARY

Aging in place Continuing to live in one's home; not having to move to another location to receive services as care needs change.

THE LIVED EXPERIENCE

"This is my home. We are all like a family, and I will die here. The girls that help me during the day, we treat one another like family members. We have some days when we are grumpy, some days we are happy, and we don't hold our feelings back, like you would do with your own family at home."

An 85-year-old resident living in a long-term care home

A mobile, youth-oriented society may find it difficult to fully comprehend the sadness and insecurity older adults feel when moving from one residence to another. In addition to the stress of relocation and the initial anxiety of adapting to a new setting, older adults often move to a more restrictive environment at a time of crisis. This chapter discusses care across the continuum and related implications for nursing practice. The major challenge older adults and their families or care partners may encounter at a time of transition are the choice and control an older adult has over relocation, assistance to the older adult with making personally appropriate choices, strategies to ease the transition to a different care setting, and the creation of environments that enhance care outcomes in whatever situation the older adult encounters.

AGE-FRIENDLY COMMUNITIES

"Home" is defined as basic shelter, a place to establish security, and the place where a person "belongs." However, a home means more to people than just basic shelter and security. Habitat for Humanity (2021) asked Habitat homeowners, volunteers, and staff what a home meant to them. One person responded by saying the following:

"Home is a safe haven and a comfort zone. A place to live with our families and pets and enjoy

with friends. A place to build memories as well as a way to build future wealth. A place where we can truly just be ourselves. And whether our houses are big, small, fancy or modest, they are our shelters and our sanctuaries." (Linda; Habitat for Humanity, 2021)

A home should provide the highest possible level of independence, function, and comfort for the older adult. Most older adults prefer to remain in their own homes, "**aging in place**," rather than relocating, particularly to a nursing home setting. Being able to age in place depends on appropriate support for changing care needs, so that the older adult can stay wherever they want. Developing age-friendly communities and creating more opportunities to age in place enhances the health and well-being of older adults.

In a project organized through the World Health Organization (WHO), 33 cities, including 4 Canadian cities, implemented and evaluated age-friendly principles. The response to this project was overwhelming, so the WHO created a global network of age-friendly communities (World Health Organization, 2021). In Canada, the Age-Friendly Communities Initiative—which is based on the principles of the WHO program—is led by the Public Health Agency of Canada in collaboration with other federal, provincial, territorial, and nongovernmental partners. Several provinces have age-friendly programs, and many municipalities both formally and informally adopted age-friendly initiatives by assessing their communities and designing community-level interventions to enhance the potential for older adults to remain in their homes and familiar environments. The eight domains of age-friendly communities are depicted in Box 28.1. Age friendliness is determined not only by the physical environment but also by the social environment and by the health and social services available. A checklist of essential features for each element is provided by the WHO (see the Resources section at the end of this chapter). Box 28.2 describes a study that was conducted as part of the Age-Friendly Cities project in Québec.

BOX 28.1

EIGHT KEY DOMAINS OF AGE-FRIENDLY COMMUNITIES

1. Outdoor spaces and buildings
2. Transportation
3. Housing
4. Social participation
5. Respect and social inclusion
6. Civic participation and employment
7. Communication and information
8. Community support and health services

Sources: Government of Canada. (2016). *Age-friendly communities.* https://www.canada.ca/en/public-health/services/health-promotion/aging-seniors/friendly-communities.html; World Health Organization. (n.d.). *The WHO age-friendly cities framework.* https://extranet.who.int/agefriendlyworld/age-friendly-cities-framework/.

HOUSING OPTIONS IN LATER LIFE

Some older adults, by choice or by need, move from one type of residence to another. A number of housing options exist, especially for people with sufficient financial resources. Options range from remaining in one's own home; to senior retirement communities; to shared housing with family members, friends, or others; to care communities such as assisted-living settings; and (for those with the most needs) to long-term care (LTC) or nursing homes (Fig. 28.1). There are many different models of housing, and older adults and families may seek assistance from gerontological nurses when choosing what kind of living situation will be best for them. The terms used to describe the different models vary between jurisdictions across the country; the legislation and regulations vary as well. Information about housing options and care homes in Canada is available on the Government of Canada website (https://www.canada.ca/en/financial-consumer-agency/services/retirement-planning/cost-seniors-housing.html).

INDEPENDENT LIVING OPTIONS

With the aging of the "baby boomers," architects and engineers are focusing on home designs that adjust to

---

BOX 28.2
RESEARCH FOR EVIDENCE-INFORMED PRACTICE: OLDER ADULTS' HOUSING NEEDS AND THE MEANING OF HOME IN OLDER LIFE

Problem: Most older Canadians want to age in their own homes. Alternative housing options are available, including seniors' communities. Some research indicates that available alternatives do not always meet older adults' needs. The aim of this study was to examine the meaning of home and older adults' housing needs from their perspective.

Methods: A multimethod study was conducted in Québec. One part of the study was composed of 49 focus groups, including older adults, caregivers, and service and health care providers. The second part was a case study about nonprofit community-based housing for older adults that was conducted using 11 in-depth interviews. Thematic analysis was completed.

Findings: One of the main study themes was the social aspect of the meaning of home. Participants wanted to have access to services and amenities—access to public transportation and being able to walk to services such as grocery stores, banks, and clinics. However, zoning regulations and the manner in which communities are now built mean that this access is unlikely. Concentrating housing and services for older adults in one area was seen as problematic. Participants were reluctant to live in seniors' neighborhoods, describing these areas as "ghettoized." They wanted to live in neighborhoods with people of all ages. Pedestrian safety and being able to walk to green spaces were important.

Implications for Nursing Practice: Collaboration between health care providers, provincial and municipal governments, and nongovernmental organizations is necessary for achieving age-friendly communities that meet older adults' needs. Concentrating services and housing for older adults may seem efficient, but doing so could isolate those older adults.

Source: Bigonnesse, C., Beaulieu, M., & Garon, S. (2014). Meaning of home in later life as a concept to understand older persons' housing needs: Results from the 7 Age-Friendly Cities pilot project in Québec. *Journal of Housing for the Elderly, 28,* 357–382. doi: 10.1080/02763893.2014.930367.

Independence

- Home ownership
- Single-room occupation (SRO)
- Condominium ownership
- Apartment dwelling
- Shared housing/co-housing
- Adult lifestyle communities
- Life lease

Independence to partial dependence

- Public/subsidized housing
- Residence with family
- Supportive housing/living
- Assisted living
- Residential facility
- Retirement homes/ residences/communities

Partial dependence to complete dependence

- Extended care
- Hospice care
- Complex continuing care
- Residential respite care
- Long-term care homes (special care homes, personal care homes, nursing homes)
- Acute care facilities
- Rehabilitation facilities

Independence ◄──────────────────────────────────► Dependence

Fig. 28.1 ■ Continuum of residential options based on the level of assistance needed. *Source:* Adapted from Ebersole, P., Touhy, T., Hess, P. et al. (2008). *Ebersole and Hess' Toward healthy aging: Human needs and nursing response* (7th ed., p. 438, Fig. 17-1). Mosby.

the changes that accompany aging, thereby enabling older adults to stay in their homes safely even if they experience age-related changes. These new designs are marketed as "transgenerational" or "universal" designs and can benefit everyone, not just older adults. Designs and modifications may include safety fittings in the bathroom, walk-in showers, wider doorways, remote-controlled devices for lights and window coverings, raised countertops, polyurethane or cork flooring, and adjustable-height sinks, among other features. Available online, *Safe Living Guide—A Guide to Home Safety for Seniors* (Public Health Agency of Canada, 2015) includes strategies for home adaptations that improve safety and accessibility. Additional information, including information about financial assistance programs, is available from the Canada Mortgage and Housing Corporation (CMHC) website at https://www.cmhc-schl.gc.ca/en/co/acho/index.cfm.

Social Housing

Social housing, also referred to as subsidized housing or public housing, includes municipally owned and operated housing; nonprofit and for-profit properties; provincial cooperative housing; and privately owned housing, all of which receive government rent supplements for low-income tenants. The subsidies ensure that the tenant does not spend more than 30% of income on rent (Government of Alberta, 2021). Social housing is an important option for older adults, because poverty is an issue for 12.5% of older Canadians (Healthcare of Ontario Pension Plan, 2017). The rates of poverty are higher among women, people who live alone, immigrants, and Indigenous peoples (see Chapter 24).

Since 1996, social housing programs and their administration have been the sole responsibility of the provinces and territories. Some programs reserve social housing units for older adults. Unfortunately, the waiting lists for social housing are long. Statistics Canada (2019) reported results from the 2018 Canadian Housing Survey showing that over 280,000 Canadian households had at least one member on a waiting list for social and affordable housing. Two-thirds of these households were on a waiting list for 2 years or longer (Statistics Canada, 2019).

Life Lease

Life lease is an arrangement in which a resident neither owns nor rents a home but has a lifelong lease for one. The lease requires a single upfront payment and monthly fees for the management and upkeep of the property. The lease contract gives residents the right to occupy their units and use common areas and facilities until they die or move. Some life lease projects are co-located with assisted-living facilities or LTC homes, and leaseholders can access care services through these facilities for a fee. Life lease buyers are often older adults who are looking to move into a smaller home (Government of Ontario, 2019).

Life lease projects are run by for-profit or nonprofit organizations. The exact number of life lease projects in Canada is not known, because there is no requirement for registration. Manitoba is the only province with legislation specific to life lease housing. Advocates for older adults are lobbying for legislation to ensure that residents' rights are protected. Issues for legislation include protecting civil and human rights; regulating the provided care services; prohibiting illegal promises of automatic admission to LTC homes; and addressing a number of consumer protection issues.

Adult Lifestyle Communities

Adult lifestyle communities or neighbourhoods are also known as retirement communities, resort communities, and 55-plus communities. Housing is typically in the form of condominiums—as high rises, townhouses, or detached homes. The communities are designed for newly retired persons and often include recreation facilities (e.g., golf courses, trails, swimming pools, fitness centres, and clubs). Most of these communities are "gated," may have security, and have age restrictions that limit ownership and residency to persons of a certain age (such as 50, 55, or 60 years of age).

Shared Housing

Shared housing among adult children and their older relatives is a preferred choice for many because of cultural preferences or need. The sharing may relieve the economic burdens of maintaining a home after widowhood or retirement on a fixed income. Cultural influences predict the frequency of multigenerational residences. Among Asians and South Asians, shared housing is often an expectation. Relocating from one's own home to the home of an adult child can have many benefits; without adequate preparation, however, it can also be stressful for both the family and the older adult. Interventions to support healthy relocation and transition are discussed later in the chapter. Box 28.3 presents some factors to consider when a family is planning to add an older adult to the household.

A variation of multigenerational housing is the "granny flat." Granny flats can be apartments added to existing homes or small housing units on family property that provide privacy and the sharing of time and resources. Such arrangements allow an older adult to live separately from the family but close enough to the family to obtain assistance if needed.

Cohabitation or Cohousing

Another model of shared housing is that of opening homes to others, or *cohabitation*. Older adults often live in houses that they purchased in their younger years and that have ample space geared to family life, but about one-half of the space is underused. The cohousing model is more formalized in the United States and Europe, where there are services to match older adults who are looking for houses to share. People who

---

BOX 28.3
PLANNING TO ADD AN OLDER ADULT TO THE HOUSEHOLD

QUESTIONS TO ASK

- What are the needs of the new household member and of the family?
- Where will space be allotted for the new member?
- How will the new member be included in existing family patterns?
- How will responsibilities be shared?
- What resources in the community will assist the older adult in the adjustment phase?
- Is the environment safe for this new member?
- How will family life change with the older relative in the household, and how do family members feel about it?
- What are the differences in socialization and sleeping patterns between the older adult and other family members?
- What are the older adult's strong needs and expectations?
- What are the older adult's skills and talents?

NECESSARY MODIFICATIONS

- Semiprivate living quarters for the older relative if possible.
- Regularly scheduled visits to other relatives to give each family member time for respite and privacy.
- Adult day health programs and activities arranged for the older adult to help them keep contact with members of their own generation. Consider how the older adult will feel about giving up familiar surroundings and friends.

POTENTIAL AREAS OF CONFLICT

- Space (especially if someone has given up their space to the older relative).
- Possessions. Some older adults may want to move their possessions into the house; others may not find them attractive or may insist on replacing them with new things.

- Entertainment and times when older adults and young persons feel the need or desire to exclude the others from social events.
- Responsibilities and chores. Older adults may feel useless if they do nothing, and they may feel that they are in the way if they do anything. Younger family members may feel that their position is being usurped or may be angry if they are expected to wait on the older adult.
- Expenses. The increased costs of home maintenance, food, clothing, and recreation may not be shared appropriately.
- Vacations (whether to go together or alone). Younger family members may feel uneasy about not taking the older adult out and may be resentful if they must.
- Child rearing (disagreement over child-rearing policies).
- Child care. Grandparental babysitting may be welcomed by the family but resented by the older person. If it is not allowed, however, the older person may feel a lack of trust in their capability.

DECREASE AREAS OF CONFLICT BY DOING THE FOLLOWING:

- Respecting the older person's privacy.
- Discussing space allocations.
- Discussing the older person's furnishings before the move.
- Making it clear in advance when social events include everyone or exclude someone.
- Clearing decisions about household tasks (with everyone's responsibility geared to their ability).
- Having the older person pay a share of expenses and maintain a separate phone (reduces strain and increases the person's feelings of independence).

share homes report feeling safer and less lonely. Studies on home sharing focus on its effects on well-being, finances, health, social life, and daily satisfaction. Most successful is the intergenerational model, in which an older adult shares their home with a much younger person.

Cohousing is a model in which older adults own or rent individual homes that are clustered around a "common house" where residents share a kitchen, dining room, playroom, laundry room and workshop area. Each home is self-sufficient, but residents often share meals in the common area. Cohousing in Canada includes multigenerational communities as well as older adults' communities. This model is a growing option in North America (Canadian Cohousing Network, 2021).

COMMUNITY SERVICES FOR AGING IN PLACE

Adult Day Services

Adult day services are community-based group programs designed to provide social and health services to older adults who need supervised care in a safe setting during the day. These programs also offer caregivers respite from the responsibilities of caregiving. Most adult day centres operate during normal business hours 5 days a week, but some offer services in the evening, overnight, and on weekends. The three types of adult day centres are social (meals, recreation, some health-related services), medical–health (social activities and more intensive health and therapeutic services), and specialized (assistance for older adults with dementia or developmental disabilities). Adult day services are provided by publicly funded and volunteer organizations, and some communities offer ethnoculturally specific programs. Fees vary, and subsidies are available in many programs. Adult day services can make it possible for older adults to remain in the community and postpone moving to LTC homes (Jarrott & Ogletree, 2019). Use of adult day services is associated with reduced use of hospital services (Kelly, 2017). Access may be limited in rural and remote areas (Morgan et al., 2015).

Home and Community Care

Home care helps older adults live in the community by providing health services at home rather than in a hospital or an LTC home. In 2015–2016, close to 1 million

> **BOX 28.4**
> **GOALS OF HOME CARE**
>
> - Help people maintain or improve their health status and quality of life
> - Assist people in remaining as independent as possible
> - Support families and care partners in coping with a family member's need for care
> - Help people stay at or return home and receive needed treatment and care, rehabilitation, or palliative care
> - Provide caregivers with the support they need
>
> *Source:* Health Canada. (2016). *Home and community health care* (Goals, para. 3). https://www.canada.ca/en/health-canada/services/home-continuing-care/home-community-care.html.

Canadians received home care services (Gilmour, 2018). Older adults, women, and those living alone, as well as those in poorer health, are most likely to receive home care (Gilmour, 2018). Home care is delivered by nurses and other regulated health care providers, non-regulated workers, volunteers, friends, care partners and family members. The goals of home care are listed in Box 28.4.

Home care provides nursing, personal care, physiotherapy, occupational therapy, speech therapy, social work, dietitian services, homemaking, respite, Meals on Wheels, friendly visiting, medical supplies and equipment, and case management. Services can be delivered via information and communication technologies (e.g., telehomecare).

Home care is often seen as a desirable way for an older adult to receive health care while aging at home and as a way to decrease government expenditures on institutional-based health care (Box 28.5). Home care meets the following three needs: short-term acute care, long-term supportive care, and specialized services such as rehabilitation and palliative care. Some people receive short-term acute home care services as a substitute for (or a complement to) acute hospital-based care. These persons receive a higher proportion of professional services. Other home care recipients, most of whom are older, receive long-term home care that helps them to maintain their functioning and avoid admission to acute or LTC care. These seniors are more likely to receive supportive services from nonprofessional staff.

BOX 28.5

RESEARCH FOR EVIDENCE-INFORMED PRACTICE: NO PLACE LIKE HOME: A SYSTEMATIC REVIEW OF HOME CARE FOR OLDER ADULTS IN CANADA

Problem: Little is known about home care for older adults in Canada. Specifically, there is limited research on the characteristics of home care recipients, gaps in services, and interventions designed to support client needs.

Methods: Researchers conducted a systematic review to examine home care users, challenges and gaps in home care, and interventions that are used to support home care services for older adults.

Findings: Researchers identified four main themes from the literature: (1) older adult client-level predictors; (2) unmet home care needs; (3) interventions; and (4) home care issues and challenges experiences by home care staff and clients. No studies focused on home care needs of older Indigenous adults or among immigrant or refugee older adults. Many older adults who received home care experienced a cognitive impairment, mobility issues, and other chronic conditions. Those who lived in urban areas, those who were older, and women were more likely to use services. Many older adults who received home care services suffered from depression and mental illness. Home care was shown to reduce costs related to hospitalizations. Lastly, there is a need for more education and training among home care staff regarding topics such as falls prevention, physical activity, and nutrition.

Implications for Nursing Practice: This research reinforces the importance of home care services, the types of clients receiving care and services, and the need for more research.

Source: Johnson, S., Bacsu, J., Abeykoon, H., et al. (2018). No place like home: A systematic review of home care for older adults in Canada. *Canadian Journal on Aging, 37*(4), 400–419. doi: 10.1017/S0714980819000375.

Providing adequate access to home care services is a challenge across the country because of rising costs and limited funding; a shortage of health care and social care providers; and a lack of high-quality information for evaluation and quality improvement. These issues are compounded in rural, remote, and northern settings.

Under the *Canada Health Act*, home care is an extended service, not an insured service. Home care programs vary from province to province. In Ontario, it is estimated that 150,000 people receive an additional 20 million visits/hours of home care services annually (Home Care Ontario, 2014).

SUPPORTED LIVING OPTIONS

Supportive Housing

Supportive housing consists of apartment buildings designated for older adults; they provide on-site personal support services such as homemaking services and on-call staff. Social and recreation programs and dining services may be provided. These programs are often operated by charitable or nonprofit organizations. Supportive housing may be provided in conjunction with social housing for older adults. Depending on the provincial model, government funding for care services for frail older residents is available. Residents are tenants whose rights are determined by provincial tenancies acts.

Retirement Homes

Retirement homes are nonmedical community-based settings that provide housing to seniors and provide services such as meals, medication supervision or reminders, activities, transportation, and assistance with activities of daily living (ADLs). Most of these residences provide a rented single room or rooms (suite) and access to shared facilities. They are designed for older adults who do not need care in a LTC home but who need more support than is available in shared housing. This kind of residence is known by different names across the country, including assisted living, retirement homes, seniors' residences, personal care homes, and retirement residences.

Most retirement homes are operated by for-profit corporations, and some are operated by nonprofit or charitable organizations. They are not part of the health care system, and costs are not covered through provincial health insurance. Residents are tenants who pay separate fees for accommodation and care. Most retirement homes offer two or three meals per day, light weekly housekeeping, and laundry services, as well as optional social activities. Many homes have transportation services and Internet access. Some also have exercise facilities, movie theatres, pharmacies, and swimming pools. Rent varies, depending on the market. In addition, health care services can be purchased, which can significantly increase costs but also allows individuals with financial resources to remain in the setting longer as their functional abilities decline.

The governance, regulation, and funding of retirement homes vary across provinces and territories. British Columbia and Ontario have provincial regulations that apply specifically to retirement homes. The Canadian Accreditation Council (2018) publishes standards for the accreditation of retirement homes.

Many older adults and their families prefer retirement homes to LTC homes because retirement homes are more homelike and offer more opportunities for control, independence, and privacy. However, many tenants in retirement homes have chronic health care needs; with time, these residents may require more care than the home is able to provide. Services (e.g., home health, hospice, homemakers) can be brought into the retirement home, but there is some question as to whether such services are an adequate substitute for 24-hour supervision by a registered care team.

Nurses should be familiar with retirement home options in their communities and be knowledgeable about the rights of the tenants. Nurses should help the person living with dementia and their family or care partners to investigate the available services as well as staff training when making decisions as to the most appropriate housing and support for older adults living with dementia. (See Chapter 21 for further information about dementia.)

More research is needed on care outcomes of tenants in retirement homes and the role of both unregulated and regulated health care providers in these homes. However, the nonmedical nature of retirement homes is the primary factor in keeping costs down. Consumers are advised to inquire as to exactly what services will be provided and by whom if a resident becomes frail and needs more complex or frequent care. The Advocacy Centre for the Elderly provides a consumer guide to choosing a retirement home at http://www.advocacycentreelderly.org/ace_library.php.

HEALTH CARE SETTING–BASED LIVING OPTIONS

Long-Term Care Homes

LTC homes (also called nursing homes, care homes, and personal care homes) provide around-the-clock care for people who need specialized care that cannot be provided elsewhere. According to the Canadian Institute for Health Information (CIHI), there are 2,039 LTC homes in Canada (Canadian Institute for Health Information [CIHI], 2021a). Most LTC homes operate on a for-profit basis; 46% are publicly owned and 54% are privately owned (CIHI, 2021a).

LTC homes provide care for persons with various circumstances and health conditions—persons recently discharged from hospitals, frail persons, persons living with dementia, and older adults at the end of life. There are more than twice as many women as men residing in LTC homes. Just over half of LTC residents are aged 85 years or older (CIHI, 2021b). Inability to perform ADLs is one of the main reasons for moving to an LTC home, and most residents require significant assistance with ADLs and with the instrumental activities of daily living (IADLs). More than two-thirds of the residents are cognitively impaired. The prevalence of dementia is high. In Ontario, 90% of residents have some form of cognitive impairment, 86% need extensive assistance with ADLs, 80% have neurological diseases, 76% have heart and circulatory diseases, and 61% take 10 or more prescription medications (Ontario Long Term Care Association, 2019).

The development of new models of care provision are priorities in this setting (see Chapter 27).

Costs of Care

Like home care, LTC is an extended service, not an insured service. Canada offers nonprofit LTC and for-profit LTC homes, both operating under the same regulation. Provincial and territorial governments provide partial funding for LTC home services. In all provinces and all territories (except Nunavut), residents pay facilities fees to cover the costs of accommodations and lodging. On average, about 70% of costs are publicly funded, but this varies significantly across the country (Norris, 2020). The three payment models for facilities fees are (1) a per diem based on public pension incomes available to residents, (2) a per diem that is subsidized depending on the resident's income, or (3) a per diem that is subsidized depending on the resident's assets and income. In addition to the facilities fee, the resident pays medical and personal expenses (e.g., dentures, hearing aids, specialized wheelchairs, foot care, personal hygiene products, and over-the-counter medications). Insurance for LTC is available for purchase in Canada.

Regulations and Quality of Care

LTC homes are highly regulated environments, and the related laws, regulations, and standards vary across provinces and territories. Although LTC homes recognize the need to ensure quality, the lack of additional funding to meet new regulations and standards and the increasingly complex needs of LTC home residents can make achieving quality a struggle. Criteria and standards often create a bureaucratic structure and a punitive environment for health care staff employed in LTC homes. LTC homes are inspected regularly on an unannounced basis to determine compliance with regulations and to investigate quality-of-care indicators. In most jurisdictions, data on quality indicators and complaints are publicly available on provincial government websites.

Regulations have also been created to protect the rights of the residents living in LTC homes. Residents have rights under both federal and provincial laws. For example, Alberta's *Nursing Homes Act* can be found at https://www.qp.alberta.ca/documents/Acts/N07.pdf. The health care staff of the home must inform residents of these rights and must protect and promote those rights. The rights to which the residents are entitled should be conspicuously posted in the LTC home. Box 28.6 lists LTC residents' rights as set out in Ontario's *Long-Term Care Homes Act*.

BOX 28.6

BILL OF RIGHTS FOR LONG-TERM CARE RESIDENTS IN ONTARIO

1. Every resident has the right to be treated with courtesy and respect and in a way that fully recognizes the resident's individuality and respects the resident's dignity.
2. Every resident has the right to be protected from abuse.
3. Every resident has the right not to be neglected by the licensee or staff.
4. Every resident has the right to be properly sheltered, fed, clothed, groomed, and cared for in a manner consistent with his or her needs.
5. Every resident has the right to live in a safe and clean environment.
6. Every resident has the right to exercise the rights of a citizen.
7. Every resident has the right to be told who is responsible for and who is providing the resident's direct care.
8. Every resident has the right to be afforded privacy in treatment and in caring for his or her personal needs.
9. Every resident has the right to have his or her participation in decision making respected.
10. Every resident has the right to keep and display personal possessions, pictures, and furnishings in his or her room, subject to safety requirements and the rights of other residents.
11. Every resident has the right to do the following:
    i. Participate fully in the development, implementation, review, and revision of his or her plan of care
    ii. Give or refuse consent to any treatment, care, or services for which his or her consent is required by law and be informed of the consequences of giving or refusing consent
    iii. Participate fully in making any decision concerning any aspect of his or her care, including any decision concerning his or her admission, discharge, or transfer to or from a long-term care home or a secure unit, and obtain an independent opinion with regard to any of those matters
    iv. Have personal health information kept confidential and have access to his or her records of personal health information, including his or her plan of care
12. Every resident has the right to receive care and assistance toward independence based on a restorative care philosophy to maximize independence to the greatest extent possible.
13. Every resident has the right not to be restrained, except in the limited circumstances provided for under this Act and subject to the requirements provided for under this Act.
14. Every resident has the right to communicate in confidence, receive visitors of his or her choice, and consult in private with any person without interference.
15. Every resident who is dying or who is very ill has the right to have family and friends present 24 hours per day.
16. Every resident has the right to designate a person to receive information concerning any transfer or any hospitalization of the resident and to have that person receive that information immediately.
17. Every resident has the right to raise concerns or recommend changes in policies and services on

BOX 28.6
BILL OF RIGHTS FOR LONG-TERM CARE RESIDENTS IN ONTARIO—cont'd

behalf of himself or herself or others without interference and without fear of coercion, discrimination, or reprisal, whether directed at the resident or anyone else.

18. Every resident has the right to form friendships and relationships and to participate in the life of the long-term care home.
19. Every resident has the right to have his or her lifestyle and choices respected.
20. Every resident has the right to participate in the Residents' Council.
21. Every resident has the right to meet privately with his or her spouse or another person in a room that assures privacy.
22. Every resident has the right to share a room with another resident according to their mutual wishes, if appropriate accommodation is available.
23. Every resident has the right to pursue social, cultural, religious, spiritual, and other interests, to develop his or her potential and to be given

reasonable assistance by the licensee to pursue these interests and to develop his or her potential.

24. Every resident has the right to be informed in writing of any law, rule, or policy affecting services provided to the resident and of the procedures for initiating complaints.
25. Every resident has the right to manage his or her own financial affairs unless the resident lacks the legal capacity to do so.
26. Every resident has the right to be given access to protected outdoor areas in order to enjoy outdoor activity unless the physical setting makes this impossible.
27. Every resident has the right to have any friend, family member, or other person of importance to the resident attend any meeting with the licensee or the staff of the home.

Note: This list is an example from Ontario-legislated rights of residents of long-term homes. Nurses should check the laws in their province or territory for specific rights.

Source: *Long-Term Care Homes Act, 2007*, S.O. 2007, c. 8. http://www.e-laws.gov.on.ca/html/statutes/english/elaws_statutes_07l08_e.htm#BK5.

The Culture Change Movement in Long-Term Care Homes

Across North America, the movement to transform LTC homes from the typical medical model into homes that nurture quality of life for older adults and support and empower health care staff is changing the face of LTC. Encouraged by the Pioneer Network, a US national nonprofit organization that serves the culture change movement, many homes are changing from a rigid institutional approach to a person-centred approach (https://www.pioneernetwork.net). "Culture change" is the term given to the national movement for the transformation of older adult services. The movement is based on person-directed values and practices, where the voices of older adults and those working most closely with them are solicited, respected, and honoured. Core person-directed values are relationship, choice, dignity, respect, self-determination, and purposeful living (Pioneer Network, 2021).

Older adults in need of LTC want to live in a homelike setting that does not look and function like a hospital. They want a setting that allows them to make the

decisions that they are used to making for themselves, such as when to get up, take a bath, eat, or go to bed. They want health care staff who know them and understand their individuality and their preferences. Box 28.7 presents some of the differences between an institution-centred culture and a person-centred culture.

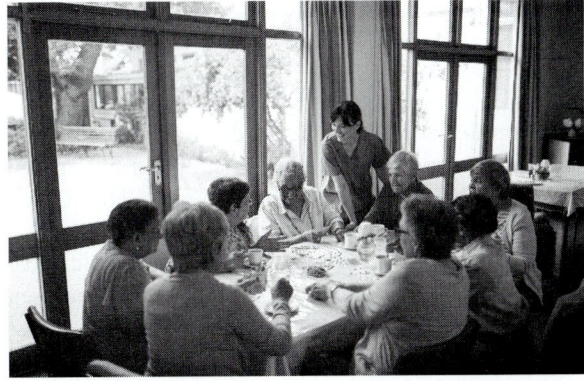

A person-centred approach to long-term care settings allows older adults to feel respected and valued. (**Source:** iStock.com/shapecharge).

Examples of philosophies and programs of culture change are the Eden Alternative, founded by Dr. Bill Thomas (http://www.edenalt.org), and The Green House Project (www.thegreenhouseproject.org).

The Eden Alternative is best known for the addition of animals, plants, and children to LTC homes. However, truly transforming an LTC home requires the involvement of all levels of staff, as well as changes in values, attitudes, structures, and management practices.

The Alzheimer Society of Canada (2014) developed PC P.E.A.R.L.S., an evidence-based guideline that outlines key elements to sustain culture change in order to provide person-centred care in LTC homes. Some of the principles of culture change activities are as follows:

- Person and family engagement: Ensure families and friends are involved, supported, and engaged in the life of the person living with dementia.
- Care: Focus care planning on each resident's abilities and include routine pain assessment and management in order for the person to enjoy an improved quality of life.
- Process: Embed person-centred care principles into the strategic and operational plan to sustain culture change.
- Environment: Promote a physical and social environment that supports the resident's abilities, strengths, and personal interests.
- Activity and recreation: Engage each resident in stimulating and meaningful activities, tailored to the person's interests, preferences, and abilities.
- Leadership: Embrace strong leaders who are champions of person-centred care and ingrain these principles in their organization's philosophy and values.
- Staffing: Support staff training, continuity of care, and the fostering of intimate and trusting relationships between families, residents, and staff.

The full guideline can be found at https://alzheimer.ca/en/help-support/im-healthcare-provider/providing-person-centred-care.

Making LTC Home Decisions

Gerontological nurses are frequently asked to help older adults and their families make decisions about choosing an LTC home. It is important for nurses to be aware that the vast majority of older adults want to remain at home and that the idea of moving into a nursing home is seen as the last resort when all other care options have been exhausted. The decision to move to an LTC home, therefore, is often difficult to make and surrounded by a sense of loss and grief. Elders in Indigenous communities prefer to not leave their community to receive care, given their traumatic historical experiences in health care facilities and mistrust of non-Indigenous health care providers (Life, 2018; Jacklin & Walker, 2019).

In situations where this decision does have to be made, older adults and their families aim to select a home with high standards and quality of care. A study by Wilkinson et al. (2019) looked at overall quality performance of LTC homes in Ontario. Authors reviewed the overall quality performance of LTC homes and identified whether organizational factors impacted quality performance. They found that nonprofit homes performed similarly to private homes on measures of quality performance. Larger LTC organizations scored higher on quality performance. Authors described how this difference could be the result of more resources and more innovative ways of operating (such as computerized medical records) (Wilkinson et al., 2019).

The most appropriate method of choosing an LTC home is to personally visit the home, meet with the director of nursing or resident care, observe care practices, and discuss the potential resident's needs.

IMPROVING TRANSITIONS ACROSS THE CONTINUUM OF CARE

Older adults have complex health care needs and often require care in multiple settings across the continuum of care. "Care transition" refers to the movement of care receivers from one health care practitioner or setting to another as their condition and care needs change. Transitional care requires a set of clinical and communication activities that should occur when older adults move from one care setting to another. An older adult may be treated by a family practitioner; hospitalized and treated by an intensivist or nurse practitioner; discharged to an LTC home and followed by another practitioner; or discharged home or to a retirement home, where the family practitioner may or may not continue to follow them. Many health care providers practise in only one setting and are not familiar with the specific requirements of other settings; language and health literacy issues and cultural differences exacerbate the problem:

Successful care transitions require multi-disciplinary communication and coordination, comprehensive planning, including patient/caregiver education and clinician involvement, and shared accountability during all points of transition. When gaps occur in care transitions, individuals are susceptible to fragmentation in care, poor quality of care, unfavourable experiences, compromised patient safety, and adverse medical events. (Canadian Institutes of Health Research, 2020).

Transitions between settings happen often. There is increasing evidence that older adults experience serious care deficiencies when undergoing transitions. Older adults who are at high risk for transitional care problems include persons with multiple medical conditions or mental disorders, isolated persons (without family or friends), non-English speakers, immigrants, and persons on low incomes.

A significant number of older adults who are admitted to an acute care hospital end up in another setting, typically an LTC home. Many people wait for a long time in an acute care hospital until there is space available for them in an LTC home or until home care becomes available so that they can go home. Some hospitals have converted some of their acute care beds to provide alternate level of care (ALC). Older adults with dementia account for about half of all ALC days, and those with dementia are three times more likely to have ALC days than those without dementia (CIHI, 2021c). Unnecessary functional decline is a common outcome for seniors who are receiving ALC in hospital (Rojas-García et al., 2018).

Integrated care was developed as an alternative to LTC homes for frail older adults who want to live in their communities independently and with a high quality of life. Integrated care programs are seen as a possible way to reduce unnecessary waiting in hospital. Examples of integrated care in Canada includes the Program of Research to Integrate the Services for the Maintenance of Autonomy in Quebec (MacAdam, 2015) and the Comprehensive Home Option of Integrated Care for the Elderly in Alberta (The Good Samaritan Society, 2021). These programs provide a comprehensive continuum of primary care, community and home-based care, social care, and specialty care, provided by a case manager and an interprofessional team.

Minimizing the number of care transitions is associated with more consistent nursing care and better quality of life for older adults (Boscart & Brown, 2018). In addition to taking on the roles of case managers and transition coaches, nurses play a role in many elements of successful transitional care, such as medication management, family caregiver education, comprehensive discharge planning, and adequate and timely communication among providers and sites of services.

Relocation

At times, relocation is necessary. Relocation is a stressor and sometimes a crisis, both for the older adult and for their family or care partners. Nurses in hospitals, the community, and LTC homes frequently care for older adults who have experienced several relocations. The first issue to address in any move is whether it is necessary and whether it will provide the least restrictive lifestyle appropriate for the individual. Assessing the impact of relocation and determining methods to mitigate any negative reactions are additional nursing actions.

Research indicates that relocation is associated with increased morbidity and mortality but that it does not necessarily result in serious effects on mental or physical health (Sullivan & Williams, 2017). The research calls into question the validity of a commonly accepted nursing diagnosis of *relocation stress syndrome*, a catastrophic reaction to relocation. Research indicates that individuals are better able to meet the challenges of relocation if they have a sense of control over the circumstances and have the confidence to carry out the needed activities associated with a move. Advance notice, preparation, choice, and self-efficacy (i.e., "the beliefs in one's capability to organize and execute the courses of action required to manage prospective situations" [Bandura, 1997, p. 2]) may be an important variable in a positive adjustment to a relocation. The Self-Efficacy Relocation Scale, developed by Rossen and Gruber (2007), can be used to assess the self-efficacy of individuals who are relocating, identify potential pre-relocation adjustment issues, and guide interventions to promote positive relocation outcomes.

To assist older adults with relocation decisions and adjustments, nurses should become aware of resources that are available to the older adult; assess the older adult's relocation needs; individualize a realistic relocation plan; promote coping while making a relocation decision; help the person prepare for the move; and facilitate continuity of care (Hertz et al., 2016). After relocation, nurses should tailor interventions to the older adult's values and preferences; promote the person's sense of control, autonomy, and mastery; provide social support and activities; promote the person's coping with relocation; orient the person to their new surroundings; maintain continuity of care; and ensure that the person's physical and psychosocial needs are met (Hertz et al., 2016). Often, family members or care partners will need support when an older adult moves into an LTC home. No matter the circumstances, family members often feel that they have in some way failed the older adult. (See Chapter 25 for a more in-depth discussion of these issues.)

IMPLICATIONS FOR GERONTOLOGICAL NURSING AND HEALTHY AGING

This chapter and this book in general discuss the care of the older adult in a variety of care settings. Many theories, frameworks, implications, research, evidence-informed practice recommendations, and resources for gerontological nursing and healthy aging have been presented. Nurses with competence in the care of older adults will be in great demand as the population ages. Gerontological nurses have always assumed a leadership role in improving care for older adults and in promoting healthy aging. Through their expertise, commitment, dedication, advocacy, and compassion, gerontological nurses who care for older adults in all settings will continue to be leaders in creating models that truly change the culture of existing systems. Our hope is that nurses find joy and fulfillment in nursing older adults. Irene Burnside (1980, p. 32), quoting Martin Buber, wrote, "No one can say thank you the way an old person can." May you hear many "thank yous" in your practice.

KEY CONCEPTS

- A familiar and comfortable environment allows an older adult to function at their highest capacity.
- Eight elements of age-friendly communities enhance the ability of older adults to remain in their homes and familiar environments.
- Nurses must be knowledgeable about the range of housing and residential options for older adults so that they can assist older adults and their families or care partners in making appropriate decisions.
- Access to supports needed by the older adult to remain in the community, including home care and adult day programs, is inconsistent from region to region. Accessibility issues are compounded in rural and remote regions and for Indigenous peoples.

■ Long-term care homes and home care are integral parts of the health care system, providing subacute, chronic, long-term, and palliative care.

■ Culture change in long-term care homes is a growing movement to integrate models of person-centred care and improve care outcomes and quality of life for residents.

■ Nurses play a key role in ensuring optimal outcomes during transitions of care.

■ Relocation has variable effects, depending on the individual's personality, health, cognitive capacities, sense of control, opportunities for choice, self-esteem, and preferred lifestyle.

ACTIVITIES AND DISCUSSION QUESTIONS

1. Pick three objects in your living space that are important to you, and explain why they are significant. What would be the effect on you if you were unable to move them to a new home?

2. Using the World Health Organization checklist of essential features of age-friendly cities (see the Resources), look in your neighbourhood or community for one or more of the eight elements of age-friendly communities. Compare your findings with those of a classmate.

3. Ask an older relative about the items or conditions in their home that make them feel secure and comfortable.

4. How might your life be affected, positively or negatively, by having an older family member join your household? What might change for you and for the older relative? How would this experience compare with that of moving the older relative to a retirement or long-term care home?

5. Discuss with an older adult their various moves and how they made the person feel. How did the

person adjust? What are some of the cultural needs for adjustment?

6. Discuss how the care needs of an older adult in a retirement home might differ from those of an older adult living in a long-term care home. What is the role of a nurse in each of these settings?

7. Contact three retirement homes in your community, and make inquiries to each regarding a possible move to the home by an older adult. What questions did you ask? What is the cost? What are the provisions for health care? What activities and assistance are available? Which home would you recommend for your grandmother, and why?

8. From your experience in the acute care setting, what would you suggest to improve transitions to other care settings? Discuss any experience you or your friends or family may have had with transitions after hospital discharge.

9. If you were the director of nursing, what would your long-term care home be like (for instance, in its design, staffing, quality of care, and training)?

RESOURCES

Alzheimer Society of Canada. (2014). *PC P.E.A.R.L.S. 7 key elements of person-centred care of people with dementia in long-term care homes.*
https://archive.alzheimer.ca/sites/default/files/files/national/culture-change/pcpearls_full_e.pdf.

Canadian Institute for Health Information. *Long-term care homes in Canada: How many and who owns them?*
https://www.cihi.ca/en/long-term-care-homes-in-canada-how-many-and-who-owns-them

Eden Alternative
https://www.edenalt.org

World Health Organization. *Age-friendly environments program.*
https://www.who.int/teams/social-determinants-of-health/demographic-change-and-healthy-ageing/age-friendly-environments

World Health Organization. *Checklist of essential features of age-friendly cities.*
http://www.who.int/ageing/publications/Age_friendly_cities_checklist.pdf

World Health Organization. *Global age-friendly cities guide.*
http://www.who.int/ageing/publications/Global_age_friendly_cities_Guide_English.pdf

For additional resources, please visit *http://evolve.elsevier.com/Canada/Ebersole/gerontological/*

REFERENCES

Alzheimer Society of Canada. (2014). *PC P.E.A.R.L.S. 7 key elements of person-centred care of people with dementia in long-term care homes.* Author. https://archive.alzheimer.ca/sites/default/files/files/national/culture-change/pcpearls_full_e.pdf.

Bandura, A. (1997). *Self-efficacy: The exercise of control.* W.H. Freeman.

Boscart, V. M., & Brown, M. (2018). Transitional care for seniors: What do care partners and seniors really experience? *Journal of Nursing and Care, 7*(4). doi:10.4172/2167-1168.1000469.

Burnside, I. (1980). Why work with the aged? *Geriatric Nursing, 2*(3), 29–33.

Canadian Accreditation Council. (2018). *Standards.* https://www.canadianaccreditation.ca/accreditation-process/standards/.

Canadian Cohousing Network. (2021). *What is cohousing?* https://cohousing.ca/about-cohousing/what-is-cohousing/.

Canadian Institute for Health Information. (CIHI). (2021a). *Long-term care homes in Canada: How many and who owns them?* https://www.cihi.ca/en/long-term-care-homes-in-canada-how-many-and-who-owns-them.

Canadian Institute for Health Information. (CIHI). (2021b). *1 in 9 new long-term care home residents potentially could have been cared for at home.* https://www.cihi.ca/en/1-in-9-new-long-term-care-residents-potentially-could-have-been-cared-for-at-home.

Canadian Institute for Health Information. (CIHI). (2021c). *Dementia in hospitals.* https://www.cihi.ca/en/dementia-in-canada/dementia-care-across-the-health-system/dementia-in-hospitals.

Canadian Institutes of Health Research. (2020). *Transitions in care.* https://cihr-irsc.gc.ca/e/50971.html.

Gilmour, H. (2018). Unmet home care needs in Canada. Statistics Canada. Catalogue No. 82-003-X. *Health Reports, 29*(11), 3–11. https://www150.statcan.gc.ca/n1/en/pub/82-003-x/2018011/article/00002-eng.pdf.

Government of Alberta. (2021). *Affordable housing programs: Housing options for families, seniors and individuals with special needs, and building construction standards for affordable housing.* https://www.seniors-housing.alberta.ca/housing/seniors_self_contained_housing.html.

Government of Ontario. (2019). *Life lease housing.* https://www.ontario.ca/document/life-lease-housing.

Habitat for Humanity. (2021). *What does home mean to you?* https://www.habitat.org/stories/what-does-home-mean-to-you.

Healthcare of Ontario Pension Plan. (2017). *Seniors and poverty—Canada's next crisis?* https://hoopp.com/docs/default-source/newsroom-library/research/hoopp-research-article—senior-poverty—canada-next-crises.pdf.

Hertz, J., Koren, M. E., Rossetti, J., et al. (2016). Management of relocation in cognitively intact older persons. *Journal of Gerontological Nursing, 42*(11), 14–23. doi:10.3928/00989134-20160901-05.

Home Care Ontario. (2014). *Home care.* https://www.homecareontario.ca/home-care-services/facts-figures/home-care.

Jacklin, K., & Walker, J. (2019). Cultural understandings of dementia in Indigenous peoples: A qualitative evidence synthesis. *Canadian Journal on Aging, 39*(2), 220–234. doi:10.1017/S071498081900028X.

Jarrott, S., & Ogletree, A. M. (2019). Adult day services outcomes: Delphi review of an integrated participant assessment system. *Journal of Applied Gerontology, 38*(3), 386–405. doi:10.1177/0733464816675423.

Kelly, R. (2017). The effect of adult day program attendance on emergency room registrations, hospital admissions, and days in hospital: A propensity-matching study. *Gerontologist, 57*(3), 552–562. doi:10.1093/geront/gnv145.

Life, P. (2018). *Outside the nursing-home narrative.* In S. Chivers & U. Kriebernegg (Eds.), *Care home stories: Aging, disability, and long-term residential care* (pp. 191–202). Transcript Verlag. doi:10.14361/9783839438053.

MacAdam, M. (2015). PRISMA: Program of research to integrate the services for the maintenance of autonomy. A system-level integration model in Quebec. *International Journal of Integrated Care, 23*(15), e018. doi:10.5334/ijic.2246.

Morgan, D. G., Kosteniuk, J. G., Stewart, N. J., et al. (2015). Availability and primary health care orientation of dementia-related services in rural Saskatchewan, Canada. *Home Health Care Services Quarterly, 34*(3–4), 137–158. doi:10.1080/01621424.2015.1092907.

Norris, S. (2020, October 22). *Long-term care homes in Canada—How are they funded and regulated?* https://hillnotes.ca/2020/10/22/long-term-care-homes-in-canada-how-are-they-funded-and-regulated/.

Ontario Long Term Care Association. (2019). *This is long-term care 2019.* https://www.oltca.com/OLTCA/Documents/Reports/TILTC2019web.pdf.

Public Health Agency of Canada. (2015). *The safe living guide—A guide to home safety for seniors.* https://www.canada.ca/en/public-health/services/health-promotion/aging-seniors/publications/publications-general-public/safe-living-guide-a-guide-home-safety-seniors.html.

Rojas-García, A., Turner, S., Pizzo, E., et al. (2018). Impact and experiences of delayed discharge: A mixed-studies systematic review. *Health Expectations, 21*(1), 41–56. doi:10.1111/hex.12619.

Rossen, E., & Gruber, K. (2007). Development and psychometric testing of the relocation self-efficacy scale. *Nursing Research, 56*(4), 244–251. doi:10.1097/01.NNR.0000280609.16244.de.

Statistics Canada. (2019). *First results from the Canadian Housing Survey, 2018.* https://www150.statcan.gc.ca/n1/daily-quotidien/191122/dq191122c-eng.htm.

Sullivan, G. J., & Williams, C. (2017). Older adult transitions into long-term care: A meta-synthesis. *Journal of Gerontological Nursing, 43*(3), 41–49.

The Good Samaritan Society. (2021). *CHOICE© Program.* https://gss.org/services/choice-program/.

Wilkinson, A., Haroun, V., Wong, T., et al. (2019). Overall quality performance of long-term care homes in Ontario. *Healthcare Quarterly, 22*(2), 55–62. doi:10.12927/hcq.2019.25903.

World Health Organization. (2021). *About the global network for age-friendly cities and communities.* https://extranet.who.int/agefriendlyworld/who-network/.

INDEX

Page numbers followed by f indicate figure(s); t, table(s); b, box(es).